NUTRITION AND SUPPLEMENTATION
for sport and physical performance

MASSIMO SPATTINI

NUTRITION AND SUPPLEMENTATION
for sport and physical performance

From BODYBUILDING to MARATHON passing through CROSSFIT

THE SUPPLEMENTS
from A to Z

II EDITION

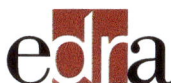

Original title: Massimo Spattini - Alimentazione e integrazione per lo sport e la performance fisica II edizione
©2021 Edizioni LSWR* – All rights reserved

Book Publishing Manager: Costanza Smeraldi
Paper, Printing and Binding Manager: Paolo Ficicchia
Translation: Life, Tirana, Albania
Copyediting: ALTER EDOM s.r.l., Noventa Padovana (PD), Italy

©2022 Edra S.p.A.* – All rights reserved

ISBN: 978-88-214- 5474-5
eISBN: 978-88-214-5475-2

The rights of translation, electronic storage, reproduction or total or partial adaptation by any means (including microfilms and photostatic copies), are reserved for all countries.
Photocopies for personal use of the reader can be made within the limits of 15% of each volume upon payment to the SIAE of the compensation provided by the art. 68, paragraphs 4 and 5, of the law of 22 April 1941 n. 633. Photocopies made for professional, economic or commercial purposes or for any use other than personal use can be made following a specific authorization issued by CLEAredi, Licensing and Authorization Center for Editorial Reproductions, Corso di Porta Romana 108, 20122 Milan, e-mail permissions@clearedi.org and website www.clearedi.org.
Knowledge and best practice in this field are constantly changing: As new research and experience broaden our knowledge, changes in practice, treatment, and drug therapy may become necessary or appropriate. Readers are advised to check the most current information provided (i) or procedures featured or (ii) by the manufacturer of each product to be administered, to verify the recommended dose or formula, the method and duration of administration, and contraindications. It is the responsibility of the practitioners, relying on their own experience and knowledge of the patient, to make diagnoses, to determine dosages and the best treatment for each individual patient, and to take all appropriate safety precautions. To the fullest extent of the law, neither the Publisher nor the Editors assume any liability for any injury and/ or damage to persons or property arising out of or related to any use of the material contained in this book.
This publication contains the author's opinions and is intended to provide precise and accurate information.
The processing of the texts, even if taken care of with scrupulous attention, cannot entail specific responsibilities for the author and / or the publisher for any errors or inaccuracies.
The Publisher has made every effort to obtain and cite the exact sources of the illustrations. If in some cases he has not been able to find the right holders, he is available to remedy any inadvertent omissions or errors in the references cited. All registered trademarks mentioned belong to their legitimate owners.

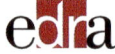

Edra S.p.A.
Via G. Spadolini, 7
20141 Milan
Ph. 02 881841
www.edizioniedra.it

Printed by "LegoDigit" Srl., Lavis (TN, Italy), February 2022

* Edra S.p.A. belongs to the LSWR GROUP LSWR GROUP.

To Cinzia,
the lighthouse that guides me
and shows me the best way
to reach the end of each of my journeys

Foreword

The fundamental role of nutrition in maintaining and promoting health is certainly not new: just think of the role of fasting and dietary moderation in cultural and religious traditions. To give an example, in the tenth speech of the *Book of Grades* (late 4th-early 5th century, probably from in a Syriac-speaking community) it says: "Intemperance in relation to food is harmful to the bodies even when they are healthy". But perhaps the most famous are the sentences of rabbi Moshe ben Maimon, known to most as Maimonides (1135-1204), including: "One of the rules of the health regime is also that the attention must be paid to the quality of food ". Maimonides himself then gave advice on the quantity and the method of physical exercise also in relation to nutrition.

In more recent times, the Venetian nobleman Luigi Cornaro described a similar "integrated" approach to health in his *The Discourses and Letters of Louis Cornaro on a Sober and Temperate Life. In which, with the example of himself, he demonstrates by what means a man can keep himself healthy up to his old age*, published in 1620. I would like to quote here one of the first sentences of his pamphlet, which I find quite current: "O miserable and unhappy Italy, don't you see that crapula kills so many of your people every year, that many could not die at neither in the times of very serious plagues, nor from the iron or the fire of many arms". The role of nutrition and exercise in maintaining and promoting health are therefore ancient concepts. But also searching for the most suitable nutrition for the athlete is nothing new: when Dromeo from Stymphalus won two running races in 484 and 480 BC in Olympia, after a diet based only on meat, the high-protein diet gradually became common, even though it was expensive for an athlete who was not particularly wealthy.

This first "fashion" was followed by many others, always aimed at "maximizing" the performance: for example, Carmides of Sparta, a speed Olympian in 668 BC, declared that he only ate dried figs. And so, from extreme diet to extreme diet, we arrive at the famous supplementation based on brandy and eggs (and strychnine) by Thomas Hicks at the Olympics marathon in St. Louis, in 1904, and also the consumed beer during the stages of the Tour de France in the thirties of the last century. Although, especially in recent years, the science of sports nutrition and related supplementation has evolved, unfortunately we still see preconceived and outdated beliefs (an athlete does not need to eat in a different way, an athlete does not need supplementation, more than 0.8 g of protein per kg of body weight are not needed in a sportsperson, etc.) or dangerous leaps forward with respect to science with statements that refer to an almost magical value of supplements that are often not even verified by a sufficient "corpus" of studies carried out on humans.

In this still confused panorama, the work of my friend Massimo Spattini is meritorious, he not only updated, but also expanded the new edition of this volume. I have known Massimo for more years than I am pleased to remember and during all this time we have shared the passion for the "cast iron"... but while he continued his path as a doctor and popularizer, I moved to a more "secluded" position, dedicating myself to research. Despite this fact, and given the many interests we have in common, we often meet on various occasions and it was during one of those that Massimo asked me to participate in the new edition of his book, with a chapter and this presentation. This text is, to all intents and purposes, a weighty work that could frighten you due to its size, but it is easy to read and, due to its structure, it is also useful for consults in case of doubts or questions on a topic related to nutrition in a particular sport or for a specific supplement.

In fact, these pages show not only Massimo's great transversal culture for everything related to nutrition and well-being, but also his enormous passion, which has led him over the years to deepen these topics by studying, participating at conferences and meeting with researchers from all over the world. This book is a path of studies, career and life that Massimo has admirably managed to condense (even if the number of pages would suggest the opposite) in these pages, which are not only updated on the basis of the most recent research and scientifically accurate, but are also declined with a practical and applicative style, which I'm sure, will find everyone's approval.

Antonio Paoli, MD, FECSS, FACSM
Full Professor of Physical Exercise and Sport Sciences
Department of Biomedical Sciences, University of Padua, Italy
Extraordinary Professor of Sports Nutrition and Strength Training
Catholic University of Sant'Antonio de Murcia (UCAM) – Murcia, Spain
President of the Italian Society of Motor and Sports Sciences (SISMeS)
President of the European Sport Nutrition Society (ESNS)

Introduction

My interest in supplements was born over 47 years ago when, at the age of 17, I started practicing Physical Culture and buying *Sportman* magazine, which dealt with physical efficiency, pre-athletics and dietetics, which I subsequently edited myself for a few years. The magazine, in addition to containing advertisements for sports equipment, also advertised supplements for sports use, such as protein powders, weight gainers (i.e. mixtures of proteins and carbohydrates), cod liver oil, wheat germ oil, brewer's yeast etc., all supplements whose goal is to improve the muscle mass and the athletic performance. The idea of obtaining results by assisting training with the use of powders and pills (obviously completely natural) was certainly stimulating, but I was aware that the basis had to be the nutrition and therefore I began the path of my studies in Medicine and Surgery, of which Science of Nutrition is a branch.

From studying Medicine I learned the notions of biochemistry, which helped me to understand how certain nutritional molecules can influence the biochemical processes that regulate our organism; however, I learned much less about nutrition aimed at athletic performance and, I would say, almost nothing about the use of supplements. In order to deepen my research on the subject I had to devote myself to reading texts and magazines mainly from the USA and started experimenting on myself the effects of various supplements. I participated in various scientific studies carried out at the Institute of Medical Clinic of the University of Parma under the guidance of Professor Mario Passeri, on the use of various supplements such as arginine and creatine, and finally presented a thesis for the School of Specialization in the Science of Nutrition entitled "The effects of dietary branched chain amino acids supplementation on the hormonal values of track and field athletes". My interest in amino acids led me, already in the eighties, to establish relationships with the Aminoacid Profile company, in Los Angeles, which performed the serum aminogram test, making it possible to replicate it in collaboration with an Italian company (Italiana Ingredienti), which specialized in the evaluation of nutritional composition. At the same time, I established relationships with the Doctor's Data laboratories in Phoenix for the performance of the mineralogram on the hair to further customize an integrative approach that took into account mineral imbalances, in order to able to set up a personalized nutritional approach taking by into account the constitutional biotypes that were identified on the basis of the ratios between the various minerals, thus indicating their oxidative capacities (hypo, hyper, mixed).

My studies on the amino acid profile of whey led me to the design of an amino acid pool that considered the need for essential amino acids, the aminogram of blood serum and the amino acid profile of muscle proteins. All this resulted in the development of a supplement produced by LPA, a company for which I also designed an advanced formula where, in addition to BCAAs, we added glucogenic amino acids such as glutamine, alanine and glycine (at that time, glutamine was still not discussed as a supplement). This formulation was then taken up, and is still proposed, by other companies in the sector. In the nineties I studied a product that contained lipoic acid and pyruvate for Powerhouse Nutrition, which was the first marketed supplement based on lipoic acid in Italy and in the world, proposed not only as an antioxidant or normoglycemic, but also as a stimulator of the oxidative metabolism of fatty acids through the activation of the Krebs cycle. In the same years, again for Powerhouse Nutrition, I created a three-phase protein blend (fast, medium and slow absorption proteins) with whey protein isolate, soy protein and casein, with the aim of promoting an immediate but also constant anabolism. This formulation was subsequently abandoned by the company as, given the poor palatability of soy, it had not been successful, however the concept of the multiphasicity of protein assimilation has been taken up by the major American supplement companies during recent years, following the studies that have shown its greater efficacy, which I had already postulated at the time.

My scientific beliefs on food supplementation linked to athletic performance were not accepted in the scientific community at the time, and in all the conferences I attended, I found myself discussing with speakers who argued that food supplementation was absolutely useless, except the reintegration of mineral salts and carbohydrates drinks. During a sports medicine conference, while I was reporting on the protein needs of athletes, arguing that the 0.8 g of protein per kg of body weight reported by the LARNs were not enough, I was even interrupted by the moderator, who cited specious timing reasons.

At that time the world of Sports Medicine was still not introduced to the world of Food Science; in this sense, the lecturer of the Specialization Course in Sports Medicine I attended at the University of Chieti, used the following sentence to conclude the lesson, referring to the athletes of the Under 21 National Football Team: "When we played in Thailand, the boys ate snake without knowing it and they digested it very well... they are young... in the end they digest everything, even the stones... what is the problem?". Now, apart from the fact that snake meat is an excellent source of protein with low fat and, therefore, easily digestible, it is the type of approach to the problem that is criticized, precisely because it is not considered a problem.

The same federations or sports clubs have never invested, or did at least very little investment, in making use of the collaboration of nutritionists or by promoting a correct eating style and even less the correct supplements, fearing that the first was too coercive and the second favored the use of doping. In this regard, I would mention a study which showed that among the habitual consumers of food supplements, there is a greater number of people who resort to the use of substances by considering them doping. Ergo: using food supplements favors the use of doping drugs. It is easy to see that this conclusion is nonsense, it would be like saying that it is easier to drown if you know how to swim, while it should be clear that swimmers drown more because they go into the water, unlike those who, not knowing how to swim, avoid the water.

In the same way it is understandable that an obese person who is addicted to fast food and beer is unlikely to be a consumer of supplements and even less a user of doping drugs, because they will not be involved in performance aimed at athletic performance. Over the years I have followed athletes from various sports who had come to me because they understood how proper nutrition and supplementation could be the tool to achieve high performance for as long as possible, because, if it is true that "young people could even digest stones", as the years pass we need to pay more attention to everything we do.

I will mention three of them, with whom I shared, I hope they allow me to say, a friendship: Samir Bannout, Mr Olympia of bodybuilding in 1983 and participant in Mr Olympia Over 40 in 2013, Fabio Cannavaro, part of the national football team from 1997 to 2010 and 2006 world champion and Golden ball 2006, and Stefano Tilli, 10"16 in the 100 meters outdoor flat in 1984, world record holder in the 200 meters indoor flat in 1985 with 20"52 and finalist of the 100 meters in the quarterfinals at the Sydney 2000 Olympic Games with 10"27. These athletes have been able to maintain such a remarkable longevity in sport at very high levels because they have adopted adequate dietary and supplementary regimes that have allowed them to still be today, albeit former athletes, in a perfect shape and health, which they acquired by nutrition and lifestyle education.

I also believe that the use of supplements is important not only for their real effectiveness, but also because their use contributes to and helps with the regularity of the rhythm of life, and becomes a kind of ritual that favors the maintenance of correct habits. Taking a supplement is a bit like a form of ritual that leads to awareness of what you are doing and your goals, before a workout or before a meal. I have always been fascinated by the so-called "placebo effect", that is the intake of a neutral substance which, when proposed as a medicine, is able to exert a positive effect in 30% of cases.

It is the amazing demonstration of the power of the mind and I believe that is a part of positive thinking, which is a very powerful tool that we should make more use of. But this is another matter and I do not want to enter here into dissertations that could take an unscientific turn which, no matter how interesting, is not gutted in this context. For this reason, the book will deal only with supplements about which there we have a large scientific bibliography, that will be reported and will not follow the fashions of the past or the present which have not been supported by scientific evidence; obviously I will also take into account my forty years of experience and what has already obtained solid validation in the "field".

However, each one of us, in "science and conscience" will be free to use the supplements that "feel" they work better, being in possession of solid scientific knowledge where we can base our choices. Another valid reason for taking supplements is that even if the diet you follow is theoretically the ideal one, you would not be able to take all the necessary nutritional substances in any case, because food these days does not have the same nutritional value it once had.

In fact, this comes from the intensive farming that has depleted the land, worked with artificial fertilizers and sprayed with pesticides and herbicides, producing low-quality food used to raise livestock, grown with hormones and antibiotics. The food is then transported over long distances, preserved and stored on supermarket shelves for a long time, thus becoming "dead food", losing most of its nutrients and its electrochemical potential, i.e. its energy, as time passes.

Furthermore, nowadays, the stresses that our body undergoes due to the environment are increasing exponential: pollution, radiation, electromagnetic fields, preservatives, dyes, pesticides, heavy metals and thousands of chemicals that did not exist before. We therefore need more food with high nutritional value, but instead our diet, being industrialized, is increasingly poor. Consequently, a right integration should be part of every correct diet for all people, for both preventive and curative purposes, and not just for athletes. Nutraceuticals, phytonutrients, antioxidants and alkalizers could also be included in this discussion, but the attention of this book is mainly aimed at athletes and the nutritional substances that can improve their performance.

They are not limited to simply filling a gap, they actually represent a natural possibility, such as that offered by the choice of one food rather than another, to optimize certain biochemical processes which are essential to maximize athletic performance. I believe that the real fight against doping consists precisely in finding the best possible nutrition and supplementation for everyone to optimize their performance. As long as it continues to be argued that supplements are "useless", athletes will always resort to doping.

In this book I have availed myself of the collaboration of other professionals. In particular, among the others, I refer to Antonio Paoli, whose training from ISEF (Istituto Superiore di Educazione Fisica) graduate to a specialist in Sports Medicine, and finally full professor of the Department of Biomedical Sciences of the University of Padua, means that he represents, on a global level, one of the world's leading institutional academic experts in reference to nutrition and sport. In addition to the forward, Antonio Paoli personally edited the chapter on the ketogenic diet, which is a particular area of his competence. The "woman's world", on the other hand, was mainly dealt with by Fabrizio D'Agostino, the president of SIFA (Società Italiana di Fitness e Alimentazione), a graduate in Motor Sciences and Nutritional Biology, the creator of the SIFA Dieta software, which allows you to translate into practice most of the notions contained in this book.

Being sure that I have done good work I wish you pleasant reading.

Table of contents

1. The energy production system (energy metabolisms) 1
- The aerobic and anaerobic energy systems 2
- Aerobic capacity 5
  - Alactic anaerobic capacity 6
  - Lactate anaerobic capacity 7

2. Calculate your calorie needs 9

3. Nutrition for the athletes 13
- Quantitative aspect 16
  - How much protein for an athlete? 16
- Qualitative aspect 18
  - Sugars, glucids or carbohydrates 18
  - Proteins 19
  - Fats or lipids 21
  - Fibers 23
  - Minerals 25
  - Vitamins 29
  - Water 31
  - Refreshment drinks 32
- Chronological aspect 32
  - How to keep fit during the summer holidays 34

4. Nutrition for the mass 39
- The 10 dietary rules for gaining muscle mass 46

5. Nutrition for strength
by Andrea Angelozzi and Massimo Spattini 49

6. Nutrition for endurance sports 55
- Carbohydrates 56
- Lipids 56
- Proteins 57
- Water and electrolytes 58
- The diet of the competition period 59
  - The recovery ration 60
  - How much should you eat? 63
  - Which foods are to be preferred? 63
- The metabolic efficiency 64

7. Nutrition for slimming 69

8. Nutrition for concentration
by Marco Tullio Cau 77

9. Nutrition and supplementation for vegetarian/vegan athletes 83
- Protein deficiency 84
- Calcium deficiency 84
- Iron deficiency 85
- Zinc deficiency 85
- Taurine deficiency 85
- Vitamin B12 deficiency 85
- LC-PUFA (Long Chain Polyunsatured Fatty Acids) deficiency 86
- Iodine deficiency 86
- Vitamin D deficiency 87

10. Nutrition and supplementation for the senior athlete 89

11. Nutrition and supplementation for the diabetic sportsperson 95

12. Nutrition in bodybuilding
by Marco Guercioni 101
- Muscle building phase (bulk phase) 103
  - From Kcal to macronutrients 105
  - Number of meals and the protein quantity 107
  - Meal timing 107
- First, we build mass, then we lose fat (cut phase) 108
  - From Kcal to macronutrients 110
  - Meal timing 111

13. The carbohydrate refill
by Massimo Spattini and Valeria Galfano 113

14. Nutrition and aerobic gymnastics
by Giovanni Montagna 121
- Introduction 121
- Aerobics for weight loss? 122

15. Nutrition and dance
by Alessandra Cascone e Barbara Hugonin 127
- Dancers in dance schools 129
  - The differences between the sexes during puberty 129
- Nutrition for the training of professional dancers 131
  - Nutrition for the competition or for the performance on stage 133
  - Food supplements and ergogenic aids 133
- Malnutrition and injuries 134
  - Low bone density and fractures 134
  - The triad of the female athlete 134
  - Relative energy deficiency in dancers 136
- Obsession with thinness and behavioral disturbances 136
- Nutrition for the post-injury rehabilitation 137
- Conclusions 137

16. Nutrition and soccer ... 139
- The quantitative aspect ... 140
  Factors to be considered with particular attention ... 140
- The qualitative aspect ... 140
  How much protein for the soccer player? ... 141
- The chronological aspect of carbohydrate intake ... 141
- Water supply ... 142
- Soccer and supplementation ... 143

17. Nutrition and cycling ... 147

18. Nutrition and CrossFit ... 151
- The Paleodiet ... 152
- The Zone Diet ... 154
  Physiological benefits for athletes entering the Zone ... 156
  List of foods by their main macronutrient ... 157
  The rules for entering the Zone ... 158

19. Nutrition and swimming
by Giovanni Montagna ... 163
- How many and which carbohydrates for the swimmer? ... 164
- How many and which fats for the swimmer? ... 165
- How many and which proteins for the swimmer? ... 168

20. Nutrition and downhill skiing ... 169

21. Nutrition and high-altitude sports ... 173

22. Nutrition and combat sports ... 177

23. Nutrition and supplementation for weightlifting
by Antonio Squillante ... 181

24. Nutrition, supplementation and training during the menstrual cycle
by Francesco Guardato, Antonella Berardi Nazzarena and Massimo Spattini ... 187
- The woman today ... 187
- Biphasic protocol for the gynoid subject:
  diet and workout ... 189
  Follicular phase: from the 1st to the 14th day of the cycle ... 191
  Luteal phase: from the 15th to the 28th day of the cycle ... 192
- Food supplements for the gynoid subject ... 196
- Training for the gynoid subject ... 198
  The follicular phase ... 198
  The luteal phase ... 199
- Biphasic protocol for the android subject: diet and training ... 199
- Food supplements for the android subject ... 203
- Training for the android subject ... 204

25. Nutrition and supplementation for the premenstrual syndrome ... 207
- Foods and PMS ... 209
- Vitamins and minerals ... 211

26. Nutrition and supplementation for cellulite
by Fabrizio D'Agostino 213

27. Nutrition and physical activity for pregnant women
by Fabrizio D'Agostino 221
- Nutritional requirements in non-pathological pregnancy 222
- Foods to be avoided during pregnancy 226
- Physical activity in pregnancy 227

28. Nutrition and circadian rhythms
by Ivan Martellato and Vittoria Troianiello 229
- Introduction 229
- Central clock and peripheral clock 230
- Circadian misalignment 230
- Circadianity of the nutrition 231
- Optimal supplementation and circadianity 235

29. Intermittent fasting 237
- Fast for 12 hours a day 238
- Fast for 16 hours 238
- Fast for 2 days a week 239
- Fasting every other day 239
- 24-hour weekly fast 240
- Skip the meal 240
- The warrior's diet 240
- Intermittent fasting and circadian rhythms 241
- Intermittent fasting and weight loss 243
- Intermittent fasting and the physical performance 244

30. The ketogenic diet
by Antonio Paoli 249
- Biochemical/physiological bases and applications 249
  What is ketosis? 249
- What is a ketogenic diet? 254
- The ketogenic diet and fat loss 255
- Not just low insulin 256
- The safety of ketogenic diets 257
- The ketogenic diet and sports 259
  Weight categories 259
  The ketogenic diet and endurance performance 260
  The ketogenic diet and strength performance 262
  The ketogenic diet and hypertrophy 262
- Conclusions 263

31. Supplementation for strength 265
- Creatine 266
- Betaine 266
- Proteins and amino acids 266
- Hormonal stimulators 267
- Caffeine 267

32. Supplementation for muscle mass 269

33. Supplementation for endurance sports 273
- Omega-3 essential fatty acids
  (DHA: docosahexaenoic acid; EPA: eicosapentaenoic acid) 274
- Magnesium 275
- An essential amino acids pool 276
- Phytonutrients and free radicals 277
- Carnitine 278
- Taurine 278
- Inosine 279
- Guarana 279
- Arginine 279
- Coenzyme Q10 280
- Lipoic acid 280
- Iron 281
- Caffeine 282
- Water 282

34. Supplementation for slimming 283
- Lipotropics 284
- Thermogenics 285
- Coleus forskohlii 286
- Lipoic acid 287
- Replacement meals 287
- Multivitamin-multiminerals 288
- Water 288

35. Supplementation for concentration
by Marco Tullio Cau 289
- Caffeine 290
- Guarana 296
- Rhodiola rosea 299
- Tyrosine 303
- DMAE 305
- Vinpocetine 307
- Ginkgo biloba 308

36. Supplementation for the immune system 311

37. Pre- and post-workout supplements in the gym 317
- Pre-workout 317
  - Creatine 318
  - Beta-alanine 319
  - BCAA 319
  - Taurine 319
  - Nitric oxide (NO) stimulators 320
  - Caffeine 320
- Post-workout 321
  - Powdered carbohydrates 322

Powdered proteins.. 322
   Creatine.. 323
   Leucine... 323
   HMB... 323
   Betaine... 324
   Glutamine.. 324
   Arginine alpha-ketoglutarate 324

38. Supplementation and stress 325
- Supplements in hypercortisolism 327
- Supplements in hypocortisolism 328

39. Supplementation and joints.. 331

40. Supplementation and inflammation
by Giovanni Montagna... 335
- Which are the main substances that control inflammation? 335
- What supplements can help us to keep
  the chronic inflammation under control? 336

41. Supplementation for the sexual performance
by Marco Tullio Cau 339
- Nitric oxide.. 340
- Tribulus terrestris 340
- Cordyceps sinensis.. 340
- Ginkgo biloba.. 341
- DHEA.. 341
- Citrulline and arginine 342
- Pycnogenol 343
- Yohimbine... 343
- Ginseng 345
- Icariin 345
- Peruvian maca.. 346
- Other substances 346
- Conclusions 347

42. Supplementation for the heart
by Paolo Conforti 349
- Vitamins.. 350
- Coenzyme Q10 (CoQ10) 351
- Omega 3 351
- Beetroot juice and "NO-boosters" (arginine and citrulline).............. 352
- Taurine 353
- Carnitine 355
- Probiotics 356

43. Nutrition and supplementation for American football
by Antonio Squillante 359

44. Supplements, from A to Z 367
- Acetyl carnitine (ALC) 368
- Acetylcysteine (NAC) 371
- Agmatine 374
- Alpha-glycerilphosphorylcholine 376
- Antioxidants 378
- Arginine 381
- Arginine alpha-ketoglutarate (AAKG) as a precursor of nitric oxide (NO) 386
- Ashwagandha (Withania somnifera) 390
- ATP 394
- Bacopa 396
- Beta-alanine 398
- Beta-ecdysterone 402
- Betaine 403
- Branched amino acids 406
- Caffeine 412
- Capsaicin 417
- Carnitine 420
- Carnosine 425
- Cellfood® by Giorgio Terziani 428
- Citrates 431
- Citruline 434
- Citrus aurantium 438
- Coenzyme Q10 441
- Colostrum 445
- Conjugated linoleic acid (CLA) 448
- Cordyceps sinensis 450
- Creatine 453
- Cyclodextrins 459
- D-aspartic acid 461
- DHEA (dehydroepiandrosterone) 462
- DMAA 465
- DMAE 467
- DMG 469
- Echinacea 472
- Eleuterococcus 473
- Ephedrine/Ma Huang/pseudoephedrine 476
- Essential amino acids 478
- Exogenous ketones 481
- Fenugreek 484
- Forskolin (Coleus forskholii) 486
- Fucoxanthin 488
- GABA 489
- Ginkgo biloba 491
- Glucosamine and chondroitin sulfate 492
- Glutamine 495
- Glutathione 499
- Glycerol 501
- Green tea 504

Table of contents

- Guarana 506
- HMB 508
- 7-Keto-DHEA 510
- KIC: alpha-ketoisocaproic acid 512
- L-alanyl-L-glutamine 514
- Leucine 516
- Lipoic acid (ALA) 519
- Magnesium 523
- Maltodextrin 528
- MCT 530
- Melatonin 533
- Mucuna 538
- NAD$^+$/NADH 540
- Omega 3 544
- Ornithine 552
- Panax ginseng 554
- Phosphatidic acid 557
- Phosphatidylserine 560
- Pycnogenol 562
- Probiotics 566
- Protein powder 570
- Reishi (Ganoderma lucidum) 583
- Rhodiola rosea 587
- Ribose 592
- SAM-e (S-Adenosyl-Methionine) 594
- Sodium bicarbonate 596
- Super-amide 598
- Taurine 601
- Tribulus terrestris 603
- Turmeric (Curcuma longa) 604
- Tyrosine 609
- Vitamin C 612
- Vitamin D 614
- Vitargo® 619
- Waxy maize (waxy corn starch) 621
- Yohimbine 623
- ZMA 625

Acknowledgments 629

Note: References are available at www.massimospattini.com into "Books" section.

CHAPTER 1

The energy production system (energy metabolisms)

Readers might not want this, but I just could not, before talking about calories, carbohydrates, fats and proteins, not deal with the energy metabolisms. This is the basis of the physiology of muscle contraction and it has become fundamental in understanding the use of macronutrients for energy purposes.

When a muscle contracts and exerts a force, the energy used to command the contraction comes from a special molecule present in the cells, known as adenosine triphosphate (ATP). ATP is the body's source of energy as much as gasoline is the source of energy for a car engine. The more quickly and effectively the muscle cells produce ATP, the more work the cells will be able to do before they tire. Even if there is a certain amount of ATP stored in a muscle cell, its availability is limited.

This means that the muscle cells must continuously produce ATP in order to continue working. Muscle cells feed the ATP reserve using three different biochemical pathways: 1) aerobic, a system which is mainly used in endurance sports that produces ATP through the oxidation of fats and carbohydrates in the Krebs cycle; 2) anaerobic lactacid, a system which is mainly used in speed sports, which produces ATP by transforming glucose into lactic acid; 3) anaerobic alactacid, a system which is used in explosive power sports, which uses the pre-established reserves of ATP and those immediately resynthesized from creatine phosphate (CP). An important concept that should be fixed immediately is that even if they are separated, they still work simultaneously and the predominance of one over the others will depend on the intensity and duration of the exercise.

Table 1.1 Energy mechanisms

Alactic anaerobic	Anaerobic lactate	Aerobic
Without O_2	Without O_2	With O_2
CP	Sugars	Sugars, fatty acids
High power	Medium power	Low power
From 0 to 15"	From 15" to 90"	From 90" and after

The aerobic and anaerobic energy systems

The word *aerobic* means "in the presence of oxygen". The aerobic energy system for the ATP production is predominant when cells are supplied with enough oxygen to meet the energy production needs, as occurs, for example, when the muscle is at rest. Most cells, including muscle cells, contain structures called mitochondria. Mitochondria are the sites of aerobic energy production (ATP). The larger the number of the mitochondria in a cell, the greater the ability of that cell to produce aerobic energy.

The other two energy systems are the primary sources of ATP when the cells receive insufficient oxygen to meet their energy needs. In the absence of a sufficient oxygen supply, such as when a muscle cell needs to produce a great force very quickly to lift a large weight, the cell switches to the anaerobic energy system, which provides a rapidly available source of ATP.

Anaerobic means "in the absence of oxygen". The anaerobic production of ATP occurs inside the cells, in the cytoplasm, but outside the mitochondria.

Many cells, such as those in the heart, brain and other organs, have extremely limited anaerobic capacity. Therefore, these cells must be continuously supplied with oxygen, otherwise they will die. Unlike the heart and the brain, skeletal muscles have a considerable anaerobic capacity. An athlete must know how the aerobic and anaerobic energy is produced, both in terms of the substances (nutrients) used for the production of ATP, and in terms of the intensity of the exercise, where rest and maximum effort represent the extremes of the possible intensity.

The body uses an extremely complex chemical process to produce ATP. However, even a basic knowledge of the process can greatly help the athlete in setting up a training program and the related nutrition and supplementation. Lipids (fatty acids) and carbohydrates (glucose) are the two substances (substrates) that the body's cells use to produce most of the ATP. Proteins, which are made up of various combinations of amino acids, are not a preferential energy source; in an athlete who has a balanced diet, proteins play a minor role in the energy production.

However, when a diet does not provide a sufficient amount of calories, the body is able to use the proteins stored in the muscle tissues to produce the necessary energy through a biochemical process called "neoglucogenesis", which involves the dismantling of the proteins and their transformation into glucose, although this is certainly not an ideal process as it is catabolic. At rest, when the cardiopulmonary system is easily able to supply the adequate amount of oxygen to the mitochondria of the muscle cells, both fatty acids and glucose are used to produce ATP, but mainly fatty acids.

In other words, at rest, most of the necessary ATP is produced aerobically, using both glucose and fatty acids. In fact, at rest, the body consumes approximately one Kcal per minute. About 50% of these calories per minute come from the fat tissue, even if the person is not trained. Fat in a well-trained athlete provides up to 70% of the caloric expenditure at rest (considering that, however, about 100 g of glucose per day are used by the brain alone).

When the intensity of the exercise increases, the cardiovascular system makes all possible efforts to increase its supply of oxygen to the mitochondria of the working muscles, in order to aerobically produce the necessary amount of ATP. By continuing to increase the intensity of the exercise, at a certain point, determined by both the athlete's training level and genetic characteristics, the cardiovascular system becomes unable to supply sufficient oxygen to the working muscles; then the muscles use the anaerobic system to rapidly produce ATP.

The exercise intensity at which an adequate supply of oxygen is no longer available is called the *anaerobic threshold*, which is reached before the maximum effort. The anaerobic system, however, cannot be used for an extended period. The primary source for the anaerobic production of ATP is glucose, which is contained in the muscles and in the liver as glycogen, a large molecule made up of glucose chains. A second source for ATP production is creatine-phosphate (CP), a molecule from which a molecule of phosphorus (P) can be quickly separated to reconstitute an ATP molecule from an ADP (adenosine diphosphate) molecule.

However, as with the ATP reserve in the muscles, there is an extremely limited availability of creatine phosphate. Some research (J. Bergstom and others) has shown that, even in a well-trained athlete, the muscles only store an amount of creatine phosphate and ATP, which together are called phosphagenes, sufficient for 10 seconds of maximum effort, and this basically reflects the capacity of the alactic anaerobic system. Glycolysis, i.e. the breakdown of glucose, which is the prelude to both pathways, is a chain of nine reactions, each catalyzed by a specific enzyme, and occurs in the cytosol.

During these reactions, a molecule of glucose ($C_6H_{12}O_6$), containing 6 carbon atoms, is gradually transformed into 2 molecules of pyruvate, each containing 3 carbon atoms. The pyruvate molecule, the final product of glycolysis (during which 2 molecules of ATP are produced), can undergo further demolition: 1) aerobically through the reactions of the Krebs cycle and the electron transport chain (respiratory chain) that occur within the mitochondria and are extremely dependent on each other; 2) anaerobically through the fermentation process that occurs in the cytosol and which to the formation of lactic acid.

At this point I would like to say a couple more words to describe the Krebs cycle, because the understanding of the latter (great concern of all students in the biochemistry exam) can be very useful to understand the complicated mechanisms that lead the organism to the use of an energetic substrate rather than another. The Krebs cycle is the basis of the aerobic pathway and the pyruvate molecule, before starting the Krebs cycle, enters the mitochondrion, loses a molecule of CO_2 and becomes an acetyl group containing 2 carbon atoms. The acetyl group binds to a molecule of coenzyme A, through which it enters the Krebs cycle.

The acetyl group bonded to coenzyme A (AcetylCoA) binds to a molecule of oxaloacetate (composed of 4 carbon atoms) forming citric acid (composed of 6 carbon atoms). Citric acid undergoes a subsequent series of oxidations (it loses 2 carbon atoms in the form of 2 CO_2 molecules, generates one molecule of ATP, 2 of NADH, one of $FADH_2$; the reducing power of NADH and $FADH_2$ will be used to produce ATP in the respiratory chain) until the oxaloacetate molecule is reformed, which restarts the cycle by binding to another acetyl group.

Well, I believe that the availability of oxaloacetate represents an important traffic light for the use of fats or carbohydrates. Oxaloacetate is formed from two pyruvate molecules that normally derive from the glycolysis of glucose. If there is a low availability of glucose, there will be a low production of pyruvate, which leads to a slowdown in the functionality of the Krebs cycle. Hence the phrase: "fats burn in the fire of carbohydrates". If there is not enough oxaloacetate, it cannot bind to the acetyl group coming from the oxidation of fatty acids and therefore these acetyl groups follow a different path and give rise to ketone bodies.

But even before the formation of ketone bodies, the body tries to compensate for this oxaloacetate deficiency by converting the neoglucogenic amino acids into pyruvate. In reality, both mechanisms, the production of ketone bodies and neoglucogenesis, are not the ideal biochemical metabolisms for the athlete as the former induces an increase in metabolic acidosis which is already tendentially high in the overtrained athlete (if a particular metabolic adaptation does not occur, it requires a specific diet and a certain time) and the second is a protein catabolism that does not help the muscles.

To summarize, as long as a muscle cell is aerobic, it uses both fat and glucose to produce ATP, but at least a quantity of carbohydrates is still needed to avoid ketosis and neoglucogenesis.

The aerobic system produces much more ATP than the anaerobic system, since between the Krebs cycle and the respiratory chain there are 36 molecules of ATP compared to 2 of the anaerobic glycolysis. In addition, the waste products of the aerobic production of ATP are water and carbon dioxide (CO_2); both are tolerated quite well by the body, so the aerobic energy production does not cause muscle fatigue.

Since water is a waste product of the aerobic production of ATP, it is essential to replace the water eliminated by drinking a lot every day. The more you exercise, the more water you need to drink. When a muscle in exercise exploits the anaerobic metabolism, it uses glucose (and to a limited extent the phosphagen system) to produce ATP.

However, not only the anaerobically produced ATP is much less than that produced aerobically for each molecule of substrate used, but also the waste products of the anaerobic production of ATP include lactic acid. As the levels of lactic acid and other waste products in the muscle increase, it will be increasingly difficult to allow the muscle to contract continuously. It is believed that the lactic acid is the main cause of sudden pains (burning) in a muscle that is being exercised. In addition to the formation of the lactic acid, the muscles send other signals when they can no longer produce aerobically the necessary amount of ATP.

One of these is hyperventilation, defined as breathing faster than necessary, which represents the sign that the anaerobic production of the ATP is predominant. When sufficient oxygen is not available, the muscle signals to the brain about the need to increase the rate and the depth of breathing. However, since the limiting factor is not breathing but the extraction of oxygen from the muscle, hyperventilation is a futile process. The chemical process that the body uses to produce ATP depends on certain proteins in the body, which are called enzymes. Enzymes are needed to start the chemical reaction that produces ATP, both aerobically and anaerobically.

The enzymes that metabolize fat are different from those that metabolize carbohydrates. In addition, to metabolize carbohydrates anaerobically the organism uses enzymes which are different from the ones used to metabolize carbohydrates aerobically. Thus, when exercising at an intensity below the anaerobic threshold, the aerobic enzymes that metabolize fat and carbohydrates are dominant in ATP production. But when the exercise is done near the anaerobic threshold, anaerobic enzymes play a dominant role in the production of ATP.

The aerobic training leads to an increase in the capacity of the aerobic system, but has a small effect on anaerobic enzymes. Therefore, aerobic training significantly increases our ability to burn fat. Anaerobic training, on the other hand, will mainly lead to a functional improvement of the anaerobic enzyme system. All this represents another application of the principle of the specificity of training.

Aerobic capacity

The aerobic system starts working after about one minute from the start of an exercise, but reaches its maximum in around 20 minutes. The aerobic capacity indicates the time for which it is possible to maintain the rhythm indicated by the anaerobic threshold, which represents the maximum physical effort that the body can sustain without lactic acid accumulation.

The total ability to consume oxygen at the cellular level is known as maximum oxygen uptake or VO_{2max}. This function affects our maximum aerobic capacity. VO_{2max} depends on two factors: 1) the distribution of the oxygen to the muscles that are working through the blood or cardiac output and 2) the ability to extract oxygen from the blood in order to distribute it to the capillaries and to use the oxygen in the mitochondria (elements of aerobic energy production which are present in most cells). The maximum oxygen consumption is represented by the following formula:

$$VO_{2max} = \max \times \text{cardiac output} \times \text{max oxygen extraction}$$

VO_2 (the volume of the consumed oxygen) is measured both in milliliters of oxygen consumed per kilogram of body weight per minute (mL of oxygen/kg/min), and in liters of oxygen consumed per minute (liters of oxygen/min). We can now indicate how much oxygen is used at rest and compare it with a hypothetical maximum aerobic capacity of an athlete weighing 70 kg. If your resting heart rate is 60 bpm, the SV unit volume is 70 mL/beat (remember that: cardiac output = heartbeat × volume unit) and the oxygen extraction is 6 mL of oxygen/100 mL of blood; therefore the VO_2 at rest is:

$$VO_2 = 60 \text{ bpm} \times 70 \text{ mL/beat} \times 6 \text{ mL oxygen}/100 \text{ mL}$$

This is equivalent to 252 mL of oxygen/min. Divided by 70 kg, the resting VO_2 is about 3.5 mL/kg/min. During a maximal exercise our athlete has a heartbeat of 180 bpm, a unit volume of 115 mL/beat and an oxygen extraction of 15 mL of oxygen/100 mL of blood. Therefore, the maximum VO_2 is:

$$VO_{2max} = 180 \text{ bpm} \times 115 \text{ mL/beat} \times 15 \text{ mL oxygen}/100 \text{ mL}$$

which is equivalent to 3.105 mL of oxygen/min, or 44.4 mL/kg/min. Although the example refers to a hypothetical athlete in average conditions, it clearly illustrates that our bodies have an enormous capacity to increase oxygen consumption; in this example there was an increase of more than 12.5 times. While the increases in both heart rate and unit volume justify the increase in cardiac output during exercise, the increase in oxygen extraction (also referred to as arterio-venous oxygen difference) is caused by various stimuli.

Numerous changes occur during the exercise to make it easier to withdraw oxygen from the hemoglobin molecules and its subsequent use for the production of the aerobic energy in the muscles. These changes include increases in temperature, acidity and in the level of carbon dioxide in the bloodstream.

The resting VO_2 value of 3.5 mL/kg/min is also referred to as the *metabolic equivalent*, or 1 MET. Activities are often described in terms of MET; for example, volleyball has a 3-6 MET field and aerobic dance a 6-9 MET field. To determine the VO_2 equivalent to a given MET value just multiply the latter by 3.5. Doctors often prescribe exercises based on the MET value, especially for those patients undergoing a cardiac rehabilitation program.

With aerobic training, not only does an increase in VO_{2max} occur, but it also causes an increase in the percentage of maximum effort at which the anaerobic threshold occurs. In practice, this means that an individual is capable of producing ATP aerobically with an intensity that increases with the level of training. Furthermore, an aerobically trained person can generally perform more intense activities than an untrained person. As soon as an individual reaches a good level of aerobic fitness, their VO_{2max} increases.

The maximum oxygen consumption, like the training heart rate, is influenced by age, hereditary factors and the level of the physical fitness. For example, after the age of 30, a slow but progressive loss of aerobic capacity occurs (at the age of 65 it can decrease up to 35%). Some individuals develop a considerable aerobic capacity, so they are able to sustain a high-level workout. The greater a person's aerobic fitness, the higher the VO_{2max}.

Another interesting physiological relationship occurs between the oxygen consumption and the number of calories (Kcal) burnt during an exercise. The amount of oxygen consumed during an exercise can be converted into the number of calories used in each minute. For example, when a liter of oxygen is used, we spend approximately 5 Kcal. Therefore, a woman who runs at an average pace with a heart rate of 135 bpm and who uses about 20 mL of oxygen/kg/min (1.16 liters/minute) will burn approximately 5.8 Kcal per minute. A man who uses about 1.4 liters of oxygen/minute will burn about 7.0 Kcal/minute. Movement physiologists use this energy conversion ratio to calculate the approximate number of calories burnt during an exercise.

Alactic anaerobic capacity

The alactacid anaerobic capacity basically depends on the reserves of ATP and CP in the muscle and cannot be improved that much by training because they do not require particular enzymatic adaptations, however it can be partially improved by a "speed resistance" training where high intensity sets (90-95%) are performed with a very short recovery time between repetitions and wider recovery time between sets. These substrates generally run out in the order of about ten seconds; however, it is possible to increase the amount of phosphates stored in the muscle with the use of supplements, for example creatine.

Lactate anaerobic capacity

When an intense effort lasts for more than about 10 seconds, the phosphate reserves are depleted and the alactacid anaerobic system is no longer sufficient to produce energy; at this moment the lactic acid anaerobic system comes into play. To obtain energy, this system uses glycogen, but since glycolysis occurs in the absence of oxygen, it leads to the transformation of pyruvate (which cannot be metabolized aerobically, given the intensity of the effort) into lactic acid. The lactic acid produced in this way is accumulated inside the muscle cell and slows the breakdown speed of muscle glycogen by interfering with the mechanism of muscle contraction, which becomes painful; thus, the phenomenon of fatigue takes over.

Muscle acidity caused by lactic acid at pH values of 6.5 (normal muscle pH is 6.9) prevents contraction by inhibiting the release of calcium ions (Ca^{++}) which are essential for the muscle contraction, making the action of 1-phosphofructokinase ineffective (PFK), deactivating pyruvicodehydrogenase, a complex of enzymes involved in glycolysis, and destructuring the elastic proteins titin and nebulin, which are functional in the return phase of the actin filament sliding on myosin.

The lactacid anaerobic system has an average duration of 30-40 seconds in maximal mode, also considering the initial alactacid phase; in the case of more prolonged efforts the athlete is forced to reduce the intensity of the effort or stop it. The capacity of this system depends on the amount of lactic acid that the muscle is able to tolerate, which can be increased by training. Training in anaerobic lactacid optimizes the action of glycolytic enzymes and increases the tolerance threshold to lactic acid and the muscle endurance. The use of supplements that can exert a buffering effect by decreasing acidity or by improving the enzymatic efficiency of glycolysis can also help.

CHAPTER 2

Calculate your calorie needs

Calorie intake is essential for improving physical performance, increasing muscle mass or losing fat. The daily energy expenditure is made up of the calories necessary for the basal metabolism plus the calories consumed by essential daily activities, such as dressing, washing, etc. and those related to the practiced physical exercise. Basal metabolic rate can be measured using a specific equipment, such as the indirect calorimetry, which is based on the oxygen consumption of a person who has put on a mask, inside which one can breathe. If this equipment is not available, the Harris and Benedict formula can be used to measure the resting basal metabolic rate. This method is certainly less accurate and can easily underestimate the basal metabolic rate.

Harris and Benedict RMR formula for men:
66.5 + (13.75 x weight in kg) + (5 x height in cm) – (6.78 x years of age) = Kcal

An example for a 40-year-old man who weighs 73 kg and is 175 cm tall:
66.6 + (13.75 x 73) + (5 x 175) – (6.78 x 40) = 66.6 + 875 + 1003.75 – 267.2 = 1678.15 Kcal

Harris and Benedict RMR formula for women:
655 + (9.56 x weight in kg) + (1.85 x height in cm) – (4.68 x years of age) = Kcal

An example for a 36-year-old woman who weighs 61 kg and is 163 cm tall:
655 + (9.56 x 61) + (1.85 x 163) – (4.68 x 36) = 655 + 583.16 + 301.55 – 168.48
= 1371.23 Kcal

If this formula seems complicated to you, you can use a much simpler one:

**weight in kg x 1 Kcal/kg x 24 hours = Kcal of the basal metabolism
(for women use 0.9 instead of 1)**
An example for a man weighing 73 kg: 73 x 1 x 24 = 1752 Kcal
An example for a woman weighing 61 kg: 61 x 0.9 x 24 = 1317.6 Kcal

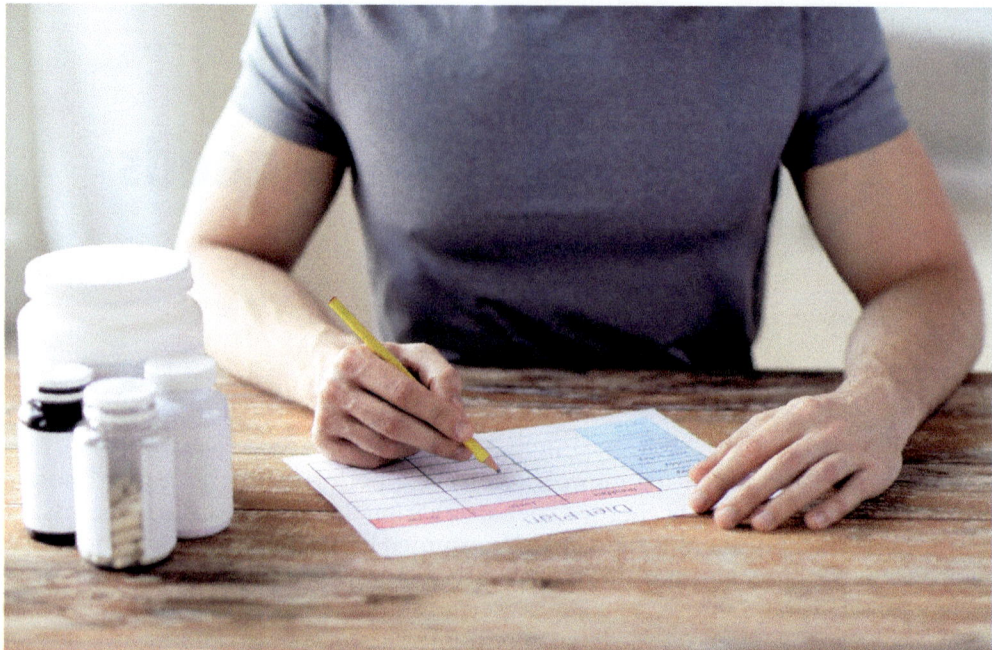
Figure 2.1

The reason why it is also possible to use these formulas, even though they are very approximate, is due to the fact that the daily caloric consumption is linked to many variables, therefore the measurement with indirect calorimetry is purely indicative in order to establish the real caloric requirement. In this regard, I can refer to when I made arrangements with the Parenteral Nutrition Unit of the Cremona Hospital, many years ago, with an intent to being able to customize the dietary approach to the maximum, taking into account the real metabolism, by using the indirect calorimetry, which consists in measuring the consumption of oxygen and carbon dioxide inhaled and exhaled in the unit of time.

Normally, in that setting, they administered nasogastric or intravenous replacement meals to bedridden patients who were unable to feed naturally. In this case it was obviously essential to be able to calculate their basal metabolic rate (BMR), which corresponded to the daily need for calories, in order not to cause conditions of malnutrition or overeating. As for the athletes, things were different: after some experiments I realized the uselessness of this approach as I immediately verified that athletes who during the measurements of the calorie consumption (in this case carried out during a cycle ergometer test, at a certain percentage of maximum heart rate) had almost identical values and similar characteristics (weight, height, age), in fact needed completely different caloric levels to maintain their body weight, despite of the physical activities with a superimposable calorie consumption.

The reason for this is linked to the macro and micro movements (NEAT = Non-Exercise Activity Thermogenesis): we indeed fact consider working in the office as sedentary, but a person who is really stuck at their desk must be considered differently than someone who, for example, constantly drums their fingers, gets up and sits down continuously by changing position, goes to the bathroom every 30 minutes, talks incessantly, gesticulating and maybe are also particularly nervous and short-tempered. The same can be said for an instructor in the room or during a course: there is the one who demonstrates the exercises by performing them personally and the one who explains them only verbally. There is a big difference! There are special portable devices capable of measuring daily energy expenditure.

One of these is ARMBAND®, a band that is put around the arm and kept on throughout the day. In this way, by monitoring movements, body temperature, heart rate and linear acceleration of the body, the calorie consumption can be estimated quite accurately. In reality, it is always an estimate and, in fact, the only effective method to measure caloric needs is to monitor the change in the percentage of body fat. Any decrease or increase in fat tissue will mean a calorie deficit or surplus, bearing in mind that 1 kg of fat is equivalent to 7500 Kcal. This means that if in two weeks there is an increase of half a kg of fat tissue, the daily caloric requirement compared to the diet you are following is about 250 Kcal lower per day.

However, it is always good to start either from a measurement or from a theoretical calculation and, in this case, in addition to the basal metabolic rate, it is also necessary to take into account the daily work and physical exercise. Regarding daily work, there are various levels of physical activity (light, moderate, heavy) which, multiplied by the BMR, give the daily calorie consumption, which must be added to the calorie consumption of the physical exercise.

The calculation of the calories consumed during exercise depends on the type of activity being carried out, the intensity, loads and weight of the person. A physical exercise can consume from 5 to 20 calories per minute, with an average of 7-11 Kcal. The typical aerobic training of 30-40 minutes consumes about 300 Kcal, while training with weights, lasting an hour, consumes about 500-600 Kcal (obviously related to the lifted loads). However, there are some fairly accurate tables to calculate the calories consumed during a specific sport activity (McArdle WD, Katch FI. *Exercise physiology: energy, nutrition and human performance*. Philadelphia: Lippincott Williams and Wilkins, 2001; Ainsworth et al. The compendium of physical activities: classification of energy costs of human physical activities. *Medicine and Science in Sports and Exer-*

Table 2.1 Physical activity levels (PALs) to be used to estimate the energy needs by gender and age groups

	DAILY PALs		
Adults	Light activity	Moderate activity	Heavy activity
Men	1.55	1.78	2.01
Women	1.56	1.64	1.82
Elderly	Light activity	Moderate activity	Heavy activity
Men	1.45		
Women	1.48		

cise, 25, n. 1 Jan 1993). Once you have calculated the daily calorie consumption and added the calorie consumption for the exercises, taking into account the hours and days of training, you can make a weekly average.

In reality, up to this point we should have been talking about estimation and not calculation; this will only be a starting point for calculating the daily calorie requirement. In order not to run the risk of making too many mistakes using these mere theoretical calculations, it is advisable to use a food anamnesis that consists in calculating the calories of our daily diet, which tends to keep our stable body weight, and average this value with the theoretically calculated one. In the end, the field test, i.e. the measurement of the body fat after a few weeks, will be the definitive data to be taken into consideration to calculate the real daily caloric requirement.

CHAPTER 3

Nutrition for the athletes

It is certainly obvious that supplements can represent a very important help for the athlete, but they cannot be separated from nutrition, which is the foundation on which the athlete's nutritional approach must be based. For many years the concept of nutrition for the athlete has been relegated only to a quantitative discourse, starting from the assumption that "the athlete trains and consumes more calories and therefore needs more food". In some cases, this can also be the determining factor; I am thinking, for example, of the cyclists who participate in the "Giro d'Italia", during which they have to worry about replenishing the enormous quantities of energy with equally enormous quantities of food without paying too much attention to quality (even if, as we will see in the specific chapter, it shouldn't be exactly like that.)

However, in reality the athlete's performance during the "Giro" is not linked only to nutrition, but above all to the performance skills that have been created and strengthened during the training period and in which qualitative nutrition plays a fundamental role. If this is intuitive and valid for an endurance sport such as cycling,

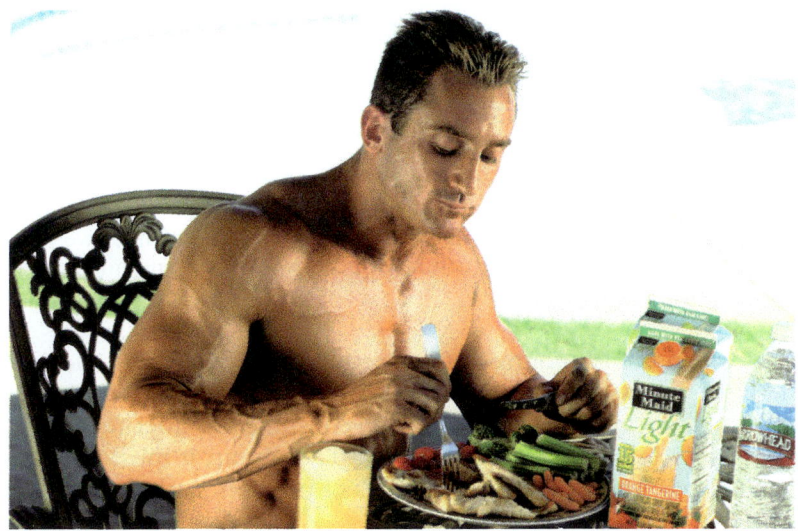

Figure 3.1

it is even more so for a power sport where the increase in strength and muscle mass, necessary to express the maximum of competitive performance, is built over time and it needs a power supply with specific characteristics.

Sports performance is influenced by the type of habitual diet; in fact, unbalanced nutrition (not for a day or a week) can become a critical factor for performance. Sports dietetics applied systematically and not occasionally offers two advantages:
- improves the physical capacity and the technical ability of the athlete;
- allows the athlete to acquire correct eating habits from which to benefit even in the following years.

Too often, they read brochures and texts on sports nutrition which insert the following misleading statement in the introduction: "In short, there are no substantial differences between the diet indicated for athletes and the diet for those who are not athletes". This sentence could be the cause of a lack of sporting result by an athlete. Such a statement cannot be accepted, especially when it comes to the nutrition for non-recreational sports, such as competitive or amateur ones, even though we all know that many times those who play sports as a hobby make a considerable effort. In this short chapter, I will try to talk in a simple but comprehensive way about the relationship between nutrition and physical activity, mentioning the role that controlled and targeted dietary supplementation can play for the well-being and the health of the athlete (young or adult), because too often the word integration is associated with doping and exasperation of the athletic gesture, but nobody connects it with the expression "health and prevention from injury".

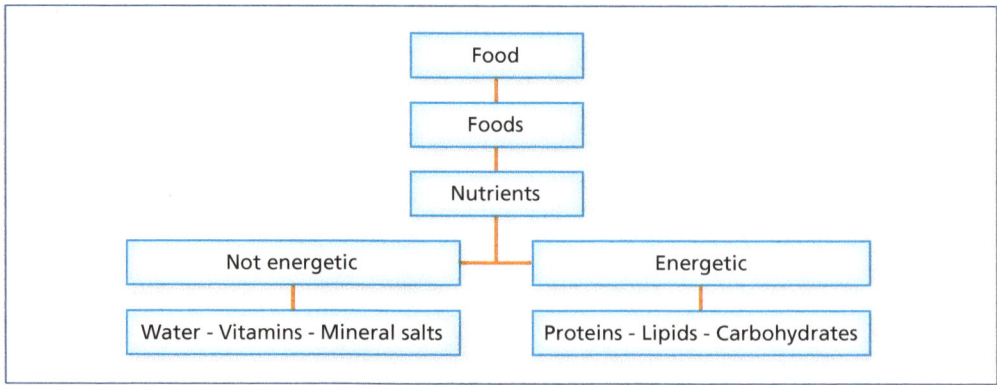

Figure 3.2 It is possible to distinguish the family of nutrients into two main groups: macronutrients, used by the body for structural or energy purposes, and micronutrients, responsible for maintaining the homeostasis.

If we do not feed ourselves correctly from a qualitative and quantitative point of view, we will not obtain the desired results (on the contrary, we could obtain a decline in performance) because we will consume our internal resources. It is therefore essential to take care of our food 365 days a year; it must be varied, balanced, rich in nutrients (with the right quantities of proteins, carbohydrates, fats, vitamins and minerals), but above all personalized.

Table 3.1 Micronutrients and macronutrients: main functions and the distribution in foods

Substance	Function	Food
Sugars (glucids or carbohydrates)	They provide energy 1 g = 4 Kcal	Milk, fruit, cereals (pasta, rice, bread, wheat, cornflakes), vegetables, honey, sweets
Proteins	They build and repair the muscular mass 1 g = 4 Kcal	Meat, fish, cheese, eggs, legumes, milk, etc.
Fats (or lipids)	They build up to provide slow-release energy 1 g = 9 Kcal	Butter, cream, margarine, milk, meats, fish, cheese, eggs, lard, bacon, olive and seed oils, nuts, etc.
Fibers	They perform functions of regulation and assimilation in the intestine level	Fruits, vegetables, cereals, wholemeal, legumes
Vitamins	They regulate all the vital functions of the body	Fresh fruit and vegetables, milk, cheese, egg yolk, cereals, meat
Mineral salts	They perform various structural functions of the organism and regulate its functions	Fresh fruit and vegetables, milk, cheese, egg yolk, cereals, meat
Water	Essential for all vital functions	Almost all foods, water

Energetic foods: provide the energy needed to carry out various activities (breathing, heart rate, maintaining body temperature, running, work, etc.): these are **fats, carbohydrates and eventually even proteins**.

Structural foods: contribute to the body composition of muscles, bones and organs: they are proteins, fats, minerals and water.

Regulatory foods: facilitate and condition the chemical reactions and regulate the functioning of our organs and tissues: they are water, vitamins and minerals (sodium, calcium, phosphorus, iron, magnesium, iodine, etc.).

Therefore, the nutrition must not be taken care of only for the purpose of slimming or in any case for esthetic reasons, since it also affects various other aspects:

- performance improvement;
- prevention of trauma and damage to the structures that make up the body (ligaments, joints, etc.);
- improvement of attention, reaction speed, decision-making skills depending in what you are doing;
- acceleration of recovery processes after trauma and after intense competitions and/or trainings;
- improvement of metabolism, biochemical processes (especially those for the detoxification of the body);
- improvement of the general state (the health first of all).

The weight and the body composition of the athlete must be carefully evaluated, as, too often, the ideal weight deduced from anthropometric tables is associated with the right one for the individual subject (perhaps it is valid for a sedentary person), without paying attention to the ratio of lean mass/fat mass and to the constitutional morphology.

Chapter 3 ▸ Nutrition for the athletes

In the athlete of any discipline it is necessary to evaluate the ideal weight, i.e. the weight agreed between the athlete, the sports doctor, the coach, the nutritionist, which coincides or has coincided with the optimal performance and which is associated with a subjective sensation of psychophysical well-being. There are three aspects that must be evaluated in an athlete's diet:
- quantitative;
- qualitative;
- chronological.

Quantitative aspect

- Nutrition is linked to the energy expenditure, which depends on the basal metabolism, work activity and training.
- The energy expenditure during the training depends on the sport and how it is interpreted (300-700 Kcal/h with the average consumption of 500-600 Kcal).
- In demanding conditions, with particular climatic conditions (rain, wind, snow, etc.) an energy expenditure of 1000 Kcal/h can be reached.
- The breakdown of nutrition into macronutrients (proteins, carbohydrates and lipids) is usually the following:
  carbohydrates   50-55%
  proteins   20-25%
  fats   25-30%
- New scientific studies are re-evaluating the percentages reported above, moving towards the following subdivision:
  carbohydrates   40-50%
  proteins   25-30%
  fats   25-30%
- It is also important to take it into consideration when you want to achieve a maximum athletic performance (carbohydrate discharge and recharge methods to increase glycogen stores, even if they are outdated).

How much protein for an athlete?

To calculate your protein requirement, you must first start with the calculation of your body composition so that you can extrapolate the amount in kilograms of the lean mass (there are skin-specific methods, bio-impedance meters, special scales, DEXA, etc.). At this point the calculated weight is multiplied by a coefficient of the physical activity shown in the following table.

The calculated result will give the grams of the proteins that must be ingested daily. First of all, let's see what proteins are used for:
- replacement of worn muscle mass;
- building new muscle mass;
- trophism of the ligaments;
- synthesis and resynthesis of hormones and enzymes;
- for energy purposes (depending on the type and intensity of the effort, they can also provide 17% of the expended energy).

Chapter 3 ▸ Nutrition for the athletes

Table 3.2 Evaluation of the amount of dietary protein that must be taken in order to estimate the optimal protein intake

Protein requirement (g/kg of lean mass)	Activity
1.1	Pure sedentary (television and slippers)
1.3	Quiet work, without training or regular sporting activity
1.5	More active work with fitness activities (some walking); obese subjects: over 30% (men) and 40% (women) of fat mass
1.7	Stressful jobs; managers and career women; subjects who train at least three times a week or systematically practice a sport
1.9	Working and daily aerobic or weight training (barbells or machines)
2.1	Heavy daily training (barbells or machines)
2.3	Intense training for competitive purposes, supplemented by heavy daily weight training, or double intense daily sports training

The estimated requirement for an athlete is about 1.5 grams of protein per kilogram of body weight, although when a certain strengthening or an increase in muscle mass is sought, it can reach 2.3 g/kg of body weight, naturally in healthy subjects. When setting the amount of protein (especially in people who do not tolerate the amounts indicated above), it must, however, be remembered that carbohydrates in particular and fats (such as the amount of calories consumed during the day) have a protein-sparing effect.

Young athletes engaged in high-intensity physical activity should learn more about their dietary needs to optimize their growth.

For example, their protein requirements range from 1.8-2.0 g/kg of body weight.

The timing of the protein intake is also very important. Research has shown that consuming a drink containing carbohydrates and proteins within one hour of the end of exercise stimulates the release of insulin and growth hormone, resulting in an increase in muscle mass and in a greater energy recovery.

Table 3.3 Estimation of the protein requirements based on the type of activity carried out. Data expressed in g/kg of body weight

	Need	Strength sport with development of muscle mass	Cross-country sport (long distance running, cycling, walking, etc.)
Basic necessity	0.9	0.9	0.9
Muscle mass development	0.2	0.2	–
Protein heritage growth	Up to 0.3	0.1-0.3	0.1
Use for energy purposes	Up to 0.8	0.2	0.3-0.8
Increase in turnover	Up to 0.4	0.1-0.4	0.1-0.2
Total daily needs		1.5-2	1.4-2

Qualitative aspect

The question that arises is: which foods are preferable to consume?

Sugars, glucids or carbohydrates

Sugars are the most readily available source of energy for an athlete.

Many organic compounds belong to the large group of sugars, united by the chemical structure which includes carbon, plus hydrogen and oxygen combined with the ratio of water (H_2O); for this reason, they are also defined as carbohydrates.

Foods that contain carbohydrates are: fruits (in the form of fructose and glucose), cereals, pasta, other wheat products, rice, corn, potatoes (in the form of starch), vegetables, milk (in the form of lactose).

Snacks, biscuits, sweet beverages and other foods sweetened with sucrose (a disaccharide composed of glucose and fructose), despite being rich in carbohydrates, have no other nutrients: use them rarely, indeed very little amounts. If you want to eat sweets, it is better to prepare them with xylitol instead of sucrose. Xylitol, also called wood sugar, is a polyol with a sweetening power similar to that of sucrose but with 40% fewer calories and a glycemic index (the capacity of a food, with the same carbohydrate content, to raise blood sugar) equal to half of sucrose; among other things, since it is not metabolized by the oral bacterial flora, it does not contribute to the onset of caries.

After their digestion is completed, sugars are transported by the blood circulation to the liver, where they are converted into glucose. Glucose, on the other side, is transported by the circulation as a supply of energy for the muscles and the brain. A small amount of glucose is converted into glycogen and remains stored in the muscles and liver, the rest is transformed into fat and deposited in the subcutaneous tissue. An athlete lacking carbohydrates will experience that the consequent lack of glycogen makes the physical activity difficult: the feeling of fatigue, after prolonged exercise, is often due to the lack of blood sugar and because of the exhaustion of glycogen reserves.

A diet that is too low in carbohydrates makes the physical activity difficult if not impossible.

However, carbohydrate intake must be focused on those with a low glycemic index, which release glucose slowly and steadily and subsequently ensure a "glycemic stability".

High glycemic index sugars, on the other hand, cause a sharp rise in the blood sugar level, and therefore an energy peak, temporal and very short as it stimulates a high release of insulin into the circulation, which will cause a drop in the glucose level in the blood: exactly the opposite of what an athlete in a competition needs!

However, normally, except for certain situations such as the "definition" phase in bodybuilding or during diets aimed at returning to the "weight" category, most athletes, especially in aerobic disciplines, tend to favor the consumption of carbohydrates. In reality, an unbalanced intake of these nutrients, especially in the form of refined cereals, compared to other macronutrients, causes a condition of hyperinsulinism with harmful effects on health. In addition, cereals are acidifying (as well as meat and dairy products) and therefore favor a situation of chronic acidosis that generates fatigue and stiffening of the muscles and the related tendons, ligaments and connective tissue, predisposing the athlete to cramps, strains and tendon-muscle and ligamentous ruptures.

SUMMING UP:

Right choices: less insulin reaction
- biggest part of the fruit
- most vegetables that are rich in fiber
- selected cereals (oat flakes, hulled oats, barley, quinoa, buckwheat)
- low glycemic index foods

Wrong choices: increased insulin reaction
- most refined cereals (bread, pasta, etc.)
- 00-01 flour types
- some fruits (for example grapes, raisins, ripe bananas, figs, dried fruits)
- some vegetables (corn, cooked carrots, potatoes)

Proteins

Protein affects the growth and the maintenance of the muscle tissue. They are the major source of building material in our whole body: muscles, internal organs, skin, etc.

They play a decisive role in the production of proteinic hormones, and also other hormones, including testosterone.

Once digested, the proteins are broken down into amino acids, which make up the blood amino acid pool or are used to make up other proteins.

The human body uses amino acids when it needs new proteins to repair cells or for muscle growth: it needs about 21 amino acids to synthesize new proteins.

11 of them are produced by our organism: they are called *non-essential amino acids*. Another 8, which cannot be produced by our organism, are called *essential amino acids*: they must necessarily come from food; 2 of them are called conditionally essential (arginine and histidine) because they are essential in certain situations, such as in the growth phase.

In order for the body to properly utilize proteins, all essential amino acids must be present at the same time in the correct proportions. If only one of them is missing or deficient, the protein synthesis will proceed at a low level or it will not happen. That is why protein sources containing all essential amino acids must be introduced into every meal. In reality there are some amino acids defined as semi-essential that can replace the essential ones: cysteine can replace methionine and tyrosine can replace phenylalanine.

An animal organism is in a neutral nitrogen balance state when the amount of nitrogen introduced in the diet (through the intake of amino acids) is equal to that excreted in the urine and feces. The maintenance of nitrogen balance in sedentary adults is ensured by 1 g daily per kg of body weight of high biological value proteins, while the need for an athlete can exceed 2 g. The positive nitrogen balance situation occurs when the introduction of nitrogen exceeds the elimination.

Table 3.4 Essential and non-essential amino acids in humans

Valine*^	Phenylalanine ^	Tyrosine	Aspartic acid
Isoleucine*^	Threonine ^	Glycine	Aspartic acid
Leucine*^	Tryptophan ^	Alanine	Arginine ^
Lysine^	Histidine ^	Serine	Proline
Methionine^	Cysteine	Asparagine	Glutamine

* = branched chain amino acids, BCAAs; ^ = essential amino acids

The body will find itself in a positive nitrogen balance condition whenever the nitrogen intake is higher than/equal to the actual nitrogen demand (during growth, in the case of a high-calorie diet). On the other hand, the organism will find itself in a negative nitrogen balance situation when the nitrogen elimination exceeds the introduction, i.e. when the nitrogen supply is lower than the actual requirement (or the capacity to use) by the organism.

The amount of protein needed to ensure the neutral nitrogen balance depends on the content and proportion of the essential amino acids that constitute it. It is precisely this content that gives proteins the so-called "biological value". An athlete must always be in a positive or neutral nitrogen balance to preserve their muscle mass, to make sure to always synthesize the best hormones, enzymes and other compounds that require an amino acid base, and improve their physical performance.

Proteins cannot be stored like carbohydrates (in the form of glycogen) or lipids (in the form of fat tissue), even if, in a certain sense, the muscle can be considered the store of amino acids, and therefore their intake must be constant.

Insufficient amounts of protein in diets cause a slow recovery from workouts, low energy levels, low disease resistance and a tendency to muscle catabolism.

An athlete who follows an intense training and fails to take the necessary amount of protein to rebuild or grow muscle tissue will soon fall into overtraining. Recovery will be insufficient and they will harm themself by training. This is the catabolic process (as opposed to the anabolic process).

The body works on a priority system: if the internal organs ask for proteins to repair and rebuild their tissues, the muscles will be deprived of the proteins which are necessary for their growth.

Remembering that essential amino acids are the main requirements in the diet, the best foods that contain complete proteins are: beef, chicken, fish, turkey, dairy products, eggs (especially cooked egg whites) and soy beans. Animal proteins have a higher biological value than those of vegetable origin, being richer in essential amino acids, but, given the complementarity of the two protein sources, a 2/3 animal and 1/3 vegetable proportion, which could also become 1/2 and 1/2, is to be considered optimal for an athlete. This does not mean that a vegan cannot have a good protein synthesis, as in fact all the essential amino acids are present in vegetable proteins, but, being less concentrated, it is necessary to take a greater quantity and the correct combinations.

SUMMING UP:

- Proteins provide essential amino acids which are fundamental for the synthesis of muscle proteins, enzymes and hormones.
- In certain situations, such as strict diets or intense workouts, they can also acquire true energy functions.
- The protein intake for the athlete must be calculated on the basis of body weight (1.5-2 g/kg) and not as a caloric percentage and must be divided into the various meals of the day.
- The ideal contribution is made up of 2/3 of animal origin and 1/3 of vegetable origin.

Fats or lipids

According to a popular misconception within athletes and "health conscious" people in general, fats should be removed almost completely from any diet.

Fats are the most concentrated source of energy in the diet: when oxidized, they provide more than double of the calories (9) per gram compared to those provided by carbohydrates (4) or proteins (4).

Furthermore, they can be stored in the form of adipose tissue as reserve energy: it is estimated that the average caloric reserve represented by the fat tissues of a normal weight individual is around 75,000-100,000 Kcal, sufficient to cover 50 days of fasting. Not everyone knows that, in addition to being a "life jacket" or "love handles", fats can be accumulated in intra- and intermuscular spaces in the form of vacuoles, which are easy and ready to use. By educating our body (through a targeted diet) to effectively accumulate these fats, we will obtain longer lasting energy savings with minimal additional weight.

Beyond the energy supply, they provide essential fatty acids, transport fat-soluble vitamins, participate in the formation of fundamental cellular structures (such as membranes), surround and protect vital organs (heart, liver, kidneys, spleen, brain, spinal cord), and subcutaneous fat limits heat loss by maintaining the body temperature.

Based on their melting point, they are divided into fats (solid at room temperature) and oils (liquid at room temperature). As we have seen for essential amino acids, there are also some essential fatty acids that our body cannot produce and which must be introduced in our diet.

As for proteins, it is recommended that the intake of fats should be divided between animal and vegetable sources, because the latter, which is rich in essential fatty acids (vitamin F), has the ability to reduce the level of triglycerides and cholesterol in the blood, thus preventing atherosclerosis.

A big part of the bad reputation of fats is played by cholesterol. However, it must not be forgotten that cholesterol is essential for the formation of bile salts (to digest fats), it is an essential precursor of various adrenal hormones (DHEA, pregnenolone, aldosterone, cortisol), of the male and female gonadal sex hormones and also of vitamin D; moreover, cholesterol is an essential constituent of cell membranes and it is essential for the health of the brain. However, we have all heard that high cholesterol increases the risk of heart attacks and strokes.

First of all, it must be pointed out that when total cholesterol levels are very high, this does not depend on dietary factors but on genetically predetermined dysfunctions; moreover, the relationship between cholesterol and atherosclerosis deserves to be reviewed on the basis of recent acquisitions. Blood cholesterol is carried by the VLDL (Very Low Density Lipoprotein), LDL (Low Density Lipoprotein) and HDL (High Density Lipoprotein) lipoproteins. As for LDL, there are some subtypes: *large and buoyant LDL, small and dense LDL,* and an intermediate type between the two. The most atherogenic lipoproteins are the sd-LDL as they remain longer in circulation, oxidize more easily (and it is the oxidized cholesterol that is atherogenic) and pass the endothelial membrane of blood vessels more easily, thus contributing to the formation of atherosclerotic plaque. Unfortunately, their identification is not foreseen in normal laboratory tests.

Atherosclerosis is a multifactorial pathology with an inflammatory etiopathogenesis characterized by the presence of plaques due to cellular alterations and oxidative phenomena promoted by the increase in oxidized sd-LDL. It has been seen that it is not so much the amount of cholesterol in the diet, but the high content of refined carbohydrates and trans fatty acids that increase the level of triglycerides and sd-LDL lipoproteins and cause a reduction in HDL. In various studies it has even been shown that frequent consumption of eggs (14 per week) promoted the increase of HDL and the reduction of sd-LDL (the best form of egg intake is soft-boiled or ox-eye, so that the cholesterol of the yolk is not cooked and oxidized).

A diet that provides fat in the correct proportions favors an increase in HDL and lb-LDL at the expense of triglycerides and sd-LDL. When the body has a good amount of unsaturated fatty acids, a large amount of the cholesterol is carried in the form of complex molecules called HDL, which counteract the deposition of cholesterol on the arterial walls. For this reason, it is called "good cholesterol".

Therefore the polyunsaturated, monounsaturated and saturated fatty acids must be taken in the proportions of 1/3 each as: the polyunsaturated ones, among which the so-called essential (linoleic-omega-6, alpha-linolenic-omega-3), are fundamental for the proper functioning of the cell membrane and for the prevention of atherosclerosis; the monounsaturated (oleic-omega-9) have a neutral or moderately benign effect against atherosclerosis and protective against tumor diseases; the saturated, being always associated with cholesterol in the animal kingdom, are fundamental for hormonal production, especially for testosterone.

Alpha-linolenic acid, which is the progenitor of the omega-3 family, is present in linseed oil and its derivatives, and those such as EPA (eicosapentaenoic acid) and DHA (docosahexaenoic acid), are present in abundance in marine animals, especially fish from the cold seas of the North (salmon, mackerel and herring). Omega-6 prevails in our diet, especially the arachidonic acid which is present in foods of animal origin, and linoleic acid, which has a vegetable origin (present, for example, in sunflower and corn oils), which, unlike omega-3, if in excess (especially arachidone), can cause an inflammatory effect.

While unsaturated fatty acids increase the insulin sensitivity, saturated fats lower it, and this is a valid reason to limit them but not to eliminate them completely, as some can easily be used for energy purposes, such as for example, short-chain (present in butter) and medium-chain (present in coconut) fatty acids, and they also favor the production of sex hormones which are almost always associated with cholesterol.

I would therefore say that the proportions mentioned above: 1/3 polyunsaturated (linseed oil, soybean oil, hemp oil, fish oil), 1/3 monounsaturated (olive oil, peanuts, avocado), 1/3 saturated (mostly contained in products of animal origin, such as meat and dairy products, but also vegetables such as coconut) represent the ideal formula. The only fats that must be absolutely eliminated are the hydrogenated ones because they have no function in the human physiology and if they become part of the cellular membrane, they can alter its functionality.

During rest, fats produce about 2/3 of the energy needed by the body. When the energy demand increases, sugars intervene, changing this proportion in their favor. However, it is again the fats that intervene in the prolonged phases of activity.

In sudden effort, as well as in untrained sports, 80% of the "fuel" is provided by sugars and 20% by fats. With training, the sportsperson, who has become an athlete, learns to make better use of the fats which are stored in their body. It has been verified that, after four hours of intense effort, the supply of energy sources is broken down as follows: 65% from fats, 30% from sugars, 5% from other sources. This is an advantageous adaptation because the athlete can save sugars, the reserve of which is of a limited quantity, for the final stages of a race, such as a sprint.

SUMMING UP:

- Polyunsaturated fats provide the linoleic acid (omega-6) and alpha-linolenic (omega-3), EPA and DHA that cannot be synthesized by the human body and therefore it is essential to include them in our food (linseed, soy and sunflower oil, salmon, mackerel, etc.).
- Saturated fats are important for the production of sex hormones.
- On a physical level, they can act as cushions in traumatic events (protect the organs and viscera) as well as being thermal insulators.
- They provide a considerable amount of energy (9 Kcal/g) and are the most used substrate in aerobic conditions.

Fibers

Fibers are a particular category of complex carbohydrates that humans cannot digest or that are digested only minimally because we do not have certain digestive enzymes that herbivorous animals have. They are represented by a series of substances which are present mainly in the walls of plant cells (cellulose, hemicellulose and lignin) and in a variety of gums, mucilage and algae. Dietary fiber performs important physiological actions, including that of retaining large quantities of water (fiber of insoluble type: cellulose, hemicellulose, lignin), especially at the gastrointestinal level, increasing the transit speed and the volume of stools.

The other function is to form viscous gel-like solutions in the gastrointestinal tract (soluble fibers: pectins, mannans and mucilage) with a mainly metabolic function, controlling and regulating glucose and cholesterol levels. Soluble fibers (for example, oat beta-glucan, inulin, pectin) improve the insulin sensitivity, reduce the post-prandial glycaemia and cholesterol, improve glucose tolerance, regulate intestinal functions, stimulate the immune system (this is probably due to a prebiotic effect, i.e. modulation of the intestinal bacterial flora).

In addition, soluble fibers, especially oat fibers, have physicochemical properties that modulate the mobility of the upper gastrointestinal tract by delaying stomach emptying and by slowing or preventing the absorption of specific macronutrients, such as glucose and fat, and by promoting the sense of satiety. There is no such thing as a well-defined and precise need for fibers. The current consumption of fiber is around 15-18 grams per day or even less; it is thought that humans in the Paleolithic consumed at least four times as much. It would be appropriate to bring the consumption of fiber to at least 25 grams for women and 35 grams for men, as recommended by various international scientific societies. To increase fiber, it is advisable to increase the consumption of foods that are naturally rich in it, such as whole grains, legumes, vegetables and fruit. The consumption of fiber also affects the energy level of the individual, modulating their glycemic levels and avoiding the phenomenon of "craving" (compulsive hunger induced by glucose imbalance).

A high-fiber breakfast reduces fatigue. 142 adults were studied, none of whom regularly ate a high-fiber cereal breakfast. They were then divided into two groups: one who maintained their usual breakfast and another who was given a high-fiber breakfast for 14 days. Subjects who ate the high-fiber breakfast were significantly less fatigued than those who ate a low-fiber breakfast.

Among the foods that are rich in fiber, it is advisable to favor fruits and vegetables, as they provide vitamins, antioxidants, phytonutrients, minerals and trace elements in quantity.

Sportspeople who train intensely often have problems with intestinal disorders linked to poor digestion of food due to the execution of workouts while still being in the digestive phase. This can easily lead to intestinal dysbiosis, which is an altered bacterial flora, also favored by the intake of refined foods for athletes (jellies, maltodextrins, protein powders) that are consumed for convenience but do not provide the amount of fiber necessary for the correct development of the bacterial flora.

Exhausting physical activities can cause the leaky gut syndrome, that is, the formation of micro-lesions on the intestinal wall that cause the inability to selectively absorb the nutrients that come from digestion. All this is caused by the fact that if physical activity is intense and prolonged or occurs immediately after meals, the blood circulation that should support the digestive processes moves from the intestine to the muscles, causing a nutritional deficiency in the cells of the intestinal wall that favors the onset of leaky intestine. Well, in this case, "resistant starch" can be useful.

Resistant starch or RS is that part of the starch, about 1/10 of food starch, which resists the digestion process by intestinal enzymes and reaches the colon intact, where it can be fermented and used as a nutrient by the intestinal bacterial flora. The bacteria transform this fraction of starch into short-chain fatty acids that can be used for energy purposes but with a lower caloric efficiency than starch, or be used directly by the bacteria themselves.

This, in addition to the fact that resistant starch is only partially converted into fatty acids, means that it brings fewer calories than expected. Of these, it seems that butyric acid also exerts a preventive effect against colon cancer. The fact that resistant starch favors the development of a correct intestinal bacterial flora is important for the immune system as the intestine has the largest immune cell apparatus, which consists in Peyer's plaques, and bacteria modulates its functioning, thus protecting the organism from infectious diseases.

Resistant starch is found mainly in legumes, barley, oats, potato starch, green bananas, plantains, or is formed through the retrograde process that occurs through the gelatinization and cooking phase of the starch after cooling down. So, in this case, it might be useful to cook our rice and potatoes and consume them only after they have cooled down.

Starting from the example of the resistant starch, we must consider that today it is believed that 70% of the fibers that are present in traditional foods, which by definition are edible substances of vegetable origin that are not normally hydrolyzed by enzymes of the digestive system, can actually be fermented by the bacterial flora of the colon and they can produce short-chain fatty acids that provides a significant caloric intake.

Determining its real energy value, considering the influence exerted on the absorption of other micronutrients, is certainly a difficult problem that the FAO commission has decided to overcome by setting the average energy value of dietary fibers at 2 Kcal/g. Thus, the concept that dietary fiber does not bring calories is dispelled and, consequently, the calorie content reported in nutritional labels and in the preparation of diets, must also consider the contribution provided by dietary fibers.

Minerals

Minerals perform many important functions, taking an active part in the cellular life processes such as the formation of teeth and bones, and in regulating the fluids of our body. They are divided into macrominerals or mineral salts, i.e. calcium, chlorine, phosphorus, magnesium, potassium, sodium and sulfur, and microminerals, i.e. chromium, iron, fluorine, iodine, manganese, molybdenum, copper, selenium, zinc, bromine, cobalt, silicon, boron.

The former must be introduced in quantities ranging from 100 mg to 1 g per day, while the latter must be taken in smaller quantities, from less than 1 mg to 100 mg. Then there are the trace elements, the real need for which has not yet been established, but it is in micrograms.

The most important mineral salts for the muscle physiology are: sodium, potassium, calcium, magnesium and phosphorus.

As for the functions and foods in which the various minerals are contained, we refer to the relative table.

Mineral salts

The functions of these minerals are many, but I will point out some elements:
1. they don't provide calories;
2. they are fundamental (the first four) for muscle contraction and for the maintenance of the electrical activity of the heart, as well as for regulating the blood pressure and flow in the various districts and organs of the body.

Sodium

Sodium (Na) should not be taken in excess because, as you well know, it can cause hypertension in predisposed subjects, and water retention (to which bodybuilders are particularly... sensitive, as it causes the unpleasant sensation of muscle fogging and poor definition). Normally, with the diet, one also takes in more sodium than necessary, so supplementation is not recommended. The daily sodium intake for an athlete must be between 2 to 6 g.

But the athletes often sweat, especially during summer in hot, humid conditions and during prolonged efforts, so they can lose more salt than a normal subject.

Therefore, sodium intake must be carefully kept within a certain range based on these factors, to avoid a deficiency that can give rise to:
1. nausea, somnolence and other cenestopathic disorders;
2. less ease of muscle contraction;
3. loss of potassium due to the compensatory attempt of the sodium-sparing hormone, aldosterone, which retains sodium in the kidneys and precisely eliminates potassium;
4. hypotension and decreased vascular tone.

From all this can derive a poor training, a "drained" muscular aspect and fatigue. Also in this case, the key is in the balance.

Potassium

Potassium (K) is the main intracellular cation. Its fate is linked to that of the sodium (in a kind of balance, one up and the other down); furthermore, potassium binds to muscle proteins and above all to glycogen. This can be of a fundamental practical importance, especially if glycogen levels vary rapidly (discharge and recharge diet): in this case, if the K intake is not appropriately modified, there is a risk of hypo- or hyperkalaemia.

Potassium deficiency is extremely deleterious for the athlete, causing: disturbances in heart and muscle contraction (up to paralysis) in the worst cases, profound fatigue and "empty muscles" in less severe cases. In general, the athlete's diet must contain a good amount of potassium (from 3 to 8 g); in this particular case, the healthy body is able to cope with a slight excess, so the "better to abound" rule may apply. Finally, in some very special conditions, a slight excess of potassium can even be exploited (temporarily) to block aldosterone and promote a natural sodium loss for the purpose of pre-contest definition in bodybuilding.

Calcium

Calcium (CA) is essential for the muscle contraction, as it is like a spark plug that gives the spark to burn the fuel.

Hypocalcemia would therefore be dramatic for the athlete, but in normal individuals it never occurs, because, unlike sodium and potassium, calcium has a very abundant reserve (bones), so conditions of slight excess and especially deficiency, are tolerated for a long time at the expense of the bone itself, which can be "nibbled" slowly (hence the "osteoporosis").

This condition is typical for older women; hopefully young males (who have very powerful calcium accumulation mechanisms) are free of it.

However, recent studies have shown unequivocally that even a minimal calcium deficiency in the juvenile period will show itself as osteoporosis (fragile bones that break from nothing) at the age of 60-70, when it will be too late to do anything about it.

So, for sporty women it will be of vital importance to have:
1. a sufficient supply of vitamin D, which is calcium-absorbing and fixing;
2. a sufficient intake of calcium itself (at least 800 mg per day, according to the aforementioned studies).

The fact is that dairy products, typically rich in calcium, are also acidifying, thus promoting the release of calcium from the bones for buffering purposes. Therefore, a well-established diet should provide calcium from alternative sources (some particularly rich vegetables, such as spinach, etc., or dried fruit and nuts, such as almonds).

Magnesium

It will be treated separately in a specific paragraph in the chapter dedicated to supplements.

Phosphorus

Phosphorus (P), bound in the form of organic and non-organic compounds, is typically distributed within cells.

Generally, its importance is "neglected" because it does not participate like the other four in the events of the formation and conduction of the electrical impulses that cause the muscles to contract.

Phosphorus (in the form of ATP and phosphocreatine) is simply the fuel of the muscles, which is provided by calorie foods.

In the case of the power athlete, a sufficient supply of phosphate is essential because the accumulation of ATP, and above all of phosphocreatine, represents the physiological adaptation of the muscle subjected to a certain number of heavy repetitions, with the visible result of the increase in the muscle "mass" itself.

Apart from supplements such as inosine, etc., it is necessary, especially in the training phases, to provide the right amount of phosphorus in order to build up a better reserve of ATP.

As with potassium, a slight excess is well tolerated. The mere calculation of the phosphates consumed with the diet may not be enough, because these substances are difficult to absorb from the intestine, and the degree of absorption varies depending on the type of food to which the phosphorus itself is bound.

Trace elements

They are elements with various bioregulatory and structural functions, present in small but essential quantities.

Clinically, **iron** is the most important, so the discussion about phosphorus is also valid in this case: not the quantity, but the quality of dietary iron is essential.

The iron linked to oxalate and phytate complexes is poorly absorbed, the iron linked to meat is better, and the iron linked to eggs; vitamin C, alcohol, etc. is even better, as they promote absorption. However, from what has been said before, it appears that many of these foods cannot be consumed in excess by athletes for caloric and dietary balance reasons.

In this case, a dietary supplement is needed as, for example, in vegetarian sportswomen. Women, obviously, having menstruations, are subject (in one case out of three!) to iron-deficiency anemia. Since this is asymptomatic for a long time (before becoming symptomatic it should reach very low levels), it will be a duty for every female athlete to check the level of iron and hemoglobin in the blood with laboratory tests and, in terms of diet, provide the right amount of iron.

However, some scholars have noted that sporting males are subject to "myolysis" (partial destruction of muscle fibers) and rupture of red blood cells, again due to hypoxic and mechanical stress.

In the long run, this can lead to anemia, also highlighted in some famous champions as a chronic and progressive cause of an athletic inefficiency.

Table 3.5 Main trace elements: distribution in food, functions sustained in the body and deficiency symptoms

Minerals	Foods	What is it for	Symptoms of deficiency
Calcium	Milk, yogurt, cheese, vegetables dark green leaves, dried legumes, sardines, clams, mussels, chicory, hazelnuts	Formation of bones and teeth, blood clotting, conduction of nerve impulses, muscle contraction	Rickets, Growth stop, convulsions
Chlorine	Table salt, milk, meat, seafood, eggs	Formation of gastric juice, acid-base balance	Decreased appetite, apathy, muscle cramps
Chrome	Vegetable oils, fats, shellfish, whole grains	Contributes to energy and glucose metabolism	Decreased ability to metabolize glucose
Copper	Liver, seafood, poultry, cereals, legumes, cherries, nuts	It is an element contained in enzymes involved in digestion and in the formation of elastin	Anemia
Fluorine	Seafood, rice, spinach, onion, lettuce, tea and coffee	Maintenance of the bone and dental structure	Increase in the cases of deterioration of the teeth
Iodine	Milk, fish and fruits of sea, vegetables, algae	It is an element contained in the thyroid hormones	Hypothyroidism
Iron	Liver, meats, cereals, fruits seafood, eggs, legumes, dark green leafy vegetables	It is an element contained in hemoglobin and is linked to energy metabolism	Hypochromic anemia
Magnesium	Cereals, green leafy vegetables, milk, meat, legumes, almonds, cocoa, pumpkin seeds	Activation of enzymes, protein synthesis	Growth stop, spasms, behavioral and sleep disturbances

Continues

Continued

Minerals	Foods	What is it for	Symptoms of deficiency
Manganese	Milk and its derivatives, whole grains, legumes, berries, fruit, tea, ginger	It is a contained element in enzymes for fat metabolism, it promotes bone growth, supports the thyroid gland and erythropoiesis	Bone loss, nausea and vomiting, low cholesterol and sex hormones
Molybdenum	Milk and its derivatives, liver, cereals, legumes, dark green leafy vegetables	It is an element contained in some enzymes, especially hepatic ones	Not certain
Phosphorus	Milk, cheese, red and white meat, fish, legumes, nuts	Formation of bones and teeth, acid-base balance	Demineralization of the bones, weakness, loss of calcium
Potassium	Milk, meat, most fruits, cereals and potatoes, legumes, vegetables, tomatoes etc.	Water balance, nervous function, acid-base balance	Muscle weakness, paralysis
Selenium	Brazil nuts, fish, red and white meats, milk, cereals	Coenzyme of glutathione peroxidase	Bone and muscle pain, thyroid hypofunctionality
Sodium	In almost all foods, except fruit	Acid-base balance, nervous function, water balance	Apathy, decreased appetite, muscle cramps
Sulfur	Foods with protein value	It is a component of tissues and cartilage	Articular pains, skin problems, decreased detoxifying capacity
Zinc	Liver, seafood, milk	It is an element contained in enzymes that deal with the metabolism of nucleic acids, digestive enzymes and the enzyme that carries carbon dioxide in the red blood cells	Hypogonadism, growth stop

Vitamins

Vitamins do not represent a source of energy for our organism, nor do they participate in the structural component of our body. Our body is not able to produce them, and even though the need for our body is minimal, it is essential.

Vitamins are divided into fat-soluble and water-soluble: the former are stored by our organism, creating a reserve in case they are not taken daily.

The water-soluble products cannot be stored in any way and must therefore be taken daily.

Fat-soluble vitamins participate in particular reactions – such as vitamin A, which plays the role of forming and maintaining the skin, mucous membranes, bones and teeth – and are present only in some foods.

Water-soluble vitamins play roles such as catalysts in metabolic pathways and are present in various quantities in all foods.

Table 3.6 Main vitamins: distribution in food, sustained functions in the body and deficiency symptoms

Vitamins	Foods	What is it for	Symptoms of deficiency
Water-soluble vitamins			
Vitamin B1 or thiamine	Pork, liver, shellfish, whole grains and derivatives such as bread and pasta, brewer's yeast	Good functioning of the nervous system and digestive system	Beriberi, muscle weakness and cramps, mental confusion, heart failure
Vitamin B2 or riboflavin	Meat, liver, milk, eggs, cereals and derivatives, vegetables green leafy, mushrooms	Maintains the mucous membrane, frees energy from carbohydrates, proteins and fats	Diseases of the skin, eyes and growth
Vitamin B3 or Vitamin PP or niacin	Meat, poultry, liver, tuna, cereals, legumes, milk, yeast	It is part of the electron carriers	Pellagra, injuries to the skin located mainly in areas exposed to light, diarrhea, irritability, mental confusion, dementia
Vitamin B5 or pantothenic acid	Meat, liver, kidney, fish, eggs, whole grains, green vegetables, nuts, yeast	Metabolism of the of carbohydrates, proteins and fats, hormone formation	Neuromotor, cardiovascular and gastrointestinal disorders
Vitamin B6 or pyridoxine	Liver, fish, cereals and wholemeal bread, spinach, peas, bananas, yeast	Metabolism of proteins, utilization of fats	Dermatitis, convulsions, dizziness, anemia
Vitamin B7 or inositol	Brewer's yeast, liver, nuts, citrus fruits, egg yolk, whole grains	Stimulates lecithin production, reduces blood cholesterol, decreases fat deposits in the liver, helps maintain the memory	Hypoglycemia, skin excoriation
Vitamin B8 or Vitamin H or biotin	Liver, kidneys, egg yolk, green vegetables, peas	Synthesis of fatty acids, frees energy from carbohydrates, general amino acid metabolism	Flaky dermatitis, muscle aches and weakness
Vitamin B9 or folacin or folic acid	Liver, kidney, green leafy vegetables, brewer's yeast, wheat germ	Nucleic acids synthesis, formation of red blood cells	Megaloblastic anemia, diarrhea, hyperhomocysteinemia
Vitamin B12 or cyanocobalamin	Meat, liver, kidneys, fish, molluscs, eggs, milk	Synthesis of the genetic material, maturation of red blood cells, utilization of fats, functioning of the nervous system	Anemia, red blood cell malformation, pernicious anemia, peripheral nerve degeneration
C vitamin or ascorbic acid	Citrus fruits, melon, strawberry, tomatoes, potatoes and green leafy vegetables	Maintaining bones and teeth in good condition, maintenance of collagen and blood vessels, increases the body's natural defenses against infectious diseases	Scurvy, bleeding of the gums, bleeding with intact vessel, dry skin, teeth fall
Fat-soluble vitamins			
Vitamin A	Liver, egg yolk, vegetables, fruit, butter	Formation of visual pigments, maintenance of the normal structure of the epithelium	Visual disturbances, night blindness, changes in the skin and mucous membranes

Continues

Continued

Vitamins	Foods	What is it for	Symptoms of deficiency
Vitamin D or calciferol	Tuna, salmon, fish oil, liver, milk and dairy products. It is synthesized in the exposure of the skin to sunlight	Controls calcium absorption, bone growth and mineralization, regulates glucose and testosterone metabolism	Rickets, bone and tooth calcification disorders, muscle contractions and spasms, prostate cancer
Vitamin E or tocopherol	Vegetable oils, margarine, wholemeal bread, liver, green leafy vegetables	Prevents the oxidation of polyunsaturated fatty acids, enhances the resistance of red blood cells to lysis	Fragility of red blood cells
Vitamin K or naphthoquinone	Green leafy vegetables, milk; it is synthesized by intestinal bacteria	Essential for blood coagulation and for the deposit of calcium in the bones	Hemorrhages

Water

The replacement of water is a physiological mechanism that allows the body to maintain its homeostasis. The water introduced through drinks, that present in foods and that produced by the oxidative metabolism of macronutrients must be balanced with that eliminated through urine, feces, sweating, breathing and transpiration. A state of optimal hydration is associated with a lower risk of injury and dehydration, and a faster recovery from physical exertion.

Red blood cells carry oxygen to the muscles involved in exercise by flowing in the plasma, which is primarily made up of water. The nutrients, described in the previous pages, reach the muscles thanks to the plasma stream and therefore thanks to the water. The final products of muscle work are also eliminated through the body fluids. The volume of the plasma is important: in fact, if the loss of body water is high, the volume of the plasma decreases and there is a risk of cardiovascular damage. A loss of 2% of body weight in water is enough to reduce the sports performance capacity.

Sweating during an exercise is the most striking event that must be balanced with a continuous intake of liquids. Especially in long-term sports, such as running, cycling, cross-country skiing, marathons, it is necessary to drink small quantities continuously: for example, a glass of mineral water at regular intervals (every 20 minutes), anticipating the onset of thirst. The evaporation of sweat is the essential mechanism for cooling the body surface. Physical activity rapidly raises the body temperature.

If there is no rapid and effective cooling, what happens is the same as an engine launched at maximum speed and not cooled adequately, which overheats and damages every mechanical part. The normalization of body fluids, despite the attention in drinking, always occurs slowly. In fact, hydration levels return to normal even as late as 48-72 hours after sporting performance.

- Water makes up about 60% of the body mass; in the muscles it rises to 65-75%.
- The water requirement in adults is at least 2.5 L/day for men and 2 L/day for women (the amount depends on the climate, physical effort, etc.).
- A 4-5% reduction in body water content has a negative effect on the performance, up to a 40% decrease in muscle capacity.
- Water is often underestimated, but instead it is essential for:

– digestion, absorption and transport of nutrients, as well as for the excretion of metabolites;
– the functionality of the lymphatic and blood circulation;
– the constitution of cells, organs and tissues;
– the lubrication of some tissues (for example eyes and lungs);
– the lubrication of articular joints;
– the maintenance of the body temperature in the phenomenon of thermoregulation.

The recommendations concerning water requirement foresee 1 mL of water/Kcal; this requirement can increase to 1.5 mL/Kcal in case of intense and prolonged activities. An active muscle produces 100 times more heat than an inactive muscle; if this heat were not distributed externally, the body temperature would increase by 1 °C every 5-8 minutes during the exercise, leading to hyperthermia or collapse after about 15-20 minutes. Hence, the importance of the phenomenon of sweating; however, by losing more than 10% of the body water, one runs into a state of dehydration that can be fatal. Water is essential for health and performance, which increases by 6.5% in those who consume large amounts of fluids during exercises.

Refreshment drinks

Let's see the ingredients of a rehydration and recovery drink that can be taken during and after sports performance:

- simple and complex carbohydrates (usually a mix of glucose, maltodextrin and fructose) to replenish and preserve muscle glycogen reserves and to maintain a constant energy during the performance, if it lasts more than an hour;
- minerals (sodium, calcium, magnesium and potassium) to compensate, in part, the amount eliminated by sweat and to facilitate their recovery; they prevent the onset of cramps during and after the performance; stimulate (in the right relationship with carbohydrates) the passage of water from the intestine to the blood;
- protective vitamins: vitamins C and E with antioxidant effects;
- temperature: not cold;
- an isotonic drink will be preferable before and during the performance, while afterwards, a hypertonic (i.e. more concentrated) drink can also be taken;
- rapidly absorbed whey proteins, which, by stimulating insulin, favor a faster recovery of glycogen and activate the protein synthesis.

Chronological aspect

It refers to the distribution of meals throughout the day, based on the start time of the athletic performance, workouts, duration and recovery times.

At least three hours must pass between the end of the meal and the start of sports effort (except for the administration of easily metabolized supplements or in any case in times of emergency). The pre-race meal, if misinterpreted, can negatively affect the performance itself.

Before an athletic performance, a meal with a high glycemic index or simple sugars such as sucrose, which is the cooking sugar, or glucose, can be counterproductive because they can cause, after a short time, a state of hypoglycemia (low blood glucose levels) by a stimulating action on insulin. Therefore, meals with a low glycemic index, consisting of all three macronutrients, are more preferred.

A doubt that still remains is whether the pre-competition meal is positive on an energetic or mental level, as it has not yet been established whether what is ingested shortly before the start of a physical effort is actually available for the immediate use.

The fact is that if your athlete feels tired and immediately after drinking an energy supplement they feel better, or at least on a psychological level (in one study it was found that even just rinsing the mouth with a sweetened drink without ingesting it increases the energy level), only for the fact that taking an energy drink just before the race gives them more vigor and also more safety, give it to them without any problem.

During the time between the end of the last meal and the start of the competition, it is useful to sip waiting rations consisting of: fructose + glucose + maltodextrin + water with the addition of mineral salts and branched chain amino acids (the solution must be isotonic); they provide some immediate and long-lasting energy.

After the race it is advisable to consume a dose of carbohydrates to restore the glycogen storage. The post-race or training meal can also provide 30% of the daily amount of carbohydrates.

The evening is the best time to have a meal rich in carbohydrates, thus stimulating serotonin, which stimulates relaxation and physiological sleep.

SUMMING UP:

Nutritional rules for those who train
The diet must gradually adapt to nutritional needs, increasing or decreasing the calorie intake depending on the intensity of training and the quality of muscle work. The athlete needs a varied, balanced diet capable of satisfying the personal tastes. The calories and nutrients must be calculated and distributed throughout the day so that the weight is always the same (if it corresponds to that of the maximum performance) or brought to the weight which is defined by the coach and the sports dietician.

Nutritional rules:
- distribute the food in small meals throughout the day;
- consume foods that contain high quality proteins: meat, fish, lean cheeses, milk (pay attention to intolerances); limit fatty cheeses, fatty meats and sausages;
- moderate the consumption of foods rich in saturated fats (at least remove the fatty parts, especially if they are made of meat from farm animals) and prefer those of vegetable origin (extra virgin olive oil, dried nuts);
- take adequate amounts of foods that contain carbohydrates with low glycemic index and foods that are rich in fiber, fruits, vegetables, whole grains;
- pay attention to the consumption of sugars with a high glycemic index: use fructose instead of common sugar to add to drinks (tea, coffee), however limiting the quantity; reduce or eliminate sugary drinks;
- take the acid-base balance into consideration and consume vegetables in such quantities that can buffer the acidification caused by protein foods and cereals, and possibly supplements based on potassium, magnesium and calcium citrates;

- limit but not eliminate the use of salt in the kitchen;
- limit the consumption of alcoholic beverages;
- consume as much as possible food from organic farming and from wild animals;
- absolutely avoid foods containing hydrogenated fatty acids and trans fatty acids.

The diet must not be based solely on the sporting event, but must be regular throughout the week.

In the event that the performance or training takes place:

In the morning – The dinner of the previous day must be abundant, rich in carbohydrates, avoiding foods that are difficult to digest. A plate of pasta al dente, preferably wholemeal, a light second course (white meat or fish), cooked vegetables and extra virgin olive oil will therefore be fine to provide the fats necessary for the performance. Breakfast, to be consumed at least two hours before the performance, may contain: fruit juice or seasonal fruits, tea, wholemeal toast or wholemeal rusks with sugar-free jam or acacia honey, or an oatmeal; an easily digestible protein source (excellent protein powders or amino acid pools that do not strain the digestion) or scrambled egg whites, all accompanied by a source of healthy fats (nuts, almond cream or peanuts).

In the afternoon – In this case, breakfast must be abundant and also include salty foods, such as bread and ham and whole eggs or toast; lunch will have to reflect the dinner of the previous point, also adding a pice of fruit (if tolerated) and consumed at least three hours before, so as to be assimilated and not steal blood from the muscles due to digestion.

In the evening – Breakfast and lunch will be eaten as in the previous example, but an hour and a half before the start, the athlete can consume a waiting ration consisting of Parmigiano Reggiano and fruits, or lean cold cuts and fruits, or protein-carbohydrate bars, or a drink consisting of fructose and easily digestible protein powder, with a pleasant taste, especially useful for those who feel the competition a lot and whose stomachs "tightens".

In any case (whether in the morning, afternoon or evening):

During exertion (if it exceeds 60 minutes) in rest times or during the interval, the body must be supplied with water, fructose and maltodextrin-based drinks, and possibly with a suitable amount of easily assimilable proteins.

After exertion, nutrition must help the recovery; an immediate intake of rapidly absorbed proteins and carbohydrates in liquid form is useful and the subsequent meal must be complete with all macronutrients, with particular attention to vegetables and liquids, which serve to compensate for the loss of salts and water..

How to keep fit during the summer holidays

For a sportsperson, holidays are undoubtedly a wonderful time, indispensable for relaxing and recharging psycho-physical energies which are largely exhausted by the pressing pace of work and training, aimed at always maintaining the necessary physical shape. Often the holidays, especially the summer ones, also represent an incentive to increase adherence to diet and training, to reach *peak condition*; the problem is that, when they finally arrive, they inevitably bring with them that relaxation which, from the point of the physical form, turns out to be more than deleterious. In a short time, the results obtained in the course of a whole year dissolve and all our efforts appear to be useless.

So, what are the possible strategies to avoid this situation? For simplicity, let's establish four "moves" that will help us keep the perfect shape even on vacation:

1. Prevention is a fundamental point: we must not get close to "breathless" holidays, we must not do exasperated workouts or too restrictive diets. A constant and progressive training is much more suitable in order to maintain the results, accompanied by a balanced diet, started well in advance so as not to have to "tighten the belt" at the last moment, with the risk of the dangerous rebound effect. It may be useful to start about ten days before the holiday period, to slow down the pace a little, avoiding commitments that are not of a fundamental importance in order to gradually prepare ourselves, both psychologically and physically, for a total relaxation that normally accompanies us during the holidays.
2. The essential thing in order to maintain physical shape from an esthetic point of view is the nutrition, while, from the athletic performance point of view, is the training. If we suspend training for a week, we do not create any problems with regard to athletic performance, on the contrary, this could even improve due to the supercompensation processes that occurs in the recovery phase; the same principle does not apply, however, to an equivalent period of food transgression, which could have a devastating effect on the physical fitness as regards to the body composition: if we eat too little we lose muscle mass, if we eat too much, we gain weight. In this regard, I remember a vacation in the USA, when, in Las Vegas, following a false movement that occurred while I was performing side lifts in the hotel room using the trolley as a tool, with the air conditioning at maximum, I got a contracture and pain from the intense cold", which left me completely blocked in the lumbar area, to the point of not even being able to walk. The consequences of the trauma, while not having opportunity to access any treatment and being a "on the road" trip, lasted for the entire duration of my stay in the USA, that was over a month. I was prevented from training, but, strictly adhering to a "congruous" diet, I was able to maintain a perfect physical shape that was not affected not even a bit by the lack of training. Conversely, I have well imprinted in my mind a photograph of the "before and after" during a week-long Mediterranean cruise holiday, during which, despite the daily workouts in the ship's gym, I was constantly tempted by the continuous buffets available. I understood the result at the end of the cruise, when the photographer of the ship gave me a souvenir photo from the last day, and by comparing it with the one of the arrival, it looked like I was Superman and then the Michelin Man: I could hardly recognize myself because of how large I was. How to follow an adequate diet even on vacation, where the temptations and opportunities are many and it is often difficult to find suitable foods? Obviously, a little good will and the ability to adapt to various situations are needed both from a practical and an economic point of view. A rule that will help you keep fit and that will also be good for your

wallet is to eat in restaurants only once a day. Of course, if breakfast is included in your reservation, it will have to be used. In case you are spending an "on the road" holiday, a hearty breakfast will allow you to have a frugal lunch (for example, boiled eggs, turkey breast, some wholemeal bread and fruit). Sachets of dried fruits (walnuts, almonds, cashews) and balanced bars for snacks are also excellent. At dinner you can also relax with a full meal accompanied by a glass of wine or a beer. If, on the other hand, you are a guest in a holiday village or in a hotel, it might be useful to have a small breakfast in your room as soon as you wake up using the coffee maker and consuming a balanced bar or a little oat and protein powder, so then you can take advantage of the hotel's breakfast as an "early lunch" based on eggs, ham, rye bread and fruit. After that, small snacks every three hours based on dried fruits or bars allow you to arrive at dinner not particularly hungry, but still with the right appetite to enjoy your meal at the restaurant. If breakfast is not included, then you can have a mini-breakfast in your room, a full lunch at the restaurant and a dinner with the right foods bought in a market. The "just one meal at the restaurant" rule is very simple and obviously works if you stick to the correct food choices. Eating small amounts is not enough, you have to eat the right things.

I remember that a patient of mine, who during the post-summer vacation checkup was found to have gained several kilos, could not find an explanation, since he had been on vacation on a boat and claimed that he had eaten very little and limited him drinking. To my question about what he had drunk in particular, he replied: "all light stuff: orange juice, coke.... In this regard, particular attention should be paid to soft drinks, especially in the USA, where the portions are oversized and the cost is negligible. Just think that in supermarkets a gallon of coke (3.5 liters) costs less than plain water.

3. If we have said that skipping a few days of training does not cause too much damage, extending the period of inactivity will certainly affect our physical fitness, so there are many solutions: book your holidays at facilities equipped with a gym or organize to be able to carry out exercise with elastic exercise bands and body weight in your room, even better by taking advantage of the possibility of doing sports that are appreciated as fun. If the time available to exercise is limited for your daily schedule, take advantage of any situation: for example, personally I never take the elevator even if the hotel room is located on a top floor, and I go up the stairs, two steps at a time. Obviously, the possibility of exercising during the holidays is also conditioned by the habits of your holiday companions. If your partner is not as interested in physical activity, you should organize yourself by getting up an hour earlier in the morning and practicing it before breakfast, so you will have already fulfilled your duty and then you will be available to your partner.

4. One thing my patients often ask me about is the use of supplements on vacation: the question is whether to take them or not. My answer is yes! Maybe not all of them, but, for example, if you are taking a multivitamin, vitamin C, glutamine that supports the immune defenses, it is not advisable to stop them suddenly, especially in the moment of such a marked change as is the fact of getting away from daily places and habits. In reality, the sudden interruption of normal work rhythms,

the transfer to a different climate, new schedules and different foods and, absurdly, also excessive relaxation, can represent a stress that is not recognized by the organism, which does not implement the necessary countermeasures; we can so easily find ourselves with a deficit in the immune system that predisposes us to diseases. How many times has it happened to you to get sick and to have a feverish episode just when you were relaxing on vacation? Well, continuing to take supplements is a way to make this step less traumatic and, in addition to those mentioned above, I also recommend taking beta-carotene to protect yourself from the damage of the solar radiation, melatonin to deal with any jet lag at a dosage of 5 mg per day for the first five days, and even more if it was already part of the supplements you were using. I also recommend whey proteins to be used in case you cannot reach the necessary protein quota with normal foods. Well, I hope these simple instructions can be of help, and remember that it's all a question of "balance": by finding the one that suits you, you can have fun and relax without giving up your hard-earned fitness!

THE ACID-BASE BALANCE

Often, in articles dedicated to health, we read about the acid-base balance. It is advisable to clarify it, otherwise there is a risk of confusion. What we all know is the acid-base balance of the blood, which must necessarily be between 7.35 and 7.45, that is, moderately alkaline, and which can undergo only small variations, under the penalty of death, as a pH acid (less than 7) is not compatible with life. The acid-base balance to which, at least the one we refer to, is that of the connective tissues, the so-called "extracellular matrix", to which even science has recently assigned the dignity of an organ.

The extracellular matrix is the environment that surrounds the cells of every organ and tissue and, through it, the cells receive nutrients, eliminate toxic substances and also receive electromagnetic information faster than those mediated by the nervous or hormonal system. To function at their best, cells need an alkaline environment, because only a pH of 7.4 is the best condition for the transport of nutrients within the cell. In order to maintain an alkaline environment, it is necessary to:

- drink a sufficient quantity of water, as dehydration causes acidification, favored by the stagnation of acids outside the cells, which cannot be properly drained;
- take an adequate intake of alkalizing mineral salts (such as potassium, magnesium, sodium, calcium, iron), which can be taken with your diet (fruits and vegetables are alkalizing due to their high potassium and magnesium content);
- avoid stress, as hyperactivation of the sympathetic system increases the acidity due to the vasoconstrictor effect, which in turn limits the supply of oxygen to the tissues causing hypoxyacidosis;
- practice moderate physical activity, since physical exercise, especially the aerobic one, promotes drainage by improving microcirculation. Muscle hypertonia must be avoided, as postural contractures and tensions exert a compressive effect on blood vessels, favoring the stagnation of acids produced by cell metabolism and by an intense physical activity.

Continues

Continued

At this point it is clear that, while practicing a regular physical activity, it has a positive effect on the pH because it improves the blood circulation and reduces stress levels. On the other hand, an intense anaerobic physical activity, which produces high amounts of lactic acid, such as bodybuilding and crossfit, and extreme endurance sports such as cycling and marathon, but also mixed sports such as football, lead to a high risk of incurring acidosis. Therefore, those who practice sports at a good level must be particularly careful to keep the pH of their extracellular matrix at levels around 7.4 otherwise, turning towards acidity, in addition to the deterioration of the performance, could more easily cause injuries, muscle injuries, joint problems, inflammation and catabolism.

Consequently, for the advanced sportsperson it may be useful, if not necessary, to resort to practices that go beyond simply drinking more and to favor alkalizing foods, also because with regard to this last factor, nutrition is often conditioned by need that go in the opposite direction, such as the increased need for carbohydrates (such as pasta and rice) in endurance sports and the increased need for animal proteins in power sports. A valuable aid for athletes, especially if practicing sports in hot and humid conditions that cause copious sweating, is the use of isotonic drinks containing sodium.

It is also recommended to take mineral salts based on potassium citrate and magnesium citrate, which combine the basifying power of minerals with that of the citrates. It is also advisable to use the extractor to make fruit juices and, above all, vegetable juices, which are not always able to be taken in the necessary quantities. Also, functional food juices such as açai, pomegranate, blueberry and noni, in addition to having a basifying effect, are particularly rich in antioxidants.

Having machinery that is capable of delivering purified, filtered and alkaline water can also be very useful for alkalizing and detoxifying the body.

Many consume bottled water which, if made of plastic, can pollute itself; moreover, if we consume it with the addition of carbon dioxide, its pH becomes extremely acid (do not be fooled by the label, which reports the pH at the source and not the real one). The fact remains that in the mains tap water there is a high content of chlorine (used for disinfection) and an innumerable quantity of chemical substances, which are added for pipeline problems. For this reason, more and more people drink filtered water to which they add alkalizing minerals in order to increase its pH, alkalizing minerals in form of powder or drops, are added to increase its pH, taking into consideration the dangers of the acid-base imbalance.

Among all the waters on the market that are proposed for this purpose, I believe that the "HADO alkaline hydrogen water" has the best characteristics, since it contains calcium hydrate [$Ca(OH)_2$], potassium hydrate (KOH) and hydrate of magnesium [$Mg(OH)_2$]. The hydrating capacity of HADO water is linked to the size of the molecule clusters, which are very small (called microclusters), so they are able to penetrate very easily deep into the tissues and even reach the most difficult to reach parts of our body. In this way it greatly improves the supply of oxygen to the tissues, as well as the removal of waste, thus optimizing the moisturizing, oxygenating and detoxifying effect.

CHAPTER 4

Nutrition for the mass

My studies on nutrition science have always led me to the conclusion that the excessive weight gain in the off-season period aimed at increasing the muscle mass, is inappropriate.

To set up a diet for mass gain, it is necessary to start with a theoretical approach, calculating the basal metabolic rate, the energy expenditure during work and training and adding the minimum number of calories that are necessary for growth.

The only cases in which it is possible to obtain an increase in the muscle mass without adequate nutrition are those in which you are completely new to weight training or when it is a question of recovering muscle mass previously acquired but lost due to a suspension of training, using the so-called "muscle memory". In all other situations, when an individual is no longer a beginner, two fundamental parameters must be respected: calorie intake and protein intake.

A sufficient caloric intake is necessary to promote the increase of the muscle mass, because, in addition to providing the energy to support a hard workout, a positive caloric balance is the "conditio sine qua non" to have a positive nitrogen balance, i.e. a protein synthesis in order to make anabolism prevail over catabolism. The problem is that if the caloric balance is in excess, in addition to protein synthesis, it will also stimulate the fat synthesis, which will then be deposited as an energy reserve in the visceral and subcutaneous adipose tissue. Therefore, to set up a diet for mass gain, it is necessary to start from a theoretical approach, calculating the basal metabolism, the energy expenditure during work and during training, and adding the quantity of calories that is necessary for growth (which normally does not exceed 10%).

All this must then be verified "in the field" by monitoring the body fat with the skinfold meter and with an impedance analysis. Basal metabolism and calorie consumption related to physical activity are in fact statistical data, not applicable a priori to everyone, and it is therefore advisable to check the individual response and find the right calorie intake depending on the changes in body composition. A minimal body fat gain is acceptable during a bulking phase; however, we should take care in order not to exceed 10-15% body fat for men and 15-20% for women, which can lead to being forced to more drastic diets to reach the "perfect shape", which would lead to a probable loss of the hard-earned muscle mass.

We talked about the quantity of calories, but in reality quality is also fundamental. The calories must come mainly from carbohydrates rich in fiber with a low glycemic index and from "good" fats, which are monounsaturated (which have the advantage of being more easily usable for energy purposes) and polyunsaturated (which are able to improve the sensitivity to insulin, a very important factor for regulating the body composition).

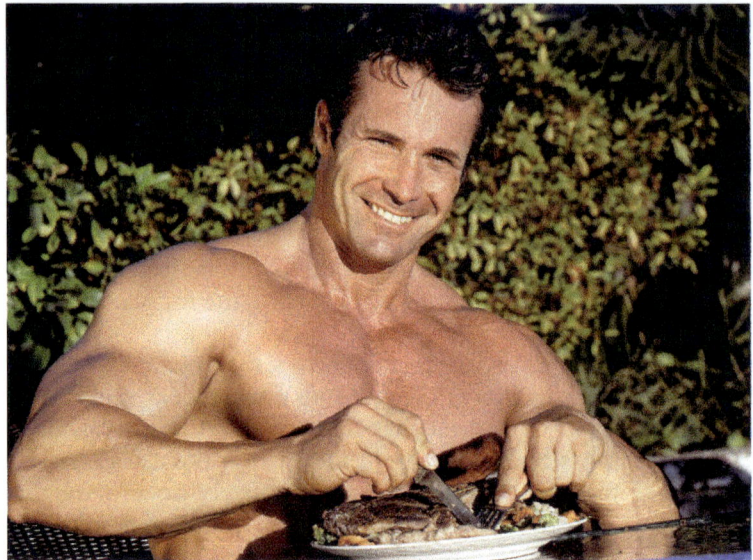

Figure 4.1

At this point, an endless diatribe opens: we can certainly say that a specific amount of protein is needed to promote muscle protein synthesis (and this we will see later), but how should we divide the rest of the calories between carbohydrates and fats?

We know that some fats, or essential fatty acids, are really "essential" for the body and must be necessarily included in the diet; the same goes for the essential amino acids of proteins, while carbohydrates can be supplied through neoglucogenesis from proteins and from glycerol that comes from triglycerides.

Fats are also important for the absorption of fat-soluble vitamins, for proper intestinal motility, as precursors of sex hormones and other types of hormones. We could reasonably say that to cover this need we should consume about 1 g of fat per kg of body weight divided equally between saturated, monounsaturated and polyunsaturated. This amount corresponds to 20-30% of a normal calorie maintenance diet.

Once the proteins have been administered, also according to the body weight, the rest of the calories must be provided by carbohydrates. If the goal is to increase the body mass, is it necessary to set a high-calorie diet and should these calories be provided by fats or carbohydrates? In general, especially in young athletes who have a good sensitivity to carbohydrates (therefore, a good insulin sensitivity), I would like to say that if proteins constitute the metallic component of the tap, fats are the seals and carbohydrates are the jet of water that can be adjusted according to the need.

However, this is not always the case: there are individuals who, due to their genetic, metabolic and chronomorphological characteristics (the polymorphism of the regulatory genes of the carbohydrate metabolism, hyperoxidators, hyperlipogenetics) do not tolerate carbohydrates well, and others who do not tolerate fats well (the polymorphism of the genes that regulate the metabolism of hypoxidizing and hypolipolytic fats). It is therefore necessary to make these assessments through genetic tests, mineralograms, hormonal and morphological assessments, before deciding whether to go towards more carbohydrates or more fats.

In the event that, for these reasons, we opt for carbohydrates, their percentage on the diet should be between 50 and 60% and, obviously, the choice should fall on those carbohydrates with a low glycemic index and those that are rich in fiber. If one opts for fats (but cases of people who respond well to this approach are rare), the surplus compared to 1 g per kg of body weight should be administered in the form of monounsaturated fats (olive oil, nuts).

Now we arrive at proteins: how many, which ones, how? I believe that now no one can think that the old LARN recommendation of 0.8 g of protein per kg of body weight may be sufficient to increase the muscle mass. I am reporting various studies on the subject below:

- **Celejowa (1970):** negative nitrogen balance in male weightlifters with 2 g/kg (250% RDA).
- **Laritcheva (1978):** positive nitrogen balance in male Soviet weightlifters with 1.3-1.6 g/kg (160-200% RDA).
- **Consolazio (1975):** consistent nitrogen retention and an increase in lean mass after 40 days of training with 2.8 g/kg compared to 1.8 g/kg (350% vs 175% RDA).
- **Dreagan (1985):** 5% increase in strength and 6% in lean mass in Romanian weightlifters, passing from 2.2 to 3.5 g/kg (275% vs 440% RDA).
- **Tarnopolsky (1988):** balanced nitrogen in bodybuilders with 0.9 g/kg (112% RDA).
- **Lemon (1991):** maximum daily protein requirement for endurance athletes level of 1.6 g/kg (200% RDA) and for all other cross-country skiers 1.2-1.4 g/kg (150-175% RDA). For power sports athletes, it is proven to be a neutral nitrogen balance with 0.9 g/kg (112% RDA) is possible, while for the muscle strengthening phases there is a need for an increase in the daily protein intake which must not exceed 2.0-2.2 g/kg (250-275% RDA).
- **Lemon (1992), Tarnopolsky (1992):** no further increase has been shown to increase muscle strength or lean mass when exceeding 1.8 g/kg (230% RDA).

Recent research indicates that to stimulate protein synthesis, for about 2-3 hours, it is necessary to provide at least about 3 g of leucine (amino acid that stimulates mTOR, which activates protein synthesis) per meal. This amount of leucine corresponds to about 20-40 g of protein depending on the type of protein (20 g of whey protein, 30 g of protein from 150 g of chicken, 40 g of protein from 200 g of beans). However, the total daily amount of functional protein needed to increase the muscle mass does not exceed 2.2 g of protein per kg of body weight. Obviously, on the basis of what has been said before, it is clear that in reality the quantity of proteins is also a dependent on their quality. In one study it was shown that at a dosage of 20 g of whey and wheat proteins, those who used wheat failed to stimulate muscle protein synthesis and they were able to do so only at a dosage of 40 g. By adding leucine to wheat proteins, balancing the amount of leucine with that of the whey, protein synthesis could be stimulated, thus demonstrating that leucine is the limiting amino acid necessary for stimulating muscle protein synthesis.

This concept must be kept in mind especially by vegetarians and even more by vegans, who, by not consuming proteins of animal origin and limiting themselves to those of plant origin, struggle to reach the quantities of leucine that are essential for increasing the mass. If it is true that a quantity of 20-40 g of protein is necessary, it is equally true that higher dosages will not give a greater response, and it is therefore useless to consume protein mega-meals, just as it is useless to consume protein meals too often, as there is a period of refractoriness during which there is no response.

If it is true that 20 g of protein can be enough to stimulate protein synthesis, it is also true that a total quantity is needed, corresponding precisely to 2.2 g per kg of body weight, necessary to make up for the increased protein demand due to increased turnover and increased fixation of the proteins themselves in the muscles. In order to always keep the protein synthesis activated, the best thing is to distribute the protein quota in five to six meals spread out, about every three hours.

Preference must be given to the proteins of animal origin: red meats, fish and poultry are particularly balanced in the content of the amino acids glycine, arginine and methionine.

According to some researches, the supplementation of arginine, ornithine and some lipotropic factors (methionine, choline, betaine) seems to increase the formation of creatine, which reacts with the phosphorus molecule to form the creatine-phosphate, which constitutes a very important energy substrate during muscular contraction. This would explain why supplementation with ornithine and arginine helps the muscle growth and, through this mechanism, leads to an increase in energy, as well as by stimulating the production of the growth hormone (GH).

Carbohydrates are very important in the athlete's diet because they constitute the energy substrate used during intense muscle contraction.

As seen previously, the protein quantity needed to build a particularly muscular physique should be around 2.2-2.3 g of protein per kg of body weight. But why? How and when should it be taken? And most importantly, what kind of proteins do we need to build our physique? It seems obvious that for an athlete there is an increased protein requirement, but, in reality, there is a bit of confusion and above all the opinions go from one extreme to the other.

In general, the traditional scientific community, the one linked to archaic concepts, which I like to call "archaeological medicine" because it is able to approve only concepts that have already been demonstrated and validated for at least 50 years, continues to talk about a need of 0.75 g of protein per kg of body weight, without making distinctions between sedentary people and people who practice intense physical activity. In fact, for decades, there have been scientific studies that show the opposite, that is, athletes need a greater protein intake to maintain a positive nitrogen balance, to avoid catabolism in order to avoid losing the muscle mass.

There are some studies on "elite" weightlifters who have demonstrated the need for as much as 3.5 g of protein per kg of body weight in order to maximize protein synthesis and therefore increase the lean muscle mass; however, these were athletes who trained several times a day, every day. On the other hand, making a general consideration of the various studies we have examined in this regard, the demonstration of the real need for a greater protein intake for athletes emerges more or less in these terms: for endurance athletes, 1.6 g of protein per kg body; for speed sports, 1.8 g of protein per kg body; for strength sports, at least 2 g of protein per kg of body, and 2.3 g of protein per kg of body for those who are finalizing the training for hypertrophy.

Why is this protein surplus necessary for strength sports?

First of all, strength sports require an increase in muscle mass and proteins are the muscle building blocks; consequently, it is obvious that a protein surplus is needed to build new muscle mass. It has been shown that during an intense physical exercise there is also an energy consumption of muscle proteins, which therefore must be covered by a greater protein intake. Furthermore, in an athlete, there is also a greater protein "turnover" not only at the muscle level, but also in all the other body parts that are mechanically involved in the physical exercise (ligaments, joints, bone tissue, blood system), and this leads to a further increase in the need for protein.

Finally, considering that the value of 0.75 g per kg of body weight was valid for a normal person in proportion to their muscle mass which is relative to their weight, you understand well that the muscle mass in a strong athlete, being in proportion to their weight, is in certainly in greater percentage than that of a normal person, and therefore the protein requirement will be increased according to this proportion. Here are some various reasons that justify the need for a greater protein intake when you want to improve your muscles.

At this point, having demonstrated the need for more proteins, one wonders: how should they be taken?

The main food sources of proteins that we can find in nature are mainly represented by foods of an animal origin, such as meat, fish, eggs, dairy products; however, a fair amount of protein is also present in vegetables, especially legumes (20%), but also cereals (6-10%). Proteins of an animal origin have a higher biological value, as they are richer in essential amino acids that the body cannot synthesize on its own and which, consequently, are indispensable for an optimal protein synthesis, just as vowels are indispensable to form words.

The disadvantage of proteins of animal origin is that they are often associated with significant amounts of saturated fats in foods (red meat, eggs, cheeses), while vegetable ones are associated with unsaturated fats, which as we know, have a beneficial effect on the body. It has been shown that a greater consumption of meat is linked to a greater incidence of cardiovascular and cancer diseases, but this does not seem to depend on the protein component, but on the presence of saturated fats or on the fact that the development of an intestinal bacterial flora favors the conversion of L-carnitine (which is present in the meat) into TMAO (trimethylamine N-oxide), a compound that is capable of causing atherosclerosis.

Nowadays there are some preparations on the market, supplements in the form of mixtures of protein powders, which give the possibility to increase protein intake without increasing the intake of fats and which also certainly represent a great practical solution for the need of eating more meals throughout the day. But where does this need come from? Isn't it enough to have all the proteins we need in the three main meals? Aside from the obvious reasons for the digestive capacity, there is a very important reason for splitting the protein intake into numerous meals: stimulating protein synthesis! And it has been shown (Litvinova, 1976) that by distributing the food intake over five meals instead of three, the rate of muscle protein synthesis increases. Assuming it takes about three hours to digest a meal, if you only eat three times a day you are feeding for nine hours and fasting for 15, and when our body fasts it enters a catabolic phase where it "auto-cannibalizes" the muscles and it certainly doesn't build their mass. By going to six meals a day, our body is nourished for 18 hours and it is in a fasting situation for only six hours. As we have said, muscle mass is subject to continuous protein "turnover".

Within about six months, 98% of our body's proteins are recycled. Old proteins are destroyed (catabolism), while new ones are reformed (anabolism). Meals stimulate protein synthesis, while fasting reduces it. When we eat proteins, the amino acids contained in them stimulate the growth factors that are able to trigger the mechanism of protein synthesis. It is obvious that the hormonal and the metabolic (as well as mechanical) conditions also need to exist to translate this protein synthesis into the formation of the new muscle mass, but this task belongs to the training.

To translate, it means that you cannot increase the muscle mass while sitting in front of the television and by eating more protein: the adequate stimulus given by intense muscle activity is still the "conditio sine qua non". A certain threshold of amino-acidemia must therefore be reached to stimulate these growth factors, and the whey protein, which is the basis of the most modern formulations of protein powder mixtures, is the one that is absorbed more quickly and that is able to cause a pharmacological level of amino acids called hyperaminoacidemia, capable of increasing the protein synthesis. But if it is true that whey proteins greatly raise the levels of amino acids in the blood, it is equally true that they are metabolized very quickly, and in a short time the amino acidemia is drastically lowered; vice versa, caseins (other milk proteins) are absorbed more slowly and by doing so, they maintain a fair level of amino acids, which, even if it fails to stimulate the protein synthesis to the maximum, is still able to curb the catabolism. For this reason, if you choose protein powders especially as meal replacement snacks between main meals, it is good to choose a combination of whey protein and casein. If we were only using whey protein, eating every three hours might be insufficient and the number of snacks would have to be increased to maintain a stimulated state of protein synthesis.

A widespread belief among athletes is that muscles grow at night during the night's rest. In reality, during the overnight fasting, the muscles release amino acids into the bloodstream, thus entering the catabolic phase. One way to remedy this situation is to consume a nice protein shake based on casein or a combination of casein and whey, just before going to bed; the progressive absorption of amino acids will buffer the catabolism. And if we usually get up in the middle of the night to go to the bathroom, in this case it might be a good idea to consume another mixed shake of whey protein and casein.

However, as soon as you get up in the morning, it is always a good thing to consume a good portion of whey protein in order to immediately raise the amino acidemia and give the anabolism a good boost. This explains the reason for a fractional intake of proteins and also the reason for choosing whey proteins or caseins. In fact, breast milk, which gives a very strong anabolic boost to the baby who grows dizzyingly fast, is a combination of whey protein and casein, specifically 80% whey protein and 20% casein. This way, it has the anabolic effect of whey proteins and the anti-catabolic effect of the casein.

Another important aspect to know is that if even on non-training days you need as much protein as on training days. In a study by Bandegan et al. they examined some bodybuilders who had performed their last workout 48 hours before the test. These subjects were fed various doses of protein during the days they were resting and what emerged was that, despite the "no training" days, the bodybuilders maintained a constant and high protein requirement. The estimated average of the protein requirement was found to be between 1.7 and 2.2 g/kg per day, even on off days. This means that, even if you don't train every day, the muscle recovery process and construction, induced by the previous training, remains constant.

But let's see in practice how we should behave in the various meals of the day, while using protein supplements.

Breakfast

As soon as you wake up it is advisable to consume at least 30-40 g of whey protein to restore the levels of amino acids in the blood as soon as possible. Then a "normal" breakfast based on egg whites (allowed one or two yolks), cereals and fresh and dried nuts.

Mid-morning snack

After about three hours, as solid foods take longer than protein powders to digest, you can take one or two protein bars or a combination of whey protein and casein. The bars are already combined with carbohydrates; in the case of protein powders, it is good to combine them in a smoothie with one or two fruits (20 to 30 g of protein, depending on body weight), adding a tablespoon of linseed oil or a handful of almonds and walnuts.

Lunch

After two or three hours, you can have a typical meal with a first based on carbohydrates (pasta, rice), a second based on meat or fish, and vegetables in large quantities plus one or two tablespoons of olive oil. The second should not exceed 200 g in order not to overload the digestive system, which takes longer to digest solid foods.

Afternoon snack

About three hours after lunch you can repeat the mid-morning snack; in this case, easy-to-digest and already balanced meals can be the ideal solution, especially if this is the snack that precedes the workout. Meals rich in casein are preferred, which carry out the anti-catabolic action during the training.

Snack after training

It is rule n. 6 of the Decalogue, which we will see later, and it is very important, because we need to restart the anabolism which was blocked during the training. In this case, a dose of 30-40 g of whey protein plus fast-absorbing simple carbohydrates, such as glucose, perform the purpose by immediately blocking the catabolism induced by training and by stimulating the insulin which favors both glycogen and protein re-synthesis mechanisms.

Dinner

Within one hour of the training, it is good to have a normal meal such as lunch, perhaps with a lower carbohydrate content if a large amount of carbohydrates has been taken in the snack after training, as we do not need their energy support, and any excess would lead to their transformation into fat. However, it is not advisable to completely eliminate the carbohydrates since they probably still serve to restore the glycogen stores, and their association with proteins has a significant anti-catabolic and protein-saving effect. Some recent studies seem to indicate that to achieve maximum results, it would be good to reduce the intake of fat provided by this meal. In an experiment published in the *Medicine and Science in Sports & Exercise* journal, two groups of athletes performed two training sessions per day; between the two sessions, one group ate a meal rich in carbohydrates and the other a meal rich in fat. By monitoring the gene activity, the researchers found a reduction in the p70S6K1 enzyme in the group that had eaten high amounts of fat between the two workouts. This particular enzyme is able to stimulate the protein synthesis, so its reduction hinders muscle growth. In conclusion, perhaps it would be better to avoid consuming fat during the meals that are close to the training.

Snack before going to bed

A casein-based protein drink (30-40 g) is ideal for stopping the night catabolism for as long as possible; you can possibly include a fruit that is not very caloric (pineapple, strawberries, kiwi), to bring a little fructose which will favor the formation of glycogen in the liver, which will help to keep blood sugar constant with a further anti-catabolic effect.

P.S. Don't set the alarm to get up at night; I think that a restorative sleep is better, but if you have to get up, or if you wake up during the night, a 20-30g glass of a mix of whey protein and casein can only be good for your hungry muscles!

The 10 dietary rules for gaining muscle mass

1. **Get the right number of calories.** The calories provided by food are very important because if there is a defect, we will not be able to have an adequate muscle growth and if there is an excess, we will accumulate fat. As we have seen, there are some fairly precise formulas to calculate the total calorie requirement, which obviously depends on age, gender and work activity. However, there is a very simple formula, albeit a bit approximate, to calculate your calorie needs, and it consists in multiplying your body weight by 30 if you want to lose weight; by 35

if you want to keep the weight; by 40 if you want to gain weight. For example, an individual who wants to gain weight and is actually weighing 80 kg will have to multiply 80 × 40: the result (3200) is the calories that should allow them to gain muscle mass without gaining weight.

2. **Provide a sufficient amount of protein.** Protein is the building block of the muscle mass. Whether you want to increase your musculature or you want to define it, you have to increase the consumption of protein foods: meat, eggs, fish dairy products. An adequate muscle mass cannot be developed or maintained without a sufficient protein intake; the best and most bioavailable ones are those of animal origin, however, those derived from legumes are not to be despised. As a general rule, you should consume about 2.3 g (maximum 2.5) of protein per kg of body weight per day, which equates, for our 80 kg athlete, to 800 calories in the form of protein, which provides 4 calories per gram. Hence, protein must make up at least 25% of a diet's total daily calorie requirement for bulking.

3. **Eliminate simple sugars in favor of complex sugars.** Carbohydrates are very important for those who play sports. They are, in fact, the primary energy source. If proteins are the building blocks, carbohydrates are the masons. In your opinion, to build a house is it better to have strong available masons who get tired immediately, or less strong but very resistant masons who work for hours without getting tired? Certainly, the second option! For the same reason, it is better to prefer complex carbohydrates that give longer lasting energy than simple carbohydrates, which provide energy which, if not exploited, increases fat and predisposes to diabetes. The amount of carbohydrates needed in a diet for bulking is about 5-6 g per kg of body weight.

4. **Prefer unsaturated fats to saturated ones.** Fats are not to be demonized! They are, in fact, the cement that is needed to hold the bricks together. Fats are an indispensable element for cell membranes and for the formation of sex hormones. It is good to consume mainly unsaturated fats, which have a protective effect against cardiovascular diseases and improve insulin sensitivity by improving anabolism and lipolysis. It is recommended to consume about 1 g of fat per kg of body weight, choosing sources such as fish from the cold seas of the North (salmon, mackerel, tuna) or seed oils such as linseed, sesame, corn, olive oil.

5. **Splitting meals.** It is much better to divide the total amount of nutrients into several meals: for example, three main meals and three snacks. By consuming a meal about every three hours, our body maintains a higher metabolism and always has the right amount of nutrients to optimize protein synthesis at all times.

6. **Consume a meal with easily absorbed proteins and simple sugars after training.** The moment in which simple carbohydrates are granted is after training, when they are used to restore the glycogen reserves in the muscle. Before training, in fact, there is the risk of causing a subsequent hyper-stimulated hypoglycemia which damages the performance. We have already explained how proteins are essential for muscle building. After a hard workout it is important to provide proteins with a high biological value, to replenish the muscle that picks them

up immediately and then grows. Whey proteins are ideal because they are easily assimilated and rich in leucine.

7. **Supplements.** The magic pill certainly doesn't exist (and you don't even have to look for it), but there are supplements that can help a lot. If I had to narrow down the choice, I would definitely recommend creatine. This supplement is exceptional for the increase of strength and muscle mass; 3-6 g per day, to be taken before and after training, are enough to guarantee excellent results. Another supplement not to be missed is a good multivitamin and multi-mineral vitamins and minerals by themselves will not immediately make you gain strength and muscle mass, but they are essential for the proper functioning of all the body's biochemical processes. In addition, antioxidants protect cells from the damage caused by free radicals, which unfortunately are produced in large quantities during intense workouts.

8. **Drink at least 2-3 liters of water per day.** It is often forgotten that our body is made up of about 65% water, and therefore water is the plastic element par excellence. In fact, well hydrated muscle cells have a greater protein synthesis. Furthermore, a good water supply is essential to drain the largest amount of nitrogenous waste produced by a high-protein diet through the kidneys. It is advisable to drink non-carbonated, low-hardness water with low fixed residue and alkaline pH. It is not true that you should not drink during meals! You simply don't have to drink too much so as not to excessively dilute the gastric juices. It is not true that you should not drink during training, on the contrary, it may be useful to take a slightly sugary and isotonic drink; the important thing is that it should not be cold.

9. **Do not drink alcohol and carbonated drinks.** Alcoholic beverages contain empty calories which cannot be used for dynamic energy purposes and which are easily converted into fat. Furthermore, alcohol acts negatively on the protein synthesis. According to a study conducted by Anthony Duplanty of the University of Texas (Denton), alcohol reduces the signaling of mTORC1 in muscles, which is important for the activation of muscle protein synthesis. Carbonated drinks promote stomach dilation and tend to limit the intake of other drinks, such as plain water, which is important to consume in large quantities.

10. **Once a week… diet-free!** Once a weak, treat yourself to diet-free meal or for a whole day, for example on Sundays. It is a good way to avoid feeling too enslaved to a diet that is perhaps too monotonous, it allows social relations and the ability to tolerate other foods. Without exaggerating, however, because any caloric surplus, while already being in a basic diet for mass which is high in calories, would easily be deposited as fat. Personally, I recommend making the main meals a little freer and skipping snacks, so you are less forced to respect schedules and possibly to carry food with you. Also, after a day of transgression, you will be happier to return to the rules, which no longer seem so unpleasant.

CHAPTER 5

Nutrition for strength

by Andrea Angelozzi and Massimo Spattini

Muscle strength development is defined as the ability of a muscle group to resist a training load. It is a fundamental parameter for athletes who perform power sports (powerlifting, weightlifting, speed, throwing, wrestling sports, bodybuilding), as, by improving the maximum strength, it is possible to release more power in the execution of the exercise and therefore have a better performance.

Strength training is preparatory and functional both for the increase of the muscle mass and for the improvement of some state of health indicators (reduction of fat

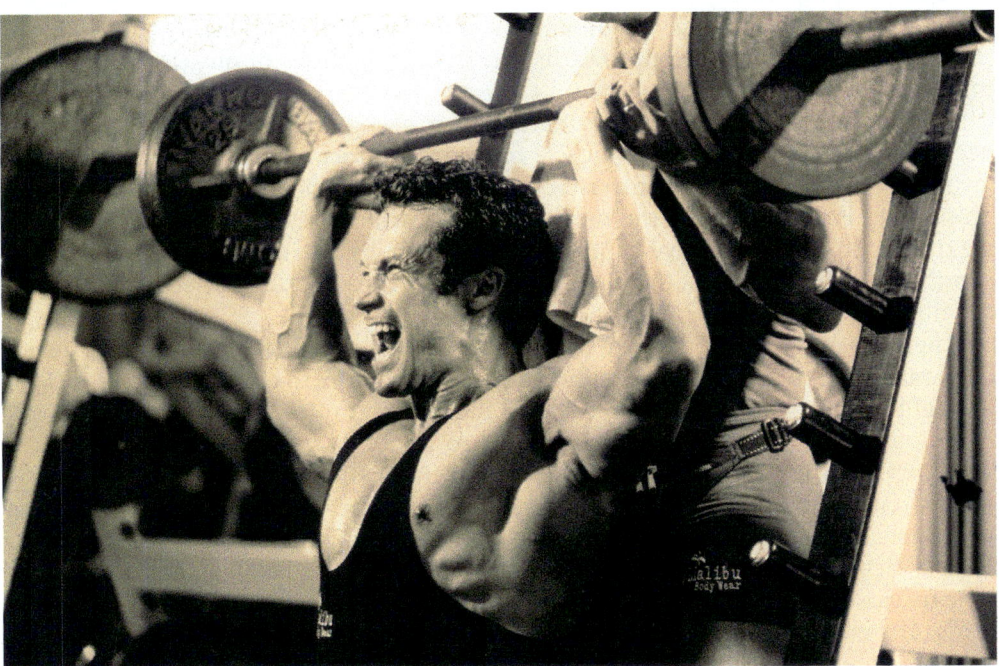

Figure 5.1

mass, increase of anabolic hormones, increase in ossification levels, improvement of insulin resistance, etc.).

Strength training can be included in the programming of all competitive sports, especially for those of an anaerobic type, since, by increasing the training load, body composition is improved; in addition, the increase in the muscle mass and bone mass makes the structure more solid, reducing the risk of injuries. This is very important, especially in the context of sports that exploit the alactic acid anaerobic metabolism, in which the performance ends within a maximum of 10 seconds.

The increase in strength has always included the execution of "basic", multi-joint exercises, such as squats, deadlifts and flat bench presses, which are the exercises that stress our body the most and that are able to induce the production of micro-secretions of the anabolic hormones par excellence (testosterone and GH) during the training. This increase in testosterone and GH causes some important metabolic changes, in fact it allows the muscle cells to induce a better protein synthesis, promotes muscle recovery during the post-training phase and allows an increase of strength over time. Regarding this matter, training management is of a fundamental importance to avoid overtraining, which is characterized by the production of stress hormones and happens frequently in powerlifting or Olympic weightlifting competitive athletes.

Analyzing the strength training from a biochemical point of view, it can be seen that the part mainly involved in the metabolism is the anaerobic alactacid, therefore it uses the creatine-phosphocreatine system with an increase in the production and consumption of ATP. Generally speaking, this happens if maximal or submaximal exercises (1-3 MR) are actually performed, but the anaerobic lactacid system will also be used in a preparatory program where they carry out long, high-volume sessions (both as regards to the total weight and the total number of series). For this reason, the nutrition must be directed towards increasing the stores of muscle creatine and muscle glycogen.

Another aspect to take into consideration for strength is the neuromuscular connection, therefore the ability of muscle fibers to contract quickly and efficiently, allowing the coordination of the muscles involved in expressing the technical gesture. This ability is controlled by the nervous system, which in the process of making a maximum effort sends nerve signals to the muscle by recruiting as many fibers as possible. A good fluidity of the nerve signal and of the conduction between the various fibers allows for greater efforts.

There are many diets proposed for strength gain. Assuming that strength is developed mainly by training, or by adapting the body structure to carry out exercises with a weight which is always close to 100% of the maximum (theoretical and effective), nutrition in this case must act as a support so the body won't be lacking energy, it must improve the recovery not only after a training session but during an entire period of strength training, it must improve and increase the muscle mass and regenerate worn structures (muscles, tendons, joints, bones) to maintain a good state of health.

The diets found on the web or the ones that are proposed by trainers advise a caloric increase (200-300 Kcal) every two to three weeks based on the serial increase in loads. There is no scientific evidence to support this and also logically there are no relationships between an increase in workloads and an increase in energy expenditure (with the same training volume). Let's take an example: if I am a very strong athlete and I bench press 120 kg for 5 reps at my maximum limit, I will consume more or less the same calories as a weaker athlete who lifts less weight but who has the same body composition. Calorie consumption is linked to the subjective intensity of the effort for the athlete's body weight.

For this reason, the diet related to the increase in strength, must be proportioned according to the classic nutritional parameters: evaluation of the basal metabolism with indirect (Harris-Benedict/Katch and McArdle/impedancemetry) or direct (calorimetry) methods, calculation of the daily energy expenditure and an assessment of the energy expenditure due to training.

Once you have calculated your energy expenditure, you must divide the various nutrients. The distribution must take into account the level of training of the individual subject; a trained person accustomed to working with high loads will need a higher quantity of calories than a novice athlete, since he will certainly be able to sustain a much higher volume of training than a novice. On the contrary, a beginner athlete will have to increase the calorie level based on the improvement of the muscle mass, body size, and training, in a way to accompany the improvement of the athletic performance with the improvement of the structures used to perform the athletic gesture.

In addition, nutrition and above all supplements will be aimed at increasing the values of anabolic hormones to promote the muscle recovery and to increase the muscle mass. Physically, there is a linear relationship between the increase in muscle fibers (both in number and in section) and the increase in strength (translated into practice in the increase in kg lifted). In these cases, the body will adapt to the type of effort and will mainly generate white, fast fibers with glycolytic metabolism, which use glycogen (and therefore glucose) as an energy substrate. The diet will be aimed at increasing the synthesis of ATP and creatine. This concept already suggests that people who want to focus on the development of their strength must give up the definition because in order to lift more weight, you need to have a greater energy availability and to obtain it, you need to consume greater quantities of nutrients.

Furthermore, if we analyze the structure of the great weightlifters, powerlifters and weight throwers, it is clear that a certain amount of fat tissue is present in their conformation. This excess fat has its own function, as it increases the load on tendon and muscle structures, joints and bones, creating a continuous training load and therefore it is useful for the development of strength. Let's think about the subjects who have to carry a ballast of 10-20-30 kg; the force-weight vector (mass × acceleration of gravity) falling on the bone structure will be greater and therefore the counter-resistant and/or the static force will be greater (which is the physical quantity that allows the best development and increase of power and strength in a workout) in order to oppose with a consequent physiological adaptation in terms of both muscle section (hypertrophy and/or muscle hyperplasia) and neuromuscular adaptation to the training load.

Furthermore, a certain amount of fat, especially an intramuscular one, could exert a sort of a "cushion" effect that helps to release an elastic return force which favors the explosiveness of movement. This happens above all in sports where the same body weight can act as a propulsive component (shot put), and not in other sports where the body weight represents a ballast (high jump).

As with hypertrophy, strength is also needed to heal the muscle mass and increase it, so it is important to make the anabolic phase prevail while minimizing the catabolic one. The proteins must be quantified on the basis of the kg of body weight and balanced according to the training effort. Many studies have shown that a protein intake per kg of body weight must be greater than 2 g and often exceed 3 g. On average, the ideal protein balance should not be excessive because the unused proteins are expelled with a rather laborious process, so it makes no sense to take too many proteins if they are not used properly.

This is why protein must be used as a support and a recovery nutrient and it must correspond to no more than 30% of the total calories, with an ideal range of 20-30%. The choice of protein source will fall on foods with a high biological value of proteins, therefore foods of animal origin, such as white meats, red meats (especially for the high content of creatine and carnitine) and cow's milk.

The intake of carbohydrates and fats is also very important. If proteins have to support, sustain and facilitate muscle recovery, carbohydrates have the fundamental task of providing energy, increasing ATP synthesis and acting in synergy with amino acids (deriving from proteins) in stimulating the mTOR protein machine and therefore in maximizing the protein synthesis.

The choice of carbohydrates will fall on slowly absorbed complex carbohydrates, but also on simple carbohydrates that are needed during training and in some cases to better convey nutrients and some supplements (such as creatine). The fats will perform the function of helping the synthesis of steroid hormones (saturated fats and cholesterol), modulating the inflammatory response (polyunsaturated fats of the omega-3 and omega-6 series: EPA, DHA, GLA), as well as conveying the fat-soluble vitamins, increase the nerve impulse transmission capacity and favor the turnover of membranes and cellular structures.

To sum up: the strength diet must necessarily be a high-calorie diet, calculated as a function of the basal metabolic rate multiplied by the physical activity level (PAL) of a heavy activity (i.e. 2.01). The breakdown of macronutrients should be made up of proteins (20-30%), 15-20% from fats and 50-60% from carbohydrates. The increase in calories will go hand in hand with the increase in muscle mass, so it is necessary to adjust the caloric level approximately every 30 days based on the changed energy expenditure.

The meal frequency will follow a pattern that is similar with the hypertrophy diet, therefore the distance between one meal and another will be two hours, trying to take an adequate amount of proteins, fats and carbohydrates during each meal, and maintaining a ratio of carbohydrates to proteins of at least 2:1.

In general, this is the breakdown of macronutrients; obviously, you have to make changes based on your body composition, size and structure.

Making a somatotype analysis, therefore a body size analysis, the indicated scheme would be ideal for an ectomorphic subject (which has a structure that is not very suitable for the development of strength: long limbs, unfavorable levers, little propensity to hypertrophy), obviously creating a caloric surplus of at least 20% compared to the daily caloric expenditure and possibly increasing the protein intake towards 30%, given that these subjects have serious difficulties in stimulating hypertrophy. They also have a very rapid metabolism that easily reduces carbohydrates aimed at providing enough energy for a workout with large loads.

For endomorphic subjects, i.e. those who have a propensity for the development of mass (both muscle and fat) and who have a constitution which is suitable for the development of strength (short limbs, large muscle masses, low center of gravity), the distribution of macronutrients should vary slightly. As for the protein fraction, in this case, a caloric intake of about 20% could be sufficient, perhaps by increasing the fat fraction to 30%; carbohydrates in this case should not exceed 50% and their distribution should be associated with the main meals, before carrying out a training session.

This is because endomorphs usually have a high insulin response and, therefore, there is no need to stimulate it frequently; the choice of carbohydrates will therefore fall on starchy, slow-release foods, so that glycemic and insulin stimulation is as constant as possible, in order to avoid creating glycemic decompensation or drops that can lead to situations of mental fatigue.

As described, the suitable nutrition to increase strength must be an aid to accelerate muscle recovery, prevent energy losses and improve the neuromuscular communication. Nutrition alone is not sufficient to increase this fundamental parameter and therefore it can be said above all, training is the one that leads to the progressive improvement of both the technique and the increase in workloads, allowing the athlete to increase the ability to lift even heavier loads.

MUSCLES, NUTRITION AND RED MEAT

Just recently, as you may have noticed, there has been a great deal of hype about the news that red meat has been found to be carcinogenic by the WHO (World Health Organization). The perceived message was that sooner or later, all those who consume meat would have bowel cancer. In a period in which "veganism" appears "politically correct", this news has been ridden by most, misrepresenting the reality, which instead classifies processed meats as carcinogenic, i.e. those treated with salting, fermentation and smoking (frankfurters, sausages, bacon, etc.); red meat, on the other hand, is classified as "potentially carcinogenic", not excluding that the cases of cancer found are actually linked to other factors.

Another less publicized but also negative news towards red meat has been added to the first one. It is linked to a study that would show that red meat can promote cardiovascular diseases due to its high content of L-carnitine, metabolized by the bacterial flora and transformed into the TMAO compound (oxide-trimethylamine), which is capable of causing atherosclerosis. It was also found that subjects who consume meat have higher levels of TMAO than vegetarians who take L-carnitine as a supplement.

This would suggest that a diet based on red meat would induce the development of an intestinal flora which is capable of converting L-carnitine into TMAO, promoting cardiovascular disease. Bad news for athletes who have always been major consumers of beef!

However, this study is not conclusive in showing that red meat causes cardiovascular disease, it simply highlights an association.

Continue

Continued

For example, to better clarify the concept, we can say that statistically, people who can swim, die more often from drowning, but the cause of their death is not knowing how to swim, but the fact that they go more easily in areas where the water is deeper. In addition, TMAO has also been found in foods such as soy and fish, which are believed to decrease the cardiovascular risk, and some studies show that L-carnitine can prolong the survival of individuals who survive a heart attack. But why is beef so important for those who want to gain muscle mass?

First of all, beef is rich in proteins, about 30 g per 100 g of meat, with a high biological value and easy to absorb. In fact, these proteins can be used to promote the protein synthesis by stimulating the increase of the muscle mass in youngsters and by preventing the loss of the muscle mass in the elderly. It is also rich in B vitamins, essential for the conversion of food into energy, and in zinc, which promotes testosterone production. Beef, especially the one that comes from pasture farms, is particularly rich in CLA (conjugated linoleic acid), which belongs to the family of polyunsaturated fatty acids derived from the essential omega-6 fatty acid, linoleic acid.

CLA is able to modify the body composition, favoring both the increase in muscle mass and the loss of fat, and promotes the increase of testosterone by reducing its conversion into estrogen thanks to its ability to inhibit the aromatase enzyme, which is responsible for the conversion of testosterone to estradiol. Furthermore, red meat is particularly rich in creatine, which stimulates both the increase in strength, thanks to its ability to increase the synthesis of ATP, and the increase in muscle mass, stimulating the production of myosin and decreasing the production of myostatin, which blocks muscle growth.

The underlying mechanism for the effect that favors the chronic inflammatory stimulus which leads to atherosclerosis would seem to be the bacterial endotoxins produced by the bacteria that are carried with the meat. They are usually annihilated by cooking, but not their endotoxins. Furthermore, a diet rich in meat predisposes to a bacterial flora that is capable of transforming carnitine into TMAO, which in the presence of inflammation predisposes to cardiovascular diseases.

The key to reading all this is that if you don't want to give up the great athletic benefits that you can get from red meat, you need to counteract the inflammation with a large amount of flavonoids and antioxidants which are found, for example, in fruits and vegetables. You can also take prebiotic food substances (also present, for example, in red wine) which can modulate the formation of a more favorable intestinal microbiota (bacteria), which does not metabolize carnitine into TMAO.

CHAPTER 6

Nutrition for endurance sports

When we talk about nutrition as a function of endurance sports such as the marathon, we only think about the consumption of foods in order to meet caloric needs, but we must also achieve other goals:

- higher energy;
- constant lucidity;
- abbreviated recoveries;
- reduction of fat mass;
- increase in lean mass;
- prevention of injuries and diseases;
- a more restful sleep.

Sports performance is influenced by the type of the usual diet, in fact an unbalanced diet (not for a day or a week) can become a critical factor for the performance.

Regularity and consistency in eating properly, offer the sportsperson two great advantages:

- to improve the physical capacity and the technical ability;
- to allow you to acquire correct eating habits from which to benefit, also in the future years.

Too often, for energy needs, we rely only on theoretical calculations and tables to determine how much a sportsperson should eat, but there are many variables, both subjective (age, sex, weight, training) and objective (altitude, temperature, humidity degree, the type and the intensity of the effort) which can affect the balance between the energy intake and expenditure, and the hydroelectrolytic homeostasis.

Let us also remember that not all workouts have the same intensity, therefore, it will be useful to calculate a sort of an "average" between the expenditure in the intense workouts and the so-called "exhaust" workouts. As I've said before, it is an approximate calculation which however provides us with a starting point; then it will be necessary to evaluate, from time to time, based on the sensations of the athlete during training, competitions, recovery, etc., whether to increase or decrease the consumed calories.

Carbohydrates

Carbohydrates are the main muscle fuel for intense physical exertion, although new research is evaluating the use of intramuscular triglycerides (IMTG) in high intensity efforts. The reserves, made up of glycogen, present both in the liver and in the muscle tissue, are mobilized to keep a constant value of glucose in the blood (glycaemia), within a certain range. The decrease in blood sugar or the drastic reduction in muscle glycogen can accelerate the onset of fatigue and worsen performance. Even this last statement can be revised, as some studies show that even with a low amount of muscle glycogen, the athlete has no deficit on the athletic performance, of course, if educated through both nutrition and training to better use the fat.

If an interval of one to two days is foreseen between one effort and another, normal meals with medium-high content of low glycemic index carbohydrates (which do not cause a rapid rise in blood sugar) are indicated in the recovery phase, such as whole grains, fruits and vegetables. Research has shown that the intake of low glycemic index (GI) carbohydrates before a prolonged muscle commitment is capable of exerting several positive effects:

- more stable blood sugar levels for longer exercise times;
- moderate insulin response with less interference on the lipid metabolism;
- performance improvement;
- less lactic acid production compared to a high GI meal;
- a delay in the onset of fatigue.

Usually, if an athlete has a caloric expenditure of up to 4000 Kcal (16,700 Kj), about 600 g of carbohydrates (2400 Kcal, which is 60% of the calorie expenditure and which is equivalent to about 850 g of pasta) are recommended to replenish the glycogen deposits. Such a high share, even if distributed in different meals (at least six a day), could cause intestinal swelling, flatulence, nausea, etc. However, it should be kept in mind that women are less dependent than men on the intake of carbohydrates in the diet, as it has been shown that in prolonged aerobic exercise they use more lipids and less carbohydrates and proteins than males, and that they do not respond well to carbohydrate loading to replenish their glycogen reserves.

We would therefore ask ourselves whether to re-evaluate the classic carbohydrate load in which the carbohydrate intake reaches up to 75% and instead opt, as an energy source, for fats (presented below), which could become the main fuel, and thus spare of part of the muscle glycogen for the final sprints.

Lipids

Lipids are the second source of energy (or perhaps the first in aerobic conditions) for muscles during exercise. The use of fats depends on the degree of training and the type of the exercise: in fact, endurance training increases the ability of the muscle to use fat as an energy source and increases the sensitivity of adipocytes to stimuli that mobilize free fatty acids. Most research shows that fats are the main energy substrate only in prolonged exercise at 40-60% of the maximum aerobic capacity, since in high-intensity exercise the availability of carbohydrates, which are metabolized more quickly than fats and with less consumption of oxygen, is the limiting factor for the performance; however, getting back to what was previously said, intramuscular triglycerides which are stored in the form of easily usable droplets can be used at high intensity, as shown by some researches.

Very often it is not recommended to take fats during exercise because they would tend to slow down the gastric emptying. This may be true if you take large quantities of fatty foods, and in any case mainly saturated fatty acids, because monounsaturated foods in adequate quantities do not cause these problems, plus they are easily usable by the active muscle. In addition, promising indications seem to come from the use of medium-chain triglycerides, which do not delay the gastric emptying and are metabolized at the same rate as glucose.

When you opt for an increase in fats at the expense of carbohydrates to fill the caloric needs caused by an intense and prolonged endurance activity, it is advisable to privilege among these the consumption of olive oil, as it is a monounsaturated fat that improves the insulin sensitivity, is easily used for energy purposes and has some anti-inflammatory properties.

Referring to fats, one cannot fail to mention the omega-3s (such as fish oil), which have a vasodilator function and allow you to increase the oxygen supply to the muscles, with benefits from different points of view, such as performance, energy and circulation (less fatigue of the heart). Furthermore, recent research has shown that a fish oil supplement in the diet, rich in omega-3, reduces bronchial narrowing and the production of inflammation mediators in athletes with exercise-induced bronchoconstriction.

Intense exercises have been shown to increase the inflammation, decrease the anti-inflammatory immune defenses, and also increase the oxidative stress.

Fats are powerful immune system mediators and can modulate the immune depression from strenuous exercise. Some studies have shown that a diet which is low in fat and high in carbohydrates (fat 15%, carbohydrates 65%, protein 20% of the daily calories), the classic followed by endurance athletes, increases the inflammatory state and decreases the anti-inflammatory immune factors. It also consumes antioxidants and has negative effects on the lipoprotein fraction in the blood. By increasing the intake of fats to 42%, there are no negative effects on the immune system or on the lipoprotein fraction given by the physical activity, and it also improves VO_{2max} by 60-80% during endurance performances in cyclists and runners.

Proteins

During exercise, the oxidation of amino acids, especially in the branched chain (leucine, isoleucine and valine), contributes to the production of energy. The researchers found that between 6% to 15% of the calorie expenditure in one hour of intense exercise is covered by the protein catabolism. The latter involves a decrease in the concentration of some amino acids in the blood, resulting in two situations, an altered relationship between branched-chain amino acids and other amino acids, and the formation of ammonia, both associated with the fatigue onset.

During endurance training, the protein requirement increases and the requirement is between 1.4 and 1.8 g/kg of body weight.

Proteins cannot be stored like carbohydrates (in the form of glycogen) or lipids (in the form of fat), and therefore their supply must be constant.

An insufficient protein intake in the diet causes a slow recovery from workouts, lower energy levels, lower resistance to diseases, and a lower muscle tone. Even the majority of the hormones, enzymes and blood proteins that are responsible for the transport of molecules are made of amino acids (the building blocks of proteins), so an insufficient amount in the diet would also be detrimental to these important structures, predisposing to a slower metabolism, slowed digestion, anemia, etc. An athlete who goes through intense training and fails to get the required amount of protein to rebuild the muscle tissue, will be overtraining. Given their reconstructive function, proteins should also be included in the last snack of the day (before going to sleep), to decrease the catabolic effect of the overnight fasting.

The importance of proteins was also demonstrated in a study of marines who were subjected to intense military exercises. After the exercises, they were given a snack containing proteins + carbohydrates + fats, or just carbohydrates + fats. The following effects were found in the group in which proteins were also included:

- 33% fewer medical visits;
- 28% fewer visits for bacterial or viral infections;
- 37% fewer visits due to muscle and/or joint problems;
- 83% fewer visits due to heat stroke.

This indicates the importance of an appropriate dietary protein quota.

Branched-chain amino acids are an optimal source of nitrogen (N) for the muscle in the recovery phase, when the protein synthesis is increased. Also, glutamine, whose concentration in the blood decreases in over-trained athletes or in conditions such as physical exhaustion, seems important for muscle protein synthesis. However, it should not be forgotten that the energy deficit itself induces the protein catabolism and that the intake of carbohydrates and fats is equally important to avoid a negative nitrogen balance.

Branched chain amino acid supplements (5.76 g of leucine, 2.88 g of isoleucine and valine per day) have been shown to prevent muscle loss in subjects on a 21-day trek at an average altitude of 3250 m.

Water and electrolytes

During any athletic performance (even in the cold or in the water itself, as in swimming) there is always a loss of water due to sweating, evaporation or breathing, so it is essential to replenish the lost fluids. Electrolytes are also lost with sweat, but to a lesser extent than with water; however, compensating for copious sweating with water alone can result in decreased sodium levels in the blood (hyponatremia), which is just as dangerous as dehydration.

This situation occurs more often in sports with a very long duration (ultra-endurance), especially in less experienced sportsmen, who drink beyond their needs (due to the very long duration times). Therefore, rehydrating solutions must replace not only fluids, but also electrolytes that are lost in sweat. The addition of small quantities of quick and medium-release simple carbohydrates improves the absorption of water itself, contributes to the maintenance of the glycemic homeostasis, saving endogenous glycogen reserves with effects on the protein catabolism, fatigue and general physical performance.

The rehydrating solution proposed by Brouns consists of:
- carbohydrates: 30-100 g/L
- sodium: 400-1100 mg/L

with the possible addition of:
- chlorides: 500-1500 mg/L
- potassium: 12-225 mg/L
- magnesium: 10-100 mg/L
- calcium: 45-225 mg/L

Carbohydrates can be chosen from glucose, fructose, sucrose, maltose, maltodextrin and soluble starches (always to be customized). For fructose, the quantity must be less than 35 g/L. These solutions are absorbed at a maximum speed and are normally taken by athletes in quantities not exceeding 600-800 mL per hour. Slightly hypertonic solutions have no influence on the water balance, because they slightly reduce the absorption of liquids, but have the advantage of providing more carbohydrates, while strongly hypertonic solutions are not recommended, because they induce the secretion of liquids in the gastrointestinal tract, thus reducing their net absorption and causing possible gastrointestinal problems.

Adequate intake of fluids improves the performance and helps to reduce the fatigue.

The diet of the competition period

On the day of the competition, the athlete undergoes a real stress that affects the whole organism: rational dietetics must find its full expression precisely in this circumstance, because, even if it cannot improve the maximum performance of the athlete, it can at least avoid the loss of form and minimize the fatigue reactions that occur during and after the effort. Beyond the contrast between sports characterized by a short effort (power sports) and sports that use a prolonged effort (endurance sports), the only concept that deserves to be privileged above any other is that of the respect for the fundamental laws of nutritional balance. The last meal before the competition, which should be consumed preferably three to four hours before the start of the tests, must provide several fundamental contributions: a) the intake of meat or fish must provide amino acids of high biological value, in order to ensure a good neurovegetative tone (some amino acids are the precursors of brain neurotransmitters that increase the attention threshold); b) the intake of carbohydrates, which are directly and easily absorbed, must ensure a certain constancy of blood sugar; c) the water intake, relatively high and well distributed throughout the day and the race, will allow for faster mobilization and elimination of the fatigue toxins; d) the significant but reasonable intake of salt (2-4 g) is necessary for the constitution of a good reserve of sodium chloride, which is useful for the hydromineral metabolism and for the muscle contraction during exercise.

The pre-race meal, if misinterpreted, can negatively affect the performance of the race itself.

A meal with a high glycemic index (simple sugars such as sucrose) before the competition and/or training can be counterproductive because it is followed, after a short time, by a state of hypoglycemia due to a stimulating action on insulin.

The recovery ration

The day after the race, the athlete suffers real muscular and nervous aggression, following the abnormal energy expenditure and the real wear and tear of the organism, which now requires repair and purification from the metabolites of fatigue. Let's review the various physiological elements occurring after the competition's stress.

In the 24 hours following the test, the body has an increased need for water, which is lost essentially through perspiration: without taking into account the water that is present in foods, the replenishment rate is around 2 L and over, spread throughout the day. The abundant sweating has inevitably also exhausted the sodium and potassium reserves, elements that must be immediately replenished to improve the urinary excretion of toxins. In the same way, the carbohydrate compartment, especially if techniques for enriching the glycogen reserves (carbohydrate load) have not been carried out, must be reconstituted, while the lipid compartment does not show excessive need for recovery, as the fat reserves are practically inexhaustible. For their part, the protein catabolism products which are present in the blood are above normal values, reflecting a considerable protein wear. Since the detoxification processes have a priority value, they will take place within 24-36 hours, so avoid including excessive animal proteins during this time interval. The most useful vitamins at this time are represented by vitamin B6 (which favors the work of the protein reconstruction, improves the metabolism of the myocardium, and allows a rapid return of ammonia and exercise nitrogen to the norm) and vitamin B12 (antitoxin factor par excellence). However, they should not be administered in excessive doses and they should preferably be associated with glutathione (the most powerful antioxidant and detoxifier in our body).

The stress that the entire hormonal sphere presents after the competition is extremely interesting. It can be translated above all in a hypersecretion of the adrenal hormones: the diet following a sports competition must therefore provide the raw materials necessary for the body to process its own hormones (amino acids, cholesterol, mineral salts, vitamins).

In the event of the competition or training taking place:

In the morning - The previous day's dinner must include a good amount of carbohydrates, avoiding foods that are difficult to digest. Whole grains are fine, a second based on white meat or fish, and cooked vegetables seasoned with extra virgin olive oil. Breakfast must be consumed at least 2-3 hours before the performance, and may contain carbohydrates in the form of seasonal fruits and/or wholemeal toast or wholemeal rusks with sugar-free jam or acacia honey, easily digestible proteins (well cooked egg whites or protein powders or amino acid pools that do not tire the digestion) or lean sliced meat, all accompanied by a source of unsaturated fats (nuts, almond milk or peanuts).

In the afternoon - Breakfast must be abundant and it should also include salty foods, such as bread, ham and cheese or toast; lunch must mirror the dinner of the previous point and must be consumed at least three hours before, in order to be assimilated and not to sequester the blood by taking it away from the muscles due to digestion.

In the evening - Breakfast and lunch will be eaten at the usual time. About an hour and a half before the starting of the competition, a waiting ration consisting of a piece of Parmesan cheese and a fruit, or lean cold cuts and fruit, or half a slice of toast, or a protein-carbohydrate bar, or a drink that contains fructose and easily digestible protein powder, with a pleasant taste and especially useful for those athletes who have particular digestive problems.

During the effort - The supply of fluids is fundamental both for hydration and for the possibility of providing carbohydrates (usually mixtures of fructose and maltodextrin), solutions between 6 and 8%, which have proved to be the most effective from the supplementation point of view and are normally free of side effects for the intestines (excessive water recall). It is also useful to administer amino acids or easily assimilable protein powders, several times (every 45 minutes) to make a supply of amino acids that will be "sacrificed" in place of the endogenous ones. Small portions of fatty foods (for example, nuts) can be useful for providing the energy in long-running races. The brain depends on carbohydrates, which are its natural fuel, while the body uses the latter almost exclusively to provide energy in those activities that have an intensity greater than 65% of the maximum. The stores of carbohydrates in the muscles, liver and blood decrease during prolonged exercise. This can lead to extreme physical and mental fatigue. A mouth rinse with glucose solutions stimulates a group of sensory receptors linked to reward/motor control mechanisms. These rinses can improve endurance performance in those athletes who have used all their carbohydrate stores, according to Adriano Lima-Silva and colleagues, of the Federal University of Pernambuco in Brazil. In one of their studies, the subjects were placed on an exercise bike and performed a 30-minute protocol, followed by a 20 km time trial, under different feeding conditions: fed normally, 12 hours of fasting and 12 hours of fasting where the carbohydrates had already been consumed. During each session, the subjects rinsed the oral cavity with glucose solutions at regular exercise intervals. This improved the endurance capacity by 9% in the "already consumed carbohydrates" group. This technique could improve the performance and the perception of fatigue in the last stages of sports such as marathons, triathlons, workout sessions with repeats and in situation sports such as soccer or American football (*Medicine Science Sport* 2016; 48: 1810-1820).

After the effort - Immediately after a competitive endurance competition it is advisable to take a vegetable extract (black cabbage, spinach, parsley, celery, carrot, beetroot) with the addition of lemon and ginger, perhaps with coconut water, to remineralize and detoxify the acidified body from intense and prolonged physical activities, which leads to a high production of toxic metabolites.

After that, all the macronutrients must be taken in particular proportions, to accelerate the recovery from the muscle glycogen point of view and to accelerate the protein synthesis.

Studies show that the intake of carbohydrates + proteins immediately after the training is able to speed up the post-exercise recovery more significantly than the intake of carbohydrates alone. This happens because the insulin secretion is higher, with positive repercussions on the protein synthesis, the increased entry of glucose into muscle cells and the contrast on the increase in cortisol levels. According to some studies, the ratio of carbohydrates to proteins and the amount to be taken within the first hour following the training is: **0.8 g of rapidly absorbed carbohydrates + 0.4 g of hydrolyzed protein/kg of body weight.**
However, a 4/2 ratio of carbohydrates to proteins should be maintained. Immediately after the training, it would be better if the snack was liquid and easy to assimilate, so that the blood can remain in the muscles for recovery and is not conveyed to the intestine.

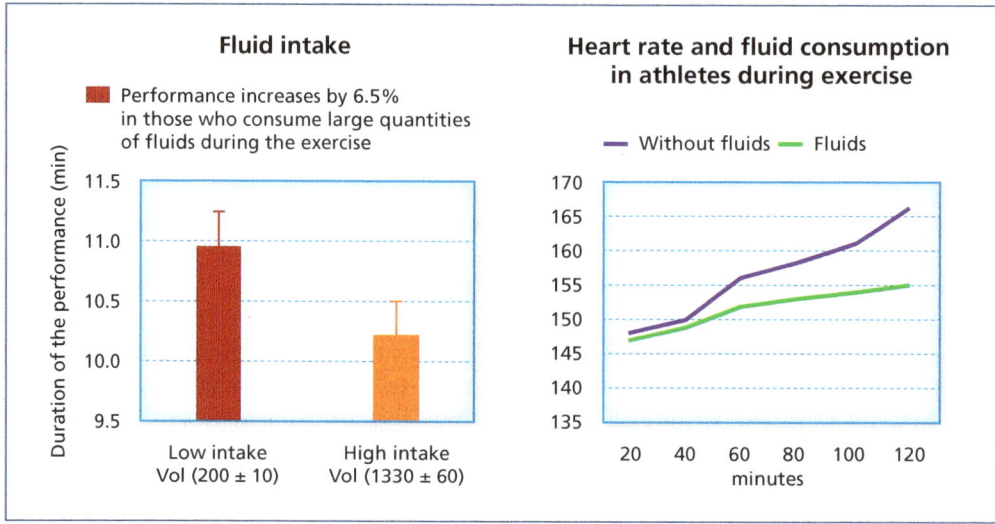

Figure 6.1 The importance of the contribution of water and electrolytes during the performance. Left: a study by Below et al. shows that athletes who had consumed greater quantities of fluids performed better, being faster than the athletes who had taken a lower quantity. Right: In another study, Hargraves et al. shows that the intake of fluids causes a lower heart rate.

SUMMING UP:

- Meals with medium-low glycemic index.
- Waiting rations consisting of: fructose + maltodextrin + proteins + fats in water; provide immediate and prolonged-release energy.
- Eating every 45-60 minutes avoids the sugar drop.
- Post-race meal: needed to accelerate the recovery and the synthesis of glycogen (medium-high GI).

Warning: After the competition or particularly intense workouts, you may be more thirsty than hungry, and at the end of the day the calorie intake may not cover the accumulated debt.

How much should you eat?

First, it is necessary to establish how much protein to consume during the day by multiplying the body weight by the adequate protein value.

Based on the training and the subject type, the following caloric percentages are established:

- proteins: 20-30% of the calories of the day;
- carbohydrates: 40-60%;
- fats: 20-30%.

However, personalization is a must because there are some athletes who perform better with more carbohydrates, and others with more fats (remembering not to go below 1.5-1.7 g of protein for every kg of body weight). However, remember that carbohydrates must have a medium-low glycemic index (except the after training ones), that proteins must come from lean meats and that fats must be predominantly monounsaturated (a proportion of saturated fats must still be represented).

Which foods are to be preferred?

Carbohydrates

Right choices give a lower insulin reaction:

- the majority of fruits;
- the majority of vegetables that are rich in fiber (raw carrots, etc.);
- selected cereals (oat flakes, hulled oats, barley);
- wholemeal al dente pasta and rice;
- low glycemic index foods.

Wrong choices give a higher insulin reaction:

- the majority of cereals (bread, pasta, refined cereals in general);
- starchy foods (cooked potatoes, polished rice);
- some fruits (raisins, ripe bananas, dehydrated fruit, etc.);
- some vegetables (corn, cooked carrots, spinach, cabbage, beetroot).

We also report that a high intake of nitrates in the diet increases the production of nitric oxide (NO) by the vascular endothelial cells; NO has a fundamental importance in the regulation of vascularized tissues. Several recent studies have discovered how the intake of beet juice, rich in nitrates, improves the endurance and reduces the blood pressure. A study conducted by Simone Porcelli of the Institute of Molecular Bioimaging and Physiology of Segrate (Italy), highlighted that cyclists that had a diet rich in nitrates have an improved efficiency with the stationary bicycle, have a reduction in fatigue during exercise and they improved their sprint. A high-nitrate diet includes raw spinach, beetroot, bananas, cooked kale, and pomegranate juice. The changes in performance were so significant that they made a difference in athletic competition.

In conclusion, adding these few foods to the diet is an easy way to improve your performance and increase metabolic health.

Fats

The addition of fats serves to reduce and modulate the insulin secretion.

- Right choices: foods that are rich in monounsaturated fats, such as olive oil, olives, almonds, avocados.
- Wrong choices: foods that are rich in saturated fat and arachidonic acid, such as fatty meats, processed meats, all those products that contain trans fatty acids, indicated on the label as hydrogenated and/or partially hydrogenated oils.

Proteins

Choose low-fat proteins: turkey, fish (including fat, except eel), chicken, ostrich, cooked egg white, low-fat cheese, lean roast beef, tofu, soy steaks, legumes.

The metabolic efficiency

If what we said before is absolutely true, namely that some subjects are better off with more carbohydrates and others with less (and this is certainly due to constitutional, hormonal and genetic factors), it is equally true that, from the metabolic point of view, there is a more suitable and functional diet for the endurance athlete, who is able to optimize the use of fats for energy purposes, as these represent the maximal energy potential that is stored in our body.

Our glucose energy stores can cover up to 1500-2000 calories, which is equivalent to two to three hours of intense exercise, while the fat stores reach 50,000 or more calories depending on the percentage of body fat. Therefore, the creation of a metabolic adaptation that allows a better use of body fat for energy purposes allows you to complete an extreme endurance performance (ultra-runner) without having to depend on the intake of large quantities of carbohydrates during the race, which, easily, can lead to gastrointestinal upset as well as become a burden to carry during the competition. In addition, during races that last several days, this metabolic efficiency allows you to need fewer calories from food, as you can easily use those that come from fat; since we need fewer carbohydrates, most of the foods we have to carry with us can be mainly represented by fats, which have about 240% more calories than carbohydrates for the same weight.

How to achieve this metabolic adaptation? The best metabolic efficiency is obtained through the manipulation of macronutrients and physical exercise.

To do this, you need to keep your blood sugar stable by eating more proteins, healthy fats, fruits and vegetables instead of foods that are rich in carbohydrates, and you must train at low intensities, especially in the initial phase. By manipulating the diet to control the blood sugar and the insulin response, we will be able to eat fewer calories during the competition, as there will be more lipolysis favored by low insulin levels, a hormone that, when stimulated, prevents lipolysis. When the insulin is high, it is impossible to use fats for energy purposes and therefore we will be less likely to consume fats during the competition, on the contrary, we will increase the use of muscle glycogen. In fact, this metabolic adaptation is useful for all sports, both short and long-lasting, especially in the competition phase. In the muscle building phase, in power sports, this approach can however be limiting as the insulin stimulus is actually a powerful anabolic stimulus that favors the increase of the muscle mass. It takes at least four weeks to achieve this metabolic adaptation, but most protocols take six to ten weeks. Before going into the details of this method, we need to know the concept of the "cross", which describes the relationship between the intensity and the use of fats and carbohydrates for energy purposes during an exercise. As the intensity of the exercise increases, the use of fats decreases and the use of carbohydrates increases; the crossover point is reached when we begin to consume more carbohydrates than fat and it can be defined in terms of speed, level, watt or heart rate.

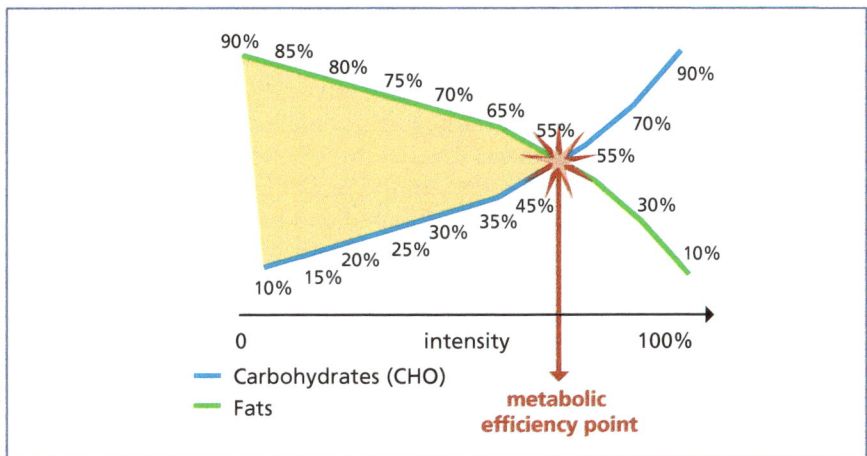

Figure 6.2

How to achieve it? First of all, we start by measuring the crossing point through a metabolimeter, which is able to measure the inhaled volume of oxygen compared to the exhaled volume of carbon dioxide. Since different amounts of oxygen are consumed in the metabolism of fats and carbohydrates, the test can determine our carbohydrate/fat oxidation ratio. To carry out the test using a cycle ergometer or a treadmill, it must be performed by fasting for 10 hours and by using a mask that enables breathing inside it. The test lasts about 30-60 minutes and it is not a maximal test: you start by walking and increase the speed of the treadmill or the watts of the cycle ergometer every five minutes until you reach the "crossing point". In this way, we will be able to check the carbohydrate/fat utilization ratio and determine the intensity at which the "crossing point" occurs. For example, a person can verify that their "crossing point" occurs when they train at an intensity of around 9-10 km/h and 130-140 beats per minute; it means that this is the area within which the athlete must remain during the training phase in order to maximize the use of fats for energy purposes.

Once the "crossing point" has been defined, it is necessary to train at high intensities below this threshold, in order to stimulate the cellular adaptation response which leads to a better metabolic efficiency in burning more fat and less carbohydrates at higher intensities. Sometimes this can be difficult because a small climb may be enough to cause an increase in intensity; in this case, to stay "in the area", you will probably have to walk. You need to train in this way for at least six to seven hours a week to get results, and this mode must make up the bulk of your training, because training above this threshold slows down the metabolic adaptation. If the training is important for 20-25%, nutrition in this case is important for 75-80%. We have already mentioned how a diet that is based mainly on carbohydrates can lead to a series of negative consequences: gastrointestinal disorders, the need to eat more frequently, weight gain, less constant energy levels, reduced mental performance, decreased ability to concentrate , slowness in the processing of auditory and visual information, not to mention the greater predisposition, in the long run, to develop diseases such as: diabetes, Alzheimer's, insulin resistance, inflammation, cardiovascular disease, cancer and obesity.

The nutritional change can be gradual and it should involve several steps. For the first period, half of the food portion can be made up of whole grains, one quarter of proteins and fats and the other quarter of fruits and vegetables. In the second phase, we move on to a third of whole grains, a third of fats and proteins and a third of fruits and vegetables. In the third phase, the diet must consist of a half of fruits and vegetables, only one tenth of whole grains and the rest of fats and proteins.

In the last phase, all cereals are eliminated and half of the diet is made up of fruits and vegetables and half of proteins and fats, so it will consist of lean proteins, good fats and a quantity of dried fruits, fresh fruits and vegetables. Legumes are allowed in small quantities. In the end, the ideal carbohydrate/protein ratio should be 1/1 or 2/1. This is not a low carb diet, but a balanced diet in which you simply don't have to consume the usual cornflakes, rusks, bread and pasta.

Breakfast could consist of black beans with an omelette with spinach and feta or, alternatively, Greek yogurt with berries and dried fruits.

For lunch and dinner, a huge salad with chicken or salmon and fruits; possibly at dinner, to promote a good sleep (carbohydrates raise serotonin, which is the precursor of melatonin) and a better recovery, you can consume a little quinoa or other low glycemic index cereals.

The snacks can be based on crudités, olives, hummus and dried fruits, or fruits and vegetables centrifuged with protein powder and linseed or coconut oil, and again, if necessary, with the addition of dried fruits.

However, if the goal is also to lose weight, snacks will not be necessary, as the body, adapting to the use of fats for energy purposes, will not undergo hypoglycemia with the relative need to eat a few hours after the last meal.

For the same reason, it will no longer be necessary to consume carbohydrate-based drinks during training, but only water and electrolytes or, if the training exceeds two hours, possibly a bar based on dehydrated fruits and dried fruits. It will not even be necessary to take carbohydrates immediately after the training, because in reality, they have been consumed to a minimal extent since we used the fat storage, training below the "crossing point", so the rehydration is enough; then a balanced snack or meal will follow. The only allowed carbohydrate-based supplement is SuperStarch® or Superamido, a hydrothermally treated form of a very high molecular weight starch that causes the glucose from the starch to be assimilated very slowly without any insulin stimulus, without weighing on gastric level and with a fast stomach transit.

With this dietary approach, by improving the metabolic efficiency, blood sugar and energy levels will be more stable, we will burn more fat and we will be able to run faster at a lower heart rate.

THE VIRTUES OF OLIVE OIL

Olives represent one of those wonders of nature that perhaps we too often take for granted. Instead, their properties deserve particular attention. Olives belong to the group of "drupes", that is, fleshy fruits with thin and membranous exocarp, fleshy and juicy mesocarp, and woody endocarp, containing only one bony seed. Other examples of drupes are peaches, mangoes, cherries, etc. There are hundreds of varieties of olives, mostly originating from the Mediterranean; olive trees tend to live for several hundred years (the record is 2000 years).

Olives can be considered powerful anti-inflammatories; they can be an excellent snack or they can be eaten during a meal. Due to their high fat content, one of the reasons that make them so tasty, many people decide not to consume them; however, most of the fat (over 75%) contained in olives is oleic acid, a monounsaturated fatty acid known for its ability to lower the risk of heart disease. In fact, in a diet, increasing the monounsaturated fat content without increasing the total fat content (thus lowering the saturated fat intake) leads to a decrease in blood cholesterol, "bad" LDL cholesterol and the LDL:HDL cholesterol ratio.

Recent studies have also shown that the oleic acid which is present in olives and in olive oil can help decrease the blood pressure by modifying the signaling mechanisms at the cell membrane (specifically, by altering the cascade processes associated with G proteins). A research which was published in the journal *BMC Medicine* concluded that the consumption of olive oil, especially the extra virgin variety, is associated with a lower risk of cardiovascular disease and mortality in those with a high cardiovascular risk. According to another research which was published in the *European Journal of Cancer Prevention*, the content of antioxidants is also important, including phenols (hydroxytyrosol, tyrosol) and polyphenols (oleuropein glucoside) along with other compounds.

In fact, olives also contain some unique antioxidants, such as oleuropein, which is found only in olives; these antioxidants reduce the oxidation of LDL cholesterol, consequently reducing the markers of the oxidative stress. The properties of the antioxidants that are present in olives have been shown to be stronger than those of vitamin E. The presence of oleic acid and squalene, which is found in a high quantity in olives, has been found to be effective for cancer prevention and may have chemopreventive properties against colon cancer. In addition to being a powerful antioxidant agent, oleuropein has an antiangiogenic function and shows a powerful antitumor and cancer-protective function.

The antioxidants contained in olives also have beneficial effects against aging. Tyrosol, for example, increases the lifespan and stress resistance in nematodes. In other laboratory studies, administration of oleuropein in cultures increased the lifespan by 15%. Oleuropein, hydroxytyrosol (another

Continues

Continued

antioxidant) and squalene (which are found in olives) can also help protect the skin from UV rays, which increase the production of free radicals in the body and promote aging. According to research published in the journal *Rejuvenation Research*, "The health benefits of the Mediterranean diet can be largely attributed to the nutraceutical properties of extra virgin olive oil (EVOO)".

The consumption of olive oil and olives in animal studies prevents the loss of bone mass and therefore osteoporosis, which is linked to aging. Oleuropein may be responsible for this beneficial effect; the phenolic compounds of extra virgin olive oil stimulate the human osteoblastic proliferation, which are the cells that form the bones. In a two-year study of 127 elderly men, the consumption of a Mediterranean diet enriched with extra virgin olive oil was associated with an increase in serum osteocalcin (a bone matrix protein) and the procollagen type I N-terminal propeptide (PINP, which is another measure for the bone health). Olive oil has also been shown to have other beneficial effects, such as an increase in insulin sensitivity, an increase in testosterone synthesis and an antimicrobial and antiviral effect.

Olives come in a range of colors – bright green, yellow, green, dark purple, or black. Their color is primarily a matter of preference and does not necessarily indicate anything about their state of ripeness or the curing process, but research suggests that the oleuropein content decreases as the olives ripen. Some types of olives turn from green to black during the ripening process, while other types remain black (or start green and stay green). Both olives, green and black, have beneficial effects on the body, but in some cases green olives may have a higher oleuropein content.

If you live in an olive oil production area, purchasing from a local producer is the ideal solution; if possible, it would be better to taste the oil before buying it. Although tasting does not necessarily constitute a guarantee of quality, it can help identify the freshest oil and avoid taking home a bottle with a rancid taste. Remember that olive oil is excellent when used for cold dishes, whereas when oil is needed for cooking, olive oil is not the ideal choice, as it is not stable enough to resist heat-induced damage.

CHAPTER 7

Nutrition for slimming

If the types of nutrition for hypertrophy, strength and endurance are more or less recognized unanimously within certain parameters that are accepted by most scholars in the sector, when it comes to weight loss, things change and opinions are mostly disparate. To support these different points of view there are numerous studies that demonstrate the validity of each of these dietary approaches. Personally, I believe that all this is essentially due to two reasons: the first is the metabolic individuality, linked above all to the individual hormonal prevalence that can influence the lipolytic processes to a greater extent than the anabolic processes; we all know that losing fat efficiently requires a perfect hormonal balance, which can more easily be altered during a weight loss diet, due to its restrictive nature.

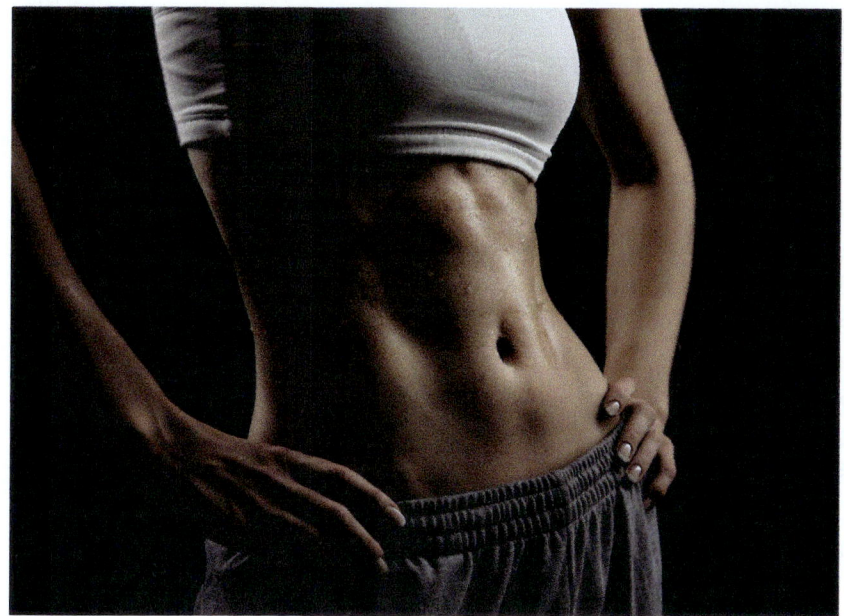

Figure 7.1

The second reason is that, all in all, you lose weight quite well (if you are not in a state of malnutrition, in which the muscle catabolism prevails) with any diet that includes moderate caloric restriction, regardless of the relationship between the various macronutrients. This is because the food shortage or the lack of a particular macronutrient was a situation that certainly occurred in the Paleolithic era, and our body has developed the ability to adapt to various situations of food shortages to survive, obviously without prejudice to the need for the supply of some absolutely essential nutrients, that is a certain amount of amino acids and essential fats, vitamins and minerals.

However, one thing is certain: to lose weight you need to create a calorie deficit with respect to the energy consumption, and this can be achieved in three ways:
- decreasing the intake of calories, i.e. by manipulating the diet;
- increasing the caloric consumption by increasing the training and thermogenesis;
- acting on both factors, exploiting their synergies.

Personally I believe that the most valid method is the latter and, considering that in order not to have a loss of lean mass and excessive performance, it is better not to

THE IMPORTANCE OF WATER IN FAT LOSS

A very important aspect when it comes to weight loss is hydration. Everyone has heard that it is important to drink water for one's health, but few have any idea how much water is actually needed to lose weight. Whenever we eat, the body consumes calories to process the nutrients we are going to digest. This phenomenon is called "diet induced thermogenesis". In this regard, water has no calories but provides enormous benefits to our body.

A study has shown that drinking 500 mL of fresh water promotes an increase of 30% in the metabolic rate, through an increase in thermogenesis which is activated after 10 minutes and reaches its maximum after 40 minutes, leading to a consumption of 25 Kcal. This means that drinking 2 liters of water consumes about 100 more Kcal. Water is just as important for appetite control. It is no coincidence that we often hear that when you are on a diet you need to drink more water, even to feel full for longer. The reason why this strategy is implemented is that in many cases what we perceive as hunger, is actually thirst. Many sensations that tend to be associated with hunger, such as stomach rumbling, low energy levels and even mental fatigue, can actually be synonymous to dehydration. Several studies have shown that people who consume more water before and after meals are prone to consume less food and lose weight.

70% of our body is made up of water and its importance for our health should already be deduced from this figure: water keeps our cells active and promotes the transport of nutrients and oxygen, keeping our muscles healthy. Epigenetics has taught us that the same as food, water is also a source of energy and information, so keeping hydrated by drinking quality water will also improve the quality of our life.

push the calorie deficit beyond 20%, I would recommend reducing the calorie intake by 10% compared to a normocaloric diet and to increase the energy expenditure by 10% by increasing the training intensity and by promoting thermogenesis with the use of specific supplements, the use of body temperature manipulation techniques and the increase of proteins which have a greater thermodynamic effect compared to fats and carbohydrates.

The reduction of the dietary calories and exercise trigger the formation of white adipose fat that behaves like brown fat (increasing the number of mitochondria which also causes the color variation). Brown adipose tissue (BAT) converts the energy of food directly to heat, while white fat does exactly the opposite: it stores energy as fat.

While it is true that each approach can be taken into consideration and can be adapted to a particular person, in my opinion, the best approach to the definition is obtained with three methods which make most people happy.

1. The **Zone Diet**, i.e. 40-30-30, is basically a good balanced diet that allows you to gradually lose weight, but hardly allows for a maximum definition. It is a little "neither meat nor fish": a little too much fat in the presence of a sustained amount of carbohydrates, and this is not good for maximizing the lipolysis.
2. The **LOW FAT-HIGH CARB** diet is the one that is generally recommended by traditional dieticians, being suitably adapted with sufficient proteins; it was the basis of the definition programs for most of the bodybuilding champions in the 80s-90s. The concept was: I want to define myself and therefore I have to follow a low-calorie diet, however, instead of lowering the diet too much, I increase the training volume and do more aerobic activities; this allows me to consume more. It is not necessary to take too much protein, so that makes it impossible to increase the muscle mass. It you already have a good result, maintain it, and this is possible with a higher level of carbohydrates that exert a much greater anti-catabolic effect than fats, which should be drastically reduced. This was the diet of Lee Labrada, Berry De Mey, Lee Haney: great bodybuilding champions of the 80s and 90s. During competitions, they even increased the level of calories compared to the off-season, but, by also increasing the energy expenditure, they still created an energy deficit.
3. Another approach is the **HIGH PROT-LOW CARB-LOW FAT**. This method was widespread in the 70s and in the early 80s (Arnold Schwarzenegger) and came back into fashion in the 2000s. It consists in significantly lowering carbohydrates and in counteracting the catabolism resulting from a low-calorie diet and the hypoinsulinism, by taking more proteins. The amino acids of proteins, and particularly leucine, stimulate the protein synthesis through the activation of mTOR, and the hypoinsulinism resulting from the reduced intake of carbohydrates promotes the lipolysis.

At this point, which method should be chosen to obtain the maximum definition? As always, I believe it is a subjective discourse; however, some considerations must certainly be taken. The HIGH CARB-LOW FAT approach undoubtedly requires a fairly low percentage of fat as a starting point, I would say no more than 9-10%, because we will not be able to make use of a "significant calorie deficit" and low insulin levels.

The advantage is that we will not lower the thyroid metabolism, which happens when carbohydrates are very low; the downside is that we will have to train a lot. It works best in young people and in people who already tend to be thin, which means, people who have an excellent insulin sensitivity and who therefore tolerate, and actually find themselves better, with a higher level of carbohydrates. We come to the LOW CARB diet. It leads to faster weight loss and people who tend to be overweight, that predisposes to insulin resistance, and those who are over 40, generally respond better to it. The muscles of the over 40s are less sensitive to the amino acid stimulation. Larger and more frequent doses of protein are needed to maintain the muscle mass.

Despite this, it's my experience that diets that are too low in carbohydrates are particularly catabolic in the long run. This is because a diet which is very low in carbohydrates can predispose to neoglucogenesis, i.e. the destruction of proteins to form glucose, as well as ketosis, i.e. the production of ketone bodies resulting from the oxidation of fats with a consequent increase in blood levels of NEFA (non-esterified free fatty acids) which suppress the GH production.

However, if we wanted to provide the numbers, I would say that in the case of the HIGH CARB-LOW FAT we could have 20-25% protein, 10-15% fat and 65% carbohydrates. In the case of the LOW CARB, we will have 50% protein, 20-30% fat, 20-25% carbohydrate. I would say that aside from the minimum amount of protein needed, everything else is variable and, as Samir Bannout told me 30 years ago in Los Angeles, quoting Mike Mentzer, while eating a fried chicken wing while preparing for Mr. Olympia, "A calorie is a calorie". This expresses a concept that has been partly overcome with recent scientific discoveries, but is still partly valid.

However, if I were to give you an indication of how to approach a weight loss program, I could give you some suggestions. When you start a weight loss diet and you have to reduce the calories, you have to decide on which nutrient to intervene and, since there are now genetic tests that are able to identify the greater sensitivity to fats and carbohydrates, it is good to use them in order to decide in a more personalized way. Generalizing, having to decide between fats and carbohydrates, since proteins should not be touched, it is best to start by cutting down on fats.

We have already referred to the fact that, if we lower the percentage of fats in the diet too much, the body activates mechanisms that tend to preserve fat deposits, and that excessive fat restriction causes the body to lose the enzymatic capacity that uses fats as an energy substrate. But this is still an effect caused by a prolonged restriction.

In reality, in the early stages of a low-calorie diet the body tends to burn, to fill the calorie deficit, especially muscle proteins by transforming them into sugars (neoglucogenesis) because the body uses these substrates more easily at the same energy level: only after about 30 days, the body learns how to burn fat for energy as a saving mechanism for the most important tissue proteins.

Therefore, in the first 30 days of a diet, it makes sense to maintain a higher percentage of carbohydrates that have an anti-neoglucogenic effect, which happens because they limit the muscular auto-cannibalism that occurs in the early stages of a low-calorie diet, and it also makes sense to keep fats at a low level, fats that cannot be used in the best possible way for energy purposes. However, after the first month, it is advisable to gradually increase the percentage of fats.

At this point, the body is ready to burn fat, and by increasing their amount we will give a further stimulus to the production of enzymes that affect the metabolism of fats, thus favoring their use for energy purposes, including those that are used as a storage. Thirty years ago, despite the fact that diets with a very low percentage of fat were in vogue, in one of my articles I supported the importance of maintaining 20% of fats in the diet, to guarantee that 5-10% of polyunsaturated fats that considered "essential", which our body cannot build from other fats, and to have a good anabolic efficiency (they are considered essential growth factors).

Fatty acids are the building materials for tissues in the body, they are the key elements of the cell membrane, which ensures intracellular exchanges and the maintenance of homeostasis.

Until recently, when we talked about building materials, we thought about proteins. Today, speaking of the raw material of which the body is composed, one cannot ignore fatty acids, especially when it comes to the brain and the nervous system in general.

Gradually, after these 30 days during which the body has now entered the lipolytic phase, I would then decrease the carbohydrates by raising the fats, especially the unsaturated ones (seed oil, fish), up to these percentages: 40% carbohydrates, 30% protein, 30% fat (practically a Zone Diet), which I would continue for at least another 30 days.

CONSUMPTION OF NUTS INCREASES THE WEIGHT LOSS

In a study published in 2008 in the *New England Journal of Medicine*, researchers found that the Mediterranean low-carbohydrate diet is an effective alternative for weight loss. It appears to be just as safe as, metabolically healthier, and more effective than a low-fat diet. The consumption of monounsaturated fats (extra virgin olive oil and nuts) improves insulin sensitivity, explaining the favorable effect on blood glucose and insulin levels. Research has shown that walnut consumption can increase weight loss.

Twenty-five years ago, nutritionists discouraged the consumption of walnuts due to their high fat content. Much evidence now shows that walnuts are a superfood that reduces the risk of cardiovascular diseases, cancer and all-cause mortality. A meta-analysis that combined the results of 20 studies involving over 819,000 people, published by Dagfionn Aune of Imperial College London, found that consuming 28 g of walnuts per day was linked to a reduced risk of coronary heart disease (29%), stroke (70%), cardiovascular disease (21%), total cancer risk (15%) and all-cause mortality (22%). Adding the consumption of walnuts to your daily diet can have a significant effect on health and as a prevention of diseases (*BMC Medicine*, 2016).

A recent study published in 2017 in the *European Journal of Nutrition* mentions "nuts", such as walnuts, peanuts, pistachios and almonds, which help by increasing weight loss and by preventing obesity. Nuts are low in carbohydrates, high in fiber and make a good addition to the low carb Mediterranean diet.

At this point, however, another problem arises: we have already been following a constant calorie restriction program for two months and our body tends to counterbalance this trend by lowering its metabolism. We must therefore fool it with diet modifications. I recommend further reducing 200-300 calories at the expense of carbohydrates from Monday to Friday and by doing this we will find ourselves on an "isometric" diet (33% carbohydrates – 33% proteins – 33% fat).

On Saturday and Sunday, we "recharge" with carbohydrates, making up for that weekly deficit of about 1000-1500 calories. Normally on Sundays I recommend enjoying a little bit of freedom: pizza and ice cream are allowed. I think one day is necessary to give a boost to the metabolism and to psychologically detach from the monotony and rigidity of the diet.

On Monday we start again, more "recharged", with motivation and energy which is stored in the form of glycogen in the muscles. And don't worry if the next day you seem heavier and less dry, it's just a water retention due to the increase in carbohydrates and possibly the salt (pizza) you consumed.

We previously mentioned that proteins shouldn't be touched. However, this statement is conditioned by the initial protein intake. If this intake is closer to 1.5 g of protein per kg of body weight, then it may be functional to increase it to 2-2.5 g per kg instead. In this sense, the studies by Butterfield et al. confirmed that athletes who ran stretches of 8-16 km courses every day, while maintaining a minimum caloric deficit, encountered a considerable negative nitrogen balance, even if they consumed 2 g of protein per kg of body weight on a daily basis.

Celejowa et al. observed 10 agonist weightlifters during a training session, who consumed on average 2 g of protein per kg of body weight. Five of them experienced a negative nitrogen balance and, of these five, three were in a calorie deficit. The conclusion of the study was therefore that, in similar conditions, with 2-2.2 g of protein intake per kg of body weight, the margin for not experiencing nitrogen losses is very minimal. The ideal protein intake, on the other hand, according to a study by Philips and Van Loon, is 1.8-2.7 g per kg of body weight for athletes who train in situations of calorie restrictions.

It must be considered that these indications do not take into account those athletes who follow weights and duration trainings and who have a very low percentage of body fat. Some studies by Helms et al., performed on thin subjects who train with weights while maintaining a restricted diet from the caloric point of view, suggested that the right protein intake varies from 2.3 to 3.1 g/kg. In this analysis, it was also established that the amount of body fat of the subjects is inversely proportional to the caloric deficit to which they must undergo, which means, the leaner you are, the lower the caloric deficit must be. If the primary intent is to maintain a lean mass, the amount of protein increases to 2.3-3.1 g/kg of the lean mass.

However, at this point, it must be taken into consideration that the decrease in carbohydrates can compromise the performance during the training, both strength and endurance, and the limit of carbohydrate reduction is certainly a subjective value. In a study, it was shown that in a diet with a fairly consistent intake of carbohydrates at the expense of proteins (1 g/kg) there was a greater loss of lean mass combined with a better maintenance of the athletic performance, compared to a diet where proteins had been increased to 1.6 g/kg at the expense of carbohydrates.

When proteins were kept at 1.6 g/kg and fat was lowered by favoring carbohydrates, both lean mass and the sporting performance were maintained. Mattler et al. found that by reducing the calories and fats, by maintaining a sufficient carbohydrate intake and by increasing the proteins to 2.5 g/kg, lean mass was preserved while maintaining the performance level in weight training athletes.

Therefore, in the light of these considerations, it is clear that in the final part of the preparation for a competition (about 2-3 weeks before, depending on the sport), when the desired level of body fat has now been reached, it may be useful to reduce the caloric deficit by increasing the calories in the form of carbohydrates and by reducing fat again, as well as by reducing the workload, thus bringing the caloric deficit from the initial 20 to 10%, or even returning to an isocaloric diet.

These final assessments are related to the fact that the prolonged period of diet, probably has lowered the metabolism level and therefore what was previously isocaloric can be highly-caloric and it can favor weight gain. However, if there were no weight problems, an excess of calories, especially in the first 15 days, would lead to an increase in muscle glycogen and, if anything, in intramuscular triglycerides, which have a functional value and a "Bulking" effect in bodybuilders, not like the annoying subcutaneous fat which, in addition to being unsightly, represents a "burden", specifically in sports where the weight/power ratio is important.

EIGHT SPICES THAT HELP YOU LOSE WEIGHT

It is often difficult to lose weight without consuming bland foods, but why do it? Why not look in the cupboatd for some spices that could aid weight loss while adding flavor to raw chicken breast or celery? Spices like black pepper and turmeric will help you stick to your diet and make it tastier.
Cardamom has several beneficial effects: it helps peristalsis by speeding up the passage of food along the intestinal tract and by improving the situations of cramps and intestinal gas. It is considered a thermogenic spice which is useful for weight loss, as it increases the body temperature by promoting the catabolism of lipids. Black pepper blocks the formation of new lipid cells, a fact confirmed by researchers from South Korea, while Dr. Barbara Mendez has shown its effectiveness in preventing weight accumulation. The bioavailability of turmeric increases when combined with black pepper.
Turmeric helps with weight loss and inflammation. It also prevents the accumulation of fat in the body's adipose tissue and helps reduce the amount of fat stored in the liver and stomach.
Cayenne pepper is another thermogenic spice that increases the body temperature, thus leading to a faster metabolism with consequent weight loss. Dr. Lauren Minchen says that adding cayenne pepper to a meal can help burn up to 100 calories while eating. It also stimulates satiety, reducing the need to nibble between meals.
Numerous studies have shown that cinnamon stimulates weight loss and lowers the risk of heart diseases. It can help in the treatment of minor digestive disorders, to lower blood sugar levels and "bad" cholesterol levels, and to prolong the sense of satiety.

Continues

Chapter 7 ▸ Nutrition for slimming

Continued

The Shahid Sadoughi University of Medical Sciences, Yazd (Iran) has performed some studies and confirmed the modulatory action of cumin on "bad" cholesterol levels and excess body fat.

Ginger can help you lose body fat, improve the blood sugar and "good" cholesterol levels. It also increases the concentration of leptin which decreases the sense of hunger, and it also increases the energy expenditure thus favoring the reduction of body weight.

Garlic is known for its nutritional value, it helps mitigate inflammation and blood pressure. A researcher from Seoul states that garlic is able to reduce the harmful effects that unhealthy foods have on the liver, thereby helping with weight loss. An Israeli study found that garlic also helps reduce the symptoms of diabetes and hinders the formation of plaque in the coronary arteries.

What you eat plays an important role in the weight loss process: if what you eat is more appetizing, you will be less tempted to make bad and harmful food choices. So why settle for tasteless foods when the addition of some spices could make your meals more enjoyable and at the same time more effective for your diet?

CHAPTER 8

Nutrition for concentration
by Marco Tullio Cau

While it is intuitive that nutrition can affect athletic performance, especially when it comes to the energy supply and muscle building, it is connected less to its effect on mental concentration, which is equally important for performance purposes, especially in the long term.

By overestimating the energy demands before a training session, a hyperglucidic diet is often used and it could cause a certain sleepiness, especially if it's made up of foods with a high glycemic index: just the opposite effect of what we would like to have in the gym (or on the track, on the platform, in the pool, etc.).

A massive ingestion of only carbohydrates generates a high glycemic load (even more "significant" than the aforementioned index) and causes an insulin peak which has, among other effects, that of *sequestering* discrete quantities of certain amino acids, such as tyrosine, phenylalanine and three branched amino acids, leaving a free field for tryptophan, an amino acid that is usually "kept at bay" by the previously mentioned.

Those yawns that we have experienced or seen during sports are because of the passage of the tryptophan molecule through the blood brain barrier, which it penetrates more easily thanks to insulin, thus stimulating the production of serotonin, which is responsible for the sensation of numbness, decreased attention and a sense of fatigue at an unsuitable time: I was recently in the gym and, after seeing a (rather heavy) rugby player chewing his jaw for a good half an hour, I asked him what he had eaten (it was 3.00 pm): "A plate of pasta", was the answer and, given the build, it certainly wasn't 50 grams...

The first studies that tested these hypotheses (Fernstrom and Wurtman, 1971 to 1975; Spring, 1984, also the interesting Wurtman et al., 2003) are now outdated, but a very recent review (Mantantzis et al., 2019), which includes over 30 studies, concludes that "CHO administration was associated with higher levels of fatigue and less alertness compared with a placebo within the first hour after the ingestion"... All this happens to a "normal" population, but if instead, we were in the middle of a hard workout, it would be even worse: branched chain amino acids are also used for energy purposes, leaving even more room for tryptophan, although large amounts of carbohydrates have not been previously ingested.

Also keep in mind that, especially in long-duration sports, the progressive depletion of glycogen, in addition to causing neoglucogenesis, will also activate a parallel increase in the release of FFA (Free Fatty Acids), which, having the same albumin carrier with tryptophan, will leave a high quantity of its free form. As a consequence, it will be able to reach the brain with the "usual" effects.

In fact, a normal carbohydrate intake and the use of BCAAs (before an activity, I repeat, a prolonged one) could help avoid the onset of "mental" fatigue, as can be seen from a series of interesting reviews by Davis, who writes: "carbohydrate intake during prolonged exercise leads to strong reductions in the tryptophan/amino acid ratio and improves the performance" and "there is a strong rationale and a large number of data supporting the favorable role of carbohydrates and branched chain amino acids to reduce serotonin and the 'central fatigue'".

Also, two trials by Blomstrand and colleagues (2006) show that during long-term physical activities, subjects who ingested a placebo had a much higher cerebral absorption of tryptophan than those who had a beverage with 6% carbohydrates; however, the same Swedish author (2001) had also reiterated the validity of using BCAAs to reduce the cerebral uptake of tryptophan and thus decrease the sense of fatigue, like Castell and Newsholme, cited below.

Davis himself, also carried out field studies: in the case of endurance stresses, specifically up to 255 minutes on a sustained effort cycle ergometer, "free tryptophan, the tryptophan/branched amino acid ratio and free fatty acids increased 5 to 7 times. These changes were attenuated in a dose-dependent manner by carbohydrate rich beverages", while in the case of marathon runners he noted that branched chain amino acids would only give an advantage after many hours of continuous work.

It should be noted that, in this trial, the lower dose of carbohydrates (6% *vs.* 12%/5mL/kg) was slightly more effective and it was administered a quarter of an hour after the start of the exercise, and subsequently every 30 minutes, and not altogether before the session, which is certainly a relevant factor.

Moreover, BCAAs are often taken to slow the cerebral absorption of tryptophan, albeit with some distinction, which we will see later ("Supplementation with branched chain amino acids can help to counterbalance the effects of the increase of free tryptophan in the blood", Castell et al.; "The intake of branched amino acids may reduce the absorption of tryptophan", Newsholme et al., 1992-6).

However, these studies that were mentioned above, seem to forget that leucine (as can be read in other chapters of this book) is an antagonist of dopamine and, if we consider that the "common" formulations of BCAA include this amino acid in ratios ranging from 2/1 to 12/1, and that it is instead valine that competes most with tryptophan, it can be understood that there is still a long way to go to fully understand the nuances of specific supplementation for concentration and fatigue reduction...

While writing this chapter, I came across a myriad of very conflicting studies about it, but going through them all is impossible here.

Therefore, I think that it is important to experiment on yourself, obviously, after having documented that each of these texts uses different doses and timings: carbohydrates alone, before or during the training session, at high and low dosages, with BCAA or without BCAA and in highly variable proportions. The results will vary according to the practiced sport, the diet in general, the individual hormonal and neural response and also the genetic one; there is no "one recipe for everyone". We should also remember that tryptophan increases its blood concentration even after a protein-rich meal (obviously), but in this case without affecting the brain's serotonin levels, due to the simultaneous presence of other competing amino acids that prevent it from passing through the blood-brain barrier.

Numerous studies (Choi et al., 2009; Fernstrom et al., 2013, just to name two) bring an interesting upgrade to the just exposed concept: lactalbumines (whey), much praised for their various properties, are the protein sources that increase the values of tryptophan more compared to caseins, wheat and corn, which are lower in many other aspects, and would therefore be counterproductive for the purposes of a high state of concentration: however, deepening the question, it can be seen that in reality, all the authors used alpha-lactalbumin, a fraction of the total, which is particularly rich in tryptophan; however, the study by Wurtman (2003), cited above, which deals with proteins that are normally present in typical (American) breakfasts, confirms the general theory that was set out in the previous paragraph.

However, a piece of valid advice is to always insert a protein source alongside the carbohydrates, perhaps branched amino acids in formulations that do not abound too much in leucine: obviously, the nutritional needs of a triathlete or a bodybuilder who performs a high intensity training are intuitively very different, but the concept of not exceeding the carbohydrate intake remains valid for everyone, also because it is desirable that the glycogen pool, determined by the intake of carbohydrates, is possibly already saturated before the last pre-workout meal, thanks to the previous meals.

Regarding this, a further warning is necessary: those who usually ingest carbohydrates in the amount of 50-70% of the daily caloric intake and want to reduce them immediately before an athletic session for the reasons listed above, must take into consideration the risk of incurring drastic drops in attention (at that point, the concentration will be lost for some time) and, in the case of very prolonged efforts, could also have drops in consciousness, which in certain sports could even be lethal (as in racing on any type of wheels), so it will be necessary to proceed step by step.

Those who have a metabolism that "leans towards fats", thanks to a diet that is normally low in carbohydrates, will not suffer too many shocks even by lowering them further (obviously up to a certain point). As mentioned, it is not necessary to give any specific advice due to the wide type of commitment of the various sports, but on a general level it is still necessary to remember how a simple lack of vitamins and minerals can contain, in itself, a reason for cognitive problems and poor mental performance, due to the incorrect brain functioning that follows: for example, some studies from the Western Human Nutrition Research Center (University of California, Davis) suggest that diets which are low in zinc, iron and magnesium, can worsen the ability to concentrate.

For space reasons, we will cite only two other studies, even though they are not specifically related to the subject: Tangney et al. show that "the concentration of all markers related to vitamin B12 is associated with the cognitive function in a general sense and with the total volume of the brain", therefore an insufficiency of the same vitamin can cause cognitive deficits and loss of brain mass; Smith et al. have demonstrated how the administration of folic acid and vitamins B6-B12 in elderly subjects was able to significantly slow down the trend of a progressive brain atrophy, while improving the results of cognitive tests.

Another basic point is (as mothers used to say!) breakfast: even the American Dietetic Association states that skipping it and not being regular with meal times can compromise the concentration and the mental performance. Starting the day with a suitable and appropriate first morning meal and having lots of small snacks every few hours, is a sure way for a superior state of mental clarity. On the contrary, skipping breakfast or, vice versa, gorging ourselves, exaggerating with calories (at any time), will give us a sleepy mood for sure.

There are numerous studies on this topic, even if they are often related to minors: an example is the excellent essay *Breakfast for Learning*, published by the FRAC (Food Research and Action Center) in Washington, which is rich in information and bibliographical references, but also that of Adolphus et al., who points out that "a higher frequency of regular breakfasts is consistently associated with a higher academic performance".

A balanced, fiber-rich breakfast promotes a higher school performance than a breakfast based primarily on refined foods. More akin to "our" interests is the work of Clayton and James (December 2015), which investigates the effects of breakfast on the energy balance and on the sports performance: the statements of Anglo-Saxon researchers fully confirm its importance: "skipping breakfast can impair the spontaneous physical activity and the aerobic performance during the rest of the day" and "currently available research suggests that breakfast may affect the work capacity more than the total amount of ingested calories".

Another study by Clayton et al. is equally useful (December 2015). It assesses the impact of breakfast on the physical activity, but in the late afternoon, finding that "not having breakfast can harm the performance throughout the day, even if you eat at lunchtime". Those who practice intermittent fasting will therefore have to carry out some tests, in order to optimize their performance and possibly make the appropriate corrections. Some studies claim that this practice reduces the mental acuity, more that it helps.

We can add that the philosophers of ancient Greece also believed in it, and in a much more extensive way: Plato was an advocate of it and used it to achieve greater mental and also physical efficiency (remember that Plato, which means "broad-shouldered", is the nickname of the famous philosopher, who was actually called Aristocles).

Ensuring a correct and constant caloric intake is the first step in staying focused and "alert", but it may not be enough, as a high concentration requires that information "flows" as freely and quickly as possible from one neuron to another through the nerve fibers which, just like electrical cables, must be insulated: omega-3s are very useful for the creation of these sheaths: not only they are present in the lipid part of myelin, but their consumption balances their *ratio* with the omega-6, which is often found in excess and therefore has a pro-inflammatory effect.

In fact, in addition to the other recognized potentials, omega-3s best express their effect on the brain, as written in the review by Sinn et al., *Oiling the Brain*, which illustrates some excellent results, and the one by Muldoon et al., who report the conclusions of many researches which show that today's modest consumption of these nutrients, negatively affects "some aspects of the cognitive performance". Furthermore, their consumption protects brain function *in toto*, as demonstrated by a long theory of studies in the antiaging field, both in acute and diachronic level.

The work of Rathod et al. is equally interesting (2016). They once again underline how an inadequate nutrition can increase the risk of cognitive deficits and how it has become a subject for many studies that evaluate the neuroprotective abilities of the aforementioned vitamin B12 and omega-3s, hoping for an overall examination to investigate and possibly exploit that synergy in their highest opinions: as proof of this, they treat the "various mechanisms through which vitamin B12 and omega-3 fats can support the brain function" in depth and from new scientific angles.

In conclusion, the road to a maximum concentration for carrying out a profitable workout passes through the union between the "right" foods at the "right" time and the use of *nootropic* substances which are discussed in the specific chapter: union makes the strength!

CHAPTER 9

Nutrition and supplementation for vegetarian/vegan athletes

In recent years, more and more people have decided to follow a vegetarian or vegan diet. At this point it is appropriate to ask whether a diet of this kind can be compatible with sporting activities. Most of the scientific evidence and even the examples of some great sporting champions show that it is possible. On the other hand, we must realize that it is certainly easier to have deficiencies, especially with a vegan diet, and therefore we must be particularly careful in considering certain factors, which we will discuss later.

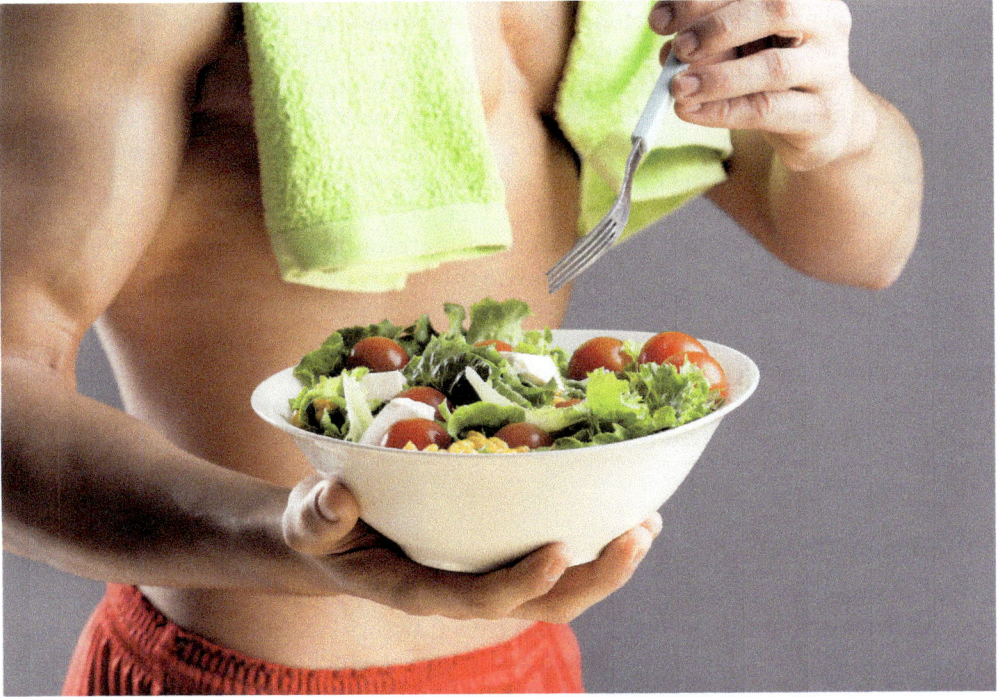

Figure 9.1

Firstly, let's explain what it means to be vegetarian or vegan. A vegetarian does not eat meat or fish, but still consumes foods of animal origin such as dairy products and eggs. A vegan, on the other hand, refrains from ingesting any food of animal origin, for example, even honey. I do not want to enter into the merits of the ethical or even ecological choices, so I will make my discussion exclusively in reference to the nutritional and health aspects. The American Dietetic Association argues that vegetarian and vegan diets, if well planned, can be followed in all stages of growth without causing imbalances or dysfunctions and do not negatively affect sports performance. The problem is precisely the correct planning. Let's see what are the deficiencies that are normally attributed to this type of diet.

Protein deficiency

Studies carried out on vegetarian or vegan adult individuals who live in industrialized countries have shown that the protein intake is equal to or slightly lower than that of non-vegetarians and it is able to cover nutritional needs if the diet is varied and includes legumes, oil seeds and nuts. Eggs and dairy products are rich in proteins, so vegetarians have no problems, but there are also foods of vegetable origin that are rich in proteins, such as nuts, legumes, seeds and quinoa, which, if consumed in an adequate quantity, also cover the protein needs of vegans. The digestibility of vegetable proteins from whole foods such as whole grains and legumes is 80%, compared to 95% of those of animal origin, and therefore it would be advisable to increase the intake by 10-15% compared to the recommendations. Furthermore, it must be considered that proteins of vegetable origin are more deficient in essential amino acids, and this is another reason why they must be consumed in greater quantities in order to have the same effect on the protein synthesis. In the case of a specific deficiency of a certain amino acid in a particular food, it is necessary to combine the latter with another that is rich in it, as the lack of an essential amino acid prevents the use of the other amino acids for protein synthesis.

This is the case of cereals that have a lack of lysine and tryptophan, while legumes are rich in them but are deficient in methionine. By combining these two foods, the concept of amino acid complementarity is exploited, which finds an example in the association of cereals and legumes. Soy proteins are among those with the highest biological value. However, it is better not to abuse with their usage, especially for the male athlete, because they are able to lower the testosterone levels if consumed in large quantities. Therefore, nutrition and even the vegan diet do not necessarily lead to a protein deficit, but you need to consume the right foods in the necessary quantities.

Calcium deficiency

It is a common belief that if you do not consume dairy products you will have a calcium deficiency, but this is absolutely not true. Calcium is found in green leafy vegetables (broccoli, lettuce, chard, spinach and arugula, which, among other things, being low in oxalates, provide a particularly bioavailable source of calcium), legumes and almonds, which do not have the characteristic acidifying power of the dairy products, that promotes the loss of calcium by releasing it from the bones to be used as a buffer substance.

Iron deficiency

Iron is very important for athletes, especially for those who practice in endurance sports; in addition, the long-term competitive activity favors its loss. Iron is present not only in meat, but also in cereals and legumes; the problem is that, in the latter, it is much less bioavailable as it is found in an inorganic form. Inorganic iron is better absorbed when it is in the ferrous state and therefore foods that are rich in antioxidants, such as vitamin C, will increase its absorption; vice versa, vegetables also have some substances such as tannins and phytates, that limit the iron absorption.

Therefore, theoretically, it is very difficult for a vegetarian to reach the amount of the absorbed iron only from the food. In reality, there does not seem to be a greater incidence of iron deficiency anemia in vegetarian populations, and this seems to be due to the fact that, in the case of chronic deficiency, such as that of a vegetarian, there is an increase in the transport mechanisms of inorganic iron as an adaptive response. However, even though there may not be fully developed anemia, it does not mean that there is no functional deficiency, especially in athletes. In this case, and not if they don't have a deficiency, the administration of Fe as a supplement causes an increase in the hemoglobin levels.

Zinc deficiency

The amount of the absorbed zinc in vegetarian diets is more or less comparable to that of the omnivorous diets, but the problem is that many foods of plant origin have some absorption inhibitors, such as phytates, which decrease zinc's bioavailability. So a possible supplement could be indicated.

Taurine deficiency

Taurine is an amino acid which is present in the cell cytoplasm and plays an osmotic role, by stimulating the entry of water into the cells. In this way, indirectly, it stimulates the protein synthesis while not being a direct part of it, as it is not a part of the constitution of proteins. Taurine, being an antagonist of the gabaergic system, which is a sedative system, also improves the attention and concentration; for this reason, it could be a useful supplement, in dosages of 1 g, divided into two intakes per day or before the training. It is an important supplement especially for vegetarian and vegan athletes, because taurine is mainly present in foods of animal origin, as it is one of their main intracellular osmolytes.

Vitamin B12 deficiency

Vitamin B12 or cobalamin is essential for erythropoiesis, for DNA synthesis and for the metabolism of proteins, fats and carbohydrates. Vitamin B12 is present only in foods of animal origin and, even though it can be synthesized in the liver, its nutritional deficiency, as in the case of a vegetarian diet (even with milk and eggs), leads to a deficiency in the long run, therefore supplementation is a must.

LC-PUFA (Long Chain Polyunsatured Fatty Acids) deficiency

If it is true that omega-3s are also present in large quantities in foods of plant origin, such as walnuts, flax seeds, pumpkin, hemp, chia etc., it is equally true that the conversion mechanism of alpha-linolenic acid (short-chain polyunsaturated fatty acid, progenitor of the omega-3 family) in EPA and DHA (long-chain polyunsaturated fatty acids) can be slowed down, especially in the over 50s. A direct supplementation of the omega-3s (EPA and DHA), endowed with anti-inflammatory and immuno-modulatory abilities, becomes essential, especially for athletes who are involved in intense trainings, which cause inflammation and depress the immune system. To evaluate the correct balance of polyunsaturated fatty acids, we should first evaluate the AA/EPA ratio (arachidonic acid/eicosapentaenoic acid); a ratio greater than 4/1 favors the inflammatory state by directing fatty acids towards the production of eicosaenoids with pro-inflammatory characteristics; the correct balance is normally achievable through a diet that consists of an intake of PUFA that makes at least 2-3% of the total calories, with an omega-6/omega-3 ratio of 4/1, and a proportion of omega-3s with a ratio of 2/1 between alpha-linolenic acid and DHA + EPA. In vegans, a dietary intake with an omega-6/omega-3 ratio of 2/1 would be desirable to favor the conversion mechanism into LC-PUFA.

In vegans, there were found significantly lower levels of EPA and DHA (less than 50% of the omnivore diet), and similar values of AA. The mechanism of conversion of alpha-linolenic acid into EPA and DHA is greater in women, probably due to the effect of estrogen, and this may be the reason why women normally cope better with a vegetarian diet. Obviously, the supplement based on fish oil (rich in DHA and EPA) may not be accepted by a person who has chosen to be a vegetarian or vegan for ethical reasons. In this case, there are some supplements that contain DHA and EPA coming from marine microalgae, which are able to synthesize them.

Iodine deficiency

Those who follow a vegetarian diet can easily consume big quantities of foods, such as brassicaceae (cabbage-broccoli-cabbage), onions and nuts, which limit the absorption of iodine. If an iodized salt is not used, it is easy to have a deficiency of this mineral, which is essential for the production of thyroid hormones and whose deficiency can cause thyroid alterations such as the goiter. The introduction of algae in the diet is certainly very useful in order to overcome this deficiency. Algae, in addition to being alkalizing, are rich in vitamins and mineral salts, including iodine. We can mention kelp among many others, which is also used as a supplement due to its high iodine content.

Vitamin D deficiency

Another very frequent deficiency in vegetarians (and not only) is that of the vitamin D. Vitamin D is produced mainly during the exposure of the body to the sun, and therefore in Westernized civilizations, where most of the activities take place indoors, this deficiency is very frequent. From a nutritional point of view, vitamin D is mainly found in foods such as salmon and mackerel, which are not included in vegetarian diets, and in eggs, which are excluded from vegan ones.

It is very important for the bone metabolism and for the regulation of the glucose metabolism. It favors the synthesis of testosterone and its levels are directly proportional to the iron levels. It is so important that this could be one of the reasons why almost all records in athletics are obtained during the summer, when the athletes have a greater sun exposure.

Without talking about vitamin D deficiencies, as it has an endogenous production, a vegetarian-type diet undoubtedly brings in lower quantities of substances such as **creatine** and **carnitine**, which are found in meat, and also the transport system of carnitine in the muscles appears to be temporarily downregulated in vegetarians. A supplementation of these substances, with proven ergogenic effects can be particularly effective in the vegetarian athlete.

In conclusion, if the choice to follow a vegetarian or vegan diet is dictated by ethical or ecological reasons, it is possible to follow it by paying a particular attention to the balance of various nutrients, selecting quality functional foods and, possibly, integrating with fortified foods or supplements without having performance deficits in sporting activities. If, on the other hand, the choice derives from health considerations, while it is true that a vegetarian diet brings greater benefits, for example, to the prevention of cardiovascular diseases or diabetes, compared to the certainly not healthy classic Western type diet, it would still be better to follow diets that take into account the principles of the proper nutrition, such as: the glycemic index and load, the correct intake of proteins and essential amino acids, the omega-3 and omega-6 ratio, the quantity of fiber, the adequate intake of fruits and vegetables (both for the content of phytonutrients and for the alkalizing effect), the choice of foods from an organic and non-intensive cultivation, the consumption of wild-caught fish, a moderate consumption of meat from livestock raised in grazing and, of course, the correct caloric intake.

CHAPTER 10

Nutrition and supplementation for the senior athlete

In the language of sport, the senior category indicates athletes who have passed a certain age. In most disciplines, this age limit is set at 35. Among the ancient Romans the *seniors* were citizens between 45 and 60 years of age, who, for military purposes, constituted the reserve. Since it is amply demonstrated that in reality, in many sports, thanks to the training methods and an adequate nutrition, maximum sports results can be obtained up to the threshold of 40 years. I will consider the senior athlete according to the ancient Romans criteria, referring to a range which we could therefore define as the middle-aged.

Proteins are the primary macronutrient of our diet, as the name implies; they are necessary for the formation of enzymes, antibodies, membrane transporters, neurotransmitters, various hormones, and are the main component of the skeletal mus-

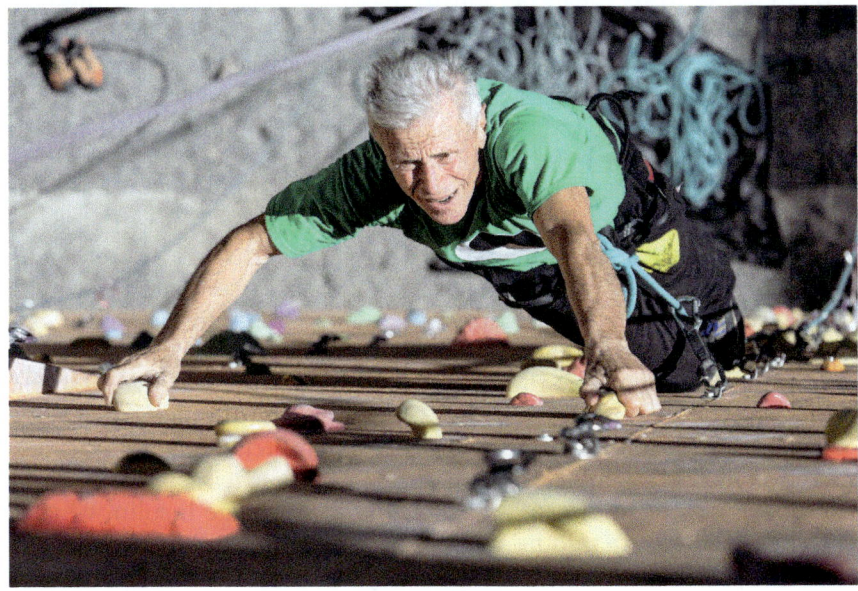

Figure 10.1

cle. Having made this necessary premise, the problem that arises is about how many proteins are needed for the organism and how many for the athlete, and if there are different needs for the middle-aged athlete. Based on a recent meta-analysis by Ramd et al., The recommendations for the protein requirements of healthy adults, regardless of age and physical activity, remain around 0.8 g of protein per kg of body weight.

While this value may be adequate to prevent the nitrogen balance deficits, it may also be insufficient to maximize the metabolism, the muscle mass and the functional capabilities in power sports, especially in an aging adult, and some studies show that this intake leads to a loss of the muscle mass in the long run.

As the level of calories needed in a middle-aged adult falls compared to a young one, the level of protein needs increases; consequently, if we think in terms of the percentage of macronutrients, the level of protein intake drops as an absolute value, so it is absolutely better to consider the protein requirement as a function of body weight. In adult men, protein synthesis is stimulated by the intake of amino acids even without other macronutrients and it depends on the dose, the amino acid profile, the type of administration (food and intravenous infusion), the age and the hormonal profile of the subject.

The increase in the protein synthesis lasts for two hours after a meal and it is particularly linked to the presence of the amino acid leucine, which is able to improve the protein synthesis by signaling that high quality proteins are available. A higher amino acid concentration favors the protein synthesis; a study by Bohe et al. has shown that protein synthesis increases linearly until the level of plasma amino acids increases by 80% compared to the baseline. After that, the system saturates and the line flattens out. It seems that the dose needed to saturate the system is between 8 and 15 g of essential amino acids, and these dosages are effective in both the young and the elderly. For example, 10 g of essential amino acids equals 25 g of protein from milk or eggs. This response can be stimulated repeatedly and, by taking 25 g of protein in five to six meals per day to maximize the protein synthesis, it would lead to a consumption of 125-150 g of protein per day, which for a 70 kg individual is equivalent to 1.8-2.1 g of protein per kg of body weight, which is more than double of the 0.8 g/kg/D of the RDA.

The catabolic phase in the post-absorption phase does not seem to increase with age; vice versa, the anabolic response to a low amino acid availability decreases (metabolism is characterized by the contemporaneity of the anabolic and catabolic functions and, depending on the prevalence of one over the other, there is protein synthesis or protein destruction). A study has shown that there is a lower anabolic response to the administration of 7 g of essential amino acids compared to young individuals. Another study showed that a dose of 2.9 g of leucine in a blend of essential amino acids can induce an anabolic response similar to that of young adults.

A study conducted by the University of Maastricht in the Netherlands showed that in the elderly, a meal containing 20 g of protein supplemented with 2.5 g of leucine increases the protein synthesis more than protein alone; or, 35 g of whey protein should be taken in order to obtain a maximum protein synthesis. This mechanism is probably linked to the ability of leucine to stimulate insulin, which prevents the protein catabolism. In middle-aged men there is often a situation of insulin resistance which is the cause of a lower anabolic response to meals. For the same reason, while the ingestion of carbohydrates with proteins increases the protein synthesis in the young, the opposite has been seen in older adults. In older adults, even non-diabetic ones, the addition of carbohydrates decreases the protein synthesis, and this suggests the desirability of a lower intake of carbohydrates and a greater intake of protein to stimulate the muscle mass in the elderly. In another study, 35 men with an average age of 59 consumed 57 g (12 g of protein), 113 g (24 g of protein) or 170 g (36g of protein) of ground beef and then ran a one-sided weight training session.

Subsequently, the protein synthesis was measured both after the meal alone, and after the meal and training. It turned out that with 170 g of beef, i.e. 36 g of protein, the protein synthesis increased more than with the other doses, both at rest and after training. Furthermore, the training had a summation effect compared to the meal alone. Summing up all the studies in the literature, we could reasonably say that for middle-aged men who are devoted to power sports, the daily protein intake should correspond to 1.7-2.1 g of protein per kg of body weight, and it should be 1.3-1.7 g for endurance sports practitioners. The moment of the protein intake in relation to training, especially for the elderly, is also important. In younger adults, it seems that it is possible to maintain a positive protein synthesis by consuming proteins up to three hours after the training, while the "older" muscles need an adequate protein intake immediately after the exercise to stimulate the protein synthesis. Creatine is undoubtedly one of the supplements that can be particularly useful in older individuals who practice resistance exercises, which means, power exercises.

In a study that included 28 men and women under the age of 65, who were involved in a total-body weight training program three days a week for 14 weeks, creatine supplementation was found to increase the isometric strength, functional tests and body composition to a significantly greater extent than the placebo (in some studies it has even been found that creatine is able to increase the muscle strength, power and the lean mass, even without exercise).

Creatine supplementation has been shown to positively affect the loss of muscle mass and strength associated with aging, both alone and in combination with training. Some data indicate that creatine concentration and its resynthesis decline with age, and these parameters can improve much more in middle-aged individuals than in young people. Another promising supplement for the middle-aged athlete is HMB (Beta-Hydroxy-Beta-Methylbutyrate), the intake of which has been strongly correlated with an increase in strength and muscle mass, and a decrease in fat mass in individuals aged 20 at 40, when associated with weight training.

The administration of HMB before exercise has been shown to be able to decrease the levels of CPK (creatine phosphokinase), LDH (lactate dehydrogenase) and urea in plasma and urine, which represent indirect measures of muscle damage. This indicates that HMB has the ability to preserve the integrity of the muscle cell membrane and to enhance the regeneration of the aging muscle. Normally recommended dosages are around 3 g, but they are based on young individuals; unfortunately, there are no data concerning middle-aged or older individuals, but, considering the greater predisposition to muscle catabolism with the advancing age, higher dosages may be needed to obtain an optimal response.

In recent years, there have been multiple cases of adults and the elderly in which prolonged vitamin D deficiency has been associated with severe muscle weakness, which improves with a vitamin D supplementation. Vitamin D receptors have also been found in the muscle and they tend to decline with age. In a clinical trial that analyzed the effects of vitamin D on the physical performance, it was found that in elderly individuals with serum levels of vitamin D3 25OH <50 nmol/L, supplementation with vitamin D improved the muscle performance of the lower limbs by 4-11% in 12 weeks. The daily intake of vitamin D, identified in 1997 as 200-600 IU, is currently considered insufficient by most experts, while doses of 2000 to 3000 IU are considered more appropriate.

Researchers from the University of Pavia (Italy) studied 130 elderly individuals, with an average age of 80, who participated in a 12-week exercise program and took supplements containing whey proteins, essential amino acids and vitamin D. Compared to the placebo group who were given fake supplements, the subjects gained about 3.5% in lean mass, reduced the body fat, increased strength and IGF-1 levels, improved the daily activities, and reduced the inflammation.

Researchers from the University of McMaster (Canada), in a 2017 study, established that a specific combination of ingredients is useful in countering sarcopenia. The combination of this mix is: 30 g of whey protein, 2.5 g of creatine, 500 IU of vitamin D, 400 mg of calcium and 1500 mg of omega-3. The study involved 49 healthy elderly individuals with an average age of 73, who were divided into two groups. One group took the supplement mix twice a day, while the other took a placebo. Neither group performed any physical activity regimes. After 6 weeks, both groups followed a training program, both aerobic and anaerobic, for an additional 12 weeks.

The results were exciting: the researchers found improvements in the overall strength and in the lean mass both before and after the implementation of the training regimen. Consuming the supplement in the first 6 weeks caused an increase of 700g in lean body mass. This is equal to the amount of muscle that these individuals would lose in a year. The results of the study clearly demonstrate the improvements that were provided to the participants by the supplement alone, or in a combination with exercises. An individual's protein needs increases with age, with older individuals requiring about 40 g of protein for a 75% increase in the protein synthesis. A study published in *The Journal of Nutrition* investigated the effect of the protein ingestion before bed on the daytime protein synthesis.

Using a randomized double-blind design, the researchers assigned 48 males to 4 different groups depending on the amount of protein they received: 40 g of casein, 20 g of casein, 20 g of casein and 1.5 g of leucine or a placebo. To be included in the study, participants had to be males over 65, had to have a BMI of 20-30 kg/m^2 and could not use protein supplements. They also had to participate in an exercise program. Furthermore, they could not be smokers, have diabetes or other illnesses, or take drugs that affected the muscle metabolism, limb mobility, clotting, or neurological, renal, and gastrointestinal function.

To prepare for the study, participants were required to maintain a regular diet and not engage in rigorous physical activities until 2 days before the study. The participants then followed an overnight fasting. The researchers took anthropometric and baseline measurements of variables such as plasma glucose levels, insulin and glucose tolerance. Each participant followed a diet which was set according to the personal caloric needs and consisting of three meals and two snacks. Participants also had to consume a drink with a certain amount of protein before going to bed. This drink consisted of water, vanilla flavoring and casein. The placebo group only received vanilla flavored water.

During sleep, the researchers used a wrist monitor on the participants to measure variables that describe the sleeping activity, such as sleep duration, wake up time, sleep efficiency, and sleep latency. Using the Pittsburgh Sleep Quality Index, sleep quality was evaluated from very poor to very good. Participants who had a short or light sleep were excluded.

At least 40 g of protein has been shown to increase the availability of amino acids in the plasma, which are then used to build the muscle proteins. Adding 1.5 g of leucine to the treatment group was based on studies showing that the protein fortification with leucine can increase the protein synthesis rates, but this study showed that the effect of leucine is mild. It is interesting to incorporate the physical activity with these interventions over a longer period of time, in order to investigate the effects on muscle mass. Overall, this study showed the feasibility of using the protein intake before bed to maintain the muscle mass in the older population.

Regarding the endurance sports, which undoubtedly require a greater calorie intake, it must be considered that middle-aged and elderly individuals begin to have deficits in the digestive system. There is often slower digestion, which causes the stomach to take longer to empty. Furthermore, the stomach often produces less hydrochloric acid and digestive enzymes; concomitantly, food intolerances develop more easily, such as, for example, that to lactose, which makes the digestion of milk and dairy products more problematic. In this way, both proteins and fats become more difficult to digest and therefore, food choices needed to increase the calorie intake must preferably be geared towards carbohydrates, especially before training and competitions.

The glycogen reserves are normally sufficient to sustain activities that last about two hours and it does not seem useful to take additional carbohydrates if the exercise does not exceed 90 minutes. On the other hand, if the exercise has a longer duration, the ingestion of carbohydrates during the execution can improve the performance. An adequate intake can be 45-50 g/hour, preferably in the form of simple carbohydrates in a 6% liquid solution, which is easier to digest and reaches the bloodstream faster than solids, helping to maintain the hydration; this is particularly important for older adults, who are more prone to dehydration. The intake of carbohydrates during exercise can cause gastrointestinal disorders and it is therefore important to proceed gradually and with caution to see how the body responds.

The diet after an endurance exercise is also important, as it affects the recovery and re-synthesis of glycogen, which is maximal immediately after the exercise. The optimal amount, if there are no metabolic disorders such as type 2 diabetes, is 0.7 g/kg of body weight in the form of simple carbohydrates, which are absorbed faster. The addition of proteins increases the glycogen synthesis, and the ideal carbohydrate-protein ratio, in the post-workout meal, is 4/1. As for supplementation, the use of carnitine and coenzyme Q10 has been shown to improve the performance, especially in those individuals with cardiac deficits, while the iron supplementation is particularly useful in individuals who suffer from iron deficiency anemia.

OMEGA-3s NOT ONLY FOR THE HEART, BUT ALSO FOR THE MUSCLES

Without a doubt, omega-3s are among the few supplements which are considered to be useful and recommended by the medical professions. In fact, omega-3s are prescribed above all for cardiopaths, for their beneficial effects on the cardiovascular level, which emerged from the observation of the low incidence of cardiovascular diseases among the Inuits and other populations that adopt a diet rich in these fatty acids, which are mainly found in fish oil.

The mechanism according to which omega-3s exert their positive effect is mainly linked to their anti-inflammatory properties, so much that in the literature and in the clinical practice there are many other uses of omega-3s for various problems, such as arthritis, asthma, colitis, reduction of the post-traumatic brain damage, etc. The omega-3 fatty acids that are particularly effective from an anti-inflammatory point of view are long-chain ones: eicosapentaenoic acid (EPA) and docosahexaenoic acid (DHA). These fatty acids are able to modulate the neutrophil and macrophage response, which are the "white blood cells" that attack the inflammation and promote tissue regeneration.

The macrophages contained in our adipose tissue change as we become fatter and produce more and more molecules that are capable of perpetuating inflammation, triggering a vicious circle that favors further fat gain. Well, omega-3s seem to be able to break this vicious circle. In one study, some guinea pigs were given a high-calorie diet that was rich in fat, with the aim of making them obese and promoting inflammation.

In one group of guinea pigs, 15% of the fat was replaced with EPA; incredibly, they presented a lower body weight and a reduced percentage of fat, with a decrease in the size of fat cells and inflammation. In practice, the EPA has increased the ability to burn fat and use oxygen. In addition to having less fat, omega-3s can be useful for having more muscle. In a study carried out on individuals with low IGF-1 levels (IGF-1 is a powerful anabolic hormone), the administration of 720 mg of EPA and 480 mg of DHA for eight weeks increased the IGF-1 levels.

In stressful chronic situations, such as very intense workouts, IGF-1 levels can be too low to allow muscle growth, in addition to the fact that in this situation it is very easy to have a high state of inflammation, both in the muscle and in the adipose tissue, making it difficult to build muscle and mobilize fat for energy. In this case, omega-3s can therefore be useful, increasing the IGF-1 and decreasing inflammation.

Omega-3s are also able to reverse sarcopenia, that is, the loss of muscle mass that occurs in the elderly (after the age of 50, approximately 1% of muscle mass is lost every year); by administering fish oil supplements containing 3.6 g of EPA and 1.5 g of DHA, roughly the equivalent of 200-300 g of salmon, there was an increase in strength and muscle mass in a population of seventy year old individuals. This result is comparable, if not to weight training, to anti-aging therapies based on DHEA, testosterone and GH. So, if you are not taking at least 300 g of fish per day and if you want to get the maximum benefits from your diet and training, I recommend that you take at least 2 to 4 g of fish oil per day, possibly the one with the highest concentration of EPA and DHA.

CHAPTER 11

Nutrition and supplementation for the diabetic sportsperson

Now, in the medical field, the fundamental role of the physical activity in the prevention but also in the treatment of numerous chronic degenerative diseases has been widely recognized, and doctors no longer limits themselves to suggesting to patients a few walks or a swimming course, but also recommend joining the gym. The problem, at this point, becomes the ability to identify which type of gym is suitable. And this is where the need for gyms that are also able to manage people with health problems arises, i.e. medical gyms.

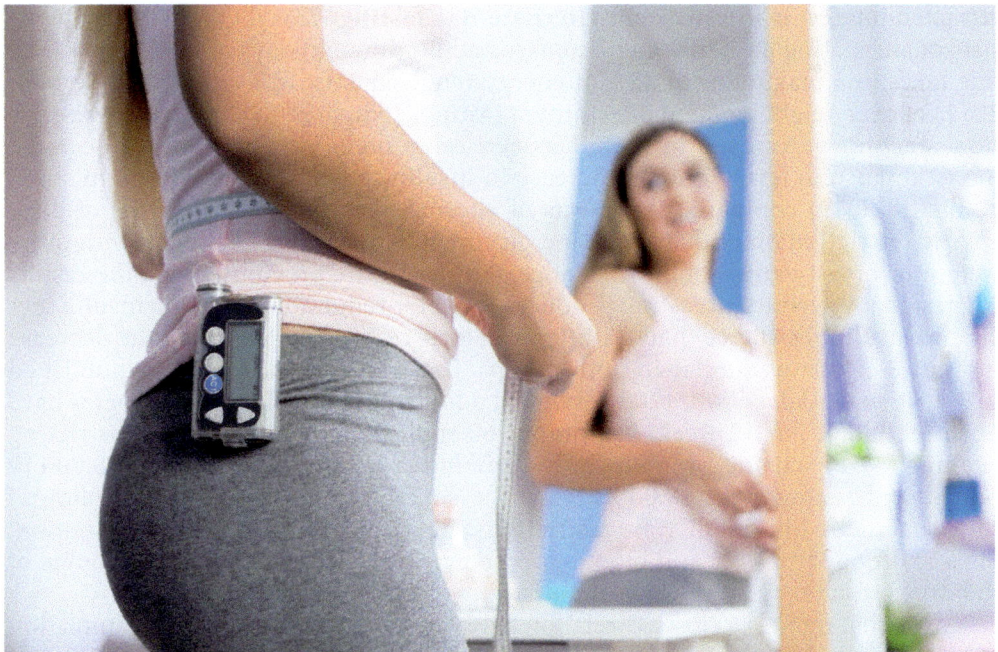

Figure 11.1

One of the rapidly increasing diseases in our society is diabetes. There are two types of diabetes: type 1, an autoimmune disease that generally occurs in childhood and requires the use of insulin, and type 2 or "non-insulin-dependent", which was once only found in middle-aged individuals and older, while today it is also present in children due to the increase in the rate of obesity. The latter type of diabetes is mainly linked to improper lifestyles and poor nutrition (which determines insulin resistance, i.e. insulin no longer performs its functions in its own way) and requires a therapeutic approach based on diet and any oral hypoglycemic drugs. Recently, in the medical field, a great interest has developed in physical exercise as an effective tool to combat diabetes or in any case to improve the conditions of the patient who is affected by it, overcoming those prejudices that considered sport as a negative element as it can decompensate the glycemic picture. For type 2 diabetes, the approach is simpler, especially if hypoglycemic drugs are not used and if there are no concomitant joint and cardiovascular diseases, as both aerobic and weight-bearing activities are able to improve the insulin sensitivity (i.e. they are able to make the endogenous insulin work better).

The nutritional approach for people with type 2 diabetes must be aimed precisely at improving the insulin resistance.

The degree of insulin sensitivity may be influenced by dietary composition. **Chronic caloric excess promotes insulin resistance** through stimulation of insulin secretion, triglyceride synthesis, and fat accumulation, with down-regulation of insulin receptors and postreceptor signaling. Current guidelines for the treatment of obesity recommend moderate caloric restriction (reducing daily energy requirements by 20-30%); however, in recent years, one form of caloric restriction that has attracted interest is **intermittent alternate-day fasting**. This dietary regimen consists of alternating days in which one feeds ad libitum and days of fasting in which one takes in a maximum of 25% of energy requirements. In a study (Harvie MN, 2011) of overweight women, intermittent fasting, compared to daily caloric restriction, was shown to result in a similar decrease in body weight, a greater decrease in fasting insulin levels, and an increase in insulin sensitivity. A very recent study (Gabel K, 2019) compared the effects of alternate-day fasting with those of daily caloric restriction on body weight and glycoregulatory factors in adults with overweight or obesity and insulin resistance. Similar to the previous study, the results suggest that intermittent fasting produces a greater reduction in fasting insulin levels and insulin resistance than traditional caloric restriction, although the decrease in body weight was similar in both groups. In a clinical study recently published in *Nutrition & Metabolism*, 120 overweight adult subjects with type 2 diabetes have been recruited. For 12 weeks a group of 60 subjects followed a Time Restricting Feeding (TRF) scheme which included *ad libitum* feeding from 8:00 to 18:00 (10 hours) and fasting from 18:00 to 8:00. The control group (60 subjects) followed the usual diet without any time restrictions. In the 12 weeks of TRF intervention, HbA1c dropped by 18% and blood glucose by 15%, which is almost the double of the drugs results.

Given that there is a close correlation between visceral obesity (the accumulation of fat at a central level, especially in the omental rather than the subcutaneous level) and insulin resistance, and that this type of fat acts as an endocrine organ that produces inflammatory cytokines and releases volatile fatty acids that worsen insulin resistance, the primary goal will be weight loss. The most suitable diet for an insulin-resistant subject is based on the control of foods that contain carbohydrates, which must have a low glycemic index and/or low glycemic load.

They are both important concepts as the glycemic index indicates the ability of a portion containing 50 g of carbohydrates to raise the blood sugar per unit of time, and it is linked to the speed of glucose absorption, which is higher for simple sugars and lower for complex carbohydrates, while the glycemic load indicates the amount of carbohydrates per 100 g of food. Certainly, a high glycemic index food, by stimulating the insulin peak, leads to a subsequent state of hypoglycemia, which in turn, by stimulating cortisol, will further worsen the insulin resistance and favor the increase of visceral fat in a kind of a vicious circle.

However, I believe that the glycemic load is even more important, it ultimately translates into the "quantity" of carbohydrates taken, which is the most important parameter in terms of insulin modulation. In simple terms, I would be more concerned about a large plate of whole wheat spaghetti which can provide up to 100g of carbohydrates, even if it has a relatively low glycemic index (55), than a slice of watermelon, which has a high glycemic index (100) but provides about 13 g of carbohydrates. The supply of fiber is very important because it is able to modulate the absorption of glucose, delaying the rise in the blood sugar and actually contributing to an improvement in the insulin resistance. Therefore, the diet should include a carbohydrate intake of around 40%, with proteins and fats at 30%.

The simultaneous presence of carbohydrates, proteins and fats must be respected in every meal in order to lower the glycemic index. In the case of hypercortisolism, often associated with hyperinsulism in these subjects, it is useful to reduce the amount of carbohydrates at breakfast, as these subjects tend to have higher blood sugar in the morning on an empty stomach, and shift the carbohydrate intake especially towards dinner. In this way, it has been seen in several studies that the insulin resistance decreases, the concentrations of leptin (an anorectic hormone that reduces appetite) and adiponectin (an anti-inflammatory cytokine) increase, cortisol levels are lowered, and the visceral and waist fat is decreased. It also brings a better physiological sleep and a better adherence to the diet (chronormorphodiet).

As for fats, it is better to include more polyunsaturated and monounsaturated fats, which improve the insulin sensitivity, compared to saturated fats, which instead worsen it. Regarding the polyunsaturated fats, it is appropriate to privilege the omega-3 series, which are DHA and EPA, mainly contained in fish from the cold seas of the North (salmon, mackerel, herring). As far as monounsaturated fats are concerned, oleic acid is contained in high quantities in olive oil, which among other things contains antioxidant substances in high quantities and has anti-inflammatory characteristics, which particularly useful in counteracting the inflammation linked to the increase in the visceral fat.

A substantial number of studies have demonstrated a relationship between dietary fat intake and insulin resistance, with particular reference to saturated fat and trans fatty acids. In animal models, a **high-fat diet has been shown to be associated with insulin resistance** (Storlein LH, 1986 – Yakubu F, 1993). Similarly, in most studies in humans, high-fat diets have been shown to reduce insulin sensitivity, even in the absence of significant changes in weight and body composition (Chen M, 1988 – Fukagawa NK, 1990 – Lovejoy J, 1992).

The amount, type (glucose vs fructose), and rate of digestion of dietary carbohydrates are determinants of postprandial glucose and insulin responses. Large amounts of protein and fat, added to glucose, have been shown to have a strong influence on postprandial hormonal responses: protein increases insulin levels and reduces glucose concentrations; in contrast, fat generally reduces both glucose and insulin levels by reducing upper gastrointestinal tract motility. In addition, dietary fats potentiate gastric inhibitory polypeptide (GIP) secretion, this may have an acute effect in increasing insulin secretion. It must, however, be emphasized that generally, in healthy subjects, the amount of protein and fat present in a normal meal is not large enough to result in a significant effect on postprandial insulin and glucose concentrations. In a study of healthy subjects, participants were given 5 mixed meals that differed in both calories and macronutrients; results showed that 90% of the variability in postprandial insulin response was determined by the glycemic index of the foods and the amount of carbohydrate in the meal (Wolever, 1996). **Fructose produces much lower glycemic and insulinemic responses than glucose** because it is converted slowly to glucose in the liver, and only a fraction of this glucose is released into the bloodstream. However, large amounts of fructose, administered to both animals and humans, have been shown to reproduce the characteristics of the metabolic syndrome and increase triglyceride and LDL cholesterol levels; therefore, the use of fructose as a method of reducing postprandial insulin is not a prudent approach (Beck-Nielsen, 1980 – Frayn, 1995).

Dietary fiber has indirect effects on insulin secretion and action. Effects on intestinal motility and transit time, gastrointestinal hormone secretion, and colonic fermentation, which produces short-chain fatty acids that suppress hepatic gluconeogenesis, have been reported. Resistant starch reduces postprandial glucose and insulin response, improving insulin sensitivity. Several studies have estimated that total dietary fiber and whole grain bread intake is associated with reduced insulin resistance values, independent of physical activity level and waist circumference. In addition, high dietary fiber intake has been found to correlate with lower insulin secretion (Damsgaard C, 2017). At the intestinal level, dietary fiber appears to be able to slow glucose absorption and, consequently, modify the metabolic response to the meal.

In case of the type 2 diabetes, we have the possibility to use supplements that improve insulin sensitivity.

Chromium: is a component of the glucose tolerance factor (GTF), which is composed, in addition to chromium, from niacin and the amino acids glycine, cysteine and glutamic acid. GTF acts as an enzymatic cofactor of insulin that helps convey the glucose intracellularly. The recommendations regarding the dosage of chromium are around 200 micrograms, but in the case of insulin resistance it can even reach 1000 micrograms per day.

Lipoic acid: used for decades in the treatment of type 2 diabetes, especially in Germany. It has a hypoglycemic effect by acting on Glut 1 and Glut 4 glucose receptors. It interacts with the sulfhydryl groups of the cell's insulin receptors, allowing a greater sensitivity for this hormone and a greater passage of glucose within the cell, and thus lowering the blood sugar levels. The useful dosage in the case of type 2 diabetes is 600 micrograms.

Berberine: stimulates the transport of glucose through a mechanism which is different from that of the insulin, perhaps by stimulating AMPK (adenosine monophosphate protein kinase), which has the same mechanism as metformin, an oral hypoglycemic drug. The useful dosage is 500 mg per day.

Vitamin D: vitamin D deficiency has been correlated with insulin resistance in various studies. It has been found that bringing vitamin D to levels above 75 mmol/L causes a significant reduction in the insulin resistance. To obtain this effect, it is required to have doses of vitamin D of at least 2000 I.U. per day.

Cinnamon: consumed at a dose of 1 g together with a meal that contains carbohydrates, it is able to lower the glycemic index.

Magnesium: 400 mg per day are able to improve the insulin sensitivity.

Moringa: extracts from the seeds and leaves of moringa have been shown to inhibit the lipid peroxidation and to stimulate the release of insulin by the pancreatic beta cells, thereby reducing the blood glucose values. Useful dosage: 500 mg per day.

Coenzyme Q10: Numerous researches have indicated that diabetic individuals have reduced coenzyme Q10 levels and it has been observed that 200 mg of coenzyme Q10 administered daily is able to lower the glycated hemoglobin (which expresses the average blood glucose for at least three previous months).

Fucoxanthin: has lipolytic, hypoglycemic, stimulating basal metabolism, thermogenesis (increased UCP-1) etc. effects. A Korean study published in Nutrition Research and Practice concluded that consumption of these kelp algae significantly promoted improved glycemic control by increasing enzymatic and antioxidant activities in patients with type 2 diabetes. Effective dosage around 5 mg per day.

Omega 3: omega 3 is known for its anti-inflammatory effect, due to which it can also improve insulin sensitivity. In people who are constantly exercising, the effect of fish oil on insulin sensitivity appears to be an additive. Unfortunately, much disagreement has been found about insulinemic sensitivity and fish oil supplementation. For example, no significant improvements in fasting blood glucose or fasting insulin are observed in type 2 diabetic patients.

Gymnema: the action of Gymnema on glucose metabolism includes an increase in insulin secretion, regeneration of the pancreatic islet, increased glucose utilization in insulin-dependent tissues, and an inhibition of intestinal glucose absorption. The effective dose ranges from 400 to 500 mg with positive effects both on post-prandial glycemia and on the reduction of glycated hemoglobin (if used for 3 months).

Banaba: has anti-diabetic and anti-obesity effects. Although its mechanism of action is not yet clear, it seems to induce an increase in cellular glucose uptake, a decrease in gluconeogenesis. The antidiabetic activity of banaba extract (standardized to 1% corosolic acid, equivalent to 10 mg corosolic acid) was evaluated and a 30% decrease in blood glucose levels was observed after only two weeks.

Green tea: green tea contains catechins, which have important insulin-modulating properties. They are protective of pancreatic islets and modulate hepatic glucose production. The protective mechanism seems to be due to the antioxidant properties of polyphenols, which would help to reduce blood glucose. The dose is 200-400 mg/day.

Coprinus comatus: it is a fungus rich in vanadium, particularly useful in diabetes. It has been found to be very effective in reducing blood glucose and glycated hemoglobin in type 2 diabetes. From this mushroom has been isolated a substance called "comatin" with hypoglycemic effects, able to inhibit non-enzymatic glycosylation and improve peripheral sensitivity to insulin. Dosage ranges from 500 to 1,500 mg of 100% pure extract.

Obviously, an adequate use of antioxidants in the form of vitamins, minerals and phytonutrients has a protective action, limiting the oxidative stress of the cells subjected to high glucose levels.

However, in type 1 diabetes things are a bit more complicated. In this case, the main risk linked to physical activity is the onset of hypoglycemic crises, as both insulin, which is used for therapeutic purposes, and aerobic exercise lower the blood sugar levels and therefore there is the possibility of a dangerous hypoglycemia during and after exercise. For this reason, diabetic patients must reduce or even eliminate the insulin dosage before the exercise. In general, the dosage of rapid pre-exercise insulin should be reduced by about 50%, taking into account the variability of the subjective response.

While planning exercise is preferable, if a person decides on impulse to go out for a run or a game of tennis, then they should plan to consume in advance 20-30 g of carbohydrates for every 30 minutes of exercise, in order to prevent hypoglycemia. Anyone with diabetes should always carry a rapidly absorbed source of glucose (for example, fruit juice or a chocolate bar) available during exercise, which should be consumed immediately if the symptoms of hypoglycemia (weakness, mental confusion) appear. Hypoglycemia deserves special attention because it can have fatal consequences. A candy bar with a glass of fruit juice removes the symptoms within five minutes.

If the person loses consciousness, it is necessary to call the Emergency Services immediately and, while waiting for help, try to introduce a glucose gel (or even a creamy dessert) into their mouth, on the inner surface of the cheeks. What about weight training? Even though it rarely causes hypoglycemia during exercise or immediately after it, because during the anaerobic lactacid training the body produces counter-insular hormones that raise the blood sugar levels, such as adrenaline, GH, cortisol, there is still a risk of a "late hypoglycemia" when these hormones diminish, especially if an adequate post-workout glucose recovery has not been made. In addition, lactic acid anaerobic sports are not particularly recommended because these alternating blood glucose values do not favor the lowering of glycated hemoglobin, which expresses the average glycemic indicator of the glycemic metabolic control.

This reasoning is true for those who practice in a competitive sport that involves a high intensity performance; if, on the other hand, we are referring to a frequenter of a fitness gym who trains with weights in a moderate manner, the problem does not exist and an anaerobic activity with weights has the same therapeutic value as an aerobic training. It is true, among other things, that proper sports, dietary education and a wise insulin management allow diabetic athletes to obtain good results, also in terms of muscle development, as insulin is still a powerful anabolic hormone at the protein level.

CHAPTER 12

Nutrition in bodybuilding

by Marco Guercioni

Recently, the nutrition for bodybuilding has had many influences from fashions from overseas and/or absolutist methods. However, these contributions have led to food for thought or have created the foundations of some theories that science and professionals in this sector have then collected, organized and proved or denied, with rationality and logic.

Working with the nutrition in bodybuilding means being able to touch the human physiology with your hands: it is related to the functioning of each system in our body and it is almost able to dialogue with them, in order to direct the esthetic condition towards the goal. How can this be done in practice? Knowing as much as possible about the subject in question: we start from knowing the energy needs, as we have seen in the dedicated chapter.

In bodybuilding, which as the name implies means "muscle building", they divide the preparation of one year into two macro-phases: one is called "bulk", or growth, which is the moment to focus on mass muscular gain; the other is called "cut" or weight loss, when, for example, close to a competition, the aim is to decrease the body fat to better enhance the muscle shapes, lines and proportions. Additional micro-phases are also set up between these moments. They serve above all to act as a link between the bulk and the cut, which are the most salient moments and they will be discussed in this chapter.

Each of the two phases requires careful control of the training, nutrition and supplementation. Here, we will deal with the nutrition part, separating the two stages of preparation that we mentioned above.

Returning to our subject, knowing his/her energy needs, we have the starting point for deciding the quantities of proteins, carbohydrates and fats to be consumed. We can summarize the nutritional preparations in the following points:

1. Muscle building phase (bulk phase):
    - from Kcal to macronutrients;
    - number of meals and protein quantity;
    - meal timing.
2. First we build, then we define (cut phase):
    - from Kcal to macronutrients;
    - meal timing.

To choose how to calculate the energy needs, a practical alternative could be to multiply the basal metabolic rate (BMR), already calculated as mentioned above, by a coefficient that represents the average activity of the subject, which includes sports (PAL, Physical Activity Level) and the non-sporting one (NEAT, Non-Exercise Activity Thermogenesis, which is made up of all the daily movements outside the sporting activity). Let's see what these coefficients are and in which cases they should be used:

- 1.25 × BMR: a sedentary subject, with a maximum of 1-2 sessions per week[1];
- 1.50 × BMR: a subject with an average activity, with 3-4 weight sessions per week;
- 1.75 × BMR: a fairly active subject, with 4-5 weight sessions per week;
- 2.00 × BMR: a very active subject, with 5-6 weight sessions per week[2].

So, if the basal metabolic rate will be 1500 Kcal and we choose to multiply it by the "average activity" coefficient, our total energy expenditure result will be approximately:

$$1500 \times 1.5 = 2250 \text{ Kcal (energy requirement)}$$

The daily caloric requirement is also defined as TDEE (Total Daily Energy Expenditure) and it represents a maintenance caloric quantity, i.e. that allows us to remain in an iso-caloric status.

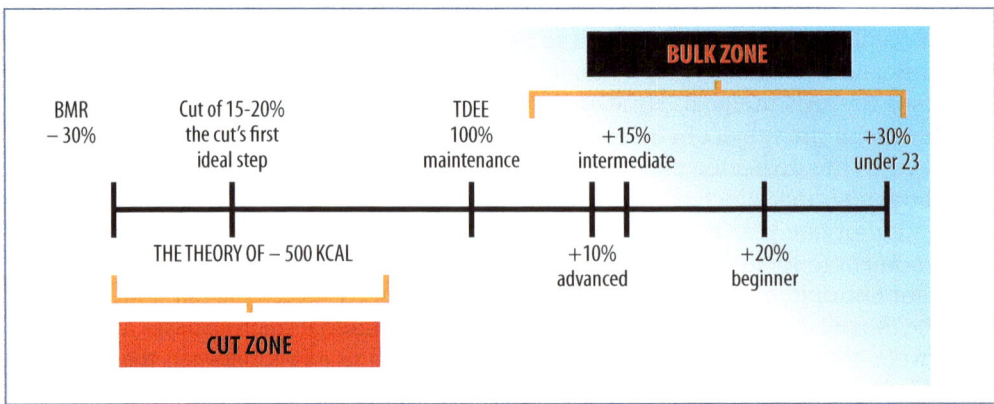

Figure 12.1 The figure represents the reference values, personally processed, of the caloric requirements according to the TDEE. They vary according to the age, the starting level of the subject and the goal.

Starting from this value, we must take into consideration the goal we want to achieve and, therefore, in which phase of the preparation we find ourselves, since, based on the fact that we will make a decision to move towards the definition or the muscle building, we will have to take into account some key points. Bodybuilding,

---

[1] This value can also be used in the case of individuals who have had problems with being overweight and obesity in the past.

[2] Reference point for all those subjects who maintain a particularly low body fat and who struggle to gain weight.

like fitness, is an esthetic sport, in which the athletic performance is a secondary parameter compared to parameters such as the body fat, muscularity, lines and symmetry. We must necessarily take these into account when we are setting up a nutritional plan.

Furthermore, the TDEE is certainly our theoretical reference point, but it is important to remember that, when dealing with bodybuilders, amateurs or agonists, it does not always perfectly reflect reality. Let me explain better: it happens, in fact, that while taking different amounts of Kcal than the estimated TDEE, the subject maintains their weight and their body composition. In reality, this happens often; obviously, if the real TDEE is higher than the theoretical one, the implications can be mainly positive. What if the opposite happens? If the real daily expenditure is lower than the theoretical one, we should first try to restore the metabolic functionality. Let's briefly see one of the possible strategies.

If the body fat is within the optimal parameters[3] for bodybuilding and fitness, there is a tendency to start from the caloric intake that was established up to that moment and then gradually increase it 100-150 Kcal per week, using carbohydrates, until we reach the estimated theoretical TDEE. In this way, we will gradually create a "work area" to which we can add or remove the right caloric quota.

If, on the other hand, the starting body composition is outside the recommended parameters and the real TDEE is lower than the theoretical one, we will be facing a situation of a metabolic inflexibility to nutrients, due to multiple and variable factors, including: insulin sensitivity, silent inflammation, hormonal changes, stress. In these cases, besides obviously investigating these points, to possibly restore the physiology of the subject, it would be necessary to bring the body fat back within the recommended parameters, by adding margins in order to cut the Kcal and/or increase the energy expenditure. Once the body fat returns to optimal values, we can try to reset the diet by returning at least to the theoretical TDEE: we could do this by adding calories from carbohydrates weekly, as mentioned above, but possibly distributing them in peri-workout moments[4]. Once we have realigned ourselves to the TDEE, if the metabolic condition of the subject allows it, we can obviously also expect to overcome it for the muscle building phase.

Muscle building phase (bulk phase)

Bodybuilding, as the word itself implies, is the sport par excellence in which the main goal is to build muscle mass. To set up a nutritional plan which is oriented towards this goal, it is useful to evaluate the level of the athlete we are referring to: beginner, intermediate or advanced. The more the subject is adapted and accustomed to the stimulus induced by the training, the lower the caloric surplus necessary to adequately deal with the bulk phase.

---

3 By optimal parameters of body fat we mean the percentages of body fat that allow you to start/continue the phase of muscle building. For men, we are talking about 12-18%, for women 22-28%. In fact, if we are beyond these values, we should first proceed with a body transformation before moving on to the actual bulk.
4 Peri-workout means all the time, before, during and after the training, that is: pre-workout, during-workout, post-workout.

On the contrary, the closer the subject is to being a beginner, the greater their potential for muscle growth: this is because they will have more room for progression in training and, therefore, for an anabolic stimulus. Potentially their caloric requirement can go even beyond 25% compared to the TDEE. In this context, a fundamental parameter which can make a big difference in results, is age. Physiologically, a young individual has higher IGF-1, free testosterone, and growth hormone than a more mature individual, and will therefore be able to handle larger caloric increases, while limiting the parallel fat gain that could occur.

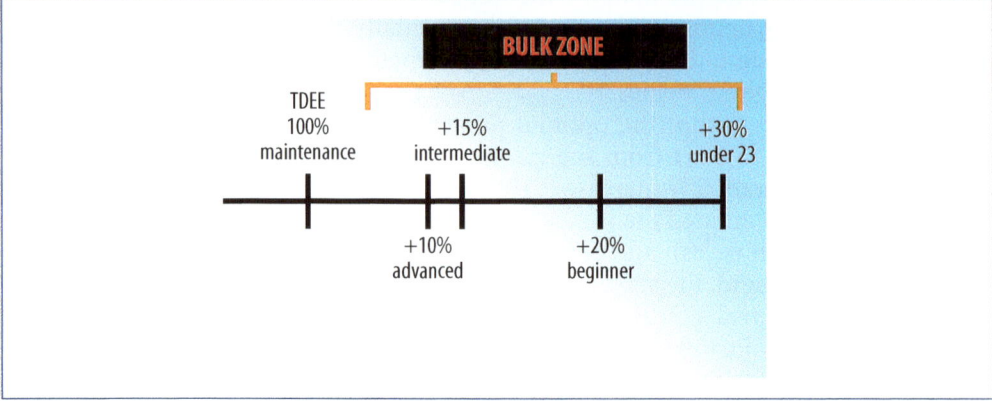

Figure 12.2 The figure represents the personally elaborated range of the caloric demand regarding the TDEE. The interval is divided according to the age and the starting level of the subject, and it is focused on the "construction" period (bulk phase).

Let's take an example:
- a man of 80 kg of weight × 180 cm tall, 30 years old;
- 4 weight workouts per week;
- average activity during the day (6000 steps per day);
- estimated body fat is 10% using the plicometry method;
- formerly overweight.

By calculating the TDEE through the formulas, we get a value of 2650 Kcal; these are the estimated Kcal that would keep him at the indicated weight. However, if, as in the case of our example subject, we are faced with a person who has suffered from obesity in the past, that is, a person who has a rather high weight set point, we must consider the fact that this person will tend to accumulate fat easily and will be inflexible at the metabolic level.

At this point, we must consider our subject's level: if we have an advanced athlete with years of training and in or near his maximum natural genetic potential, we can do as follows:

$$2650 + 10\% = 2915 \text{ Kcal}$$

If instead, our subject is at an intermediate level:

$$2650 + 20\% = 3180 \text{ Kcal}$$

Finally, if our subject is at the beginning or already has/tends to have a condition of very low body fat, we can do as follows:

$$2650 + 30\% = 3445 \text{ Kcal}$$

In order to better choose the macronutrients that we'll use, we should also take into account the body composition. Furthermore, although the TDEE is a "maintenance" level, it does not exclude the fact that there may be variations in the muscle mass and in the fat tissue; consequently, the TDEE itself is a dynamic value to be evaluated along the way.

I purposely stopped at a calorie surplus of 30%, because exceeding this level can result in an indiscriminate increase in fat and muscle that I would not recommend. It is true that both beginners and adolescents and/or "ectomorphs" could benefit from high caloric increases, since they have a sensitivity to nutrients, and consequently a response that is different than that of the advanced or mesomorphic/endomorphic subjects. However, this is another matter that will not be dealt with here.

From Kcal to macronutrients

Keeping ourselves on a practical level, knowing how much our body actually consumes at a given moment, and how much it needs, is basic and necessary. If we refer to the population in general and in the long term, for the restoration of the ideal body composition, in a perfect physiology, a calorie is a calorie. However, as it really happens in bodybuilding, when you try to overcome a limit or any obstacle "imposed" by genetic and hormonal peculiarities, it is essential to go into more detail by applying adjustments to the percentages of the daily macronutrients and single meals. It is necessary to define a linear or wavy trend for the Kcal and decide which nutrients to include according to the training time (the so-called timing) and many more factors.

If we talk about the macronutrient percentages, we have a very wide choice and it is linked to:
- the starting body composition of the subject: it would be better to set the quantity of carbohydrates and proteins in an inversely proportional way to the body fat, and vice versa for fats (Elia, 1999); this factor implies, but not absolutely, a subjective insulin sensitivity;
- the training method: the more the training will tend towards a metabolic work, the more it will require attention to the carbohydrate quota;
- the type of the daily activities that influence the energy expenditure, i.e. beware of NEAT: a very dynamic subject has a greater tolerance to high percentages of diet fats (Ruderman, 1998).

Let's report the numbers that we just mentioned:
- proteins: 15-30%;
- fats: 25-40%;
- carbohydrates: 60-30%.

We could also evaluate macronutrients by referring to them as grams per kg of body weight (abbreviated to g/kg), which in the case of a caloric surplus could be:

- proteins: 1.8-2.2 g/kg;
- fats: 1-2 g/kg;
- carbohydrates: optimal range of 3-5 g/kg.

The choice to lean towards carbohydrates or fats depends on various factors.

For example, in my opinion, fats are valid allies to be taken into consideration, precisely in the caloric load phases, particularly once the stall and/or the limit in the carbohydrate increase has been reached: this will allow us to gradually reduce carbohydrates to the bare minimum, while increasing the Kcal thanks to the increase in fat.

It will therefore be possible to exploit the advantages that this increase will have on the metabolic level. We will also find these advantages in the cut phases, in which we will be able to strategically "cut" the fats without particularly altering the carbohydrates. This will offer us some "calorie bonuses" to gradually create an imbalance in favor of the carbohydrates, as the percentage of fat goes down and the insulin sensitivity is on our side.

We know perfectly well that, in the case of training at higher volumes and intensities, this progressive increase in carbohydrates will be an excellent advantage during the definition phase; moreover, it will allow us to preserve the muscle gains of the previous phase as much as possible, protecting us from the risk of incurring protein catabolism, theoretically dictated by the low-calorie diet; moreover, it will improve the compliance with the caloric restriction compared to a low-glucose diet and this is something that should shouldn't be underestimated.

Returning to our example subject (80 kg weight, 30 years old, 180 cm tall, TDEE 2650 Kcal, body fat 10%: creating a caloric surplus of 10%, we will set a caloric target at 2915 Kcal.

Macronutrients:
- **fats:** 25-40% or 1-2 g/kg; since the body fat is at a more than acceptable level, we can start with 1 g/kg of fat;
- **proteins:** 1.6-2.3 g/kg; the lower the body fat, the more proteins we can initially set; we can start with 2.3 g/kg;
- **carbohydrates:** by difference, and given the body fat, we will be able to take advantage of the caloric boost of carbohydrates to minimize fat gain.

Making the related calculations:
- 80 g of fat = 720 Kcal
- 180 g of proteins = 736 Kcal
- 2915 Kcal (caloric target) −720 (Kcal from fat) −736 (Kcal from protein) = 1459 Kcal remaining for carbohydrates, approximated to 1460 Kcal
- 1460 × 4 (Kcal of carbohydrates) = 365 g of carbohydrates

Macronutrient summary:

- 180 g of protein = 25%
- 80 g of fat = 25%
- 365 g of carbohydrates = 50%

After starting from the minimum amount of the ideal fats during the bulk phase, we can gradually increase their percentage compared to carbohydrates. This would go hand in hand with the physiological decrease in the insulin sensitivity which is caused by the high-calorie diet, and the increase, even if controlled, of the body fat.

Number of meals and the protein quantity

Regarding the number of recommended meals, the scientific community is not unanimous, as usually happens for this type of issue. In fact, it would seem that increasing the frequency of meals during the day can be advantageous for optimizing protein synthesis in the short term, but in the long term it would not be particularly decisive.

During the phases of the high-calorie diets, increasing the time window between one protein meal and another, will hardly negatively alter the protein turnover. In the event of a calorie deficit, however, it is important to use common sense and reasoning about the fact that eating more protein meals keeps the appetite under control and helps in maintaining compliance. Furthermore, guaranteeing a fair amount of protein every 3-4 hours would help support protein turnover (Arciero, 2013; Antonio, 2015).

It should be noted that, in the case of abundant quantities of protein in the diet, in order to avoid the metabolic waste in the single meal, deferring the amount of total protein and spreading it in a balanced way in meals would still make more sense, regardless. This allows you to fall within the range suggested by the guidelines, which recommend 20 to 50 g of protein per meal.

If, on the other hand, the protein quota is low, from my experience I can say that many people are better off dividing them into 2-3 meals just to have higher satiety, but this is a matter of personal preference and habits.

Meal timing

Nutrient and meal timing are much discussed in the sports nutrition landscape, especially in the fitness/bodybuilding context. If we talk about the amateur level, they have a relative importance. However, if we are dealing with a competitive athlete, or an athlete who wants to get the most out of it, even if not in terms of competitions, then the timing must absolutely be personalized and taken into consideration.

Very briefly, thanks to the latest scientific confirmations, we can outline the different types of timing based on: the percentage of the chosen macronutrients, body composition of the subject, level of the subject (advanced, intermediate, beginner), deficit or caloric surplus, training time.

Let's take an example: an intermediate subject, with a body fat of 15%, during the caloric surplus phase (bulk); he trains at around 6 pm. We could spread the daily macronutrients in the following way:
- breakfast: fats[5] + proteins + low fibrous carbohydrates;
- snack: fats[5] + proteins;
- lunch: fats[5] + proteins + low fibrous carbohydrates;
- pre-workout snack: medium/slow release proteins + low glycemic index carbohydrates;
- peri-workout: nitric oxide stimulators + powdered carbohydrates + hydrolyzed proteins or EAA;

- post-workout dinner: proteins + carbohydrates with medium/high glycemic index + small amounts of fat[5].

First, we build, then we define (cut phase)

By "cut phase" we mean that phase in which we get rid of a part of the body fat acquired during the bulk period, to unbalance the body composition in favor of the lean mass. We all know that, when the time to lose weight in order to define the esthetic shape comes, the greatest concern is not being in shape on time, perhaps before an important event (competitive or not) or even simply for the summer period, and that one of the first things we tend to do is cut calories, which unfortunately, is often done in an extreme and uncontrolled way.

By excluding any problems of altered eating behaviors that occur with the obsessive control of one's body weight, we can actually help ourselves to lose weight more easily by using a few small tricks. When we talk about weight loss, it is necessary that this happens without altering the physiological functions and by maintaining the state of health. The optimal and recommended weight loss is 0.5 kg per week, mainly fat mass, keeping macronutrients, micronutrients and physical exercise within the optimal values. This would allow to obtain a healthy and therefore lasting weight loss (except those who adopt incorrect eating habits later), and above all, it allows to preserve the muscle mass as much as possible.

Let's make a numerical consideration, strictly theoretical: each gram of fat lost corresponds to about 7 Kcal and, considering the 500 g of "fat mass" per week that we mentioned above, ideally it would be necessary to create a caloric deficit of about 3500 Kcal per week, or 500 Kcal per day if we wanted to spread it over 7 consequent days. Clearly, this vision is of an idealistic type and it is not always applicable due to the required timing and the starting situation of the subject. For example, in the case of people with a high percentage of the starting fat mass (overweight/obesity) and a higher than normal percentage of extracellular water, a more marked caloric cut could be applied, while avoiding going below the metabolism baseline which is calculated with certain formulas.

In these types of subjects, the weight loss may therefore be more visible, even by 3 kg per week: in the early stages, first of all there will be a large loss of fluids, glycogen and hepatic triglycerides, which will stabilize at lower levels. In fact, individuals with a high percentage of adipose tissue compared to "lean" subjects also have an imbalance in the glycemic-insulin picture or, better, a greater insulin resistance. Among its consequences, it also involves a greater fluid retention in favor of the extracellular compartment, in addition to a poor carbohydrate partitioning in the muscles.

Those who find themselves in a similar situation can benefit by decreasing the amount of carbohydrates, because this would improve the insulin response and therefore, it can favor a greater initial weight loss, understood as the loss of fluids in

---

5 Please note that the quality of the fats is also important. Mono/polyunsaturated fats must be favored, without demonizing the saturated ones, which in any case have important roles at a biochemical, hormonal and cellular level. An acceptable ratio would be 70% of the total fats represented by mono and polyunsaturated ones, and 30% by saturated ones.

the extracellular compartment, which can also act as a positive stimulus to continue with the diet and increase the esthetic result.

To proceed with the drafting of the food plan we must first calculate the basal metabolic rate; this will help us especially because it represents a sort of a "cut off", lower than which we should better not go. Then we can estimate the caloric needs, counting the components related to the sporting activities (EAT, Exercise Activity Thermogenesi) and non-sporting activities (NEAT).

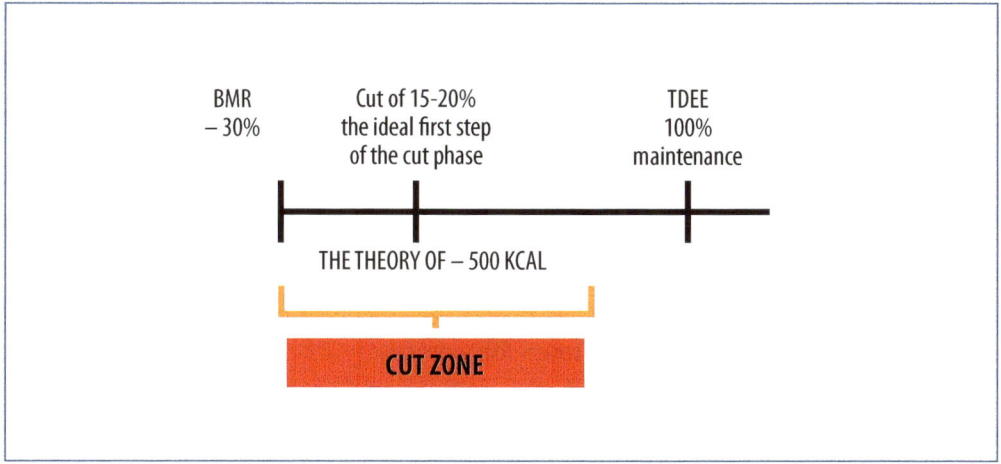

Figure 12.3 The figure represents the personally elaborated range of the caloric demand regarding the TDEE. The interval is divided according to the age and the starting level of the subject, and it is focused on the lose weight period (cut phase).

Once an estimate of the average requirement has been obtained, it will be our reference point for cutting the famous 500 Kcal or, better, a share in the range between 300 and 700 Kcal per day. For those who are used to working with percentages, you can opt for a cut of 15-25% of calories compared to the estimated TDEE or compared to the current caloric intake (if this is different from the TDEE).

Regarding this, it is good to remember that the TDEE is not a static value and that it changes according to the weight and the variations in volume and/or training intensity, without neglecting the important metabolic-hormonal changes that occur during the phase of the caloric deficit and weight loss. In fact, hormones such as catecholamines and thyroid hormones have an important impact on the basal energy expenditure (or basal metabolic rate).

Staying on the subject of hormones, it would be particularly important for overweight subjects to control the impact of meals on insulin production and to divide the daily Kcal into many meals, reaching 5 or 6. In this way the glycemic peaks, and therefore the post-prandial insulin peaks will be more controlled. This does not mean that eating more meals makes you lose weight, but that the insulin and the metabolic response improves and that, consequently, with the same total Kcal, eating more meals can optimize the weight loss and decrease the perception of the caloric reduction, therefore increasing compliance.

From Kcal to macronutrients

Taking into consideration what we have already said for the bulk phase regarding the macronutrients, we can move on to the following ranges:
- let's first set the proteins to: 2-2.7 g/kg of weight or 2.25-3 g/kg of LBM[6];
- then let's move on to fats: 0.5-1 g/kg (15-25% of the total Kcal);
- finally, by difference, let's set the carbohydrates, which in any case should be between 2.5 and 4.5 g/kg: you get the grams of carbohydrates by dividing the remaining Kcal by 4.

Example

Our subject, a man who weighs of 80 kg, with a height of 180 cm, 30 years old, 10% fat mass, with a sedentary job, trains 4 times a week.

We hypothesize that, using one of the formulas that we've already mentioned, we obtain a basal metabolism of about 1780 Kcal. For convenience, we can use the simplified formula, but noting that it may slightly overestimate. Recall that the formulas with the coefficients are:
- weight in kg $\times$ 1 Kcal/kg $\times$ 24 hours for men;
- weight in kg $\times$ 0.9 Kcal/kg $\times$ 24 hours for women.

Given the lifestyle, to indicate the daily activity (sporting or not) we assume a multiplication coefficient of 1.5:

$$1780 \times 1.5 = 2670, \text{ rounded to } 2650$$

which will be the isocaloric reference TDEE for maintenance. Assuming that we will apply the cut of the famous 500 Kcal, we get:

$$2650 \text{ Kcal (TDEE)} - 500 \text{ Kcal (ideal average cut)} = 2150 \text{ Kcal}$$

These Kcal theoretically represent the ideal ones for a gradual and controlled weight loss, always if the starting TDEE has been estimated correctly.

We have therefore chosen the following values in g/kg:
- protein 2 g/kg of weight or 2.25 g/kg of LBM = 160 g
- fats 0.5 g/kg of weight = 40 g
- we calculate the carbohydrates by the difference:

$$2150 \text{ Kcal} - (160 \text{ g} \times 4 \text{ Kcal}) - (40 \text{ g} \times 9 \text{ Kcal}) = 2150 - 640 - 360 = 1150 \text{ Kcal}$$
$$1150/4 = 287.5 \text{ g}$$

So, my macronutrients example for a 2150 Kcal diet is:
- 160 g proteins;
- 40 g of fats;
- 290 g of carbohydrates (approximate).

---

[6] LBM stands for Lean Body Mass: by lean mass we mean that body compartment that does not include fat; not to be confused with muscle mass, because lean mass includes, for example, the weight of the skeleton.

In this case we have opted for the minimum level of proteins and fats compared to the indicated range. Choosing the amount of proteins and fats within the indicated range depends on various factors: the previous share of carbohydrates, whether the subject is coming from the bulk phase or whether it is the first approach of an overweight person, a case of obesity, how many carbohydrates have already been cut, if the cut has already started and needs to go further.

In a nutshell, the higher the amount of carbohydrates before the cut/reduced during the cut, the higher the protein content must be. On the contrary, the higher the fat content before the cut (or the more fats were cut), the lower the need to increase the protein content.

Eventually, during the definition process, an increase in carbohydrates can be evaluated in this way:
- the insulin sensitivity achieved thanks to the caloric deficit and weight loss is exploited;
- the physiological decrease in leptin which occurs concomitantly is counteracted by the weight loss.

Referring to the previous example, again for 2150 Kcal, the alternative could be:
- protein 2.7 g/kg, or 215 g;
- fat 1 g/kg, or 80 g.

For the difference of the remaining 570 Kcal, if we divide it by 4, we get about 142 g of carbohydrates. We therefore see that, with the same Kcal, we have a wide range of macronutrients in which to position ourselves in order to fix our ideal balance based on personal preferences, the percentage of body fat, the time spent in the low calorie regime and the type of training.

Let's make a summary of the macronutrient range for 2150 Kcal:

Carbohydrates: 142-290 g | Proteins: 215-160 g | Fats: 80-40 g

It is interesting that when we find ourselves decreasing the carbohydrate quota, we also obtain an advantage in terms of the protein quality. A diet "for the mass" will tend to have more "indirect" proteins, i.e. not coming directly from sources with a prevalent protein content.

The decrease in carbohydrates and fats that occurs in the cut phase, while hypothetically maintaining the same amount of protein, will make us gain a greater content of direct proteins, which translates into sources with a higher biological value, i.e. we will take more essential amino acids. I specifically wanted to underline this fact to say that numerically speaking, it is not always necessary to change the protein quota when passing from a high calorie regime to a calorie deficit one.

I would like to point out that I have chosen to position myself at the extremes of the ranges referring to proteins and fats, in order to make us reflect on the fact that there we don't have just a single choice.

Meal timing

For the cut phase, it is also important to distribute the macronutrients throughout the day. The most delicate moment in this period is the post-workout one, when the levels of catecholamines are at the maximum daily peak and exceed the basal values by up to 3-4 times: it would therefore be more appropriate not to take carbohydrates in excessive quantities.

In any case, it is wise to ensure that the workout is dealt with maximal energies, by taking care to better manage the pre-workout phase and the hours before the workout, perhaps with regular and constant carbohydrates. This allows you to get to your training (in the evening, in this example) "loaded" and ready to face the volume and the intensity of your objectives. The post-workout period should be a time window that we can define as "lipolytic": first of all, we will have to ensure the protein-amino acid share, then afterwards we can calmly think about the recovery phase.

CHAPTER 13

The carbohydrate refill
by Massimo Spattini and Valeria Galfano

Glycogen loading, better known as a "carbohydrate refill", is a **dietary strategy** that leads to an unusual and high glycogen deposit in the muscles. The muscle glycogen load, associated with a **super-compensation**, represents a dietary practice aimed at maximizing the athletic performance and reducing water in the extracellular compartment, in order to rapidly and visibly improve muscle definition.

This method derives from studies conducted by Scandinavian researchers that led to the formulation of the "dissociated diet". The goal of this recharging is to improve the results of intense and prolonged performances (over 90 minutes), preventing the excessive depletion of glycogen reserves and delaying the onset of the muscle capacity exhaustion due to lack of high octane number "fuel" (more efficient for muscles that are engaged in intense efforts).

Glycogen is an important energy substrate during resistance training and its depletion compromises the muscle contraction by attenuating the release of calcium ions from the sarcoplasmic reticulum and suppressing the function of Na^+/K^+ AT-Pase, ultimately **leading to a reduction of the physical performance**.

At the subcellular level, glycogen is stored in three distinct areas: intramyofibrillar, intermyofibrillar and sub-sarcolemic space. Endurance training sports tend to preferentially exhaust the inter- and intramyofibrillar fractions. On the contrary, resistance training sports prefer subsarcolemmatic stations. Intramyofibrillar glycogen is more modified during exercise and recovery, and it could play a fundamental role in the release of calcium ions from the sarcoplasmic reticulum.

Let's look at the methods that are used to charge the muscles with glycogen.

- The **first protocol** is a simple dietary manipulation. An individual who follows a high-glucose diet for 3 or 4 days can increase the glycogen stores from the normal 15 g to about 25 g per kg of muscle. During this time, he/she should not perform any physical exercise. This method is used by athletes who are at a risk of developing hypoglycemia when they are on low carbohydrate diets.
- The **second** load **protocol** sequentially proposes intense physical exercises and a hyperglucidic diet. This method aims to exhaust the glycogen reserves through training and prepare the muscles, which will then have to be loaded through the

hyperglucidic diet maintained for 3 or 4 days. This second strategy allows you to double your glycogen stores, as long as no physical exercise is done during the recharging phase.
- The **third protocol** associates physical exercise with two special diets. Even in this case, physical exercise has the function of exhausting the pre-existing glycogen stores, in order to create the stimulus for the subsequent super-compensation. The athlete follows a diet which is almost free of carbohydrates and rich in proteins and possibly fats for 3 days, followed by a diet with a high carbohydrate content, low protein content (maximum 1 g / kg of body weight) and a very low fat intake for another 3 days. During the first phase, grueling exercises must be performed; however, in the second phase, it is necessary to rest or at least perform isometric muscle contractions (poses), which have the effect of stimulating the synthesis of glycogen. This last method allows to increase glycogen levels up to 50 g/kg of muscle.

As anticipated, the high concentration of muscle glycogen improves the resistance levels to prolonged aerobic efforts (marathon, cross-country skiing, etc.); in fact, this method has been studied and optimized especially for these disciplines. However, in more recent times, it has given way to strategies aimed at improving the **metabolic flexibility**, which promotes an adaptation to the use of fats for energy purposes. The reason is probably to be found in the weight gain caused by the carbohydrate refill, a disadvantage that is not appreciated by endurance athletes, which can easily lead to gastrointestinal discomfort problems and a decrease in sports performance.

Carbohydrate recharging, on the other hand, is very successful in the practice of bodybuilding. But what does a glycogen load do for a bodybuilding contest? The answer lies in muscle volume and definition. Glycogen is a polymer of glucose. Numerous studies, also conducted on humans, have shown that the increase in muscle glycogen, obtained through the refill of carbohydrates, is accompanied by an increase of about 3 g of water for each gram of glycogen.

By increasing the deposits, we bring the glycogen from the physiological 15 g up to 40 g per kg of muscle; an 80 kg bodybuilder with 40 kg of muscle mass will retain 1 kg of glycogen and about 3 kg of water in their muscles by the **osmotic effect**. In this way, the athlete will find, as if by magic, to have 4 kg of extra muscle and will also see more definition thanks to the reduction of the extracellular water. The effect on the muscle definition is favored by limiting the water intake, forcing the passage of water that must accompany the glycogen from the extra compartment to the intracellular one, thus rapidly and visibly improving the muscle definition. The transformation will be spectacular.

Now let's see in detail what an appropriate behavior for recharging is, in the context of bodybuilding.

In 1966, Bergström had already shown that the ability to overcompensate the muscle glycogen is closely related to the physical exercises that precede recharging.

As for **physical exercise**, in the 3 days of "discharge" it is necessary to split up the training in order to stimulate the whole body at least twice, even three times for the deficient regions, in order to obtain a greater recharge later on. Training sessions must be long and demanding in order to completely deplete the muscle glycogen (which is the fundamental "fuel" in anaerobic efforts).

At this stage, it is recommended to perform at least 20 sets with 20 repetitions per muscle group: to obtain super compensation it will be necessary to undertake a greater amount of work than what you are used to.

During this particular period, it is recommended not to train the abdominals in order not to favor the increase in the waist circumference that could result from recharging.

During the 3 days of the hyperglucidic diet, you must refrain from training in order not to consume the glycogen reserves: however, it seems appropriate to practice posing or perform a few low-rep sets for each muscle. The contractions seem to favor a further supply through the action of glycogen synthetase, a key regulatory enzyme in the glycogen synthesis.

Regarding the **composition of the diet**, in the 3 days of "discharge" it is necessary to gradually reduce the intake of carbohydrates, according to the scheme: 20% of the total calories on the first day → 15% of the total calories on the second day → 10% of the calories totals on the third day.

The first day diet must be normocaloric, in the following 2 days the overall caloric intake must be reduced by about 20%. At this stage, it is not recommended to try to reduce the body fat, since an excessively marked calorie deficit, aggravated by the absence of carbohydrates, would lead to the destruction of the muscle mass. Therefore, it seems more appropriate to reach the desired percentage of body fat at least one week before the competition.

During the 3 days of recharging, you must follow a diet rich in carbohydrates (about 80%), most of which should be complex. The consumption of simple carbohydrates is recommended only the day before the competition, since glucose (glycemic index 100) and sucrose (glycemic index 68) are more easily transformed into fat storage due to the excessive production of insulin, the lipogenic hormone par excellence. A moderate intake of fructose (glycemic index 20), less than 10% of the total calories, is allowed, as it doesn't seem to stimulate the insulin secretion. However, excessive fructose intake is strongly discouraged, as it has been linked to the onset of the insulin resistance in the liver and obesity.

Regarding the **division of calories**, it is good to consume 6 or 7 small meals a day, one every 2 hours. Each meal must include different sources of carbohydrates, in order to result in a slower and more regular absorption. On the other hand, such close meals require rapid stomach emptying, which is why it is recommended to limit the consumption of foods with a high fat content, associated with a delayed gastric emptying of the lipid phase in the duodenum.

Furthermore, in the conditions of high carbohydrate intake, the ingested fats will be accumulated more easily, at least partially frustrating the sacrifices of the bodybuilder in their path towards muscle definition. To sum up: the intake of fat must be low, maximum 10% of total calories, and it should be distributed alternately between individual meals (in every other meal).

How many carbohydrates do you need to eat for an optimal recharge?

Let's go back to the example of our 80 kg bodybuilder with 40 kg of muscle mass. During the depletion phase, the glycogen levels will be almost zeroed; therefore, to store 40 g of glycogen per kg of muscle, it will be necessary to fill the muscles with $40 \times 40 = 1600$ g of glycogen, which correspond to 6400 Kcal in the form of carbohydrates, to be divided into three days (about 2100 Kcal per day). To this calculation, we must add the necessary calories for the basal metabolism (80% of 1900 = 1520 Kcal) and for a minimum level of physical activity (about 200 Kcal), for a total of 3820 Kcal per day in the form of carbohydrates. Doing the math, referring to our 80 kg bodybuilder, we see that these calories correspond to about 12 g of carbohydrates per day, for every kg of body weight.

We must add the calories of proteins (1 g per kg of body weight) to the calories of carbohydrates: a higher share in this phase is not necessary because the subject does not train and any excess will be transformed into stored fat.

It is necessary to point out that this theoretical calculation starts from the assumption of a total depletion, which represents the fundamental stimulus for the recharging phase. If, on the contrary, our bodybuilder has not completely exhausted the reserves of the muscle glycogen, the supercompensation will reach lower levels (about 30 g/kg of muscle) and a part of the ingested carbohydrates, rather than being conveyed inside the muscle cells, will end in the subcutaneous tissue in the form of fat.

A key point to underline is that, during the immediately preceding days before the "discharge-recharge", the carbohydrate intake must be quite high, otherwise the muscle glycogen will be already depleted and the effective supercompensation will not occur during the recharge phase.

These calculations are the result of the data processing that led to the "carbohydrate refill" methodology, which was made popular thanks to an article by Massimo Spattini, published in 1987 in the *Sportman & Fitness* magazine. It is still relevant today, appearing first in online searches, and it has been confirmed by the most recent scientific literature.

An article by Valeria Galfano, published in 2019 in the scientific journal *L'Endocrinologo*, summarizes the molecular mechanisms that regulate the supercompensation.

AMPK, which is the **protein kinase activated by AMP**, is an enzyme that acts as a regulator for the cellular energy. This enzyme, by binding to the glycogen particles, can also perform the function of a cell fuel sensor; instead, muscle glycogen acts as a negative regulator for the AMPK activation: the more glycogen we have, the less it will be necessary to activate AMPK, since it is a sign of an optimal state of muscle "fuel" levels.

When the AMPK enzyme is activated for prolonged times, the concentration of muscle glycogen increases significantly; a very interesting aspect is that the activity of this enzyme increases during the physical exercises and remains high even after a few hours from the end of training.

The activation of AMPK determines two decidedly favorable effects for a bodybuilder: it improves the insulin sensitivity and stimulates the oxidation of fatty acids; in this way, the intracellular glucose is also conveyed towards the synthesis of glycogen when the reserves have returned to baseline values. Therefore, AMPK is crucial for the supercompensation process.

The chemical structure of the glycogen molecule is a branched polymer with a high molecular weight. As previously mentioned, the increase in muscle glycogen, obtained through the carbohydrate load, is accompanied by an increase of 2.7-4 g of water for each gram of glycogen. A fundamental fact for the bodybuilder is that magnetic resonance studies and the multi-frequency segmental bioimpedance analysis have shown that **the water increase occurs significantly in the intracellular compartment**, while the extracellular compartment remains almost unchanged.

Translated into practical terms for bodybuilding, this means being able to achieve a higher muscle volume and a better degree of definition.

As was often the case in other fields of medicine and pharmacology, most of the studies involving carbohydrate recharging were carried out on male subjects. Still, the well-known hormonal differences between men and women can certainly affect the mechanisms that stand behind the supercompensation and glycogen loading.

In fact, sex-related metabolic differences, which depend on the different hormonal patterns, have now been widely demonstrated. The main mediator of these differences seems to be **estradiol**, a sex hormone which belongs to the estrogens class; it is reasonable to think that, just as it influences the metabolism of carbohydrates, it can also play a fundamental role in the glycogen load. It should also be remembered that skeletal muscles in women show a greater sensitivity to insulin than in men, and theoretically, this would lead to higher storage of muscle glycogen.

In 1995, Tarnopolsky, a professor at McMaster University in Canada, conducted one of the first scientific studies to evaluate a possible difference in sex-linked glycogen load.

In this study, two groups of runners, divided by gender, consumed a hyperglucidic diet (75% carbohydrates) for 4 days. **Women consumed 6.4 g of carbohydrates for every kg of body weight and men had 8.2 g of carbohydrates for every kg of body weight.**

The results showed that men increased the muscle glycogen content by 41% and improved the timing of sports performance by 45%; instead, women did not show any increase in muscle glycogen and showed a 5% improvement in performance.

The authors hypothesized that this increase in carbohydrates in women was not sufficient to cause a supercompensation. In fact, several studies suggest the existence of a **carbohydrate refill threshold** that corresponds to 8-10 g/kg. When the carbohydrate intake reaches 12 g/kg of lean mass, athletes of both sexes reach comparable supercompensation values.

To reach these levels of carbohydrates while recharging, women need to increase their calorie intake by 34%. Therefore, to obtain benefits comparable to the male counterpart, a woman, instead of only increasing the intake of carbohydrates, must also consume additional calories. Specifically, she needs about 30% more energy for 4 days to ensure that her carbohydrate intake reaches levels above 8 g/kg per day.

Among the most peculiar aspects of preparing for the competition is the **water balance**.

During the "discharge" phase, you must not reduce the intake of liquids, in order not to incur dehydration, which is caused by strenuous workouts and low carbohydrate diets (which have a diuretic effect).

On the other hand, how should you regulate yourself when charging? It is precisely at this stage that almost all the athletes have a maximal confusion: not to drink, drink small amounts, drink a lot and, if a lot, how much? In fact, a careful analysis of the human physiology can provide a precise answer to these questions.

During the recharging phase, it is necessary to calculate the water balance, that is the "outputs" of water (sweating, *perspiratio insensibilis*, respiration and urine) in relation to the "inputs". Elaborating an estimate of the intake is a rather difficult task: to the water consumed through drinks, we must add the amounts that are contained, to varying degrees, in food (especially fruits and vegetables) and we must not forget the amounts that are "created" by the body's cells as a product of our metabolism.

Therefore, during the 3 days of recharging, it is necessary to accurately calculate the water balance, to convey the right amount of water in the muscles, in addition to glycogen, in order to "inflate" them; no more (under the penalty of clouding the definition) and no less (under the penalty of reducing the increase of the muscles volume).

Drinking too little during a diet that is rich in carbohydrates can hinder the recharging process: glucose will not be able to enter the muscles, it will remain outside the cells (drawing water into the subcutis), and it will be transformed into adipose tissue.

Thirst, a sensation finely regulated by the nervous structures located in the brain through the secretion of some hormones, will undoubtedly serve as a guide, but it is precisely at this stage that, with a careful study of your body, you can achieve surprising results.

By slightly forcing the homeostatic processes (adapters) of the organism during the very last days before the competition and by introducing a slightly reduced amount of liquids in the recharging phase, it is possible to move the extracellular water (which tarnishes your definition) inside the muscles, making them larger, vascularized and with evident streaks.

This "trick" must be calculated with extreme precision and, if done well, it will allow any bodybuilder afflicted with water retention to reverse the situation in a winning way.

Obviously, it is necessary to accurately know the amount of the extracellular and intracellular water: for this purpose, mirrors and scales are not enough, but fortunately, technology comes to our aid through the use of bioimpedance analysis.

Small errors in the water balance can be corrected with some natural methods. It is preferable to drink the calculated amount of water or a little more but, if the ultrasonic and/or the impedance analysis shows an excess of fluid in the subcutis, you can opt for a sauna and thus eliminate the surplus.

The sauna, in fact, involves sweating at the expense of the extracellular water, while the glycogen retains the water inside the cells. On the contrary, it is not recommended to seek sweating through a run or other physical activities, because it would cause water loss, for the most part, through the splitting of glycogen, thus partially frustrating the benefits of charging.

Another crucial aspect of the competition preparation is the **electrolyte balance**.

A very dangerous practice, but unfortunately often used by bodybuilders, involves the drug abuse for diuretic purposes. A side effect of diuretics is the unhinging of the electrolyte balance, with the risk of cramps, muscle depletion and other effects that are certainly more worrying from a health point of view, including arrhythmias and cardiac arrest, neuromuscular alterations, renal impairment and rhabdomyolysis.

It is much better to do things right, calibrating the intake of both liquids and mineral salts during the week before the contest.

Among these, **potassium** is of a particular importance and its need will be increased, since it enters in the muscle cell together with glucose during the recharging phase, due to the effect of insulin, which stimulates the ATP-dependent sodium/potassium pump. It is best to take the potassium through your normal diet rather than in the form of pills, as these can irritate the stomach walls; moreover, the chlorine ion, usually present in commonly used preparations, can cause water retention.

Fruits (bananas, apricots, kiwis), starchy vegetables (potatoes, plantains) and, to a lesser extent, also pasta and bread, are among the foods that are richest in potassium and which can be used in the recharging phase. However, we must not go too far with the fruit consumption because they are rich in simple sugars (fructose, glucose, sucrose) which, as anticipated, must not exceed 20% of the total calories.

The total amount of the potassium to be ingested during the 3 days of the refill must be appropriately calculated in relation to the carbohydrate intake: it will be necessary to take approximately 3 milliequivalents of potassium (about 120 mg) per 100 g of carbohydrates used for refilling purposes.

An excess (hyperkalemia) or a deficit (hypokalemia) will be equally harmful, especially for the functioning of the heart.

Another electrolyte that should be balanced is the much deprecated **sodium**. The sodium intake must be calculated starting from the amount of the extracellular water that we intend to reach at the end of the recharge: by increasing the sodium intake during the "discharge" phase and reducing it appropriately during the recharging phase, it is possible to modulate the homeostatic mechanisms, which would lead to an increased production of aldosterone with the consequent retention of water and sodium, and a loss of potassium, thus obtaining the result of preserving the muscle definition.

The sodium intake must be strictly calculated: an excess will tend to draw water into the subcutaneous tissue (sodium is a typically extracellular mineral), a deficit, on the other hand, will cause cramps that would affect your *posedown*.

Finally, **phosphorus** is important, as in the recharging phase it is actively captured by the muscle cells to form the energy compounds, risking hypophosphatemia (decreased phosphorus in the blood) characterized by neurological and muscular signs such as anxiety, irritability, decrease in strength and reflexes, all equally disastrous for a competing bodybuilder. In this case, the only way to avoid these symptoms will be a careful planning of the diet.

To conclude, it should be always remembered that the "discharge-recharge" protocols, if not properly conducted, can give rise to **unpleasant side effects**; therefore, every coach or trainer should know them and know how to properly prevent them.

Among the possible side effects, the most common is a poor digestive tolerance, which can arise especially the first time this particular regimen is adopted.

Other rarer side effects include:

- presence of myoglobin in the urine;
- pain in the rib cage;
- electrocardiographic changes.

In order to reduce the incidence and the degree of the aforementioned disorders, it is possible to introduce some changes to the charging protocols, to take a more gradual and a more similar approach to the athlete's eating habits, especially when dealing with beginners. It is essential to entrust the management of these strategies to competent and qualified personnel, avoiding resorting to "do it yourself" or obtaining incorrect information from unauthorized magazines and blogs. In these cases, the risk for the athlete becomes very high. In this regard, I will mention a case report published in 2014, of a 28-year-old bodybuilder who endangered his life a few days after a competition, due to a potassium imbalance which resulted in a hypokalemic paralysis.

From the medical history, it emerged that before the competition, the athlete had undertaken an extreme manipulation of the diet by taking excessive loads of carbohydrates, eliminating salt and drastically reducing the intake of liquids. In addition, the patient reported taking a slimming drug which he purchased on the internet. This slimming agent could probably have contained diuretics, such as spironolactone or other mineralocorticoid antagonists, which compete with aldosterone for receptors in the distal renal tubules, increasing the excretion of sodium chloride and water and the retention of potassium and hydrogen ions.

The sudden suspension of the drug, immediately after the competition, could have caused a relative excess of mineralocorticoids, which contributed to hypokalemia, in conjunction with the translocation of potassium inside the cells due to the extreme load of carbohydrates.

The figures are cited in a completely illustrative manner, based on "average" statistical data such as the basal metabolism and the percentage of muscle mass, which, unfortunately, are of little use to the individual bodybuilder, as each individual is a unique and unrepeatable set of structural and metabolic characteristics.

In order to precisely set the personalized recharge protocol for an individual bodybuilder, it will be necessary to use objectively measured data for each athlete.

CHAPTER 14

Nutrition and aerobic gymnastics

by Giovanni Montagna

Introduction

Aerobic gymnastics is practiced by people of different ages and physical characteristics, mostly women, both for recreational purposes and to improve their physical efficiency. It consists of a sequence of continuous movements, performed to the rhythm of music, which involves both the upper and lower limbs. Even aerobic gymnastics, like other endurance activities, in order to determine stable adaptations for the cardio-circulatory and neuromuscular systems, requires training sessions which, in addition to involving a large percentage of muscle mass, must: 1) **be carried out regularly**; 2) **have a sufficient duration**; 3) **be performed with an adequate intensity**.

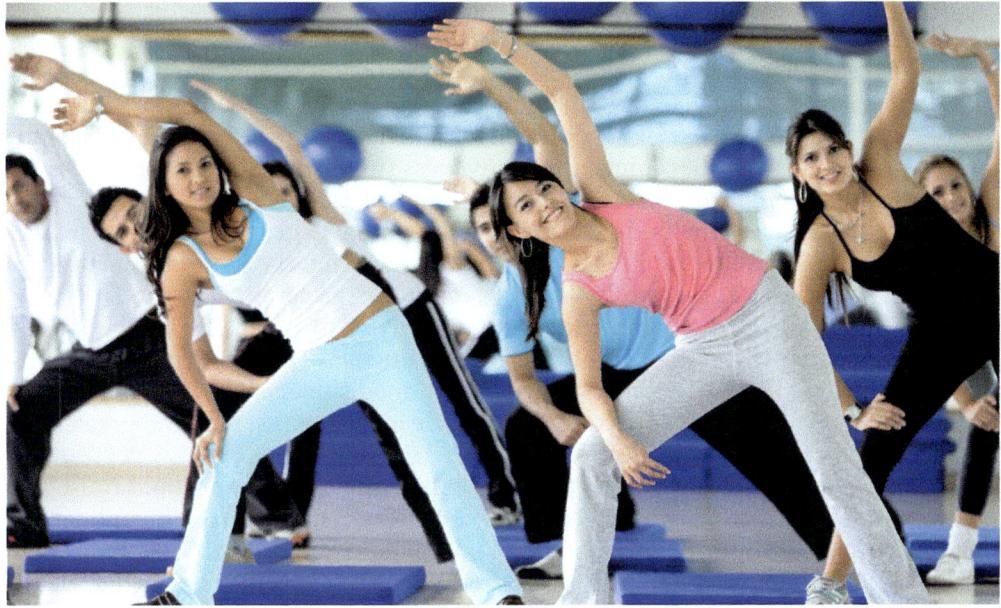

Figure 14.1.

Aerobics for weight loss?

Most people (especially girls) who take aerobics classes have approached this activity mainly for the purpose of losing weight.

However, considering the energy cost in terms of losing body weight, an unrewarding situation is highlighted (at least for those who aim to lose weight), as the real weight loss ranges from about 50 g for beginner women to about 85 g for experienced men. These values have nothing to do with the kilogram that is missing on the scale at the end of the lesson, which is determined almost exclusively by the loss of water.

This weight loss is easily replenished with a cappuccino and a croissant. At this point, think of the uselessness (for slimming purposes) of the aerobics class of a typical office worker who, as soon as she leaves work, eats a snack that is rich in carbohydrates because she feels tired and, during and after the lesson, drinks one or two bottles of beverages to replenish the mineral salts, which are normally nothing more than water with the addition of simple sugars and sodium, certainly not helpful for those who want to lose weight.

Indeed, simple carbohydrates that are taken before the physical activity are counterproductive for weight loss, as they cause the secretion of insulin (a blood sugar regulating hormone produced by the pancreas) which acts on certain fat cell enzymes by inhibiting the release of the body fat. From what has been said, it is clear that those *who decide to use aerobics as a means to lose weight cannot ignore integrating the physical activity with an appropriate diet*, while those who aim to keep fit, should not consider the lesson time as an excuse for their food "mistakes". An equally important aspect related to energy expenditure as a function of nutritional supplements is given by the analysis of the energy substrates that are used by the body to produce the necessary energy for movement (possibly, thanks to the analysis of the consumed oxygen and the produced carbon dioxide).

In fact, if we analyze the sources from which we get the energy used during the lesson, we see that most of it comes from the combustion of sugars. In fact, sugar's contribution in providing energy is 66% in men and 72% in women. This means, on the one hand, that the exercise is too intense to be classified as purely aerobic and, on the other hand, that the slimming effectiveness (in terms of fat loss) of the same exercise is greatly reduced by the fact that the intensity is high.

In fact, as we know, the body "chooses" sugars or fats alternatively as "gasoline" for its muscles, related to the intensity of the effort. When the latter is demanding, the muscles resort to sugar, while when it is mild or moderate, it is the fat that is burned. This is why the recommended motor activity to reduce fat reserves (lose weight) is essentially the long-lasting one at a low intensity (jogging, running, swimming, cycling, etc.). However, it is known that trained subjects use less glucose: the result is a slower depletion of hepatic and muscle glycogen reserves and greater resistance to effort.

The increased muscle extraction of glucose from the circulation would cause hypoglycemia if it was not compensated by the interaction of numerous hormonal activities (a decrease in the insulin secretion and an increased production of catecholamines and cortisol). Thus, an endocrine order is determined which favors the release of glucose and fatty acids into the circulation, to be used by the muscle. Thanks to these mechanisms of adaptation, the subject performs intense and prolonged physical exercises in normoglycemia.

Undoubtedly, they also include aerobics, but only if they are really "aerobic", which means long-lasting and with a low-intensity, and this does not seem to be the case for many lessons, including those that were monitored. This is why it would be useful to use a heart rate monitor that monitors the cardiac frequency in order to keep it within a "personalized" threshold based on age, sex, length of training and the wanted goal (weight loss, better cardiovascular efficiency, etc.).

Let's get to the heart of the topic: how much and what to eat. Humans and especially sportspeople, have specific protein needs to meet the constant metabolic functioning (synthesis of enzymes, hormones, transport proteins, protein catabolism, etc.). The first step is to calculate your protein needs based on the amount of your lean mass, your lifestyle and your goals. To calculate the amount of the lean mass, you need to subtract the kilograms (kg) of fat from your total weight. If you are an active person, you need to find the level of the physical activity that suits you.

The higher this index is, the more proteins are demolished and the need to replenish and rebuild the muscle tissue that is damaged by the physical activity increases. The same with the protein-based molecules (hormones, enzymes, blood proteins, etc.) that are used and consumed not only during sports, but also during recovery and everyday life.

Now comes the dilemma of the other two macronutrients: fats and carbohydrates. How to choose them, and in what quantities? All studies indicate that the best fuel for an aerobic activity is fat.

Let's start by stating that we all need a certain amount of carbohydrates, as the body must produce energy and constantly supply the brain, which needs glucose. To do this, the liver converts the carbohydrates we eat into glucose, but the liver's ability to store glycogen is very limited, and glycogen can easily be depleted within 10-12 hours: that is why we must eat carbohydrates. A normal person can store 300-400 g of glycogen in the muscles and 60-90 g in the liver: if we consume anything more than that, it turns into fat, even if the carbohydrates are fat-free. But the worst is yet to come.

Each high-carbohydrate meal causes a rapid rise in the blood glucose. To compensate, the pancreas secretes a powerful hormone, insulin, which lowers the blood sugar. This, however, stimulates the storage of stocks and triggers an accumulation of fat; moreover, by lowering the glycaemia, we feel the need to consume sugars again (hunger): we will thus go to ingest other carbohydrates, and the vicious circle will begin again.

That is not all. As previously mentioned, high insulin levels also prevent you from using the already stored fats. So, the excess of carbohydrates not only makes you fat, but it also keeps you fat. For sportspeople there is also further damage: in fact, the introduction of carbohydrates, especially those with a high glycemic index, can cause a sudden drop in the blood sugar, leaving it "empty"; if you are close to a competition or a training session, it is better not to start because it would be counterproductive and you would risk suffering from injuries.

Now let's talk about the infamous fats: each gram of fat has 9 calories, each gram of carbohydrates has 4… what is the best fuel? It seems all too obvious. In all the situations in which we train in aerobic conditions, or when we are not training but are simply taking a walk, we consume fat and not carbohydrates, so much that diets with a high fat content in cross-country athletes (cyclists, marathoners, etc.), have produced significant performance improvements. In contrast, high-carbohydrate diets have not resulted in long-term improvements.

We have just stated that what makes us fat is the glycemic jump due to the consumption of too many carbohydrates and meals that are too rich in calories (which in any case cause an excessive rise in the blood sugar level), while "good" fats alone and in the correct quantities not only do they not make us fat, but they could also help us lose weight. It is not only fat that is deposited in the form of the adipose tissue, but the excess of whatever we eat, whether it is proteins or carbohydrates, after their conversion into fat.

Paradoxically, by not modifying the blood sugar levels, fats do not stimulate insulin, and they have a lower lipogenic effect. This makes us understand that we must stop demonizing fats, since it is much easier to gain weight and have a poor performance with the use of large amounts of carbohydrates rather than fats. We will return later on the actual amount of fats to be consumed, pointing out from now on that they must consist mainly of mono and polyunsaturated fatty acids such as those contained in extra virgin olive oil, nuts, olives, etc.

Now we come to the crux of carbohydrates. It is now established that every food we consume and every food combination we adopt has its hormonal implications that are far more important than the caloric ones. It is precisely on the hormonal effects of foods that scientific research in the field of nutrition is being directed, as these substances are able, if well-modulated, to make us lose weight and make us work at a maximum efficiency. So why not take advantage of everyday foods to improve our quality of life?

The credit for shedding some light on this topic goes to Dr. Barry Sears (although certainly someone before him had the same intuitions), who with his books has managed to divulge and make it accessible to a wider audience what a food causes, on a hormonal level, when it is ingested and absorbed.

Based on his studies and research, it has been seen that a ratio between proteins and carbohydrates (P/C) oscillating between 0.5 and 1 (however, it also depends on the genetics of the subject) allows the body to have a hormonal production and balance capable of improving the functioning and the efficiency of the organism, both from the physical and psychological point of view, with a greater mental clarity (it will serve to better fix the choreography, both for the instructor and the student), an increased resistance and adaptation to effort, improved aerobic capacity, better oxygenation, weight loss if desired (also influenced by the consumed amount of fat, as we will see) etc.

Furthermore, by doing so, the body is taught to become more efficient in burning fat, both while exercising and when resting, which is very useful for weight loss but also to save glucose that can be used more in the brain, by the red blood cells and where it is needed. Therefore, once you have established the amount of protein you need, just take into account the P/C ratio = 0.5-1 to calculate the daily amount of carbohydrates, which must mainly consist of low glycemic index carbohydrates, because they increase the blood glucose level slowly, with a moderate influence on the insulin secretion.

The most favorable carbohydrates are those who are rich in fibers, less refined and low in starch and glucose, for example: fruits such as apples, pears, apricots, peaches, melons, watermelons, etc.; vegetables such as broccoli, cauliflower, asparagus, spinach, green beans, leafy vegetables etc.; some cereals, such as oat flakes. The unfavorable ones include pasta, bread, rice (if you really can't do without them, take small portions of the whole wheat ones), cereals, corn, potatoes, ripe bananas, papaya, cooked carrots and all packaged fruit juices.

Let us now return to the amount of fats. If a person wants to lose fat (whether or not an athlete), a starting carbohydrate-protein-fat ratio of 40%-30%-30% in caloric terms will be established until he/she reaches his/her percentage of the ideal fat mass. So, if I know the calories given by proteins (1 g of protein = 4 Kcal), which must be the same as those that will come from fats, I just have to divide the daily calories given by proteins by 9 (1 g of fat = 9 Kcal) to find the amount of fat to be consumed.

If, on the other hand, the person has an ideal fat percentage, it will be necessary to periodically evaluate whether a diet with a ratio of 40%-30%-30% causes a further loss of body fat, in order to vary the percentage of dietary fat upwards by a certain amount, based on the subject's sensations (higher or lesser energy, varying mental clarity at work and during the physical activity, tiredness after meals and/or at the end of the day, etc.), obviously respecting the indications that are already provided on proteins and carbohydrates.

For the advanced athletes, who already have the suitable body fat for their discipline, fat will be added in an adequate quantity in order not to lose weight and to allow them to perform the athletic performance and gestures always at their maximum potential. This means consuming a quantity of "good" fats, certainly higher than 30%, which should consist mainly of monounsaturated fatty acids, which, as we have seen, are the optimal source of energy for the muscle under stress.

The foods to be consumed throughout the day must be divided into at least five to six meals, three of which are the main ones (breakfast, lunch and dinner) and two or three snacks (mid-morning, afternoon and just before going to bed). It is very important to have a snack before the training, which must be consumed 1 hour and 45 minutes before the training and which must contain about 90-100 Kcal, always in the ratio 40%-30%-30% (even 50% C – 25% P – 25% G can be fine); however, it is necessary to evaluate the athlete's sensations, so that there are no sudden elevations in blood sugar with the harmful consequences reported above.

For those engaged in lessons that last more than an hour to an hour and a half (such as masters, conventions, etc.), it is preferable to take a small snack in the same proportions for every hour of physical work, in order not to encounter blood sugar drops that could compromise the continuation of the lessons due to an energetic, but also coordinative and mnemonic decrease. If the aerobics class has been tiring and the next meal is consumed after two to three hours or more, it is better to have another 90-100 Kcal snack about 20 minutes after the training. This is to speed up the energy for the recovery process and optimize the training during the lesson, to avoid both getting hungry for the next meal, and risking bingeing.

CHAPTER 15

Nutrition and dance

by Alessandra Cascone and Barbara Hugonin

The purpose of this chapter is to highlight the main nutritional issues among adult dancers, establish some nutritional tips, focus on nutrition during training and competitions/performances, highlighting some dietary supplements that could play a vital role in dance.

Therefore, dance classes can be categorized as intermittent bursts of moderate to intense activity, with a predominant strain on the anaerobic system. Some choreographies may require dancers to dance for more than 5 minutes, but these may not be performed frequently enough to induce a strain on the aerobic system.

Since an increased energy expenditure through extra hours of exercise is typically difficult to achieve due to dancers' commitments, food restriction is usually the method that dancers use to maintain a low weight and a low body fat percentage (% BF). The female athlete triad is well known and it is considered common among dancers. The triad refers to the correlation between the energy availability, menstrual function and bone mineral density (see below). Some clinical manifestations may include eating disorders, hypothalamic functional amenorrhea, and osteoporosis. The triad is particularly relevant in activities and sports where thinness and/or low body weight are considered important, such as in dance.

The nutritionist should explain that an adequate personalized nutrition program can enable each dancer to achieve their goals. Weight control interventions should be carefully crafted to avoid harmful consequences on the performance and health.

Among the physiological parameters, body composition in dance has been seen mainly in the context of ballet, where typical body fat values between female dancers range from 16 to 18% and between male dancers from 5 to 15%.

The International Society for the Advancement of Kinanthropometry (ISAK) indicates that the range of values for athletes, given by the sum of seven skin folds, ranges from 40 to 90 mm for women and from 30 to 60 mm for men. Therefore, dancers should at least reach the minimum values mentioned above, for example 40 mm for women and 30 mm for men.

Dancers should understand that an adequate nutrition (as shown in the table below), and not simply an adequate caloric intake, is necessary to maximize their dance performance, to ensure proper recovery after the training and rehearsals, and also to maintain a body composition within the healthy and adequate values. In addition, in the long term, low energy intakes can lead to poor nutritional intakes, referring particularly to micronutrients, which could result in metabolic dysfunctions associated with nutritional deficiencies, as well as in a reduction of the basal metabolism.

Referring to the data shown in the table, many researches have suggested that 30 Kcal/kg FFM/day should represent the lowest threshold of the energy availability for women, below which some reproductive disorders occur. Usually, the energy balance in healthy adults is obtained with an energy availability of about 45 Kcal/kg FFM/day. It is important to underline that an athlete in a perennial energy deficit is at a high risk for a reduced performance, impaired growth and diseases. Currently, despite these tips, dancers are known to have low energy intakes. Female dancers in dance schools and professional female dancers report that they consume respectively 70% and 80 % less than this requirement.

Table 15.1 Daily Nutrition Guidelines

Energy	≥30 Kcal/kg lean mass + energy expenditure for the training
Carbohydrates	3-5 g/kg
Proteins	1.2–1.7 g/kg
Fats	20-35% of the energy intake

As for macronutrients, there are no studies on the specific consumption required by dancers during training, although moderate intensity activities within each session are characterized as carbohydrate-dependent. As dancers struggle every day to maintain their body weight, at least 3 to 5 g/kg/day of carbohydrates have been proposed. Protein is an important nutrient for muscle growth and repair, which are essential processes following the intense training programs that dancers undergo.

Therefore, dancers should know the general guidelines regarding the protein intake for athletes, estimated from 1.2 to 1.7 g/kg/day. Fats are a necessary component within an adequate diet, as they provide energy, essential elements and fat-soluble vitamins (A, D, K, E). The optimal estimate of macronutrients for fats is 20 to 35% of the total energy intake, and intakes below 20% can compromise the performance.

Since most dancers tend to have a low energy intake and eliminate one or more food groups from their diet, the use of multivitamin and mineral supplements becomes necessary. The macronutrients that arouse most of the interest in dancers' diets are calcium and iron. Regarding the iron, on the one hand dancers and other athletes engaged in impact sports must compensate for the high level of hemolysis; on the other hand, due to a restriction of the food intake, dancers could be at risk of iron deficiencies.

It is necessary to increase the intake of vitamin C to improve the absorption of iron. Regarding to football, its adequate contribution is essential to ensure a sturdy structure that is not prone to injuries. Adequate calcium intake (and related absorption) reduces the risk of osteoporosis, which is common in dancers and can jeopardize their career. Another important micronutrient is vitamin D, which is recognized as extremely important for the bone health, immune functions and the modulation of inflammation, and it might be necessary also for an optimal muscle function and performance.

It has also been found that many athletes are at risk for a vitamin D deficiency, and particularly those who play an indoor sport, as well as dancers. Therefore, it would be advisable for dancers to monitor their concentration of iron, calcium and vitamin D and to consult with their healthcare professional and/or nutritionist to determine any appropriate nutritional interventions or/and the intake of specific supplements.

During the performance, it is necessary to pay attention to hydration, as exercise can become increasingly difficult, performance levels become slack, and dancers may experience symptoms such as general fatigue, sluggishness, headache, dizziness or nausea. Weak muscles, coupled with muscle aches and cramps, are also associated with poor fluid intake and dehydration. While the adult in average require about 2 liters of fluids per day, dancers, due to the loss of fluids during exercise, require more. During a tough training session or a long test, fluid loss can be as high as 2 L/h.

Dancers in dance schools

In ballet school dancers, from classical to modern and in other styles, the esthetic model plays a fundamental role in the nutritional planning and training. Children and adolescents are elite athletes but, unlike professionals and adult artists, there are many factors to take into consideration: growth, musculoskeletal development, menarche in women, puberty, malnutrition, insufficient sleep etc.

For an assessment of children and adolescents under 18, the body mass index (BMI) is based on the so-called growth charts.

These curves are different for boys and girls and there is very little information available on the growth and development of young dancers. Current studies, based on the observation of small groups of school and university dancers aged between 8 and 16 years, in different locations in the United States, Brazil and Sweden and in Korea, consider nutritional intake as a function of an optimal diet, body composition, bone mineral density, and measurement of the muscle function.

The interesting data concerns the distribution of the adipose tissue among female dancers aged between 8 and 16 and girls who do not dance. At the age of 8, both groups show an equal weight, while at the age of 13 non-dancers weigh more than dancers (weight of 48.5 +/- 9.6 kg for non-dancers and 40.6 +/- 8.5 kg for dancers). Hormonal factors and menarche influence the distribution of the adipose tissue and reduce the difference between the two groups by 2 kg. Dancers frequently develop late menarche; this may be due to the destruction of the accumulation of fat, which derives from the excessive exercises (13.9 +/- 2 years).

The differences between the sexes during puberty

While growing up, the differences between the sexes are important in elite dance:
- girls mature, on average, 2 years earlier than boys;
- the differences between the sexes relate to strength and motor performance.

In girls, strength and motor performance show a peak during the adolescence, and then decline, while in boys they tend to grow even after this phase. The differences between the sexes in relation to the physical performance can be attributed to a greater adiposity in girls and greater leanness in boys. Flexibility is an important component in dance, as average flexibility reports an increase in girls aged between 11 and 14, before reaching a stalemate. It is clear that growth can affect the flexibility in young dancers, and both a healthy nutritional balance and a variation of the personalized training program are equally important.

Nutritional intake in dancers in dance schools

Although it is necessary for dancers to achieve an adequate nutrition to ensure a good workout and a good performance, they must limit the nutritional intake to maintain their physical fitness, since the slim esthetic models and the concept of elegant movements influence the dance. Low caloric intake and micronutrient deficiencies such as calcium, iron and vitamin D were observed in groups aged 8 to 16 years old. The total energy intake in groups of non-dancers of the same age was 1780.2-2150 Kcal, in ballet dancers it was 1310 +/- 390.32 Kcal and in contemporary dancers it was 1454 +/- 478.59 Kcal.

These results indicate that the expenditure of the total nutritional intake is insufficient in dancers who study elite dance. After 9 months of an adequate nutritional intake, with corrections in the diet, the nutritional intake is improved from 1640 +/- 412 to 2368 +/- 182 Kcal, in order to satisfy the energy demand that is necessary for growth, to repair the tissues and for the physical activity. The body, on average, needs 30 Kcal/kg to maintain its normal functions, plus an extra 200-300 Kcal/day to satisfy the physical fatigue during the dance lessons, rehearsals and performances. Treatment consists of a good nutritional program to invest in a good health and in injury prevention: foods with a relatively low calorie intake and with a high nutritional density.

Complex carbohydrates

Complex carbohydrates should form the energy basis of a dancer's diet, as they are slowly reduced to glucose and provide a sustained release of energy over a longer period of time. They are also an excellent source of vitamins, minerals and fiber that are often lacking in a dancer's diet. These complex carbohydrates are found in legumes, whole grains and in vegetables (like starches and fibers).

Supplementation of vitamins and minerals

A balanced and energetic diet for the growing dancer includes the adequate supplementation of vitamins and minerals in order to prevent any nutritional insufficiencies. It deals with a supplement that provides 100-150% of the RDA for basic vitamins and minerals, vitamin A, vitamin C, folic acid, thiamin, riboflavin, niacin, zinc, magnesium, iodine, vitamin D and calcium. In particular, vitamin D, calcium and other supplements taken with the food intake are important during growth, to prevent various bone injuries such as fractures, bone fragility and low density, and skeletal anomalies.

Iron helps prevent fatigue. Vitamin C is important and, together with proteins, stimulates the formation of the collagen matrix. The importance of minerals and vitamins for the growth and development of tissues and for reducing the deficit before and after the supplementation is well known. There is a clear reduction in the deficit of vitamin D, vitamin C and the group of vitamins B, after the supplementation..

Proteins

During growth, the development and the nutritional requirements (partially) of the muscle structures are based on proteins. For elite athletes like ballet school dancers, it is recommended that at least 12-15% of calories should come from proteins. In a healthy nutrition program of around 2000 Kcal per day, school dancers would need around 60-70g of proteins in their diet. According to a recent study, proteins from plant-based foods are considered healthier for preventing the risks of diseases and improving the longevity of the artists' careers. The main sources of animal proteins are meat, fish, cheese, eggs and milk, while vegetable proteins are mainly found in legumes, nuts and seeds.

The body does not like to use proteins as fuel or energy. The body, as a teenager, wants to save valuable proteins for muscle building and for the production of hormones and enzymes. High-protein diets can lead to an increased calcium loss from the bones and this is a big problem for dancers during training and growth, as it increases the risk of fractures and lowers the bone density.

Fats

Fats are essential for transporting fat-soluble vitamins throughout the body, for protecting essential organs and for lubricating the joints, which are at a risk of injury. Furthermore, fats are also essential elements for the brain and for the neural tissue, especially omega-3s which, in our Western-style diet, tend to be deficient. In the diet they are found both in fatty fish, such as mackerel, sardines, herring and salmon, and in nuts and seeds.

Hydration

For the growing dancer, staying hydrated is extremely important, because poor balance and fatigue are the first signs of an inadequate hydration. Every dancer is different, but pre-professional and elite school dancers should aim for an intake of around 2800-3300 mL of fluids each day. About 20-25% comes from foods such as fruits and vegetables, but about 80% comes from beverages, such as sports beverages and water. Some ballet school dancers prefer a mix of 50% water and 50% sports beverages.

Nutrition for the training of professional dancers

The nutritional goals for meals/snacks before, after and during the training are similar to those of other sports (see the position of the American Dietetic Association, Dieticians of Canada and American College of Sports Medicine (for more information: www.eatright.org; www.dietitians.ca; www.acsm.org).

Before exercise, a meal or a snack should provide sufficient fluids to maintain the hydration and it should be relatively low in fats and fibers to facilitate the gastric emptying and to minimize the gastrointestinal stress.

It should also be moderate in proteins, relatively high in carbohydrates, preferably with a low to moderate glycemic index to maximize the glycemic maintenance, and it should be well tolerated by the dancer. The pre-event meal should contain between 1 and 4 g of carbohydrates/kg when consumed 1 to 4 hours before the exercise, to increase the availability of carbohydrates before a prolonged exercise session. At least 4 hours before the training, dancers should slowly drink 5 to 7 mL/kg of fluids. These recommendations can be followed by ingesting a sports beverage with carbohydrates or by combining water and food.

If the dancer does not urinate or if the urine is dark or highly concentrated, he should consume another 3-5 mL/kg of fluids about 2 hours before the event. It is recommended that the beverages contain between 20 and 50 mEq/L of sodium. During the exercise, especially if it lasts more than 1 hour, the primary goals for the nutrient consumption are the restoration of lost fluids and the supply of carbohydrates (from about 30 to 60 g/h) for the maintenance of the blood glucose levels. The use of carbohydrates during training has been shown to delay the fatigue, by potentially reducing the muscle glycogen depletion, keeping blood sugar as an important source of energy for both muscles and the brain, and by modulating the neurotransmitters, which could affect cognition, mood, motivation and the motor skill performance, which are essential factors for a dancer.

Dancers should drink sufficient fluids during exercise to limit the dehydration to less than about 2% of the body mass and sodium should be included in the beverages when sweat losses are high, especially when the exercise lasts more than 2 hours. The recommendations range from 150 to 350 mL every 20 minutes, depending on the intensity of the workout. The measurement of the body weight before and after the training is a practical method to ensure that the amount of fluids consumed during the training can be adequate. Ideally, dancers should neither overhydrate, which leads to transient weight gain, nor dehydrate, keeping the weight loss below 2% for each session. Fluid replacement beverages are recommended to contain 20 to 30 mEq/L of sodium and 2 to 5 mEq/L of potassium.

After the exercise, dietary goals are to provide adequate fluids, electrolytes, carbohydrates and proteins to replace the muscle glycogen and to ensure a rapid recovery. To achieve a correct recovery process, it is recommended to consume 0.8 g of carbohydrates/kg/h and 0.2-0.4 g of protein/kg/h, at frequent intervals in the first recovery period. The first meal should be taken during the first 30 minutes and again every 2 hours for 4-6 hours. The proteins that are consumed after the exercise will provide the amino acids for the construction and the repair of the muscle tissue. During the recovery from the exercise, rehydration should include replacing the loss of water and salt in sweat.

Since fluid losses will continue throughout the recovery period through urinary leaks and the ongoing sweating, the dancer will need to consume additional fluids to counteract them. Typically, in order to restore the fluid balance, during the

2-4 hours after the training they should consume a volume equal to about 150% of the post-exercise fluid deficit.

Nutrition for the competition or for the performance on stage

While performances during the competitions/stage performances do not pose a risk to fluid or nutrient deposits, as performances are generally short and have a moderate to low intensity, dancers may experience absolute exhaustion in the days before because of the long hours of rehearsal. When dancers are required to participate in lengthy rehearsals for several days, their muscles can find themselves in an almost glycogen-depleted state, especially if they are limiting their dietary intake. On the performance day, the dancers must find a plan that comfortably fits both their nutritional needs and their feelings of comfort. Since the costumes are usually tight and the choreographies are physically demanding, dancers usually don't like having a full stomach/intestine before and during the competition or stage performance. One possible strategy is to consider switching to a low-fiber diet during the last 24 hours before the event to reduce the stomach and intestinal contents.

On the day of the event, the last meal should be taken 4 hours before the show in the case of a large meal, or 1 to 2 hours in the case of a snack. Dancers should be encouraged to bring their own food and drinks with them to ensure adequate nutrition and to avoid gastrointestinal problems. In addition, dancers can suffer from anxiety and stress, which can reduce the appetite and, consequently, compromise the amount of the energy intake.

It is important to work with a plan that takes into account the nutritional needs and the practical opportunities for consuming foods and drinks during the events, especially during long ones. But, if the dancer believes that the intake of food and liquids compromises his/her performance and/or esthetics, he/she can choose not to drink or eat during the event and start the recovery strategies as soon as possible after the performance. This quickness is even more important if the event lasts several days. As performances sometimes end late at night, restaurants and bars that serve food may already be closed. Therefore, dancers must bring snacks with them, in order to eat as soon as possible after the show, to ensure a proper nutritional food.

Food supplements and ergogenic aids

Products that play a role in the dance are supplements that can be used to achieve a nutritional goal, including the prevention or treatment of a nutritional deficiency: namely, multivitamin and mineral supplements, iron, calcium and vitamin D. Caffeine can also be considered an ergogenic aid. One of its potential beneficial effects is the decreased perception of fatigue and exertion, which allows the dancer to undertake a better and a more consistent training/performance. Caffeine can also positively influence the reaction times, alertness and the processing of the visual information.

There is evidence that beneficial effects may occur with low levels of caffeine (1 to 3 mg/kg body mass). An overdose of caffeine has been associated with a reduction in reaction times and alertness, and an impaired processing of the visual information, which could offset its stimulating effect.

Malnutrition and injuries

Low bone density and fractures

For dance school students and dancers at a preparatory or a professional level, intense physical exercise, low BMI and low BMC (Bone Mineral Content), in association with various nutritional factors, can cause different types of injuries. During puberty this situation leads to a low BMC, with a high risk of fractures. Dancers between 16 and 17 years old have started dancing around the age of 5 and they have trained for about 22 hours each week. BMI, assessed by age groups, would be normal only in 42.5% of the dancers, while 15.7% of the dancers have a more or less severe thinness.

The evaluation was done for the BMI, BMC and AMBD (Apparent Mineral Bone Density). In adolescent dance students, the correlation between the BMAD and the age from menarche and onwards is positive, because estrogens have protective effects. A balanced diet is essential for proper skeletal development and to prevent the risk of fractures.

The esthetic criteria of the art of ballet encourage a low BMI and many young dancers limit their energy intake to stay slim. Energy restriction is accompanied by a lower intake of proteins and fats; in addition, many dancers are vegetarians and have a very low protein intake.

Minerals and vitamins are also quite deficient in these conditions, especially vitamin D and calcium, which are essential for bone health. Caffeine and smoking reduce the absorption of calcium by the bone tissue. Low energy intake and malnutrition delay the onset of menarche (+/- 13.9 years on average) and low estrogen levels affect the bone density.

Bone mineral content is measured with DXA (Dual energy X-ray Absorptiometry), which particularly takes into account the left femoral neck and the lumbar vertebrae (L1-L4), for the measurement of the mineralization, independent of the bone size. In dancers, 41.2% have a low BMI (grade 1 thinness) and this inadequate energy supply can lead to fractures, joint injuries, osteoporosis, postural problems and skeletal abnormalities.

The triad of the female athlete

In dance students and professional dancers, when the energy intake is inadequate and the osteoporosis is accompanied by amenorrhea, the symptoms of the "female athlete triad" occur. This concept was officially described in 1997 as a syndrome observed in very athletically active girls and women and, in 2007, it was reformulated by the American College of Sport Medicine (ACSM), to lay the foundation for a discussion on the bone health problems of the female dancers.

These three interdependent problems are: 1) energy availability; 2) menstrual function; 3) bone health. Each of these aspects exhibits a continuous variability from an optimal condition to a diagnosed problem. The ACSM defined the amount of energy left and available for normal body functions as an "energy availability", after having subtracted the amount of the energy spent with training from the energy gained through food. The table below shows the levels of vitamins and minerals in elite dancers.

Chapter 15 ▶ Nutrition and dance

A multidisciplinary, dietary, medical and psychological approach is indicated for the treatment of the triad of the female athletes, in order to provide the best possible support to dancers. The most important aspect is to inform the dancers of the relationship between the energy intake and the energy availability, promoting healthy

Table 15.2 Vitamins and minerals in elite dancers

Total population (n = 32)	Total population taking supplements (n = 11)		
Vitamins/Minerals	No. of people taking less than 100% of the RDA	No. of people with deficiencies before taking the supplements	No. of people with deficiencies after taking the supplements
Biotin	32	11	7
Iodine	32	11	7
Zinc	32	11	9
Copper	32	11	10
Linoleic acid	32	*	*
Chloride	32	*	*
Vitamin D	31	10	5
Potassium	31	*	*
Magnesium	31	11	11
Calcium	30	9	9
Molybdenum	30	*	*
Pantothenic acid	29	10	3
Manganese	29	*	*
Iron	28	7	5
Selenium	28	*	*
Vitamin B6	26	7	4
Folic acid	26	7	4
Phosphorus	25	*	*
Fluoride	25	*	*
Chrome	22	*	*
Vitamin B12	18	6	1
Sodium	12	*	*
Vitamin K	10	*	*
Vitamin A	9	4	2
Vitamin B3	8	3	0
Vitamin C	8	5	2
Vitamin B1	7	4	1
Vitamin B2	7	3	1

* Usually not included in vitamin/mineral supplements.

habits for the body and supporting constant medical checks to track the hormonal functions and the menstrual cycle.

Relative energy deficiency in dancers

In 2014, the International Olympic Committee coined the term "relative energy deficiency" (RED) to describe the effects of a syndrome, which does not only affect female athletes.

Energy availability (EA) was defined as energy income (EI in Kcal) minus the energy expenditure due to the physical exercise (EEE), divided by the lean mass (FFM in kg). The functions, regulated by energy, include the cell maintenance, thermoregulation, growth and reproduction. A low EA (<30 Kcal/kg FFM/day) is due to a low food intake or because of an extraordinary energy expenditure for training and performance.

A female professional dancer needs about 2000-2100 Kcal, while a male dancer needs about 2650-2700 Kcal or even more if the physical demands are higher. When an individual's dietary energy intake is insufficient compared to the energy expenditure due to training and performance, RED occurs. A relative energy deficiency can affect the metabolic functioning, bone health, menstrual function, the immune system, and the cardiovascular health. In addition, RED could lead to a progressive reduction in the quality of the athletes' performance due to numerous factors, such as a decreased endurance, coordination and concentration, irritability, depression and a decreased muscle strength.

Obsession with thinness and behavioral disturbances

Is thinness a perfection? In today's society, the obsession with an ideal thinness has reached epidemic proportions. In Sweden and in the United States, a joint study revealed that the demand for precise standards of thinness has increased and it is associated with a more graceful image for the movements, as well as for a perfect body. The esthetic model of the elite dance, the media, society and the impact of the social networks consider a (sometimes too much) thin body to be beautiful and perfect, and for the dancers this image represents the concept of grace and above all it is the most important goal to pursue.

Many dancers, especially young students, become really "addicted" to a diet, with a reduction in the nutritional energy intake at different levels depending on the dance school they belong to. Young dancers from more competitive schools are more likely to develop anorexia nervosa than peers from other schools. In national ballet schools, as well as in high-profile international dance companies, higher pressure, as well as higher expectations on the performance levels, can evolve into eating disorders.

Professional dancers have a greater propensity to develop an eating disorder than students in dance schools, due to a higher competitiveness and psychological stress.

Many companies select dancers from different dance schools and with different physical characteristics, but others select dancers exclusively on the basis of the school of origin, with rigid standards of weight, shape and athletic preparation, and with a particular attention to changes in the pubertal development.

Dancers who are do not have a thin constitution may be more likely to develop eating disorders. Undoubtedly, the genetic predisposition and a nutritional education suitable for the dance play an important role in preventing eating disorders. The obsession with excessive thinness is pathological, but thinness, while maintaining a healthy and proportionate body, is necessary for training and for becoming a healthy professional dancer.

Nutrition for the post-injury rehabilitation

Injuries in dance school dancers and professional performers, can result from an excessive use or a trauma to a part of the body such as the feet, joints, back, hips and pelvis. Nutritional therapy is an integral part of the injury prevention and rehabilitation process. Energy demands increase during the acute phase of the post-injury rehabilitation. In fact, the basal energy metabolism (BEM) should increase by 15-50%, depending on the severity of the damage. For example, an athletic injury and a minor surgery require a 15-20% increase in BEM, while a major surgery may require a 50% increase. The experienced dance nutritionist must balance the increased energy demand and the nutritional needs of injured and rehabilitated dancers, who are simultaneously struggling with temporary inactivity (for example, a young 14 year old dance student with a BEM of 1600 Kcal/day, who has higher energy needs during inactivity [1933 Kcal/day] and during the recovery phase [2,319 Kcal/day]). During recovery from the injury, the energy intake must gradually decrease to the pre-injury levels; dancers should eat less, but they are still athletes. Healing from an injury requires more protein, so injured dancers should take 1.5-2.0 g/kg until they subsequently drop to around 0.8 g/kg. Fats, particularly omega-3s, preferred more than omega-6s with a ratio of 3:1, are indicated in the post-injury nutritional rehabilitation, by consuming foods such as avocados, extra virgin olive oil, nuts and fish, such as salmon.

There are no particular recommendations regarding the amount of carbohydrates during the recovery phase from the injury, but the stability of insulin levels (which, as an anabolic hormone, could affect the injury healing) must always be monitored. Meals should be frequent, every 3-4 hours, and each meal should contain 1-2 servings of vegetables and fruit. Nutritional support is essential to prevent subsequent injuries and to improve the body's stamina, in both young dancers and professionals.

Conclusions

The health of the dancer requires a multidisciplinary approach that provides nutritional, psychological, postural and clinical support with a genre specificity. There are different types of dance and different types of physiques in dancers, and dance medicine is essential for finding a healthy balance and lifestyle. Many factors affect the health of dancers, such as thinness, an inadequate energy intake, intensive training, together with their consequences, such as hormonal imbalances, low bone density, eating disorders, fractures, and differences also related to the genre.

The esthetic model is an integral part of the figure of the dancer, as well as an integral part of a graceful performance, but all this can turn into an obsession to the point of inducing wrong behaviors that can develop into pathologies and cause injuries.

Dance medicine and dance nutrition are truly elite fields of specialization, since dancers are athletes, but compared to sports athletes, they have more specific characteristics and needs.

Nutritional and medical advice for children and young dancers in dance schools, and for professional performers are the only way to prevent numerous physical and psychological problems during their career. Dance is an art and its tools are the body, soul and the mind of the dancers, with physical, emotional, motivational, technical and energetic implications. A healthy mind and body must be the first goal for a dancer and for his/her career. Movement is in harmony when the body is in harmony.

CHAPTER 16

Nutrition and soccer

Soccer is a sport in which different skills are combined in the athlete: tactics, techniques, coordination, etc. These skills must be expressed and improved in every match and in each training. Of course, in order to perform in the best possible way during matches and training, the soccer player must always be in the best psycho-physical conditions, and a component that significantly influences the achievement of this state of form is the nutrition.

Proper nutrition and an adequate food supplementation are useful for the soccer player to improve their sports performance. The weight and the body composition of the athlete should be carefully evaluated, as too often the ideal weight has been associated with the right one (perhaps it is valid for a sedentary person), by not paying attention to the ratio of lean mass to fat mass. In the athlete of any discipline, it is necessary to evaluate the ideal weight, that is the weight which is agreed on between the athlete, the sports doctor, the coach, the nutritionist, a weight which coincides or

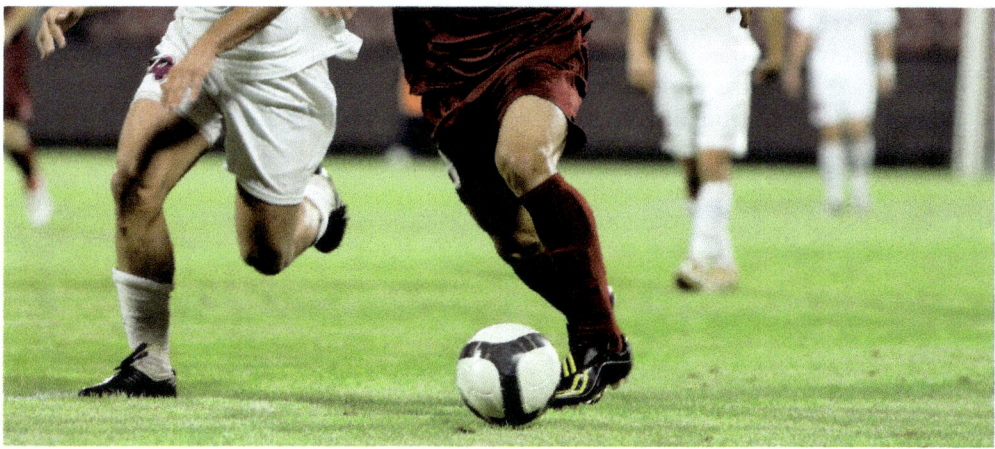

Figure 16.1

has coincided with the optimal performance and which is associated with a subjective feeling of a psycho-physical wellbeing. In soccer, the ideal weight is also related to the role of the player in the field.

In the nutrition of the soccer player (and in general also for those who practice other team sports, such as basketball, volleyball, rugby, etc.) three aspects must be considered:
- quantitative;
- qualitative;
- chronological.

The quantitative aspect

- The nutrition is linked to the energy expenditure, which depends on the basal metabolism, work activity, training and the game.
- The energy expenditure in the field depends on the role and how it is performed (300-400 Kcal/h, with an average consumption of 500-600 Kcal per game).
- In challenging matches with particular climatic conditions (rain, wind, snow, etc.) an energy expenditure of 1000-1500 Kcal can be reached.
- The daily caloric requirement of a soccer player has been estimated at around 3000 +/- 500 Kcal.

Factors to be considered with particular attention

- After the match, the player may be more thirsty than hungry and in the evening they may end up eating less than the accumulated debt. This is to be avoided, as it compromises the physical and mental recovery, resulting in a worsening of the subsequent performance or in any case a lack of improvement.
- After the game and during the interval between the first and the second half (as well as during training), it is useful to consume a beverage based on carbohydrates and mineral salts: the carbohydrates are used for energy during the activity instead of the muscle glycogen stores, which will be less significantly affected; the minerals are used to restore the electrolyte levels that are lost in sweat.
- Immediately after the game, have a pleasant beverage that contains proteins, carbohydrates, vitamins and minerals in the right quantity. All this to obviate the point that we mentioned, which means avoiding missing the recovery, an indeed accelerate it as much as possible.

The qualitative aspect

- It is related to the breakdown of the nutrition into macronutrients (proteins, carbohydrates and lipids).
- Usually the breakdown is as follows:
    - carbohydrates: 50%-55%;
    - proteins: 20%-25%;
    - fats: 25%-30%.

How much protein for the soccer player?

The estimated requirement of a soccer player is about 1.5 g of protein per kg of body weight, although when a certain strengthening or in any case an increase in muscle mass is sought, in case of energy deficit (slimming diet), during periods of very intense training, or during the rehabilitation phase after an injury, 2 g/kg of body weight can be reached.

Fats: prefer poly- and monounsaturated and untreated ones.

- Polyunsaturated fats provide linoleic (omega-6) and alpha-linolenic (omega-3) acids that cannot be synthesized by the human body, and therefore it is essential to introduce them with the food (linseed, hemp, soybean oil). Cold-water fish (salmon, mackerel) are also excellent sources of activated essential fatty acids, such as DHA and EPA.
- On a physical level, they can act as cushions in traumatic events (protect
- organs and viscera), as well as being thermal insulators.
- They bring considerable energy (9 Kcal/g) and are the most used substrate in aerobic conditions.
- Diets with fat less than 15% of daily energy intake reduce the rate of resynthesis of intramuscular triglyceride deposits (IMAT, Intra-Muscolar Adipose Tissue) that in the athlete are functional because they are involved in the production of energy between intermittent sprints. Fats should be limited if not avoided in the pre-game and immediate post-game because they slow down the digestion and absorption of carbohydrates.

The chronological aspect of carbohydrate intake

- It refers to the distribution of meals throughout the day, based on the time of the start of the match, training sessions, duration, recovery times (both during the match and between matches).
- At least three hours must pass between the end of the meal (easy to digest) and the beginning of the match (except for the administration of easily metabolized supplements or in any case in times of emergency).
- The pre-match meal, if misinterpreted, can adversely affect the performance of the match itself.
- A meal with a high glycemic index and load (for example, a plate of pasta with a dessert containing simple sugars such as sucrose) before the game can be counterproductive because it can be followed, after a short time, by a state of hypoglycemia, caused by the stimulating action of insulin. The amount of carbohydrates that a professional soccer player should consume in the pre-match meal is between 1-3 g/kg body weight. Therefore, low glycemic index meals composed of all three macronutrients are preferred but low in fat. The consumption of carbohydrates in the 30-60 minutes before the match should be avoided to avoid the risk of reactive hypoglycemia, while just before, at the end of the warm-up, you can take 20-30 grams of carbohydrates, preferably in the form of a drink.
- For those who are on the bench waiting to enter the game, or in any case during the time between the end of the last meal and the start of the match, it is useful to

sip the waiting rations consisting of: fructose + glucose + maltodextrin + water with the addition of mineral salts (the solution must be isotonic); they provide an immediate energy that lasts for a long time.
- During the match it is appropriate to take carbohydrates, whose oxidation is however slowed by the slow intestinal absorption due to the recruitment of blood flow at the level of the muscular district rather than splanchnic. To avoid receptor saturation, using only one source of carbohydrates, it is better to use mixtures that use different transporters and therefore, for example, a mixture glucose plus fructose is preferable. 30 grams per hour is the recommended amount.
- One of the priorities post-match is to restore muscle glycogen stores. The speed with which this process must be done depends on the time that elapses before the next training session or game. If the event is repeated in a short time (for example 3 games within the week and also one or two midweek training sessions) the recovery of glycogen should be started immediately after the post-match. In the two hours following the match, the intake of high and medium glycemic index carbohydrates is recommended. An insulin-independent process is present at this stage due to exercise-induced overexpression of the Glut 4 receptor for glucose without the need for elevated insulin levels.
- In this phase an intake of 1-1.2 g/kg body weight of carbohydrates per hour in the first two hours after the match is recommended, even in a fractioned way with several snacks every 20/30 minutes. This concentration represents the minimum amount of carbohydrates to be taken to obtain the maximum compensation of muscle glycogen through the activation of glycogen synthetase. Carbohydrates can be taken either in solid or liquid form, there is no difference but it depends on the preference of the player and the food must be already available in the locker room. This phase is insulin dependent and, therefore, it is preferred to use carbohydrates with low and medium glycemic index.
- In the following 24 hours the intake of 7/10 grams of carbohydrates per kg/kg of body weight is recommended. Obviously, these indications are generic because it is also important to take into account individual insulin sensitivity and in subjects "older" (close to 40 or over 40 years) this amount of carbohydrates should be reduced.

Water supply

Another very important aspect in sports activity is the hydro-saline reintegration, as even a minimal loss of the body water can negatively affect the sports performance. With 2.5% dehydration sprint time decreases, specific performance skills (dribbling skills) decrease and mental clarity is impaired. During training it is better to get used to sipping water, only for particularly intense and prolonged training with high sweating, and the game itself, is it appropriate to use sports drinks.

Refreshment drinks

Let's see what a rehydration drink to be taken before, during and after the game should consist on:

- simple and complex carbohydrates (usually a mix of glucose, maltodextrin and fructose) to replenish and preserve muscle glycogen stores; keeps energy constant during the game;
- minerals (sodium, calcium, magnesium and potassium) to partly compensate for those eliminated with sweat and to facilitate their recovery; prevents the onset of cramps during and after the match; stimulates (in the right relationship with carbohydrates) the passage of water from the intestine to the blood;
- protective vitamins: vitamins C and E with an antioxidant effect, but only in case of training or matches very intense and close together because the administration of exogenous antioxidants depresses the normal physiological response of the production of endogenous antioxidants following exercise;
- temperature: not cold;
- an isotonic drink is more preferable before and during the match, while after the match it will also be possible to consume a hypertonic one (i.e. more concentrated).

Reintegration must also be the function of favoring the compensation of biomechanical overload to increase athletic longevity which is often compromised by problems in the joints:

- aloe vera juice is useful because it is rich in mucopolysaccharides that have a significant moisturizing and protective capacity at the level of connective tissues;
- chicken broth which is particularly rich in collagen or even the direct intake of collagen peptides which have the biological action of stimulating the production of collagen by fibroblasts.
- vegetables, rich in minerals, and especially brassicas (broccoli, cabbage) rich in sulfur essential for the establishment of cross-links in osteo-articular tissues.

Soccer and supplementation

The phases that precede the game and the recovery phases after the physical effort are important moments in the life of a soccer player, on which one must act in order not to experience drops in the physical form and to count on maximum efficiency, even for several months. The association between supplementation, a suitable diet and a specific training allows us to lead the soccer player to a continuous improvement in his/her performance until his/her genetic potential is reached.

Each type and mode of supplementation must be customized for the individual soccer player (based on his/her position, lifestyle, resilience, etc.).

A "typical" plan could be the following:

- breakfast: multivitamins + multi-minerals + vitamin C + proteins 90% + glutamine, in order to reach a higher protein content, not reachable with food alone because this would involve greater metabolic and digestive work;
- lunch: vitamin B complex + iron + zinc;
- dinner: same as lunch
- before the training and/or the game: a beverage with carbohydrates (maltodextrin and fructose) + minerals + vitamin C and E + BCAA + creatine + caffeine + 650 mg of pomegranate extract.

It may also be useful to take:
- during: a beverage with carbohydrates (maltodextrin, glucose and fructose) + mineral salts;
- after the training: a beverage with simplex carbohydrates (glucose and sucrose) + mineral salts + hydrolyzed whey protein (or BCAA) + glutamine + creatine;
- about 45 minutes/an hour later: palatable and easily digestible smoothie that contains proteins, carbohydrates and fats omega 3 in the right proportions;
- 2 hours after exertion complex carbohydrates, solid lean protein, and moderate fat;
- before bed: glutamine + 90% casein protein + 480 mg of Montmorency red cherry extract for DOMS (Delayed Onset Muscle Soreness) reduction.

Additional considerations

- **Caffeine** has been shown to be able to increase repeated sprinting and jumping ability in soccer players, taken in a solution containing electrolytes and carbohydrates (1.8/kg body weight) at a dosage of 3.7 mg/kg body weight (approximately 200-300 mg) one hour before exercise, as well as giving a subjective feeling of less fatigue. In addition, in another study as well as jump performance, it has been shown to be able to improve the accuracy of steps.
- **Creatine** is another supplement that has made its appearance in the world of football in a disruptive manner, despite theoretically, that it should be a supplement more specific to strength sports. It has been seen to be able to improve performance in football players through its buffering effect on acidosis and then delaying the onset of muscle fatigue, and by favoring the resynthesis of phosphocreatine, which results in better performance in repeated sprints and jumping ability, and by increasing the speed of resynthesis of muscle glycogen after exercise in the initial 24 hours. However, it is not recommended in children or teens.
- Another supplement that can rightly find its application in soccer is **beta-alanine**, whose theoretical rationale depends on the fact that it represents the limiting precursor of carnosine synthesis, which at muscle level exerts an important buffering effect on the production of lactic acid. Given that in soccer there is a high presence of repeated sprints that use the anaerobic lactacid metabolism, beta-alanine can undoubtedly be useful by increasing the levels of carnosine. In a study carried out on 12 amateur soccer players the administration of 3.2 grams of beta-alanine improved the distance covered in a "yo-yo intermittent test" compared to the placebo group. As an undesired effect, there is the appearance of paresthesias, "tingling", which can be eliminated or significantly reduced by splitting the intake to no more than 800-1000 mg at a time during the course of the day and preferably at meals.
- **Nitrates** increase vasodilation, promote the distribution of oxygen and nutrients within contractile cells. Nitrates taken in the form of 140 mL beet juice administered at a dosage of 800 mg per day were able to improve the performance of trained soccer players subjected to intermittent high intensity exercise and a reduction in heart rate. The results of administration are acute because they are evident as early as five days after administration (Vanhatalo et al., 2009) and continue for at least two weeks after the end of intake.

- Insufficient levels of **vitamin D** (less than 30 ng/mL have been frequently observed in professional football players, especially in black athletes who physiologically have reduced vitamin D values, in the autumn and winter months. Given its influence on phospho-calcium metabolism, an inadequate level of vitamin D can cause alterations in the musculoskeletal system (also affecting muscle strength) increasing the risk of injury and delaying the recovery process from the same (Tyler Barker et al, 2013 and Shuler et al., 2012) as numerous scientific studies show. In a study on 67 players from two teams in the Greek Super League (Nikolaos E et al., 2013) a correlation between serum levels of vitamin D and muscle performance, aerobic capacity and speed was found.

A recommendation: of course, everything will have to be customized according to the needs and characteristics of the individual athlete.

CHAPTER 17

Nutrition and cycling

Cycling is a sport that involves the aerobic metabolism (mainly) but also the anaerobic one (just think of the final sprints), and therefore the substrates used, in terms of energy, are represented by both fats and carbohydrates. An adequate protein intake is useful for maintaining the body structure, for the synthesis of enzymes, hormones, transport proteins and for the super-compensation that occurs after strenuous training or competitions. Let's not forget that a portion of protein is always used for energy purposes, especially when the consumption of other substrates (carbohydrates and fats) is compromised, so as to involve a sort of "self-cannibalization" of the muscle mass (precisely to obtain energy), with a consequent catabolism that penalizes the performance and slows down the recovery time.

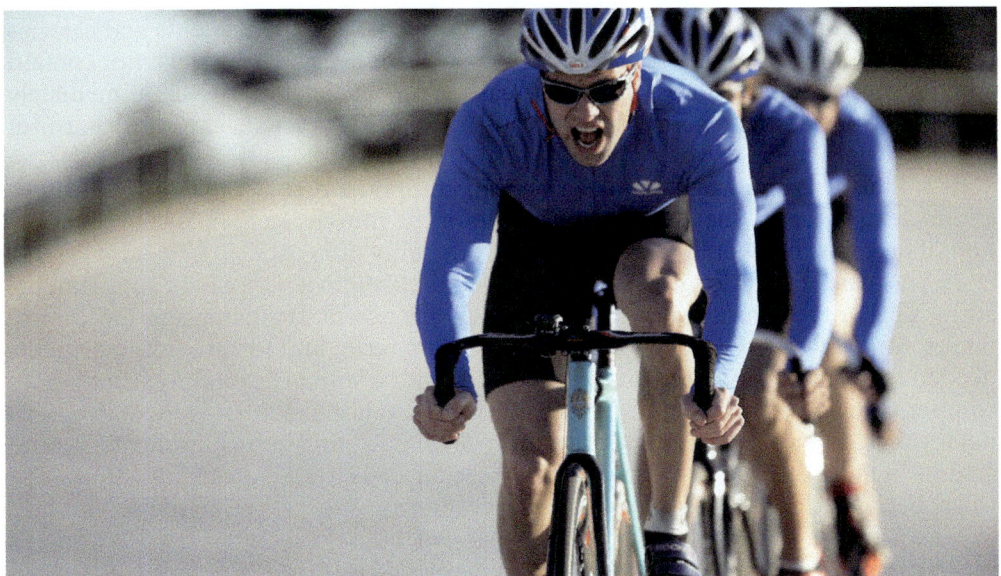

Figure 17.1

In this sport, it is very important to adapt the introduction of macro- and micro-nutrients according to the competitive or off-season period, according to the athlete's characteristics, the environmental ones, etc., as they can extremely diversify the energy expenditure and can therefore bring new food problems for each race. Therefore, it is not possible to propose a general dietary framework, but the diet must be customized for each subject and situation. It must also be considered that cyclists reach the highest levels of caloric consumption (up to 10 Kcal/hour/kg of body weight) and that their expenditure is not limited to a few minutes, it can also last many hours, with a consumption that, during stage races, can be estimated in the order of 5000-8000 Kcal/day, is difficult to be supplied only with food.

The caloric calculation must also take into account the cyclist's need to maintain a certain quality body weight, as cycling is a sport in which the movement of the body goes against the force of gravity and therefore the most favorable weight/power ratio must be sought, targeting not only the lowest body weight, but the body weight with the lowest fat mass and the highest lean mass, always in function of the best sports performance. Therefore, the most suitable combinations between the nutrition and supplementation must be sought, taking into account all the factors listed above and periodizing them according to the different preparation periods.

The diet while being away from training is not difficult to prepare and it must consist of simple foods, easily digestible and absorbable, balanced in its components and completed with a multivitamin + multi-mineral supplement for the increased metabolic demands and the increased consumption of these nutrients in the biochemical reactions; the "critical" point concerns the diet to be followed just before, during and after the performance.

An hour before the performance, supplementation with carnitine and beta-alanine may be useful to improve the use of fats for energy purposes and to dilute the feeling of fatigue, as these substances act with a dampening effect on the formation of lactic acid. If the last meal before the race has provided all the nutrients and calories in the right quantities and proportions, the pre-competition snack must not contain a high proportion of calories, it must be easily absorbable and provide immediately usable and long-lasting energy, without causing blood sugar changes that are harmful to the athlete.

It will also be important to take a protein component (preferably in the form of amino acids) that will be "sacrificed" instead of the muscle, in the place of that portion of proteins that would have been used for energy purposes.

In this case, the following prove to be useful: protein-energy bars supplemented by a mix of vitamins and minerals, which are useful for increasing the calorie intake, for providing energy in the short and long term, and for providing proteins needed for the metabolic turnover; smoothies with a suitable protein-carbohydrate composition; isotonic hydrosaline solutions with maltodextrin and fructose, essential for proper hydration and for the supply of an easy-to-use fuel; branched amino acids which also serve to reduce the formation of lactic acid during the muscle work: beta-alanine is also very useful for its buffering effect through the production of carnosine.

To overcome the hunger crises and the energy drops during bike rides (especially if they are long-lasting), it will be necessary to rely on foods that are not bulky, which have a low weight, are comfortable to carry, digestible and easy to assimilate, which do not create chewing problems and insalivation. Energy bars and saline-energy supplements will be fine; if the performance lasts for a long time, it will be useful to consume (preferably in a liquid form) a source of amino acids so that the amino acid spectrum in the blood does not drop dramatically.

Twenty minutes before the final sprint, you can take simple sugars such as glucose, which give an energy that can be quickly used thanks to the hyperglycemia caused by glucose. If this hyperglycemia at other times can be counterproductive because it can cause a reactive hypoglycemia (blood sugars drops quickly) with a sense of exhaustion and a reduced performance, in this case it is productive as we try to match the glycemic peak, which gives us a lot of energy to use at the moment of the sprint at the end of the race, which lasts a few seconds, without worrying if after the race we might have a decrease in energy.

After the competition and/or training, the glycogen stores must be recovered as soon as possible, even in the event of difficulty of taking adequate quantities of food, due to a situation of transient post-activity anorexia (especially if it has been intense). Solutions containing proteins, carbohydrates, lipids and fibers in adequate proportions are therefore useful, possibly preceded by the ingestion of branched-chain amino acids and glucose, which promptly initiate the reconstruction of damaged muscles and the replenishment of the glycogen stocks. This last stage of nutrition is also essential, as the sooner and better you recover, the more intensely you will be able to face the following trainings and competitions.

The meal that will be consumed a few hours after the race, when the muscles have decongested from the accumulated blood, must be complete in its nutrients, but also made up of foods with alkalizing and detoxifying properties, to allow for a better elimination of toxins from the body.

As for the breakdown of the macronutrients in the diet during the day, it will have to be customized according to the cyclist's metabolism, since some of them perform better with many carbohydrates and few fats and others, on the contrary, do better with more fats and less carbohydrates.

The indications that are usually given may apply to some, but not to all. For this reason, everyone must try and find the optimal combinations for themselves, naturally with the support of nutritionists who, on the dietary level, can indicate the most suitable and correct foods, and on the metabolic level, they can detect any anomalies through the evaluation of blood chemistry parameters. In this way, they can be corrected through nutrition and supplementation, or in any case they can send the cyclist to more specialized doctors.

CHAPTER 18

Nutrition and CrossFit

CrossFit is a recent sport discipline, from the point of view of the metabolic needs it is very complex as it is necessary to be strong, resistant, explosive and have a good base of an aerobic capacity, which is very difficult as each of these skills can develop at their maximum only thanks to a high level of specialization, which excludes the maximum performance in the other disciplines. As a result, the CrossFitter must train to have a very high, albeit not maximal, average capacity in all of these skills, and this often involves several hours of daily training, which very easily predisposes to an overtraining state. Obviously, given these premises, adequate nutrition and also a relative integration become essential to ensure the necessary recovery and the possibility of having performance improvements.

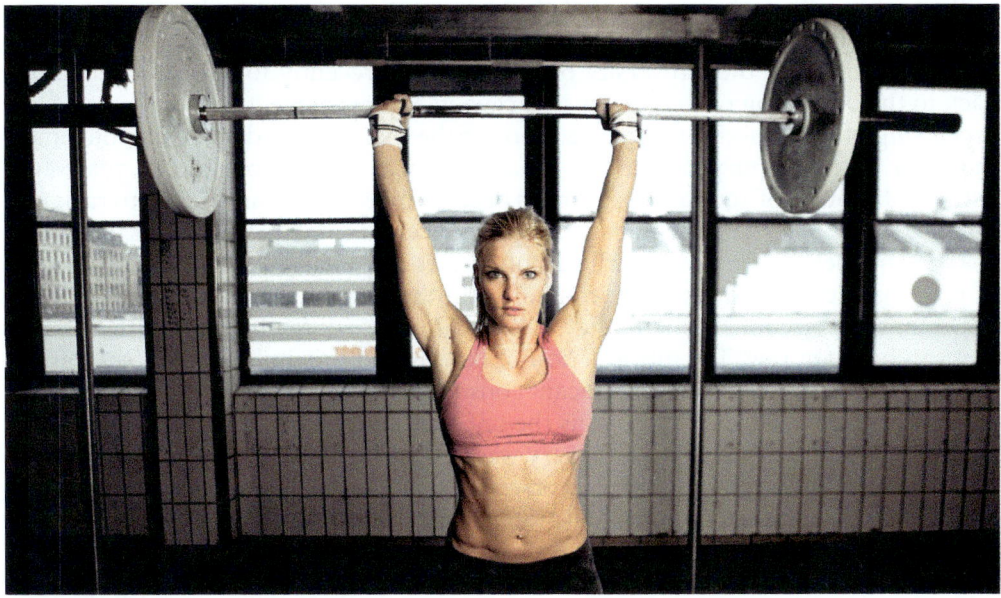

Figure 18.1

The main problem of the CrossFitter is represented by the fact that most of its work engages the anaerobic-lactacid metabolism and therefore it must absolutely counteract this tendency to acidosis with nutrition (and supplementation), in addition to providing the necessary amount of protein for the muscle development, and good quality carbohydrates to make up for the specific energy and the metabolic requirements; which could be translated into meat and fish, lots of vegetables, fresh fruit and nuts. These characteristics are typical of the Paleo Diet, which in some cases was adopted almost "religiously", by the majority of the CrossFitters. Let's see what it is.

The Paleodiet

The Paleodiet is actually the oldest diet in the world, which means, it is the diet that cavemen followed in the period prior to the discovery of agriculture, which occurred about 10,000 years ago. For about two million years, humans had been hunter-gatherers and their livelihood was based on what they could find: fruits, berries and honey as a source of carbohydrates; the need for fats and proteins was instead covered by seeds, pits, caterpillars, snails, insects, eggs, fish, crustaceans, and above all by the internal organs and the brain of the animals, which were more easily digestible than the raw meat of the muscle bands, very rich of connective tissue. Only with the use of fire, about 300,000 years ago, the muscles of the hunted animals were better exploited, being able to roast the meat and also the legumes, which were made digestible by cooking.

The forcibly nomadic humans fed themselves by collecting food where they found it, also feeding on carcasses, fishing and hunting, following the movements of their prey. This lifestyle has shaped our predecessors by genetic selection for more than a million years, although it seems that the consumption of wild grains among hunter-gatherer populations can be traced back to about 100,000 years ago. In fact, some archaeologists from the University of Calgary have recently found artifacts dating back to the beginning of the ice age in a cave in Mozambique, that demonstrate the processing of wild sorghum, a predecessor of the main cereal that is still consumed today for nutrition purposes in sub-Saharan Africa. Then, about 10,000 years ago, with the discovery of agriculture, humans became more settled and began to raise animals, not only to feed on them, but also to produce milk and its derivatives. With this change, the diet was enriched with carbohydrates (especially cereals) at the expense of proteins. Cereals, however, are not edible in their raw state and require cooking; however, even by cooking them, they still remain more difficult to digest than foods that can be eaten raw. The introduction of cereals and this imbalance in the carbohydrate/protein ratio has had significant consequences on humans. In the Paleolithic Age the average height was as high as the one that has only been reached nowadays; the average height of a Roman legionary was instead around 165 cm.

Life expectancy in the Neolithic worsened, as men fell ill more easily. When carbohydrates are in excess compared to proteins and fats, insulin resistance and inflammation develop in the body, which are the basis of the most chronic and degenerative diseases. As for milk, it should be noted that humans are the only animal that continues to feed on milk even after weaning (although, to be honest, it must be said that other animals are not able to obtain it easily, and if we give it to them, they do not disdain it).

For the newborn, breast milk is the only and the best nourishment, but cow's milk is certainly not, as it differs in percentages of the composition of macro- and micronutrients. As for the irreplaceable nature of milk and its derivatives as a source of calcium (useful for the development of bones and teeth), it must be recognized that Paleolithic humans had strong bones and teeth, without signs of osteoporosis, as evidenced by the fossil records. Without a doubt, a diet that was rich in fruits and vegetables created an alkaline environment with protective effects for the bones and health in general; vice versa, cereals and dairy products are acidifying foods, which favor the loss of calcium from the bones. Calcium, among other things, is also present in considerable quantities in all nuts, raw seeds and vegetables.

One of the most common criticisms leveled at this diet is that it is a high-protein diet; in reality, this is not the case, as carbohydrates were well present, not in the form of cereals, but in fruits and vegetables. The percentages were not fixed, but could also vary as a result of the availability of food and depending on the climate and the season. A range is indicated, in which carbohydrates go from 20 to 40%, proteins from 20 to 35% and fats from 30 to 60%. So, at certain times, it could have been a hyperlipidic diet. However, it must be considered that the fats were mostly healthy, as they were mainly from fish and nuts, and also the fats deriving from the brains and muscles of the animals were particularly rich in omega-3, the brain due to its rich lipid structure of DHA and meat because of animals that ate mainly fresh grass. Undoubtedly, a limitation of this diet is the lack of practicality and the organolepticity. We can hardly get used to eating brains, worms and industrial quantities of vegetables, which certainly, thanks to the normal fermentation processes, would produce large quantities of gas that in our civilized society can be a social problem.

However, we could implement some useful precautions for our health: starting to have many small meals instead of a few abundant ones (thus, the insulin stimulation is reduced); limiting the consumption of cereals twice a week and consuming more fruits and vegetables. As for athletes, some need more carbohydrates, and the case of the Paleodiet runs the risk of being too low-carb: we can then also consume non-Paleolithic foods, such as potatoes (alkalizing) – preferably, the American red potatoes to lower the glycemic index, the violet potatoes which are rich in antioxidants and cereals, preferably gluten-free and with a low glycemic index, such as basmati rice, or the so-called pseudo-cereals, such as quinoa, amaranth and buckwheat.

Consuming sprouted grains and legumes can also be beneficial. By doing so, the present anti-nutrients are considerably reduced; in this case, they become real vegetables that are rich in predigested starch, and phytic acid, which counteracts the intestinal absorption of various minerals, is eliminated. As for salt, the body's need for sodium should be covered by the quantity that is present in foods or possibly also using iodized salt. Regarding alcohol, some argue that perhaps even Paleolithic humans could occasionally consume fermented fruits with a relative formation of alcohol. Therefore, even for us, any alcohol consumption must only be occasional. Milk and its derivatives must also be eliminated, and obviously corn and various seed oils must be completely eliminated because they are too rich in omega-6 fatty acids, which have a pro-inflammatory effect. Trans fats, i.e. hydrogenated ones, which are present in margarines and in various packaged products, are very dangerous for our health and therefore should be eliminated. Unfortunately, 55% of the Western diet is based on foods that our ancestors did not know, such as cereals, dairy products, prepared and processed foods, sausages, refined flour, sweeteners and hydrogenated fatty acids. The consequences of this new "enriched" diet are premature aging and the increase in degenerative diseases, such as cardiovascular diseases, tumors, arthritis, diabetes, obesity and, most recently, the "metabolic syndrome". It could be objected that over time, there have been genetic modifications that have allowed humans to adapt to the consumption of dairy products and cereals, but the great spread of lactose and gluten intolerances suggests the opposite. If we want to be sure of this, in our specific case Nutrigenomics is now available, that is the possibility to identify the genetic nutritional biochemical profile of the single individual through a DNA test that is carried out with a buccal swab.

The other problem of CrossFitters is the production of cortisol, which in these athletes, given the size and intensity of the training, is almost always high. The diet aimed at controlling cortisol includes several meals distributed throughout the day, possibly spaced no more than three to four hours, and a combination of macronutrients in percentages of about 40-30-30 (carbohydrates – proteins – fats), with low glycemic index carbohydrates which raise the blood sugar just slightly, in order to avoid the glycemic fluctuations that contribute to the production of cortisol: since this is a hyperglycemic hormone, it is in fact stimulated following a possible reactive hypoglycemia due to an excess of high glycemic index carbohydrates. But these are concepts of the Zone Diet, which we will illustrate below.

The Zone Diet

This type of diet is also known as the 40-30-30 diet (protein/carbohydrate ratio = 0.75) due to the fact that it provides 40% of calories from carbohydrates, 30% from proteins and 30% from fats in every meal and/or snack. The success of the Zone Diet is due to its long-lasting effectiveness and the benefits obtained by both amateur and competitive athletes. Sportspeople must try to take care of their nutrition and lifestyle as much as possible, as they cannot afford to train without progressive improvements, otherwise this would negatively affect the possibility of getting the most out of what they are doing. If you are working hard to obtain a relevant result, you need to structure a profitable training, have a positive mental attitude and a suitable and balanced diet that will be followed in the days, months and even in the years preceding the competitive event (so why not follow it for life?).

The Zone Diet is a balanced diet, certainly suitable for at least 50% of individuals; 25% might be better off with a higher percentage of carbohydrates and 25% with a lower one. However, when it is applied to subjects who do not follow a structured diet that is suitable for them, it always produces improvements.

It has been proven in professional football, soccer and swimming teams (but not only), that those who train following this diet obtain great improvements in their performances. We know that every performance, to be taken to the highest level, requires an adaptation of the body to a constant training. This adaptation is however, achieved and mediated by hormonal systems, which allow the athlete to increase workloads by raising their stimulus resistance threshold and leading to continuous improvements; when the hormonal balances are in the correct ratio, then the athlete is said to be in the "Zone". The secret of the performance lies in understanding how the training and the diet affect these hormonal systems. A diet that is too rich in carbohydrates (often recommended for athletes and it causes a high production of insulin) prevents access to the "Zone" and therefore makes it impossible for the athlete to express himself/herself to his/her fullest potential, precisely because the hormonal systems are not in a balance.

Why then certain athletes, even if they consume a lot of carbohydrates, manage to win and still express themselves at high levels? This depends, in the first place, on genetics, which allow some people to tolerate carbohydrates well; moreover, those who constantly practice sports have the opportunity to eat a few more carbohydrates while maintaining a normal insulin secretion, as the muscles readily use the glucose that reaches the blood level; on the other hand, they haven't tried the Zone to see if it is able to improve them further.

It must be said that the body takes time to adapt to using fats instead of carbohydrates, and for this reason some athletes (and non-athletes) do not immediately benefit from the Zone Diet. However, when the body becomes fully operational, you will be able to obtain some results, such as:

- improved resistance;
- decreased fatigue;
- more efficient use of fat storages;
- increase of the immune response and improvement of the inflammatory parameters;
- reduced recovery times;
- fewer injuries;
- better lean mass/fat mass ratio.

Following the Zone, the caloric needs introduced from the outside can be significantly reduced as the athletes have access to their fat reserves as the main source of energy. Furthermore, by keeping the blood sugar constant for four to six hours, the feeling of hunger is eliminated. This does not mean that if you are not hungry you can skip the snacks; indeed, you must remember to take them, otherwise you run the risk of hypoglycemia with a decline in the athletic performance and more. The hormonal benefits of the Zone Diet mean that the precious muscle glycogen is spared, accelerating the release of fatty acids from the adipose tissue. This occurs both during training and at rest; that's why you have a quick weight loss. Oxygen is better conveyed into the bloodstream, reducing the muscle fatigue and helps to maintain better mental clarity (also thanks to the stability of blood sugar levels). In practice, to benefit from the hormonal implications of the training and nutrition, it is sufficient to indulge a snack in the Zone 30 minutes before starting and another one as soon as the activity is over. The first one allows you to enter the Zone more easily during the training and helps to burn more fat, the second allows you to continue to remain in the Zone even after the training and helps you to recover more quickly in both muscular and mental terms. Of course, for sports that exceed an hour and a half of training, a small snack will be needed every 45-60 minutes from the beginning of the performance (however, the timing is subjective). By making each meal a meal in the Zone, hormonal benefits are obtained 24 hours a day and not only during the training, and it is now established that recovery is a fundamental part of achieving improvements. So, if we optimize this process, in exchange we can have progress for our physical performance and our organism.

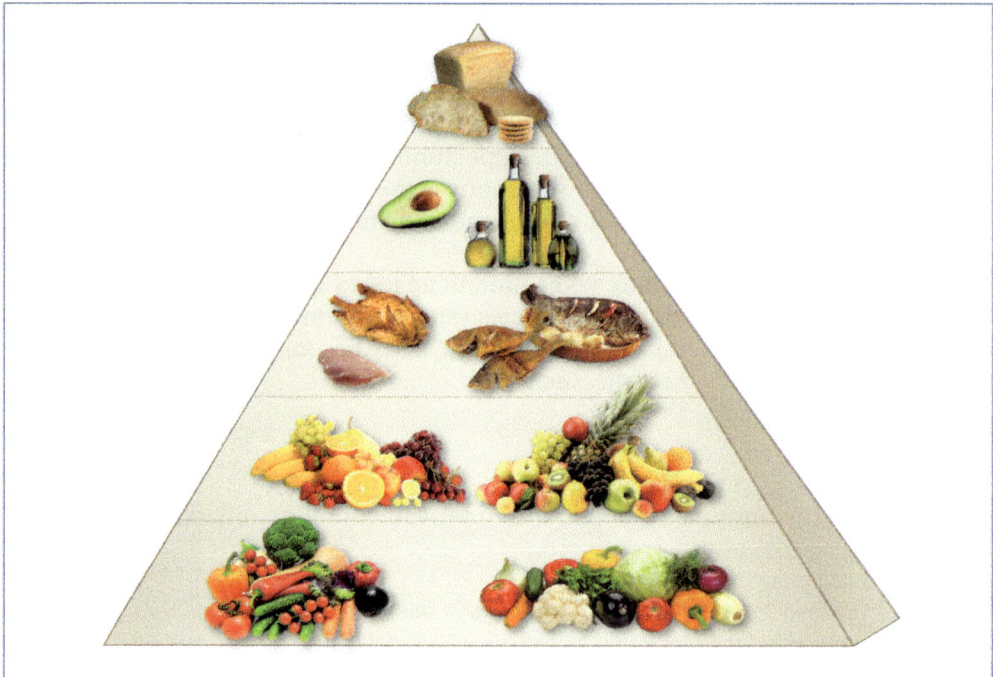

Figure 18.2 The pyramid of the Zone Diet.

Physiological benefits for athletes entering the Zone

- A constant blood sugar level in the brain that will allow a greater clarity, concentration and freshness.
- Lack of hunger and of the need for sugar, as there will be a constant sugar level.
- Fatty acids are released from the adipose tissue at a higher rate, allowing a more effective use of the stored fat, both during training and at rest.
- Thanks to the rebalancing of eicosanoids (vasodilators and bronchodilators), the transfer of oxygen is increased, therefore muscle efficiency and aerobic capacity will increase and fatigue will decrease.
- There will be an ideal secretion of hormones such as testosterone and growth hormone (GH), which are very important for improving the performance and increasing the muscle mass.
- We will achieve a control of the eicosanoid PGE2 which, if in excess, stimulates the production of cortisol, responsible for muscle catabolism.

List of foods by their main macronutrient

Carbohydrates

Cereals	Favorable	Recommended: rye, barley and spelt are slow inducers for insulin, while oats are also recommended because they contain essential fatty acids, precursors of anti-inflammatory eicosanoids (oat flakes for breakfast).
	Unfavorable	To be consumed in moderation: wheat flours (bread, pasta, rice, pizza, biscuits, slices, bread sticks), corn (cornflakes) and rice (soups, risottos, puffed rice and crackers).
Desserts	All unfavorable	They can be taken only if unfavorable bread and pasta have been avoided in the meal and the established carbohydrate levels have not been reached (better to limit them to once a week).
Fruits	Favorable	It varies, without overdoing it (apples, pears, berries).
	Unfavorable	Limit the consumption of very ripe bananas, grapes, dates, figs, persimmons.
Vegetables	Favorable	Especially leafy vegetables (radicchio, fennel, cabbage, cauliflower, lettuce, spinach, cabbage), green beans, onions, beans, tomatoes, peppers, radishes, zucchini etc. are also excellent.
	Unfavorable	Limit your consumption of cooked carrots, beets, squash, potatoes, and processed vegetables.
Sugar	Favorable	Fructose, excellent for its low glycemic index (slow insulin inducer) but to be consumed in low quantities. Xylitol is even better as a sweetener.
	Unfavorable	Sucrose (cooking sugar) and glucose.

Proteins

Meats	Favorable	Chicken, turkey, ostrich, rabbit, lean cuts of red meat, defatted raw ham, bresaola.
	Unfavorable	Fatty cuts of red meat, sausages, processed meats..
Fish	Favorable	At least three times a week, salmon is excellent, then mackerel, cod, tuna, swordfish..
	Unfavorable	Eel, tilapia.
Dairy products	Favorable	Cottage cheese, ricotta, low-fat or light cheeses (fatless than 20%). Semi-skimmed milk and low-fat plain yogurt are perfect and have the ideal proportions.
	Unfavorable	Fatty cheeses, whole milk.
Eggs	Favorable	Egg whites.
	Unfavorable	Yolk. Two whole eggs a week (never in the same meal) soft-boiled or fried, plus only cooked egg white. These indications are due to the fact that egg yolk is particu-

larly rich in arachidonic acid, an omega-6 that would unbalance the ratio with omega-3s. Personally, given my experience, I think that, if you follow a diet with little amounts of red meats and dairy products, you can reach a consumption of six eggs per week while maintaining an excellent AA/EPA (omega-6/omega-3) ratio, and at the same time favoring the contribution of substrates that favor the production of testosterone which are present in the yolk (vitamin D, arachidonic acid, non-oxidized cholesterol) and of substances such as phospholipids, which have an anti-atherosclerotic effect.

Legumes	**Favorable**	The use of soy derivatives and other legumes such as broad beans, lentils and beans is recommended.
	Unfavorable	Peas (pay attention to the carbohydrate quantity of legumes, as they could greatly affect the exact ratio between the three macronutrients and therefore sabotage the Zone Diet without the subject realizing it).
Fats	**Favorable**	Prefer extra virgin olive oil, olives, almonds, cashews, pistachios, hazelnuts, avocados.
	Unfavorable	If possible, avoid butter, lard, sausages and meats that are too rich in saturated fats.

Eliminate the hydrogenated and/or partially hydrogenated vegetable fats contained in many prepackaged foods of an industrial manufacture (see most of the snacks, some margarines, and most of those included as ingredients in industrial products etc. Read carefully the labels of the products that you buy).

The rules for entering the Zone
1. Calculate how much protein your body needs and divide it into the meals of the day. Never consume more or less.
2. Every time you eat, make sure that the ratio between the grams of protein and those of carbohydrates at each meal is 0.75 or in any case between 0.5 and 1. A ratio of 1 is more suitable for weight loss, as the percentages of the macronutrients become 33/33/33 and we automatically have a hypocaloric diet. A ratio of 0.5 is instead more suitable for athletes who finalize their training for strength and muscle building, and therefore the percentages become 50/25/25. A ratio of 0.75 may be best for a CrossFit athlete; the additional caloric needs, in addition to those provided by carbohydrates and proteins, must be filled by fats, which can therefore reach a level above 30%, with the result of creating a better metabolic adaptation of their use for energy purposes. Let me explain in a simpler way: we start from the protein requirements (for example, 2 g per kg of body weight in a 75 kg athlete is 150 g, which is equivalent to 600 Kcal), carbohydrates are added in order to respect the 0.75 ratio (225 g which are equivalent to 900 Kcal); at this point the fats are added to reach the necessary calories (in a 75 kg athlete who trains twice a day, the calorie consumption can easily reach about

3000 Kcal), and therefore, adding 1500 Kcal of fat, the diet becomes 30/20/50, i.e. 30% carbohydrates, 20% protein and 50% fat.
3. Distribute the food throughout the day in three meals and two snacks; do not consume more than 500 calories per meal and if your calorie needs are particularly high, increase the number of meals and/or snacks.
4. Never let more than five hours go by without eating (between meals and snacks). To eat you don't have to wait until you are hungry, otherwise it will be too late and you have probably left the Zone.
5. Choose protein foods with low-saturated fats.
6. Choose as a source of carbohydrates those foods that are considered favorable (vegetables and fruits which are rich in fibers and low in sugars).
7. As a source of fat, choose those foods that contain monounsaturated fatty acids. If you have a low-fat percentage, increase the amount of fat throughout the day. Avoid saturated fats and hydrogenated oils, such as margarine. The best sources of fat are almonds, walnuts, hazelnuts, avocado and olive oil. It is important to eat foods such as salmon, sardines, tuna or mackerel, or else consider supplementing with omega-3 fatty acids. Limit foods with a high content of arachidonic acid, such as organ meats, red meats and egg yolks.
8. Regularly recalculate your body composition to make dietary changes if necessary.
9. Drink plenty of water throughout the day; it is essential for the proper functioning of our body, helps fight water retention, is important for thermoregulation and is the component present in the highest quantity in our body.
10. If you leave the Zone for a short time because you missed a meal, don't worry, because you can easily re-enter with the next one and then stay there for as long as possible.

At this point, having seen the advantages of the Zone Diet, I would advise the proponents of the Paleo diet, who follow it almost "religiously", to move at least to the **Paleozone**, where the concepts of glycemic balance, the contribution of anti-inflammatory omega-3s, of the ratio between the various macronutrients, typical for the Zone, are adapted to the exclusion criteria of certain Paleo foods. But why should CrossFitters be careful not to overindulge carbohydrates and not eat large amounts like bulking bodybuilders? Well, once again the problem of acidosis comes into play, caused not only by lactic acid, but also by the hydrogen ion H+ of ATP hydrolysis, which is the real limiting factor in CrossFit performance.

In bodybuilding, maximizing the production of lactic acid is not a problem, on the contrary, I would say that it is almost a purpose, considering that the production of lactic acid is the basis of those metabolic situations that favor the production of GH and testosterone. In addition, it also creates the condition of a decreased elasticity of titin and nebulin proteins which, being anchored at the cell membrane level, favor those microtraumas during the eccentric phase, which cause the paracrine release of growth factors such as IGF1 and MGF, which in turn are essential to trigger the repair mechanisms and the muscle growth. In CrossFit, lactic acid does not allow the continuation of the performance as it blocks the contractile abilities in the muscles. A "WOD" that lasts from 15 to 20 minutes, despite being predominantly anaerobic-lactic acid, necessarily involves the aerobic metabolism which is, among other things, even more fundamental for the recovery between one performance and another. If we follow a diet that is very rich in carbohydrates, our body will necessarily develop enzymes that are responsible for glycolysis, both anaerobically and aerobically, favoring the use of glucose as an obligatory fuel at an anaerobic level and also as a preferential source at an aerobic level; this can easily lead to hypoglycemia during exercise, with energy drops at a psychophysical level, and early depletion of muscle glycogen stores. If, on the other hand, through a diet in which the balance of macronutrients favors a stable blood sugar level and a balanced insulin (insulin prevents the use of fats for energy purposes), the body progressively develops those metabolic enzymatic pathways that allow the use of fats for energy purposes. Since fats can only be used in the aerobic metabolism, they will be more easily used than on an unbalanced diet on carbohydrates. Remember that when we talk about energy metabolisms we always refer to prevalence. However, in an effort of 15-20 minutes there is an intervention of the aerobic metabolism that can be more easily supported by the greater availability of lipid substrates, by a diet that leads to an insulin calm with a lower intake of carbohydrates and a higher intake of fats. It is precisely the Zone Diet, and this also translates into a lower production of lactic acid. Returning to the other problem of CrossFitters, that is the high levels of cortisol, we can adopt the concept of the Cronormorphodieta (or COM Diet), which involves a greater consumption of carbohydrates in the evening to promote the production of serotonin and leptin, and decrease the production of cortisol. In this case, to always remain within the Zone balance, the meals before dinner should be structured with a 33-33-33 ratio or, to say it better, a protein/carbohydrate ratio equal to 1 (as fats can be increased based on caloric needs). Dinner, instead, should have a 50-25-25 ratio or a protein/carbohydrate ratio of 0.5 (as you know, the Zone Diet provides a protein/carbohydrate ratio between 0.5 and 1). Furthermore, this timing of the macronutrients intake is even more favorable to the use of fats for energy purposes during the intra-training recovery phases and, especially if the heavier training is carried out in the afternoon-evening, it favors the recovery of the muscle glycogen and it inhibits the post-workout protein catabolism, making the anabolic pathways prevail.

A brief mention of the most useful supplements for CrossFit: beta-alanine to buffer the lactic acid, phosphatidylserine to decrease cortisol, both before training; *Rhodiola rosea* for the modulation of cortisol, potassium and magnesium citrates for basifying in the morning; calcium and magnesium citrates to basify and melatonin to lower cortisol levels in the evening before bedtime.

My personal experience with competitive CrossFit athletes, at high levels or not, has allowed me to find through an examination that I carry out routinely (the hair analysis/examination of the hair bulb), significant deficiencies at the cellular level of minerals, vitamins, amino acids and even hormones. I have no hesitation in defining CrossFit at a competitive level as an extreme sport for the body's metabolic systems and it is purely utopian to think that it cannot lead to deficiencies and overtraining without the adequate nutrition and specific dietary supplements. Supplements must be often tailored for the athlete, because, when physical activity is so high, the deficiencies can be expressed not only the basis of the insufficient supplies, but also by different mechanisms of metabolization, absorption, elimination, transformation, which may depend on particular genetically characterized metabolic pathways. The rebalancing of these deficiencies through a specific intake of supplements, then verified with a subsequent examination, has always led to a significant improvement in the state of well-being and performance.

CHAPTER 19

Nutrition and swimming
by Giovanni Montagna

Those who practice sports, whether competitive or not, often focus a lot on training, unfortunately leaving out the aspect of nutrition and supplementation; yet nutrition is part of what can be defined as an *invisible training*, which is, all the rules of life that are just as important as training in the strict sense. Proper nutrition is very important for those who practice sports: it can improve the physical performance and the recovery. It is therefore essential to eat well and in a functional way. The balance and the variety of foods are fundamental. Eating correctly before a workout allows you to give the body the right sprint, to improve the physical performance and recover faster.

Nutrition must be taken care of for 365 days a year, because the body must respect a timing of adaptation to the diet itself that does not require a few days, but

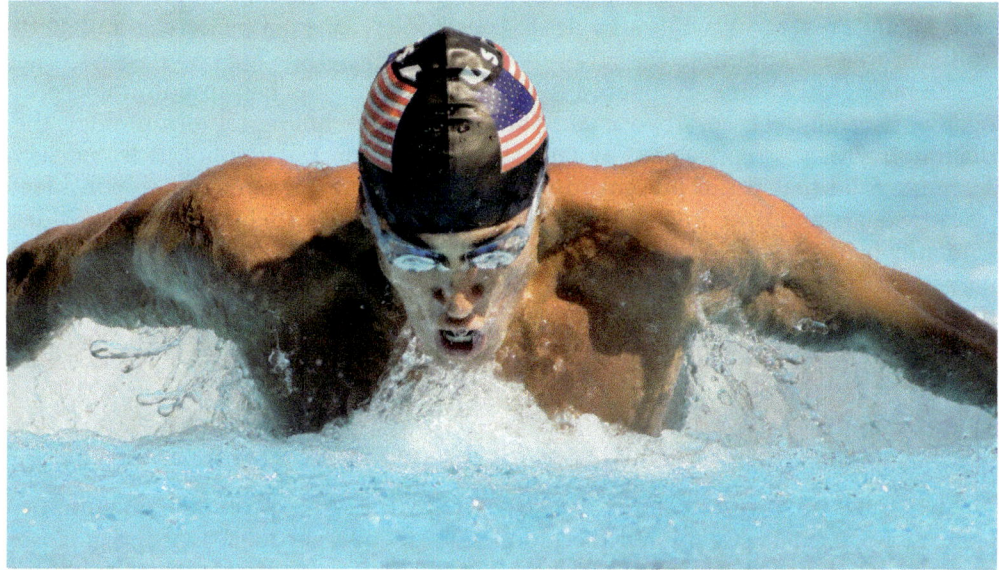

Figure 19.1

weeks and, in some cases, months. Even in swimming, perhaps more than in other sports, nutrition plays a fundamental role, as if the consumption of the food is not calculated in the right time before a competition or training in the water, in addition to a decrease in performance, there is also a danger of congestion, which can have serious health consequences. Also for this discipline, there can be a competitive period and a period away from the competitions, in which specific preparations are carried out in the pool and in the gym. The diet will be slightly different in these two periods, especially in terms of ease of digestion and the amount of nutrients taken, to bring the athlete to the optimal weight in competitive periods and/or to increase the muscle mass (if necessary) in the periods where he/she is away from competitions.

Let's first make an anthropological premise.

The human species has been eating wild animals and berries for several million years.

The average ascertained height of our ancestors, hominin hunters with decathletic bodies, was between 160 and 170 cm. Agriculture and pastoralism have been developed only in the last 10,000 years, followed by the dairy processing technology. This evolutionary process has allowed for a greater supply of food and therefore the demographic explosion. But in such a short time the human species has not had the ability to change its genetic makeup compared to the new diets which are rich in cereals and dairy products. The poor genetic adaptation to these foods manifests itself with various allergy phenomena on a significant percentage of the population. It is no coincidence that the average height of predominantly vegetarian populations is only 165 cm. From the genetic point of view, the human species, even after the second millennium, remained predominantly omnivorous and had to reconsider the role of protein foods, such as lean meats and fish, the same foods used by our ancient ancestors. It is no coincidence that people who are allergic to animal proteins (meat and fish) are a real rarity, while allergies to "new foods", for example cereals and dairy products, are very common.

The biological engine, compared to the mechanical one, has an admirable prerogative: it can in fact work by varying the fuel (or, with biological terminology, the substrate), which is represented by fats, sugars, proteins and alcohol. If we neglect alcohol, a food that is not present in nature, and if we limit ourselves to considering fats, sugars and proteins, we discover that the choice of fuel is carried out independently by the muscle cells, mainly based on the type of work and the availability of the substrate (fats, sugars, proteins). Therefore, if we want to tackle the problem of the nutrition in sports, we must take into account the metabolic choices made independently by the body and see what we can do to convey the body towards the use of a better substrate.

How many and which carbohydrates for the swimmer?

Carbohydrates provide 4 Kcal/g. In sports, carbohydrates are of fundamental importance as the nervous system and red blood cells operate particularly using glucose. Research has shown that the intake of low glycemic index (GI) carbohydrates before a prolonged muscle engagement is capable of exerting several positive effects:

- more stable blood sugar levels for longer exercise times;
- moderate insulin response with less interference on the lipid metabolism;
- performance improvement;
- less lactic acid production compared to a high GI meal;
- delay in the onset of fatigue.

Carbohydrates also play a role in the metabolization of proteins, a role which is then completed with a detoxifying function in the elimination of the nitrogenous waste. With the same function, they intervene in the demolition of fats, especially in slimming diets, where they counteract the acidity of the blood due to the formation of ketone bodies (acids derived from acetoacetic acid). Still in relation to slimming diets and the GI, recent researches have drawn attention to how the diet, in relation to the GI of foods, can significantly affect the determination of certain conditions:

- the improvement of plasma lipids and the reduction of the fat mass, while maintaining the lean mass by administering low GI diets;
- the reduction of the potential capacity of lipid utilization for energy purposes
- after consuming a meal rich in high GI carbohydrates;
- higher voluntary food intake following the consumption of a high GI meal compared to a low GI meal.

We also know that glucose is also the only fuel that the brain can use and, if a situation of glucose hunger (caused by a glucose depletion also due to the ingestion of high glycemic index carbohydrates) occurs, the brain becomes unable to think clearly and reflexes cloud over. The glycogen contained in the liver is the major supplier of glucose in order to keep the blood sugar stable during the physical activity and beyond. If we have high levels of insulin in the circulation (an event that occurs after the ingestion of high GI carbohydrates), this blocks the release of glucose from the hepatic glycogen and the risk of going into hypoglycemia is almost certain. By maintaining stable levels of blood sugar and insulin (low GI carbohydrates), this effect does not occur, and indeed we will also have greater quantities of available fats (and therefore more energy), which are easily released from the adipose tissue and used in the muscles.

How many and which fats for the swimmer?

Fats provide 9 Kcal/g. Unfortunately, the science of nutrition has excessively demonized fats, not distinguishing those that are truly harmful from those that have an energetic and healthy function. Among fats, mono and polyunsaturated ones and untreated ones must be preferred. It is not necessary to completely exclude cholesterol-bearing foods (for example eggs), as this molecule is the precursor of many hormones, including testosterone, which is very useful for maintaining a good muscle mass and for the reactivity of the performance. *Polyunsaturated* fats provide linoleic (omega-6) and alpha-linolenic (omega-3) acids, which cannot be synthesized by the human body, and therefore it is essential to include them in our food (linseed, soy and sunflower oil, salmon, mackerel etc.). However, we should take care in order to not exceed the sources of omega-6, as the modern diet is already rich in them and this can cause a greater production of eicosanoids which are harmful to both the performance and health. An optimal source of fats that the swimmer should never give up is the extra virgin olive oil, both for the quantity of oleic acid (an energy source that is easy to use for the muscle), and for the antioxidant and anti-inflammatory components found in it. Athletes who have a low percentage of body fat are usually allowed to eat a greater amount of fat, also based on their sensations during the training and the day. The presence of fats in the body also allows the **fat-soluble vitamins** to be conveyed and absorbed more easily and therefore to be used in biochemical reactions.

Experimental research has shown that the enrichment of the diet with lipids produces an enzymatic adaptation with a better metabolic utilization of the same and consequently a saving of glycogen reserves, with a better physical performance and a reduction in the sense of fatigue. A recent study conducted on swimmers at the University of Ohio tested whether the classic carbohydrate refill was more effective than a higher-fat diet in endurance athletes.

After the recharging, the following effects occurred:

- 33% increase in glycogen stores (1/3) compared to a diet with a lower carbohydrate content;
- no performance improvement was found;
- nearly double the increase in lactic acid production during exercise in swimmers.

Another interesting research done at the State University of New York in Buffalo challenges the "carbohydrate loading" theory, verifying an improvement in the performance in endurance athletes who have switched from a diet that is rich in carbohydrates to another one that has less carbohydrates and more fats. The study took place in three phases, gradually increasing the fat content until reaching 45% of the calorie intake. Each phase lasted four weeks, to allow the adjustment of the athlete's body to the new fat percentage. Endurance tests were repeated at the end of each phase. After 12 weeks, the best results were obtained when the diet included 45% calories in the form of fat:

- strength improved by 14%;
- less fatigue than in the two previous phases;
- athletes used storage fats more effectively as an energy source than in the previous two phases;
- at the haemato-chemical level, after the third phase, there was an improvement of the immune response, evidenced by an increase in white blood cells and a reduced level of the inflammatory parameters.

The thing to note and understand is that this study shows the need to give the athlete's body sufficient time to adapt to greater amounts of fat (careful choice of fats).

Why after these results (there are many others that I do not report due to the lack of space) do you not even want to take into consideration the simple fact that the old concepts on refilling carbohydrates may not be as valid, as was thought in the past? Almost all sports nutritionists still continue to feed carbohydrate-rich diets, not accepting the results of authoritative scientific research.

Perhaps not everyone knows which was the study that determined the "principle" of the famous "carbohydrate refill". The study, conducted more than thirty years ago on a group of well-trained athletes, consisted in subjecting them to a diet that was very high in protein and absolutely free of carbohydrates for several days. Within a few days, all the stored carbohydrates were consumed (with a logical decrease in performance). At this point, the athletes were tested on the treadmill and their performance was significantly reduced. Over the next three days, these same athletes were "recharged" with carbohydrate-rich meals and tested again on the treadmill. At that point, their performance improved and the researchers concluded that a diet that is rich in carbohydrates would improve the athletic performance. From this study, it can be concluded that if we do not eat carbohydrates at all, our performance could be adversely affected, which is very different from saying that carbohydrate recharging is necessary for a maximal athletic performance. Very few studies have shown that following a high carbohydrate diet for more than seven days improves the performance. On the contrary, numerous studies with elite athletes have shown that eating adequate amounts of carbohydrates (but not high) in combination with higher amounts of fats (more than those that are normally used) for seven days significantly increased endurance athletic performance; moreover, this increase in fats and the decrease in the quantity of carbohydrates, in the same athletes, brought a considerable improvement in the lipid profile, with a consequent decrease in the risk of cardiovascular diseases.

These results do nothing but confirm the considerable usefulness of fats in terms of energy and the importance of putting the body in favorable conditions for its optimal use, this is because our muscles contain a greater number of calories deriving from fat stores (about double) compared to those deriving from carbohydrate stocks (glycogen), without considering the practically inexhaustible stores of the subcutaneous fat. Just imagine what it might mean for an athlete to have the ability to access and then make the most of these large stores of energy. One of the key factors to access it, is to avoid the so-called "insulin peaks". Insulin is also responsible for the metabolism of fats: we could never store them without it. We should imagine it as a switch: when it is on, a few hours after the meal (especially if it is high in carbohydrates), carbohydrates are burned to produce energy and the excess calories are accumulated in the form of fat. When it is turned off, after the insulin has been consumed, fat is burned as an energy source. Therefore, remember that when the insulin level is low we burn fat, when it is higher our body is not able to use the stored fats.

So, summing up, we could say that excessive insulin peaks certainly make us fat and do not allow us to use the energy that is stored in the body; moreover, if we have excess fat to dispose of, we can spend hours on sport activities, but it remains where it is.

But, what stimulates the insulin? Certainly, the main stimulator is represented by carbohydrates. Clearly, not all carbohydrates stimulate insulin in the same way, and it is precisely for this reason that they are classified into "favorable" and "unfavorable". Another common cause for an insulin elevation is consuming meals that are too large.

How many and which proteins for the swimmer?

Proteins provide 4 Kcal/g. They are used for:
- replacing the worn muscle masses;
- building of hypertrophic muscle masses;
- keeping the ligaments healthy;
- the synthesis and re-synthesis of hormones and enzymes;
- energy purposes.

It should not be forgotten how modern swimming increasingly requires winter training in the gym, which in many cases involves periods of muscle-building in search of the creation of a greater muscular power, which can then be transformed into resistant strength or explosive strength. The protein requirement varies between 1.4 and 1.8 g/kg of lean mass (LM) but in conditions of intense work and in search of muscle hypertrophy, it can reach 2.3 g/kg of LM (except when it has medical contraindications). It should also be taken into account that carbohydrates and fats exert a protein-sparing effect. Lean protein food sources must be consumed during every meal of the day in the right ratio, with foods that also provide carbohydrates and fats, in order to maintain the balance between insulin and glucagon.

CHAPTER 20

Nutrition and downhill skiing

Downhill skiing is the main winter discipline. Skiers can be divided into two categories: competitors and those who practice this sport on a recreational level (which does not mean without commitment). While practicing the same discipline, they have very different needs, both in terms of training and nutrition. Let's analyze the dietary needs of the "Sunday skier". Most people are mistakenly convinced that to practice a sport only once a week, it is not necessary to eat properly or in any case with the purpose of practicing that sport. This erroneous idea puts the practitioner at risk of injuries, since, if at the metabolic and muscular level the body is not fit and ready for physical effort, as soon as it is subjected to physical and/or psychic stress it will go haywire, with serious consequences.

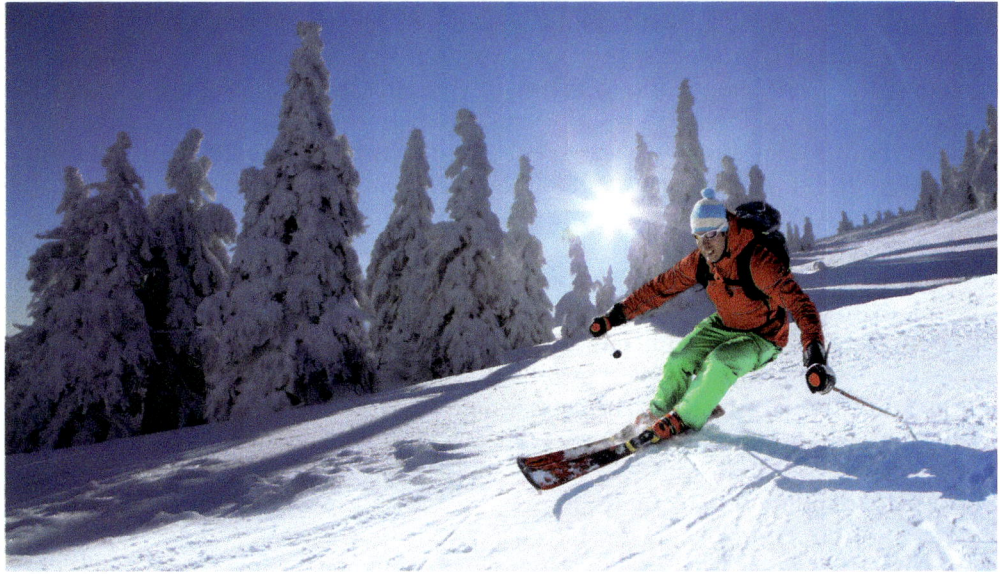

Figure 20.1

Therefore, it will be useful to follow a balanced diet during the week, which should be aimed at the day of the sporting activity. However, it is precisely on this day that we spend on skis that special attention must be paid to nutrition, especially in terms of quantity, quality and timing. The breakfast must be complete, with a good multi-vitamin and multi-mineral content (or in any case with an antioxidant complex), easily digestible and high in calories, as you are preparing to spend a day on skis in places with low temperatures. Of course, you will need to finish this first meal at least two hours before starting to ski, in order not to run into the danger of congestion.

The most commonly used foods for breakfast are: milk (to be replaced with soy milk if you have intolerance to cow's milk), yogurt (as for milk), rusks, bread, sugarless jam, peanut butter, non-dairy cereals, sugars, muesli, oat flakes, fructose for sweetening, barley coffee or tea; those who prefer a "savory" breakfast can consume eggs and/or lean meats, rye bread, walnuts, parmesan cheese and fruits, if well tolerated in the early morning (of course, they are not all to be eaten in the same breakfast, and in any case everyone must consume the calories he/she needs).

Towards mid-morning and instead of lunch, two easily digestible snacks will be useful, which provide the right calories and which do not strain the body for their digestion, so that drowsiness phenomena which leads to various injuries does not occur by the end of the day.

Protein-energy bars along with nuts can be a good choice, as they are easily transportable in a jacket pocket. During the afternoon, it is always best to keep your energy levels high by taking some handy snacks or by stopping at a bar to eat and drink something hot (easily digestible if you continue to ski).

Alcoholic beverages should be avoided, as, after providing a first sensation of heat, they have the opposite effect. In addition, those who are not used to drinking alcohol could have repercussions at the coordinative level that would almost certainly lead them to injuries on the ski slopes, or in any case represent a danger to other skiers.

As soon as you have finished skiing, you should rehydrate with a saline drink to restore the liquids that are lost through sweating, and consume few carbohydrates to recover the spent energy and to maintain your attention, if you have to go home by car.

Even though a lot of energy was spent during the day, the evening meal should not be a binge, on the contrary, it should be varied and balanced, containing all the necessary macro- and micro-nutrients. During the dinner, you can also drink a nice glass of red wine, whose cardio-protective properties (in moderate quantities) are now known to all. As for skiing that is practiced at a competitive level, it's a whole different matter. During the week, training is done as often as twice a day, so the diet must be customized with sufficient calories and nutrients for a maximum physical efficiency, as well as adequately distributed throughout the day to avoid problems with the digestion during the training sessions.

The most important meal will be breakfast, which will have to provide the calories to start the day in the best way. A useful supplement to be taken in this first meal will be a good multivitamin-multimineral, capable of providing the most commonly used and consumed micronutrients in the various biochemical reactions which are accelerated by daily physical activity. Not to be forgotten is the intake of omega-3 fatty acids (not only at breakfast, but in all meals), as, in addition to having a protective effect on the cardiovascular level, they are able to increase the response to the visual stimulus, and this is especially good in the special slalom.

Meals that precede and follow training and the competition are very important. The first ones must be light and supplemented with branched chain amino acids to preserve the muscles and reduce the production of lactic acid, which could damage performance. What follows the physical activity must contain easily assimilated proteins and carbohydrates (complete powders are useful from a nutritional point of view, diluted in water or other liquids) to restore the consumed energy supplies and to accelerate the muscle recovery.

On the day of the race, 3-4 hours before the start, you must have a complete and easily digestible meal, while an hour before and until just before the start it is good to sip a drink containing fructose and maltodextrin to keep the energy levels high. These should be taken in the doses allowed by the IOC, a thermogenic (which contains synephrine, caffeine and other natural components) to keep the level of attention high and to be more reactive between the slalom poles.

Between one run and the next, you can take two or three energy-protein bars with water or easy-to-digest meal replacement powders (based on waiting times).

At the end of the second run, you can speed up your recovery time and therefore be ready for the next week training or other competitive commitments, by consuming a drink containing carbohydrates and milk proteins (you should have a full meal later). If you consume a full meal shortly after, just take an amino acid pool enriched with leucine along with an energy drink containing a mix of simple and complex carbohydrates.

CHAPTER 21

Nutrition and high-altitude sports

In a high-altitude environment, particularly above 3000 meters, the atmospheric pressure drops and consequently the oxygen pressure also decreases, which is "pushed" less into the blood through the air that penetrates the pulmonary alveoli. This generates a situation of hypoxia in the tissues to which the body reacts by increasing the pulmonary ventilation and the cardiac output. As a result, physical activity becomes more strenuous and there is a decrease in the maximum aerobic power as you rise in altitude. When physical activity becomes sustained, due to the reduced organic performance, there is a reduction in the maximum heart rate and, therefore, a reduction in the cardiac output, resulting in less transported oxygen to the tissues.

The most sensitive tissue to the phenomenon of hypoxia is the central nervous system, so it is very easy to have drops in concentration, dizziness, headaches or, on the contrary, euphoria.

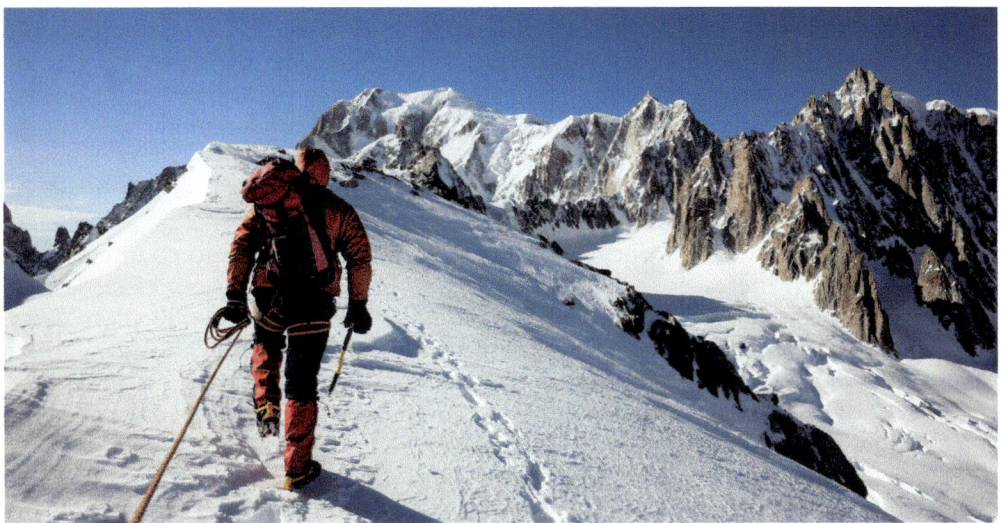

Figure 21.1

From the nutritional point of view, a diet for a high-altitude sportsperson must primarily meet three needs:
1. Bring sufficient calories as the energy demands increase, as well as due to the increased physical effort and the adaptations required in such extreme conditions, such as: shivering tremor, increased thermoregulation, increased voluntary activity (for example, beating feet to keep warm), increased heart rate, breathing and red blood cell production.
2. Contain easily digestible foods, as gastrointestinal activities slow down at high altitudes.
3. Being particularly rehydrating at the same time, as in cold environments the loss of water increases through breathing and by the induction of cold diuresis.

As for the calorie intake, it can be between 45 and 55 Kcal/kg per day for moderate physical activity, up to 55-68 Kcal/kg per day for intense physical activity (Consolatio, 1966).

A mountaineer can easily require up to 5000/6000 Kcal per day when climbing to the top. The energy intake must be provided above all by carbohydrates. This might seem in contradiction with the fact that fats have a higher caloric density and therefore also represent a food supply that is easier to transport as it is less heavy for the same caloric content; on the other hand, it must be considered that fats require more complicated digestion, drawing blood to the stomach and subtracting it from the muscular system.

Furthermore, in order to be used for energy purposes, fats need more oxygen than carbohydrates, and in high altitude conditions, when the oxygen pressure is considerably reduced, it becomes more difficult for the body to be able to transform these foods into power. At this point, it is clear that the preferred fuel must be carbohydrates, whose metabolism, among other things, produces more heat than fats (thermodynamic effect).

It appears that a minimum of 400 g of carbohydrates per day is needed in low-temperature activities; this quantity rises to the extent that these activities are carried out at high altitudes. In addition, various studies suggest that the use of carbohydrates increases during exercise and the post-exercise recovery period in conditions of moderate hypoxia compared to normoxia. This is because moderate hypoxia affects changes in the circulation of the metabolites and hormones in terms of metabolism and use of substrates during exercise and recovery. With this in mind, the intake of carbohydrates must be between 50 and 70% of the total calories.

It is also important not to neglect the protein intake in order to counteract the catabolism, which increases in these extreme conditions, but without exaggerating because proteins require a greater water intake, which is sometimes difficult to carry out. In general, the protein intake should be around 10-20% and, considering the high caloric level of the diet, in the end it is still an intake that can be even higher than 2 g/kg of body weight. This amount is necessary to counteract the catabolism in extreme physical activities.

It was found that upon returning from a high-altitude expedition, the body undergoes a muscle catabolism comparable to that of astronauts upon returning from space missions (today it no longer happens, as nutrition, supplementation and the physical activity are particularly taken care of, not only in the preparation period, but also during the staying in space).

The rest of the calories must be filled with fats, which must be mainly consumed at dinner (cheese, speck, lard), while at breakfast and during transfers it is advisable to prefer nuts and also chocolate. The latter is capable of improving the mental performance thanks to the presence of methylxanthines, substances similar to caffeine, and phenylethylamine, a molecule that binds to the same receptors as amphetamines, and therefore, it can have a positive psychotropic effect.

As we said, foods must be easy to digest and possibly also practical. They can be useful during transfers: gels, bars (including chocolate), freeze-dried meals, beverages with mixtures of maltodextrin and fructose, enriched with mineral salts and vitamins, while during the return it is advisable to consume complete meals and beverages, possibly hot ones.

The other problem to be addressed is the risk of dehydration due to a greater loss of water through transpiration and ventilation, drier air, greater evaporation from wind and/or sun, greater cold-induced diuresis, and a tendency to drink less (because doing so limits the need to urinate, which is not always easy when you are in extreme cold and also in logistical conditions).

It is therefore necessary to drink a lot of water with a good content of salts (fixed residue >1000), as waters with low fixed residue and low sodium quench thirst but increase the diuresis, favoring dehydration. The sodium intake is important because it stimulates thirst, contributes to a better hydration and prevents cramps.

Various studies have shown that supplementation with *Rhodiola rosea* and/or tyrosine can decrease the negative effects of the cold stress with a lower frequency of headaches, less fatigue and a greater endurance.

CHAPTER 22

Nutrition and combat sports

Those who practice combat sports must embody power, quick reflexes, speed, etc., all qualities that can be reached with continuous and exhausting workouts which, if not supported by adequate nutrition and appropriate supplementation, are nullified as the organism fails to recover (both physically and psychically), so the athlete cannot show his/her full potential. In addition, the risk of overtraining or injury is always lurking, often recurring in people subjected to excessive stress, who have not adequately compensated with rest.

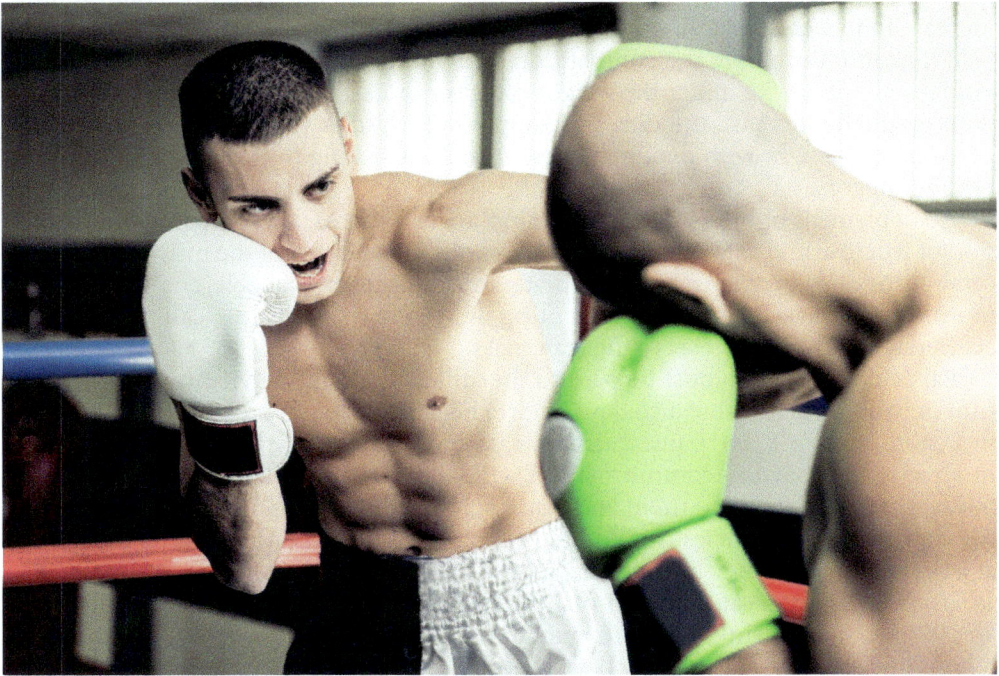

Figure 22.1

Usually, these sports require you to reach certain weight categories and often, in order to reach the weight, dietetic-nutritional errors are made. In a few words, sometimes these athletes, eight to nine days after the competition are overweight by several kilos compared to the competition weight, which they lose quickly within seven days by undergoing unbalanced low-calorie diets, saunas, restrictions of the water supply, increased physical exercise and even diuretics (dangerous and illegal in sports), arriving in the ring completely drained of energy and dehydrated. This situation that cannot be remedied in the interval between weighing and the race, with negative consequences on the performance and on the whole body. However, what should be sought is the maintenance of a healthy weight (with small fluctuations) throughout the year through an adequate diet, which must be normo-caloric and normo-glucidic (slightly high-caloric on days with intense training), and must bring the correct content of water and salts.

Indicatively, the carbohydrate quota can be around 45-50%, to be slightly increased in the two-three days prior to the race, and it should be mainly composed of slow-release complex carbohydrates; the lipid content can reach 30%, as it provides energy for the aerobic workouts as well as for the recovery during rest days and between workouts. The fats will be mainly mono- and polyunsaturated, which are more easily digested, provide essential fatty acids and are an energy source for the muscles.

The protein share is made up of the remaining percentage and it will be provided by foods containing proteins of a high biological value (therefore of animal origin, choosing the leanest sources) for at least 2/3 of the whole share. However, all this is indicative, as everyone has a unique metabolism; in addition, the percentages of macronutrients may vary according to the period of the athletic training: conditioning, increase in power, strength, speed, pre-competition, etc.

A few months before the competition, we will try to slowly drop a few kilos and even get about one kg under the weight category at least 15 days before the fight, and then gradually increase the diet and supply the muscles with the necessary glycogen to face the fight with maximal energy, without risking to exceed the limit of the weight category.

A supplement of branched chain amino acids (BCAAs), accompanied by a solution of fructose and maltodextrin, can be useful for preserving the muscles from the catabolism and providing an immediate and long term available energy. Furthermore, it has been seen how supplementing BCAAs in a slightly low-calorie diet helps accelerate fat loss and preserve the lean mass.

Particular attention must be paid to the athlete's diet in the vicinity of the match (not only hours before, but also days before) because if they are unable to eat well due to a "stomach block" and nausea, usually caused by states of particular mental tension in view of the sporting commitment, it will be necessary to act through particular foods that are palatable to them and a add suitable dietary supplementation that fills the nutritional deficiencies caused by this anxious state, in order to keep the athlete at a maximum efficiency until the day of the match.

In the short intervals between one round and another you can take small sips of an isotonic saline drink, while throughout the days between various matches that follow one another it is useful to take nutritionally complete and easily digestible liquid foods (on the market there are products in pouches with these characteristics, easily soluble and quick to consume, without over-tiring the digestive system). The constant supply of water and/or other liquids should not be forgotten, in order to avoid the dehydration phenomena and to improve the elimination of toxins that are produced in the body. If well tolerated, small amounts of creatine can improve the ability to make rapid movements in the ring and increase the speed in bringing the blow to the opponent. At the end of each match, the intake of branched chain amino acids together with fructose can accelerate the muscle recovery and quickly restore the energy reserves spent during the match. Returning to the pre-competition intake, many athletes have noticed an increase in attention and alertness by taking low doses of thermogenics (pay attention to the caffeine content, which at certain doses is not tolerated well in some athletes) containing synephrine, guarana and tyrosine with a stimulating action.

As for the off-season period, in which there are no competitions, there may be a search for an increase in strength and/or muscle mass. At this point, it is necessary to adjust the diet by increasing the calorie and protein intake without excessively increasing the volume of the consumed food to avoid stomach dilations and digestive difficulties, all accompanied by an intensification of workouts in the gym. The protein-calorie increase may consist of powdered supplements to be taken in the form of smoothies and specially formulated bars that do not contain harmful fats and substances that can be counterproductive because they are difficult to metabolize by the body. These substances can instead be contained in traditional foods, especially the ones with an industrial origin. In addition, when it comes to returning to the nutrition for preparing for the race, it will be easier to eliminate a small smoothie or a bar rather than larger portions of any food.

If you need an additional protein intake, you can rely on protein powders or amino acid pools in capsules. During this non-competitive period, supplementation with essential fatty acids of the omega-3 series has a favorable effect, since they participate in the composition of the nerves by increasing their ability to conduct the electrical signal, thus determining an improvement in the visual stimulus, in the speed of reaction and in the mind-muscle interaction, which will benefit the athlete later during the matches. A useful supplement that can increase the strength and the ability to conduct more intense and productive workouts is creatine. It must be taken only if it is well tolerated, with a good supply of liquids to avoid the onset of muscle cramps or abdominal pain, in the recommended amount (currently 3 to 6 g per day based on the degree of the physical activity), and in any case, it must always be cycled, which means, it is necessary to alternate periods of supplementation and periods where its intake is suspended. This should be done in order to benefit from the properties of creatine every time it is taken, without causing habituation of the organism.

In periods of high stress, perhaps accompanied by slight ailments which however do not prevent training, it may be helpful to take glutamine peptide with alpha-ketoglutaric acid (AKG), which have immune-stimulating properties and detoxify the organism from ammonium ions that can be formed during the muscle work and consequently affect the continuation of the training by producing a physical and mental fatigue.

Naturally, some general indications have been proposed and they will have to be personalized, as we are different at a metabolic and physical level, but also at a psychological level, where everyone responds differently to the same type of stress.

Nutrition and supplementation for weightlifting

by Antonio Squillante

Olympic weightlifters compete in the snatch and clean and jerk, divided into weight categories ranging from 55 kg to 109 kg for men and from 45 kg to 85 kg for women. The average body composition of a competitive weightlifter varies widely depending on body weight. The percentage of lean body mass (LBM) or fat free mass (FFM) tends to decrease with an increase in bodyweight. The average body fat percentage varies from 13.5 +/- 2.1% in the lighter bodyweight categories to 22.0 +/- 5.3% in the heavier bodyweight categories, with female athletes carrying more body fat than their male counterparts (+8.5 +/- 3.7). The difference in body composition between male and female weightlifters, as well as the difference between lighter and heavier body weight categories, explains the relationship between body mass (BM) and performance in weightlifting. In the sport of weightlifting, the relationship between body mass and performance in the snatch and clean and jerk is not quite linear. It is rather logarithmic, instead ($BM^{0.64}$).

In the snatch, the Olympic record in the men's 56 kg weight class – a weight category used up to the Olympic Games in Rio de Janeiro in 2016 and replaced, starting with the Tokyo Olympics in 2021, by the new 55 kg weight category – is 138 kg (Halil Mutlu, Sidney 2000). In the 62 kg weight class the Olympic record has been set at 153 kg (Kim Un-guk, London 2012). A gap of 15 kg for a body weight difference of less than 6 kg. This difference is even more noticeable in the clean and jerk, a lift that requires higher levels of muscle strength, and it tends to decrease as sheer body weight increases from the lightest to the heaviest categories, even more so if results are compared in terms of the relative strength. Lighter weightlifters have set Olympic records in the clean and jerk that equal 2.5 times their body weight, a value that is off reach for a heavier athlete. Weightlifters weighing in at 85 kg or more have hardly set Olympic records in the clean and jerk that exceed 2 times their body weight. The discrepancy in results between different body weight categories is even more noticeable in women. When compared to male lifters of similar body mass, female athletes tend to present with a lower percentage of lean body mass and, on average, 30% less strength and power.

Olympic weightlifting is purely an anaerobic sport that involves lifting heavy weights with fast, explosive movements. Heavy lifting requires complete rest between sets, anywhere from 2 to 5 minutes, with an average training session lasting about 2 hours. The average energy expenditure (EE) for an Olympic weightlifter during training corresponds to 2.78 calories per minute or, roughly, 170 calories per hour. More advanced athletes can exped anywhere between 350 Kcal and 750 Kcal per training session, on average 15-30 mL/kg^{-1}/min^{-1} or 4-8 METs (Metabolic Equivalent of Task, 1 MET = 3.5 mLO$_2$/kg/min). Daily energy requirements for a competitive weightlifter, however, also takes into consideration the amount of energy needed to support the physiological processes of protein synthesis and muscle tissue remodeling. Muscle hypertrophy is, indeed, a prerogative of resistance training and it is even more prominent in competitive weightlifters due to the demands placed on the muscle-skelatal system during training.

Studies have shown that for an athlete to perform at his/her best, energy availability (EA) must range between 35 and 40 calories per kg of lean mass. EA is the energy that remains available to support the physiological processes of maintenance and recovery (homeostasis) and it is measured as the net difference between the daily energy intake (EI) and the daily exercise energy expenditure (EEE) normalized by lean body mass:

$$EA = (EI - EEE)/LBM$$

Values below 35 calories per kg of lean body mass have been associated with a variety of maladaptations such as endocrine alterations, suppression of the reproductive axis, mental disorders, thyroid suppression, and altered metabolic responses. It is necessary for a weightlifter to consume enough calories to preserve an adequate level of energy availability (EA) throughout the day and during each week of training. Low energy availability (LEA) has been, in fact, associated with low levels of luteinizing hormone (LH) and testosteron in both men and women. In a sport like weightlifting, low levels of free and total testosterone, and dehydroepiandrosterone sulfate (DHEA-S) can have a detrimental effect on performance.

Recent studies on national and international level Olympic weightlifters reported an average daily energy intake (DEI) of 160 kJ or 39 Kcal per kilogram of body weight during periods of intense training, roughly 2.250 Kcal for a female athlete weighing in at 58 kg. With an average caloric expenditure of 370 Kcal (see below), this figure corresponds to an average EA level of 34-38 Kcal/LMB.

$$59*4*3.5 \text{ mL/kg}^{-1}/\text{min}^{-1} = 826 \text{ mL/O}_2$$
$$826 \text{ mL/O}_2 * 90 = 74.34 \text{ L/O}_2$$
$$74.34*5 \text{ Kcal} = 370 \text{ Kcal}$$

Chronic EA levels of less than 35-40 calories per kg of lean body mass have been associated with a series of overtraining-like symptoms described in the literature as relative energy deficiency in sport (RED-S). RED-S is associated with a general decline in performance, often associated with many common symptoms of acute and chronic fatigue such as weight loss, increased frequency of upper respiratory tract infection, and iron deficiency. RED-S seems to be more predominant in female athletes. In women, EA levels of less than 35 calories per kg of lean body mass have been linked with many signs and symptoms commonly seen in the so-called female athlete's triad such as amenorrhea, eating disorders, low bone density. This condition is referred to in the literature as low energy availability in females (LEAF).

Just like many other strength and power athletes, Olympic weightlifters tend to consume an average of 4-6 grams of carbohydrates per kilogram of body weight and 1.4-1.8 grams of protein per kilogram of body weight. Protein sources that are rich in the amino acid leucine, such as cod and egg white, should be preferred. Studies have shown the importance of this essential amino acid in regulating muscle protein synthesis at the molecular level, activating the mTOR signaling pathway. Meta-analysis and longitudinal studies have shown the importance of consuming 4-6 meals with an average of 20-40 grams of protein per meal (0.25 grams per kilogram of body weight per meal) in order to support muscle protein synthesis and tissue remodeling. However, a temporary caloric restriction of 500 Kcal or more per day and/or the intentional elimination of animal products might require a greater protein intake, up to 2-2.2 grams per kilogram of body weight. Carbohydrate intake might vary depending on training volume and the total calorie intake. Recent studies have shown the importance of maintaining a daily carbohydrate intake equal to or greater than 180-220 grams in order to preserve muscle function during periods of intense training.

Case study: National Championships 2019 (USA). Category: Women, 59 kg

Protein intake (PRO):
- 59×1.6 g = 95 g
- 95×4 Kcal = 380 Kcal
- $380/2{,}300 \times 100 = 16\%$ DEI

Carbohydrate intake (CHO):
- 59×5 g = 295 g
- 295×4 Kcal = 1.180 Kcal
- $1{,}180/2{,}300 \times 100 = 50\%$ DEI

FAT intake (FAT):
- $2{,}300 - 1{,}180 - 380 = 740$ Kcal
- $740/9$ Kcal = 82 g
- ~30 g/die

In order to preserve adequate liver and muscle glycogen content it is important to consume an average of 60-120 g of carbohydrates per meal. Low glycemic index carbohydrate sources such as oats, wild rice and whole grain bread and pasta must be preferred. However, in the event of two training sessions planned within 24 hours (double-session), it is necessary to maximize the physiological process of glycogenosynthesis consuming an average of 1 gram of carbohydrates per kilogram of body weight, with the addition of 0.5 grams of protein per kilogram of body weight per hour, for a maximum of 6 hours between two consecutive training sessions. Such an approach has shown to maximize muscle glycogen contents while, at the same time, preserving a state of positive protein balance. Carbohydrate intake might vary quite widely as an athlete goes from off-season training to in-season training, depending on whether or not a time of caloric restriction is necessary to reach an optimal body weight. Macronutrients distribution might change from 50% carbohydrate, 15% protein, and 30% fat in the off-season to 40% carbohydrate, 20% protein and 40% fat during the season to accomodate to for a moderate caloric deficit without sacrificing protein intake.

Case study: National Championships 2019 (USA). Category: Women, 59 kg

Off-Season:
- calorie intake: 2,300 Kcal
- carbohydrates: 6 g/kg, equal to 360 g/day
- proteins: 1.8 g/kg, equal to 110 g/day
- fats: 50 g, equal to 450 Kcal/day
- EA: 2,300-350/48 = 40-42 Kcal/FFM
- average EA per week: 40-42 Kcal/FFM/day
- CHO-PRO-FAT: 50%-20%-30%

In-Season:
- caloric intake: 1,800 Kcal
- carbohydrates: 4 g/kg, equal to 240 g/day
- proteins: 1.8 g/kg, equal to 110 g/day
- fats: 40 g, equal to 400 Kcal/day
- EA: 1,800-280/48 = 30-32 Kcal/FFM
- average EA per week: 34-36 Kcal/FFM
- CHO-PRO-FAT: 40%-20%-40%

Fat intake, therefore, varies according to the net caloric intake. Recent studies have shown a strong, positive correlation between daily intake of polyunsaturated fatty acids (PUFAs) and saturated fatty acids (SFAs) and blood testosterone levels. Because of the importance of testosterone in sports that heavily rely on muscle strength, such as weightlifting, a diet rich in SFA and PUFA is to be encouraged. Further studies have confirmed how a lower ratio between polyunsaturated fatty acids and saturated fatty acids (PUFA/SFA) tends to result in greater circulating testosterone levels. Therefore, competitive weightlifters should strive to consume a relatively higher percentage of saturated fats equal to 10% of the total caloric intake, with the remaining 15-25% of the total caloric intake equally distributed between monounsaturated and polyunsaturated fats.

In the sport of weightlifting, an athlete's body weight varies over the course of a competitive season. On average, in the off-season, body weight tends to increase by about 3-5 kilograms compared to the ideal competition weight. A slight increase in body weight is partly justified by a high training volume which tends to result in a more pronounced increase in muscle glycogen content and intracellular fluid retention. For each gram of muscle glycogen, an addition 4 grams of water are stored in the muscle cell. Therefore, for an average size athlete with approximately 1 kilogram of intramuscular glycogen stores – roughly, 30% more than a sedentary subject due to the physiological super-compensation process - there can be a difference of up to

5 kilograms between a period of high training volume and high carbohydrate intake (off-season) and a period of low training volume and low carbohydrate intake (in-season). Moreover, weight gain during the off season can also be associated with an increase in muscle mass, a hypertrophic response that is normally associated with times of high training volume and high caloric intake. When the goal is to increase muscle mass, an additional 500 Kcal per day is recommended.

In-season the average daily calorie intake is somewhat lower than the off-season to allow an athlete to reach his/her ideal competition weight. No more than 0.5 kilogram of body weight should be lost per week, for a period of approximately 6-8 weeks. A greater weight loss should require a longer period of caloric restriction, up to 10-12 weeks, rather than a greater caloric restriction per se. Studies on strength and power athletes have shown that a calorie restriction greater than 500 calories per day and/or periods of caloric restriction longer than 8-12 weeks can increase the risk of losing muscle mass (muscle waiting), even more so during periods of intense training. Muscle waiting must be avoided, as it can heavily compromise performance in competition. Training volume tends to decrease during the weeks leading up to a competition. Nevertheless, during time of caloric restriction it is still of paramount importance to maintain an average weekly EA level equal to, or greater than 35 calories per kg of lean mass. In this case, the calorie deficit is carried out at the expense of carbohydrates and fats. The daily intake of carbohydrates is reduced to 4 grams per kilogram of body weight, while fat intake is normally reduced to about 25% of the total daily caloric intake.

Studies have shown how low-fat diets – less than 20% of the daily caloric intake coming from fat – can negatively impact blood testosterone levels, potentially com-

Table 23.1 Adequate EA

	MON	TUE	WED	THU	FRI	SAT	SUN
EI	2,100	1,900	2,200	1,800	2,300	1,900	2,100
EEE	400	320	0	390	350	420	0
EA	37	35	48	31	43	32	46

National Championships 2019 (USA). Category: Women, 59 kg. Average weekly EA levels off-season (38 Kcal/kg/day).

Table 23.2 Inadequate EA

	MON	TUE	WED	THU	FRI	SAT	SUN
EI	1,750	1,550	1,850	1,450	1,950	1,550	1,750
EEE	400	320	0	390	350	420	0
EA	30	27	41	23	35	25	38

National Championships 2019 (USA). Category: Women, 59 kg. Average weekly EA levels in-season (31 Kcal/kg/day).

promising performance in Olympic weightlifting. In a very similar way, it is advisable not to increase the daily consumption of proteins above 2 grams per kilogram of body weight. Excessive protein consumption can negatively affect free testosterone levels, increasing the amount of sex hormone-binding globulin (SHBG) and, thereofe, decreasing circulating free testosterone levels.

Evidence-based practice seems to encourage the use of three main supplements in Olympic weightlifting. First and foremost, for athletes who tend to consume twice the recommended dietary allowance for protein, supplementing with isolated and/or hydrolyzed whey proteins might represent a valuable alternative to high-fat, animal products. Protein supplements that are roughly 10% leucine by protein content, which means on average 2-2.5 grams of leucine per 20-25 grams of protein are highly recommended. Creatine monohydrate is another supplement that can have an ergogenic effect. Daily creatine monohydrate supplementation with 0.03 grams of creatine per kilogram of body weight allows an increase in the reserves of creatine phosphate within the muscle cell, which facilitates the re-synthesis of adenosine triphosphate during high intensity, anaerobic type efforts. However, for athletes competing in weight categories it is important to closely monitor the effect of creatine supplementation on body weight in order to prevent any unexpected weight gain due to intracellular water retention, a common side effect of oral creatine supplementation. Caffeine can also have an ergogenic effect. Recent studies have shown how consuming 3-6 milligrams of caffeine per kilogram of body weight 45-60 minutes before a weight training session can improve strength and peak power output. The use of caffeine can mitigate the onset of fatigue, preventing the loss of muscle function normally reported during heavy strength training sessions lasting longer than 60 minutes.

There are nutritional supplements that can further improve performance in weightlifting, although their use might be contingent to a situation of high training volume and/or restricted caloric intake. Leucine (2-5 grams per day) can be used to support muscle protein synthesis with the goal of promoting muscle growth whereas hydroxymethylbutyrate (HMB), a derivative of leucine with anti-catabolic properties, which can be used to prevent muscle wasting during periods of reduced caloric intake (1-3 grams/day). Beta-alanine, a precursor of carnosine, can potentiate the buffering of hydrogen ions normally produced during intense, anaerobic training. By doing so, carnosine supplementation (3-4 grams/day in smaller doses of no more than 1.6 gram/dose) can delay the onset of muscular fatigue during prolonged periods of high intensity, high volume training. Last but not least, daily supplementation with essential fatty acids such as omega-3 fatty acids (500 mg-1000 mg, EPA and DHA in a 2:1 ratio), can mitigate the inflammatory response commonly associated with high interest resistance training, promoting recovery.

CHAPTER 24

Nutrition, supplementation and training during the menstrual cycle

by Francesco Guardato, Antonella Berardi Nazzarena and Massimo Spattini

The woman today

Nowadays, fortunately, women are slowly recovering their spaces and receiving the attention they deserve, not only in relation to preconceived and stereotyped areas, but also in terms of sectors in which studies and applications were generally reserved for men, as in the case of medicine. In fact, women are subject to hormonal variations during the menstrual cycle and during pregnancy, which would compromise the results of the pharmacological experimentation. For these reasons, drugs have always been tested only on men, just as studies on nutrition and, even more so, training studies are also performed on men. Finally, with the advent of "gender medicine" this gap is closing.

Consequently, today we have an enormous amount of information available on topics such as female biotypical morphological types, *ad hoc* diets, *ad personam* workouts and so on, which, however, are not always creditworthy. This is why it is of a primary importance to read up in detail on these key issues, first of all the correct training and nutrition.

That said, the fact remains that women and men are two very different universes, which require different specific attention, advice and preparations. Furthermore, although it may seem obvious, women are often overloaded with commitments, not only working, but also household and childcare, if she has a family. Therefore, she finds it more difficult to find moments of psychophysical relaxation or simply free spaces to devote to self-care.

Therefore, it is also essential to work from a psychological point of view: training and diet must put the person at ease and also take into account their character peculiarities, avoiding excesses that can cause negative side effects on a psychological-motivational level which would generate an excessive psychophysical fatigue.

Therefore, motivation is also fundamental to incentivize the person to follow a specific program and favor its improvement. To obtain this result, one must also be able to understand any impediments that could psychologically block the female athlete; for example, phrases like "I don't have time", "I have big bones by constitution" and others are mostly excuses to avoid lifestyle changes, because every change in habits and every change in the daily routine takes a lot of effort.

Consequently, the adherence to the program will be possible only by working on the motivation of that person, ensuring that he/she considers sports and the diet as a therapy aimed at achieving well-being and not as a constraint to adhere to esthetic models. This is how we can obtain real and lasting effects.

It appears here, at this point, the need to structure a program that is built as much as possible on the person who is in front of us, to allow them to obtain an optimal state of health. Therefore, it is essential to start from the knowledge of why the person needs to train and what his goals, his daily commitments and his habits are. Finally, when it comes to the female training, it is also fundamental to take into consideration various fundamental issues, such as the morpho-structural and hormonal typology, and the period of the menstrual cycle, as we will see in detail below; in addition, factors such as the production and circulation of various sex hormones which have a strong influence on the functionality and the structure of many body systems must be taken into consideration. In fact, the existence of a close connection between our physical characteristics and the endocrine glands of our body is undeniable: each one of us is affected by the influence of certain glands on others, and this consequently entails the existence of different body models.

It is at this point that we must begin to ask more and more specific questions, such as, for example: "Who are we working on? An athlete? A girl who does not aspire to step on the stage? A girl who has a regular period? Who has a gynoid or hypolipolytic type (veno-capillary, arterio-capillary or hormonal)? Who has an androgenic or hyperlipogenetic (metabolic androgenic, hypercortisolemic androgenic)? " and many more.

We can really start working seriously only after understanding all this.

Table 24.1 The difference between ginoid and android subjects

Gynoid subject	Android subject
• Edema and cellulite	• Metabolic syndrome
• Increased TSH	• Hyperglycemia and diabetes
• Increased LDL cholesterol	• Increased triglycerides/HDL ratio
• Alterations of the microcirculation	• Hypertension
• Menstrual disorders	• Hyperinsulinemia
• Raynaud's syndrome/phenomenon	• Increased CRP
• Accumulation of fat in the lower body	• Cardiovascular diseases
• Parasympatheticotonia	• Accumulation of fat in the upper body area
• High levels of estrogen	• Sympatheticotonia
• Problems in detoxification	• Hypercortisolemia
• Gastrointestinal problems	
• Predisposition to allergies and autoimmune diseases	

Biphasic protocol for the gynoid subject: diet and workout

Let's consider an **arterio-capillary gynoid woman with edema** (from the Greek οἴδημα, òidema, "swelling", i.e. accumulation of water) given by an increased capillary permeability, i.e. an increase in the loss of water in the extracapillary space.

Through the endothelium of the capillaries there is an exchange of gaseous and non-gaseous substances, such as oxygen, carbon dioxide, glucose, etc., with the interstitial fluid of the tissues. Depending on the location in our body, some capillaries have a greater permeability towards water and solutes (for example the kidney capillaries), others towards macromolecules (proteins, etc.).

In some cases, this selective permeability can disappear as a result of morbid conditions (circulatory stasis, etc.) which can cause alterations in the capillary permeability, especially by increasing it; this means that more liquids, gases and macromolecules will be poured from the capillary to the outer space.

Returning to our arterio-capillary subject, we proceed to carry out a careful analysis which involves the following steps, in order to understand which are the concatenated causes that determine the edema:

- postural assessment using Walker View, a highly technological treadmill capable of simultaneously carrying out both gait analysis and movement analysis of all body segments;
- BIA (Body Impedence Assessment) or bioimpedance analysis: it is an instrumental method that allows you to evaluate the body composition through the use of a low voltage electric current. The different tissues (muscle, bone, adipose, etc.) express a specific electrical conductivity, sufficient to make them recognizable. In particular, water is an excellent conductor of electricity, therefore it has a low resistance, while fat is a bad conductor, therefore it has a high resistance. Resistance is inversely proportional to the amount of body fluids, while reactance is related to fat-free mass (FFM) and body cell mass (BCM). The examination is carried out with the aid of electrodes that are applied to the hands and feet of the subject who is lying on a bed or standing on a scale, thus applying an electrical impulse which is then sent to software that processes the data and translates them into amounts of muscle mass, fat mass, intracellular water, extracellular water, total glycogen etc.;
- analysis with an infrared camera: non-invasive instrumental evaluation technique that allows you to monitor the skin circulation by measuring the body temperature based on the color that the various parts of the body absorb;
- Rima-Trendelenburg test: useful for evaluating the efficiency of the valve system of the perforating veins and possible incontinence of the saphenous vein.

Let's suppose that the subject presents with the following problems:
- paramorphism of the flexor chain: *genu recurvatum* (backward curvature of the knee), which can cause a compression of the popliteal vein and therefore an increase in the load pressure of the collateral veins, causing escape routes, i.e. the famous capillaries in evidence (telangiectasias);

- *pes cavus* (a phenomenon in which the weight of the body falls only on the heels and toes, and not in a uniform way on the whole foot), determined by a genetic predisposition and also by the frequent use of heels. This could lead to a decrease in the pump effect deriving from the calf;
- increase in the hydrostatic pressure from prolonged standing (inefficiency of the pump) due to the lifestyle of the subject who, in this case, spends several hours standing for occupational reasons.

Therefore, the goal will be to "create" a new capillary branch and decrease the excessive load on the capillaries, limiting the exercises that can cause an increase in the intracapillary pressure, such as squats, lunges, deadlifts, etc., considering that the hypergonadic gynoid subject, already has a natural tendence to have a "weak" capillary wall for the following reasons:

- high levels of progesterone, which lead to a higher protein catabolism;
- protein nutritional deficiency: generally, ginoid subjects are attracted to sugars due to their high levels of insulin (although not resistant to it), which predisposes them to hypoglycemia; this causes an imbalance between macronutrients as, erroneously, these subjects, in order to return to a low-calorie daily context, reduce proteins rather than carbohydrates;
- deficiency of the albumin synthesis, resulting from a protein nutritional defect that results in the reduction of the oncotic pressure. Albumin is an essential macromolecule for the balance between the intra- and extracapillary compartments. Its decrease (often caused by protein nutritional insufficiency) is accompanied by the loss of the sponge effect that it plays inside the capillaries (i.e. it draws the water);
- parasympatheticotonia: parasympathetic system hypertionia, which is, that part of the nervous system that deals, among other things, with storing energy, reducing the heart rate and vasodilation which, if excessive, can lead to edemas;
- hypothyroidism: the gynoid subject tends to be a hypoxidizer with higher than normal calcium levels, which slow down the thyroid metabolism and can contribute to the formation of cellulite. In addition, estrogen, which this morphotype possesses in abundance, being hypergonadotropic, increases TBG (the thyroid hormone binding protein) and, if in excess, decreases the conversion of T4 into T3. Hypothyroidism promotes the edemas so much, especially at the level of the polysaccharides of the subcutaneous tissue, that it can even cause myxedema;
- tendency to accumulate fat in the gluteo-femoral area, since estrogens in this area increase the expression of two antilipolytic proteins: perilipin, which acts as a protective layer to prevent the action of lipase, and the α_2-adrenergic receptors, which attenuate the lipolytic response. The accumulation of fat in the hips, thighs and buttocks contributes to a circulatory slowdown through the periarteriolar increase of angiotensin II receptores, a vasoconstrictor substance which in turn stimulates the increase of α_2 receptors;
- a higher activity of enzymes such as aromatase, involved in the biosynthesis of 17 β-estradiol (E2 or estradiol) from androgenic precursors.

In addition, it will be essential to stretch the posterior leg muscles and improve the proprioception of the overall body pattern.

Based on what was mentioned above, it is possible to draw up a training and a nutritional program, while taking these characteristics into consideration.

It is important to remember that, especially for the gynoid woman, the maximal strength at the turn of the menstrual phases is not the same; the same applies to mood, which is strongly influenced by hormonal fluctuations in the four main menstrual phases: **follicular phase, ovulatory phase, luteal phase and menstrual phase**.

For simplicity of exposition, we can summarize these four phases in two macro-phases: follicular phase and luteal phase.

Follicular phase: from the 1st to the 14th day of the cycle

The predominant hormones are estrogen, in particular E2. These act not only on sexual characteristics and on bone calcification, but also on the energy metabolism, as they:

- increase the expression of adiponectin (AdipoR1), a protein that is highly expressed in adipocytes with anti-inflammatory and insulin-sensitizing properties, capable of raising the levels of good HDL cholesterol, etc.;
- increase the mobilization of muscle triglycerides during a physical exertion, which promotes the breakdown of lipids for energy purposes;
- in white adipocytes, E2 increases the lipolysis by stimulating the activity of the β-adrenergic receptors, by inhibiting lipoproteinlipase and by reducing the adipogenesis;
- estrogens appear to inhibit lipolysis only in the subcutaneous deposits and thus displace the assimilation of fats from abdominal to subcutaneous deposits, increasing the latter;
- positive effects on the central control of appetite, body weight
- and fat levels, thanks to the increase in the production and sensitivity of leptin (Brown et al., 2010), a protein hormone that is mainly produced by the adipose tissue; its high concentration blocks, at a central level, the stimulus of hunger (anorexigenic action) and it also increases the lipolysis by direct effect on UCP proteins (transmembrane proteins that disperse part of the electrochemical gradient created in oxidative phosphorylation, thus determining an "energy loss that is released in the form of heat - brown tissue is rich in it);
- increase in the activity of CPT-1 (carnitine palmitoyltransferase 1), anmitochondrial enzyme which is essential in "preparing" fats to be burned as an energy source;
- improvement of the mitochondrial activity, the energy center of our body; in fact, having efficient mitochondria results in a delayed aging. These effects were observed by analyzing some activators of the mitochondrial biogenesis, Nrf1/2, TFAM and PGC1 α (Mattingly et al., 2008).

In particular, in the skeletal muscle, ER-α (alpha estrogen receptor) promotes the insulin sensitivity and the expression of GLUT4, which increases the reuptake of glucose in the muscle cells.

In addition, estrogens regulate the function of pancreatic cells and inhibit the activation of FOXO1 proteins (independent from the IRS1 and 2 signals) → glucose-6-phosphatase → gluconeogenesis and glycogenolysis → + glycolysis → + TCA. Simply stated, they help with the lipid catabolism.

Estrogens regulate the glucose metabolism through direct and indirect control of the expression of enzymes that are involved in this process:

- hexokinase (HK) → + HK → + glycolysis. HK is the first enzyme related to the glycolysis and it has the duty of phosphorylating glucose so that it can enter the cell, thus decreasing the blood glucose;
- phosphoglucomutase (PGI) → + PGI (α-D-glucose-1-phosphate ⇌ D-glucose-6-phosphate), less glucose-1-phosphate available for glycogenosynthesis, so more "space" available for the excess glucose before it is converted into fat;
- glucose transporters GLUT3 and GLUT4, less blood glucose → less insulin → less adipogenic effect.

Luteal phase: from the 15th to the 28th day of the cycle

The predominant hormone is **progesterone**, which, unlike estrogens, which improve the glucose metabolism, has the following effects:

- induction of insulin resistance (physiological);
- protein catabolism;
- activation of ASP (acylation stimulating protein), an enzyme that promotes the accumulation of fat;
- inhibiting action on aldosterone receptors, with a decrease in the retention of sodium ions and, consequently, water retention. In the premenstrual phase, there is an increase in water retention in conjunction with the drop in progesterone;
- 5% increase in the metabolic rate (an increase in body temperature by 0.5° C) through the stimulation of the thyroid gland.

As for the diet, the key points of the follicular phase will therefore be:

- greater *sensitivity to insulin*;
- better carbohydrate metabolism;
- greater oxidation of intramuscular triglycerides.

The key points of the luteal phase, on the other hand, will be:

- increased hunger;
- higher metabolic rate;
- insulin resistance which worsens the glucose metabolism and causes an increase in hunger, especially towards sugary foods;
- increased proteolysis.

Therefore, in the **follicular phase** you will need a diet:

- with medium-high carbohydrates: as mentioned above, in the follicular phase the body is able to oxidize a greater amount of glucose; for this reason, the carbohydrate intake can be kept medium-high, especially for the gynoid subjects who easily tend to adapt (decrease in metabolic rate) negatively to hypoglucidal diets

due to their hypolipolytic component (therefore it already starts from a physiological "hypothyroidism"); among other things, carbohydrates allow the stimulation of leptin, which among its various functions, increases the release of TSH (a hormone which, by acting on the thyroid gland, stimulates the release of thyroid hormones) by the pituitary;
- normoproteic and normolipidic: since in this phase the blood concentrations of progesterone are lower (which increases the excretion of nitrogen), there is no great need to implement a high-protein diet, given that, among other things, the E2 has an anti-catabolic effect; this must be combined with a diet that has a medium-high carbohydrate content, which considerably decreases the gluconeogenesis from amino acids.

In the **luteal phase**, you will need a diet that is:
- hypoglucidic, given that in this phase the oxidative capacity of sugars is lower;
- hyperproteic, to buffer the catabolic action of progesterone and the adaptive gluconeogenesis by reducing carbohydrates;
- normo- or hyperlipidic, depending on the conditions of the subject's lymphatic system, since lipids, once ingested, travel along the lymphatic system and in the event of its reduced functionality they would be oxidized with a greater difficulty; in this case, the use of short-chain fatty acids could prove to be an excellent strategy, as the latter do not travel along the lymphatic system.

Table 24.2 Biphasic diets for the gynoid subject from the 1st to the 14th day of the cycle: follicular phase

Training days	Non-training days
BREAKFAST	**BREAKFAST**
Proteins to choose from:	Protein to choose from:
• 1 egg white + 2 yolks	• 2 egg whites + 2 yolks
• 4 slices of turkey or chicken breast + 2 walnuts	• 5 slices of turkey or chicken breast + 2 walnuts
• 1 Greek yogurt	• 4 slices of smoked salmon
Carbohydrates to choose from:	• 1 Greek yogurt
• 40 g of oats	Carbohydrates to choose from:
• 40 g of spelt	• 40 g of oats
• 70 g of rye or wholemeal bread	• 40 g of spelt
Condiments to choose from:	• 70 g of rye or wholemeal bread
• 100 g of fruits	Condiments to choose from:
• 2 teaspoons of honey	• 50 g of fruits
• 2 teaspoons of jam	• 1 teaspoon of honey
3 g of beta-alanine	• 1 teaspoon of 150 mg kelp jam
500 mg of chaste tree	150 mg of kelp
SNACK	**SNACK**
1 fruit	1 fruit
3 crackers	5 capsules of essential amino acids
5 capsules of essential amino acids	

Continues

Chapter 24 ▶ Nutrition, supplementation and training during the menstrual cycle

Continued

Training days	Non-training days
LUNCH	**LUNCH**
Proteins to choose from: • 100 g of lean meat • 100 g of lean fish • 50 g of dried legumes or 220 g of legumes in a glass 10 g of EVO oil Vegetables Carbohydrates to choose from: • 60 g of basmati rice, wholemeal, red, black • 60 g of other whole grains • 120 g of wholemeal or rye bread • 180 g of potatoes	Proteins to choose from: • 100 g of lean meat • 100 g of lean fish • 50 g of dried legumes or 220 g of legumes in a glass 10 g of EVO oil Vegetables Carbohydrates to choose from: • 50 g of basmati rice, wholemeal, red, black • 50 g of other whole grains • 100 g of wholemeal or rye bread • 150 g of potatoes
SNACK	**SNACK**
Carbohydrates to choose from: • 4 rice cakes • 4 Swedish-style wholemeal crackers • 40 g of a wholemeal sandwich bread 5 capsules of essential amino acids 1 fruit	Carbohydrates to choose from: • 4 rice cakes • 4 Swedish-style wholemeal crackers • 40 g of wholemeal sandwich bread 5 capsules of essential amino acids
DINNER	**DINNER**
Protein to choose from: • 100 g of chicken breast • 100 g of turkey • 100 g of white meat • 100 g of lean fish: cod, pangasius, etc. 10 g of EVO oil Vegetables Carbohydrates to choose from: • 40 g of basmati rice, wholemeal, red, black • 40 g of other whole grains • 70 g of wholemeal or rye bread 600 mg of acetylcysteine	Proteins to choose from: • 150 g of chicken breast • 150 g of turkey • 150 g of white meat • 150 g of lean fish: cod, pangasius, etc. 10 g of EVO oil Vegetables Carbohydrates to choose from: • 4 whole grain cakes • 4 Swedish-style wholemeal crackers 3 g arginine

Training day: 50% carbohydrates – 25% proteins – 25% fats (1600 Kcal: 190 g carbohydrates – 100 g proteins – 40 g fats).

Non-training day: 40% carbohydrates – 30% proteins – 30% fats (1500 Kcal: 150 g carbohydrates – 120 g proteins – 50 g fats).

The blue text indicates a supplementation to the diet.

Table 24.3 Biphasic diets for the gynoid subject from the 15th to the 28th day of the cycle: luteal phase

Training days	Non-training days
BREAKFAST	**BREAKFAST**
Protein to choose from: • 100 mL of egg white + 2 yolks • 4 slices of turkey or chicken breast + 2 walnuts • 1 Greek yogurt Carbohydrates to choose from: • 30 g of oats • 30 g of spelt • 60 g of rye or wholemeal bread Condiments to choose from: • 100 g of fruits • 2 teaspoons of honey • 2 teaspoons of jam 600 mg of lipoic acid 1 g of carnitine 500 mg of potassium and 400 mg of magnesium	Protein to choose from: • 2 egg whites + 2 yolks • 5 slices of turkey or chicken breast + 2 walnuts • 4 slices of smoked salmon • 1 Greek yogurt Carbohydrates to choose from: • 20 g of oats • 20 g of spelt • 40 g of rye or wholemeal bread Condiments to choose from: • 50 g of fruits • 1 teaspoon of honey • 1 teaspoon of jam 600 mg of lipoic acid 1 g of carnitine 500 mg of potassium and 400 mg of magnesium (magnesium helps reduce the hunger in the 10 pre-cycle days)
SNACK	**SNACK**
1 fruit 5 capsules of essential amino acids	10 g of dried coconut without sugar 5 capsules of essential amino acids
LUNCH	**LUNCH**
Protein to choose from: • 100 g of lean meat • 100 g of lean fish 15 g of EVO oil Vegetables Carbohydrates to choose from: • 40 g of basmati rice, wholemeal, red, black • 40 g of other whole grains • 80 g of wholemeal or rye bread • 120 g of potatoes	Protein to choose from: • 150 g of lean meat • 150 g of lean fish • 100 g of fatty fish • 100 g of fatty meat 20 g of EVO oil Vegetables
SNACK	**SNACK**
10 g of dried coconut without sugar 5 capsules of essential amino acids	1 fruit 5 capsules of essential amino acids

Continues

Continued

Training days	Non-training days
DINNER	**DINNER**
Protein to choose from: • 100 g of lean meat • 100 g of lean fish • 200 mL of egg whites 10 g of EVO oil Vegetables Carbohydrates to choose from: • 4 whole grain cakes • 4 Swedish-style wholemeal crackers • 70 g of wholemeal bread or rye 400 mg of sulfoadenosylmethionine	Protein to choose from: • 200 g of white lean meat • 200 g of lean fish • 150 g of fatty fish 10 g of EVO oil Vegetables

Ginoid training day: 35% carbohydrates – 35% proteins – 30% fats (1600 Kcal: 130 g carbohydrates – 150 g proteins – 50 g fats). The proteins will be higher in order to buffer the catabolic effect of progesterone; it is also important to use olive oil and omega-3 fatty acids to reduce the inflammatory effect that exists in this phase.

Ginoid non-training day: 20% carbohydrates – 40% proteins – 40% fats (1500 Kcal: 80 g carbohydrates – 140 g proteins – 60 g fats). The blue text indicates a supplementation to the diet.

Carbohydrates remain high at breakfast to activate the thyroid metabolism and are reduced at dinner to promote a nocturnal GH secretion.

The following tables show some examples of a biphasic diet.

Food supplements for the gynoid subject

The hypolipolytic gynoid individual is a subject that tends to have an estrogenic prevalence, also partly because of a greater activity of aromatase, an enzyme that converts androgens into estrogen, with a slowing effect on the thyroid metabolism and a deficit on the detoxification function at the hepatic level and, consequently, an objective difficulty in burning fats and circulation problems at the peripheral level.

Supplements that act on the estrogen metabolism

- **Astaxanthin**: 8 mg per day. An antioxidant carotenoid with an antiaromatase activity.
- **Chaste tree**: 500 mg per day. Equipped with pro-progestin and anti-estrogenic effects.
- **Dry extract of flax seeds**: 1500 mg per day. Equipped with an antiaromatase action.
- **Indole 3-carbinol**: 200 mg per day. Contained in cauliflower, broccoli and cruciferous trees in general, it is able to deactivate estrogen.
- **Quercetin**: 100 mg per day. It is another important flavonoid with antiaromatase properties.

Supplements that promote the liver detoxification

- **Silymarin**: 200-400 mg per day. Contained in milk thistle, it is a flavonolignan complex that improves the liver function.
- **Dandelion**: 500 mg of the dry extract twice a day. It has purifying properties, as it stimulates the biliary, hepatic and renal function, which means, it activates the excretory organs (liver, kidneys, skin) which are used for the transformation of toxins.
- **Sulfoadenosylmethionine**: 200-400 mg per day. Useful both as a liver detoxifier and as an antidepressant; also effective in the treatment of osteoarthritis.
- **Acetylcysteine**: 200-600 mg per day. It is one of the precursors of glutathione, which is one of the most powerful antioxidants that the body can produce, as well as being a valid detoxifier.
- **B complex vitamins**: at least 100% of the daily DRV. They are necessary to support the liver in the metabolism of various macronutrients.
- **BCAA (isoleucine, valine, leucine)**: 5 g per day. They support the protein anabolism without straining the liver.

Supplements that promote lipolysis

- **Acetylcarnitine and carnitine**: 1 g per day. Carnitine is an amino acid that facilitates the entry of fats into the mitochondrion, where they can be oxidized to produce energy in the presence of oxygen.
- **Omega-3**: 1-3 g per day. They are able to increase the oxidation of fatty acids and improve the elasticity of red blood cells, increasing their ability to transport oxygen to the periphery.
- **Forskolin**: 100 mg per day. It works by increasing the thermogenic response, which leads to increased calorie consumption.
- **Glutamine**: 2-5 g per day. It has a positive effect on the health of the gastrointestinal tract and stimulates the GH production when taken in the evening before bedtime.

Supplements that improve the circulation

- **Escin**: 75 mg per day. It is a saponin extracted from horse chestnut that helps to reduce the resistance of the capillaries and decreases their permeability.
- **Gotu kola**: 30-60 mg per day. In the form of a total triterpene fraction, it is particularly useful for combating venous insufficiency and cellulite.
- **Sweet clover**: 500 mg of dry extract twice a day. It has an anti-inflammatory and anti-edema, diuretic and phlebotonic pharmacological activity.
- **Butcher's broom**: 100-200 mg per day. It has anti-edema effects thanks to the steroidal saponins, ruscogenins and neoruscogenins, which are able to improve the functionality of the microcirculation.
- **Beta-alanine**: 3 g per day. It is a precursor of carnosine, a molecule that counteracts the lactic acid produced by physical exercise and therefore counteracts tissue acidosis and cellulite.

- **Vitamin C**: 500 mg per day. It strengthens the capillary walls and facilitates the absorption of iron by improving oxygenation at the peripheral tissue level.
- **Vitamin B12 and folic acid**: 5 mg and 400 mg respectively can induce the erythropoiesis, improving the oxygen transport.

Training for the gynoid subject

For the gynoid subject, we propose the following biphasic training.

Based on the properties of the hormones, we can divide the training into:
- training in the follicular phase, in which strength and intense training are preferred (always paying attention to any problems of circulatory stasis of the subject);
- training in the luteal phase: mild training in LISS (Low Intensity Steady State) cardio style + leg decongestion exercises.

The follicular phase

Modified PHA Circuit/Jump Set

The **PHA circuit** is a training circuit that involves the use of distant muscles, alternating large and small muscles, and alternating the upper and lower parts to facilitate the circulation and intensify the cardiovascular work; it is precisely for this reason that it takes the name of PHA, acronym for Peripheral Heart Action. The number of exercises to be included varies between 5 and 6.

The **Jump Set** involves the execution of two exercises, alternating with a break. In the case of the gynoid subject, it is recommended to combine upper body and lower body exercises (thus maintaining the principle of PHA).

At this stage, it is advisable to practice with a good volume of work; in fact, the anti-catabolic action of estrogen protects women from catabolism, so you can use workouts that include medium-high repetitions and a controlled TUT (Time Under Tension).

It is always important to remember that, by nature, women (especially the gynoid subject) tend to have problems with edemas, therefore it is very important to dedicate a part of the training to work protocols aimed at improving the blood circulation (including walking on the carpet without shoes). Choosing the exercises is also fundamental: for example, multi-joint exercises could cause inflammation in the legs (if there is high blood permeability or if telangiectasias are present), so you can train them indirectly by concentrating the work on the buttocks.

In fact, remember that when we train a muscle, it draws a large amount of blood and fluids in both the intra- and extracellular compartment: the longer the duration of the contraction, the larger the amount of the drawn blood, and along with it, also a certain amount of metabolites such as lactic acid which, in conditions of edema, would worsen the situation.

It is therefore an obvious need to reduce the amount of these metabolites that are produced during the muscle contraction through low repetition training that does not involve the anaerobic lactacid metabolism. We remind you that at the beginning, the use of multi-joint exercises such as squats, lunges, etc. must be excluded.

In the follicular phase, in the case of ginoid subjects who do not have evident alterations of the microcirculation, it is advisable to emphasize the eccentric phase (therefore the mechanical damage) to create greater muscle damage which, in this phase, is balanced by the high levels of estrogen. It favors a greater retention of nitrogen (N), from the peak of GH and testosterone (they also favor the retention of N and stimulate the protein synthesis at the nuclear level) and from the use of intramuscular triglycerides that allow a protein sparing.

The luteal phase
Cardio LISS/capillarizing workout
Cardio LISS (Low Intensity Steady State) is a low intensity cardio workout while maintaining the aerobic threshold, i.e. with a heart rate of 65-75%; we should remember that in the symptomatic gynoid subject, running should be minimized or avoided.

Capillarizing training is a circuit that maintains the PHA principle, thus preserving the alternation of exercises between the lower and upper body parts. 4 exercises are then chosen to be interspersed with the bike recline (cardio station recommended in the gynoid as it avoids the closure of the popliteal vein and promotes the circulatory return due to its antigravitational positioning). Alternating classic pedaling with reverse pedaling performed by lifting the thigh towards the trunk, and thus involving the rectus of the abdomen, the workload at the level of the thighs is lightened ("Cyclette in the manner of Spattini").

In the luteal phase, most women tend to experience heaviness in the lower limbs. Returning to our arterio-capillary gynoid subjects, who already have problems with their legs, in this phase of the menstrual cycle these could become accentuated, so it is advisable to decrease the intensity of the workouts and support the microcirculation through capillarizing and decongestant workouts.

So the 4 weekly workouts can be divided as follows:
- 3 capillarising or decongestant workouts to reduce the swelling in the lower limbs;
- 1 total body workout, lasting 30 minutes, with repetition ranges between 12-15 and with 65-70% load; followed by 30 minutes of Cardio LISS.

In this phase, given the lack of energy and coordination (negative activity of progesterone on the motor cortex), less intense workouts are favored and in particular, capillarizing and/or decongestant protocols are used, especially in the premenstrual phase, to promote the drainage, which results less efficient due to the drop in progesterone.

Biphasic protocol for the android subject: diet and training

What changes is the type of training and the macronutrients in the diet. In fact, the android woman rarely tends to have circulatory problems, telangiectasias, varicose veins, etc. (see Table 24.1). She owes this luck to a higher concentration of male hormones such as testosterone, but also of cortisol (in fact these subjects are defined as hypercortisolemic). For this reason, multi-joint exercises such as squats, deadlifts, lunges, presses, etc. can be used in a training program.

Another characteristic of the android subjects is low glucose tolerance. There are a number of studies in this regard, in particular one carried out by Samsell et al., which focused on obese adults and children with the aim of determining whether the relationship between fat with android type distribution and fat with genoid type distribution was positively correlated to insulin resistance (IR), to the HOMA2-IR index (index that relates blood glucose values to insulin values) and to dyslipidemias, by examining a sample of android and ginoid children between the ages 7 and 13 years and BMI percentages between 0.1 and 99.6. It was noted that the high android/ginoid ratio was closely associated with IR and high levels of LDL and VLDL cholesterol (i.e. bad cholesterol). Therefore, this ratio can be used as a prognostic index for the onset of metabolic and cardiovascular diseases.

From a dietary point of view, macronutrients will change, especially in the luteal phase, in which fats can be kept higher due to some metabolic characteristics that distinguish the android subjects, that is sympathotonia (a higher activity of the sympathetic nervous system), which gives them a greater oxidative capacity towards fats.

The sympathetic nervous system is connected with the adrenal glands, which release hormones such as adrenaline and noradrenaline, that, among their various functions, stimulate lipolysis through the adrenergic receptors located in the adipose tissue. In the gynoid subject, on the other hand, there is a parasympatheticotonia, i.e. the prevalence of the activation of that part of the nervous system that is responsible for accumulating energy reserves (also remember the dominant estrogenic component which, if in excess, favors the accumulation of subcutaneous fat).

Furthermore, the timing of nutrient distribution changes throughout the day, precisely for the reason explained above, namely the high (albeit physiological) levels of cortisol, which tend to raise the blood glucose. Therefore, before consuming a carbohydrate meal, the circadian decrease in plasma cortisol levels is expected, trying to

Table 24.4 Biphasic diets for the android subjects from the 1st to the 14th day of the cycle: follicular phase

Training days	Non-training days
BREAKFAST	**BREAKFAST**
Protein to choose from:	Protein to choose from:
• 4 egg whites + 2 yolks	• 4 egg whites + 2 yolks
• 5 slices of turkey or chicken breast + 2 walnuts	• 5 slices of turkey or chicken breast + 2 walnuts
• 1 whole Greek yogurt	• 1 whole Greek yogurt
Fats to choose from:	Fats to choose from:
• 4 walnuts	• 4 walnuts
• 15 almonds	• 15 almonds
• 2 squares of dark chocolate >85%	• 2 squares of dark chocolate >85%
2 whole grain cakes	2 whole grain cakes
500 mg of *Rhodiola rosea*	1 g of omega-3

Continues

Continued

Training days	Non-training days
SNACK	**SNACK**
Fats to choose from: • 4 walnuts • 15 almonds • 2 squares of dark chocolate >85% 5 capsules of essential amino acids	Fats to choose from: • 4 walnuts • 15 almonds • 2 squares of dark chocolate >85% 5 capsules of essential amino acids
LUNCH	**LUNCH**
Protein to choose from: • 200 g of lean meat • 200 g of lean fish • 150 g of semi-fat meat • 150 g of fatty fish 20 g of EVO oil Vegetables	Protein to choose from: • 200 g of lean meat • 200 g of lean fish • 150 g of semi-fat meat • 150 g of fatty fish 20 g of EVO oil Vegetables
SNACK	**SNACK**
Fats to choose from: • 4 walnuts • 15 almonds • 2 squares of dark chocolate >85% 5 capsules of essential amino acids 1 fruit 4 whole grain cakes	Fats to choose from: • 4 walnuts • 15 almonds • 2 squares of dark chocolate >85% 5 capsules of essential amino acids 1 fruit
LUNCH	**LUNCH**
Protein to choose from: • 100 g of chicken breast • 100 g of turkey • 100 g of white meat • 100 g of lean fish: cod, pangasius, etc. 10 g of EVO oil Vegetables Carbohydrates to choose from: • 60 g of basmati rice, wholemeal, red, black • 60 g of other whole grains • 120 g of wholemeal or rye bread 600 mg of lipoic acid 1 g of cinnamon	Protein to choose from: • 150 g of chicken breast • 150 g of turkey • 150 g of white meat • 150 g of lean fish: cod, pangasius, etc. 10 g of EVO oil Vegetables Carbohydrates to choose from: • 4 whole grain cakes • 4 Swedish-style wholemeal crackers • 1 small wholemeal sandwich 600 mg of lipoic acid

Training day: 40% carbohydrates – 30% proteins – 30% fats (1600 Kcal: 140 g carbohydrates – 130 g proteins – 50 g fats).

Non-training day: 20% carbohydrates – 40% proteins – 40% fast (1500 Kcal: 80 g carbohydrates – 130 g proteins – 70 g fats).

The blue text indicates a supplementation to the diet.

Table 24.5 Biphasic diets for the android subjects from the 15th to the 28th day of the cycle: luteal phase

Training days	Non-training days
BREAKFAST	**BREAKFAST**
Protein to choose from: • 4 egg whites + 2 yolks • 5 slices of turkey or chicken breast + 2 walnuts • 1 whole Greek yogurt • 2 whole grain cakes 50 mg of CoQ10 1 g of acetylcarnitine 200 mg of potassium and 400 mg of magnesium 500 mg of vitamin C	Protein to choose from: • 4 egg whites + 2 yolks • 5 slices of turkey or chicken breast + 2 walnuts • 1 whole Greek yogurt • 2 whole grain cakes 600 mg of lipoic acid 1 g of acetylcarnitine 200 mg of potassium and 400 mg of magnesium 500 mg of vitamin C
SNACK	**SNACK**
Fats to choose from: • 4 walnuts • 15 almonds • 2 squares of dark chocolate >85% 5 capsules of essential amino acids	Fats to choose from: • 4 walnuts • 15 almonds • 2 squares of dark chocolate >85% 5 capsules of essential amino acids
LUNCH	**LUNCH**
Protein to choose from: • 200 g of lean meat • 200 g of lean fish • 150 g of semi-fat meat • 150 g of fatty fish 20 g of EVO oil Vegetables	Protein to choose from: • 200 g of lean meat • 200 g of lean fish • 150 g of semi-fat meat • 150 g of fatty fish 20 g of EVO oil Vegetables
SNACK	**SNACK**
Fats to choose from: • 4 walnuts • 15 almonds • 2 small squares of dark chocolate >85% 1 fruit 2 whole grain cakes 5 capsules of essential amino acids	Fats to choose from: • 4 walnuts • 15 almonds • 2 small squares of dark chocolate >85% 1 fruit 5 capsules of essential amino acids

Continues

Chapter 24 ▸ Nutrition, supplementation and training during the menstrual cycle

Continued

Training days	Non-training days
DINNER	**DINNER**
Protein to choose from:	Protein to choose from:
• 100 g of white lean meat	• 200 g of white lean meat
• 100 g of lean fish	• 200 g of lean fish
10 g of EVO oil	• 150 g of fatty fish
Vegetables	10 g of EVO oil
Carbohydrates to choose from:	Vegetables
• 60 g of brown rice or pasta	3000 IU of vitamin D3
• 60 g of other whole grains	
• 120 g of wholemeal or rye bread	
600 mg of lipoic acid	
400 mg of *Withania somnifera*	

Android training day: 25% carbohydrates – 30% proteins – 40% fats (1600 Kcal: 140 g carbohydrates – 130 g proteins – 50 g fats).
Non-training day android: 15% carbohydrates – 40% proteins – 45% fats (1500 Kcal: 50 g carbohydrates – 150 g proteins – 80 g fats).
The blue text indicates a supplementation to the diet.

favor the proteinic meals during the day to buffer the catabolic effect of cortisol (one of its functions is to induce gluconeogenesis starting from amino acids).

The following tables show some examples of a biphasic diet.

Food supplements for the android subject

Hyperlipogenetic android individuals are hypercorticosadrenal with hyperactivation of the sympathetic system, a tendency for an insulin resistance and an androgenic prevalence in females, predisposition to diabetes and cardiovascular disease.

Supplements and phytonutrients that are useful for improving the insulin resistance and the lipid profile (i.e. cholesterol and triglycerides in the blood)

- **Chromium**: it is part of the glucose tolerance factor and it is essential for the proper functioning of insulin. From 200 to 1000 μm per day depending on the degree of the insulin resistance.
- **Vitamin D**: after checking for any shortage or deficiency, from 1000 to 3000 IU per day. Improves the insulin response; it is fundamental especially for the android woman who denotes a lower level of estrogen and is therefore more prone to osteoporosis.
- **Magnesium**: 200 to 400 mg per day: lowers the blood pressure and promotes relaxation, with an anti-stress effect.
- **CoQ10**: 100 mg per day, especially in hypertensive and cardiopathic subjects and/or subjects who are treated with statins that destroy their formation.
- **α-lipoic acid**: from 400 to 1000 mg. The higher dosages are to be reserved for diabetic patients who have peripheral neuropathies.
- **Omega-3**: 1 g per day for cardiovascular prevention; if triglyceride levels are not within normal values, take 3 g per day.

- **Zinc**: 15-30 mg, essential for the insulin metabolism and for the immune system.
- **Selenium**: 200 mg per day; reduces the risk of the metabolic syndrome and reduces LDL cholesterol, while increasing HDL.
- **Green tea**: 200 mg or more per day of polyphenols (catechins in green tea) reduce the cholesterol levels.
- **Cinnamon**: 1 g per day; it has hypoglycemic and hypocholesterolemic properties, as well as reduces triglycerides.
- **Fenugreek**: a control study has shown positive results on the insulin resistance with 1 g per day of hydroalcoholic extract.
- **Berberine**: 500 mg 2 times a day. It has a hypoglycemic and cholesterol-lowering effect.

Supplements that act on the modulation of adrenal hormones

- **Phosphatidylserine**: 400 mg per day. Various studies have shown its ability to lower cortisol levels.
- **Vitamin C**: 500-1000 mg, it is the most important vitamin during stressful conditions, essential for the proper functioning of the adrenal glands.
- **Betasitosterol**: 300 mg twice a day. Derived from wheat germ oil, it optimizes the cortisol/DHEA ratio, especially following physical exertional stress, and it also lowers cholesterol.
- *Rhodiola rosea*: 500 mg per day. It modulates the production of cortisol and raises the levels of serotonin, exerting a relaxing action.
- **Reishi**: 500 mg 2-3 times a day. An adaptogenic mushroom that is capable of reducing cortisol production.
- **Theanine**: 100-250 mg; present mainly in green tea, it stimulates a relaxation with sleepiness, promoting the production of the neurotransmitter GABA in the brain and counteracting the stimulating effects of caffeine.
- **Ashwagandha**: 500 mg 2 times a day. It is an adaptogenic plant useful in the states of anxiety and insomnia, and it is able to modulate the production of cortisol.
- **Ginestrino**: 400-800 mg per day. It is a legume that was already known at the time of Homer. Currently it is indicated in convalescence and sleep disorders, it has a sedative effect and moderates the adrenal hyperfunctionality.
- **Passionflower**: 200-400 mg per day. It has a sedative action at the the central level of the nervous system, particularly useful in cases of insomnia due to psychophysical overmenage. It is also indicated in gastrointestinal disorders of nervous origin such as irritable colon and gastritis.
- **7 Keto-Dhea**: 25-100 mg per day. In Italy, it is considered a hormone and a medical prescription is necessary, while in the U.S. it is sold as an over-the-counter supplement. 7 Keto-Dhea reduces the activity of the enzyme that converts inactive glucocorticoids into active cortisol.

Training for the android subject

Let's now look at the training for the android morphotype.

As we said, the android subject can train harder thanks to her own testosterone levels, which give her more strength. Attention should be paid to the duration of the

workout, which should not exceed 45 minutes, in order to avoid an excessive release of cortisol.
- The follicular phase: strength.
- The luteal phase: **Giant Set** metabolic workouts. It is a type of training that involves 4 or 6 exercises performed in series, without intervals or with lengths that are reduced to a minimum, in order to increase the intensity of the training. There are different types:
  - same muscle group;
  - antagonist muscles;
  - distant muscle areas.

The follicular phase
Good levels of estrogen (lower than the gynoid subject due to testosterone). Elevated testosterone levels.
- Multiarticular exercises.
- Rep range: medium on 6-8 and high loads (75% of 1MR) for direct work on the muscle trophism.
- Split routine training.
- 4 weekly weight training sessions.

The luteal phase
Higher concentration of progesterone. Descending testosterone levels.
- Multiarticular exercises.
- Repetition range: high on 10-12 and high loads (65% of 1MR) for direct work on muscle trophism, combined, at the end of the workout, with 30 minutes of Cardio LISS.
- Split routine training.
- 4 weekly workouts:
  - 2 in the weights room;
  - 2 Cardio LISS workouts combined with exercises to strengthen the core.

Obviously, for both morphotypes, a **mobilization**, **strengthening**, **stretching** and **mobility** work will be carried out:
- anteversions of the pelvis on the fit ball: 20/30 movements;
- abdomen on fit ball with emphasis on opening and closing;
- inverse parallel crunches;
- accessory exercises for the buttocks.

There are substantial anatomical, structural, endocrine and metabolic differences between the various morphotypes. These differences lead to a different distribution and localization of the **adipose tissue**, but above all to a different response to the diet and the training, also depending on the period of the menstrual cycle. Therefore, the identification of the morphotype is the first step to take in order to draw up a correct customization of a program that must also take into account the phase of the menstrual cycle.

CHAPTER 25

Nutrition and supplementation for the premenstrual syndrome

Premenstrual syndrome (PMS) is one of the most common health problems affecting women between the ages of 18 and 45. It is estimated that about 50% of women of this age group in the Western world have symptoms of this syndrome. These are, therefore, impressive numbers.

There is some disagreement in defining PMS correctly, but there is a consensus that a woman suffers from it if symptoms recur in at least two out of every three menstrual cycles. Only if the symptoms, which can be more than 150, interfere with normal daily activity, can the person be defined as suffering from PMS.

Only 5% of women suffer from severe symptoms that prevent normal daily life.

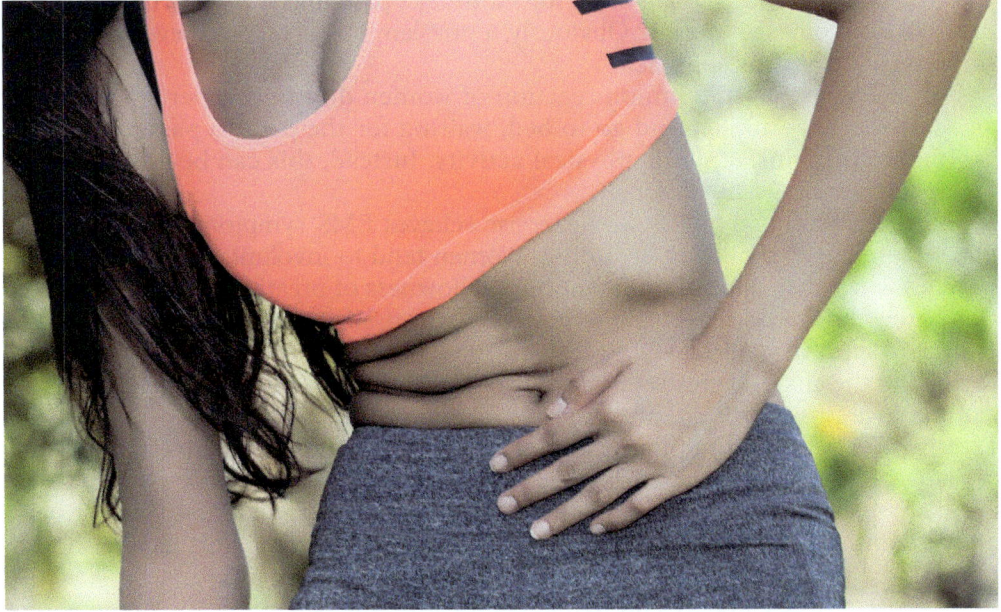

Figure 25.1

Symptoms normally begin one to two weeks before the start of menstruation and progressively improve until the start of the next menstrual cycle.

As a result, millions of women suffer from PMS symptoms to varying degrees during the middle of each month of their adult lives. This translates into a huge loss of productivity and quality of life.

Women with PMS say they don't feel "themselves" at that time. Some say they get up in the morning and feel like a different person. Others feel beaten up, tired and depressed. Others, on the other hand, feel very irritable and are ready to respond badly to their families. Women realize that they have reactions which they do not consider normal but they are not able to control.

In the United States, the case of a woman who was suffering from PMS, killed her husband and was judged by the magistrate in a condition of "incapacity to understand and intend" and was later acquitted, caused a sensation.

However, the most common symptoms can be classified into six groups:
1. Anxiety, irritability, mood swings.
2. Craving for sweets, feeling of fatigue and headache.
3. Swelling, weight gain, breast pain.
4. Depression, confusion, memory loss, insomnia.
5. Acne, greasy skin and hair.
6. Cramps, back pain, nausea and vomiting.

Other problems often worsen during the premenstrual period, for example: allergies, asthma, arthritis, constipation and cystitis. Many of these issues can coexist. Premenstrual syndrome affects every aspect of the working and family life of women who are affected by it, and who are often forced to take painkillers or anti-inflammatory drugs to overcome this period. Obviously, a problem that is repeated every month is certainly not a healthy approach.

Normally, the most common reaction of women during this period is to take an aspirin or a painkiller and go to bed, waiting for the pain to pass and hardly anyone would think of doing physical activity. Instead, this can be a solution, so get up and move!

There are various reasons why exercise relieves PMS symptoms. Premenstrual pains cause faster, shallower breathing. Women tend to involuntarily contract their muscles when they are suffering, but the shallowness of breathing and the contraction of the muscles decrease the blood flow and the tissue oxygenation, and this worsens the congestive syndrome of PMS.

Pain in the ankles, breasts, feet and belly is often due to water retention. Exercise can improve this condition. The pumping action of the muscles that occurs during exercise moves blood and fluids from the congested organs (sexual intercourse and orgasms can make you feel better for the same reason).

Exercise can reduce the back pain and cramps by strengthening the lower back and abdominal muscles. Women who exercise regularly often report having shorter periods and less bleeding.

Exercise reduces anxiety and irritability, helping the balance of the nervous system. It is a less dangerous way to unload emotional baggage and it is to be preferred over killing a husband (I personally try to make my wife do a lot of physical activity during this period…).

Most women report a sense of peace and relaxation after exercise.

This could be due to the brain's production of endorphins, which are substances that have an "opiate-like" effect, and among other things they are natural "pain-killers", i.e. painkillers that help to better tolerate the so-called "pangs" or "cramps". Physical exercises also improve the posture. Women with larger breasts tend to push their shoulders forward, but in doing so they cause muscle tension in the back and neck; this also worsens sinus congestion by reducing the circulation.

Many women with PMS have lumbar hyperlordosis, that is, an accentuation of the normal lumbar curve; this makes back pain and abdominal pain worse.

Dr. Arthur Michele, author of *Orthotherapy*, recommends exercising to improve the flexibility of the pelvic region.

Yoga is particularly recommended as it involves slow movements and a correct body position.

Foods and PMS

A diet focused to maintain normal BMI can lead to an improvement in hormonal function with a decrease in the risk of estrogen-related problems. In patients with insulin resistance, it is important to maintain a correct balance between proteins and carbohydrates, to prescribe a diet with organic foods and free hormones meat (which are mainly accumulated in fat), to decrease exposure to xenoestrogens, to inhibit the activity of cytochrome 3A enzymes that produce 16OH rather than 2OH estrogen.

The precursor fatty acids of inflammatory prostaglandins (arachidonic acid) concentrated in red meat, milk and eggs could increase PGE-2 thus increasing inflammation. Small and frequent low carbs meals are indicated, as well as high quality fats; processed food should be avoided. The worse the PMS, the more careful the patient must be. Overall, the diet must be predominantly plant-based, but with high quality proteins, possibly organic. Carbohydrates, even if reduced, should not be eliminated, especially the complexes ones; as a matter of fact, studies suggest benefits that could be due to greater transport of tryptophan, a precursor of serotonin, into the brain. Dietary fibers support the fecal elimination of estrogen by decreasing enterohepatic reuptake. The increase in SHBG, and/or the decrease in estrogen, decreases the production of inflammatory prostaglandins. Reduction in dietary fat from 40% to 20% of calories has been associated with a decrease in premenstrual water retention.

It is important to limit foods that have a high concentration of refined sugars and fats, and those that have undergone industrial manipulation and that contain preservatives and other chemicals. These foods include fizzy drinks, chocolate, alcohol, snacks, ice cream, hamburgers, hard cheeses, beef, pork, lamb and pizza.

These foods are very tasty and give immediate energy, but for the most part they are low in macronutrients and alter the hormonal chemistry.

Chocolate increases the need for vitamin B6 and intensifies the drive for sugars.

Sugars deplete the body of B-complex vitamins and cause glycemic imbalances: fluctuations in blood sugar give unstable energy levels and make painful symptoms worse.

Caffeine stimulates the nervous system, increases anxiety and mood swings. It also depletes the body of vitamin B and promotes breast pain.

It is advisable to gradually switch from normal to decaffeinated coffee, perhaps mixing them.

Dairy products (milk, cheese, yogurt, butter) interfere with the absorption of magnesium, a mineral that relieves cramps, helps glucose metabolism and stabilizes the mood. In addition, their high sodium content promotes swelling and water retention. Alcohol depletes the body of B vitamins and minerals, and alters the metabolism of carbohydrates. It is toxic to the liver and can impair the ability to metabolize hormones, causing estrogen levels to be higher than normal.

Meats like beef, pork and lamb are rich in fats that compromise the effectiveness of the liver. In addition, too much protein increases the mineral demands.

Salty foods like chips, pizza etc. increase water retention and cause breast pain and swelling.

Recently, it has been highlighted that PMS is linked to a lack of progesterone or in any case, to an unbalanced relationship between progesterone and estrogen.

Vegetarian diets lead to an increase in SHBG (Sex Hormone-Binding Globulin) thereby reducing the amount of free circulating estrogens; in addition, a low-fat diet reduces circulating estrogens. Dietary fiber supports fecal elimination of estrogens by decreasing enterohepatic reuptake.

Estrogen and progesterone must be in balance, in the sense that the deficiency or excess of one of them automatically leads to the excess or deficiency of the other. It is easier to have an excess of estrogen, as it can be found in meats and dairy products, not forgetting that pesticides and some plastics can function as estrogens (xenoestrogens).

Agnycastus is a plant whose berries exert a hormonal action on the body by increasing the secretion of LH, resulting in an increase of the progesterone levels, restoring the normal balance between estrogen and progesterone and also appears to affect dopamine and endorphins by interacting with opioid receptors. *Vitex agnus castus* was the most studied remedy (four studies, about 500 women) and was seen to consistently improve PMS better than the placebo. Single evidence also supports the use of Ginkgo biloba or *Crocus sativus* (saffron).

Curcumin is able to modulate norepinephrine, dopamine, and serotonin and influence inflammatory pathways.

Saffron can help treat the symptoms of PMS (premenstrual syndrome), a common health problem in women of childbearing age. In 2014 Direkvand-Moghadam et al., with a systematic review and meta-analysis study (17 studies that met the inclusion criteria), have shown that approximately 50% of the women suffer from it. So, 15 mg of saffron 2 times a day are more effective than placebo in the treatment of PMS symptoms, such as pain, irritability, headache, dysphoric disorder (Rajabi et al., 2020).

In addition to neurotransmitters, the production of prostaglandin E2 (a precursor to inflammatory cytokines) is likely involved in some of the physical symptoms of PMS such as pain, swelling and inflammation as well as breast tenderness, headaches, edema of the extremities and others.

Vitamins and minerals

B complex - The B complex vitamins are important for the glucose metabolism, for the inactivation of estrogen by the liver and for the proper functioning of the central nervous system. They are normally contained in foods such as whole grains, brewer's yeast, legumes and liver. Fatigue and irritability can result from a deficiency of the vitamin B complex.

Choline and inositol - They are part of the B complex and together with vitamin B6 they are particularly important for PMS. Choline and inositol increase the liver's ability to break down fats and steroid hormones such as estrogen. They are present in high quantities in soy and wheat germ oil.

Vitamin B6 - Vitamin B6 can relieve many premenstrual symptoms, such as mood swings, irritability, water retention, breast tenderness, swelling and the craving for sweets. Vitamin B6 levels decrease in women who use birth control pills. Dosage: 50-200 mg per day.

Vitamin C - It is an important antioxidant, protects the capillary walls and promotes a good blood circulation. Dosage: 3000 mg per day.

Vitamin D - It is essential for the absorption of calcium from the intestine. In addition, it decreases the skin's sebum production, which is accentuated during the menstrual period. Normally this vitamin accumulates in the liver and it is produced by the body through the exposure to sunlight, or it can be taken as a supplement. Dosage: 2000 UI per day.

Vitamin E - It is an important antioxidant; recent research shows its correlation with the reproductive system, so much so that it has been called the vitamin of fertility. This argues in favor of its efficacy and importance in hormone regulation. These effects have been confirmed by its use in fibrocystic mastopathy. Dosage: 200 mg per day.

Magnesium - A magnesium deficiency is believed to be very important as a cause of PMS symptoms, and adequate levels of magnesium help decrease the abdominal pain and control the anxious craving for sweets during the premenstrual period. Dosage: 200-400 mg per day.

Calcium - Increasing calcium levels beyond the normal recommendation of 800 mg per day "for women over 24" can alleviate the symptoms of PMS. In a study of women with PMS, adding calcium as a supplement decreased the problems of irritability and poor concentration. Dosage: 1200 mg per day.

Nutrition and supplementation for cellulite

by Fabrizio D'Agostino

It is a fact that shaping the female body is much more difficult than shaping the male one. Due to localized fat accumulations, high estrogen concentration, less muscle mass, water retention, circulatory problems and more, women need special strategies to achieve appreciable results.

In most cases, professionals such as nutritionists, dieticians, instructors and personal trainers have to address needs of women with a classic gynoid conformation, characterized by narrow shoulders and prominent thighs and hips. These women tend to accumulate localized fat in the lower part of the body, that is therefore disproportionate to the upper one, which remains unchanged and thinner despite the diet and training. It is therefore necessary to adopt a targeted strategy that takes into account dietary plans and physical workouts aimed at combating the accumulation of fat, especially localized fat. In this process, it is important to support, in all aspects, the woman who does not feel comfortable with her body, to guarantee optimal results and a greater self-esteem.

To act on the physical aspect, it is essential to have a clear understanding of the anatomical basis of the organism on which we are going to intervene with nutrition and physical activity. First, it is necessary to pay attention to the *cutis* (or skin), which represents the outermost lining of the body of mammals and in particular of humans. The skin is divided as follows:

- *epidermis*: the most superficial non-vascularized part, which is nourished from the dermis and is made up of multi-layered stratified epithelium (constantly changed);
- *dermis*: consisting of glands, vessels, hairs, hair erector muscles; obtains nourishment from the microcirculation;
- *hypodermis*: the layer below the dermis, divided into the superficial lamina, intermediate lamina and deep lamina.

The subcutaneous body fat that we can pinch with the plicometer or grasp with the fingers is confined to the surface layer of the hypodermis and it is largely represented by adipocytes, or fat cells.

A fat cell or *adipocyte* is a specialized, unilocular cell, with a nucleus that is displaced outwards, in which there is a large lipid drop where fats are packed in the form of triglycerides. The lipid drop is surrounded by filaments of a protein, called *vimentin*, which encloses the fat within the cell's cytoplasm. The adipocyte is surrounded by a glycoprotein mesh and reticular fibers which together create a support for the microcirculation and for the blood vessels that surround the cell.

However, there are some differences regarding the sites of the fat accumulation and the structure of the hypodermis. As it is well known, in fact, the white adipose tissue is distributed differently in the two sexes: in women, there is a higher percentage of body fat, which is accumulated mainly in the hips and thighs, while men tend to have deposits of abdominal fat, particularly around the viscera. Two different morphotypes are thus configured: android or hyperlipogenetic, and *gynoid* or hypolipolytic.

In the process of increasing the adipose mass due to the excessive consumption of nutrients, in men there is an increase in the volume of adipocytes, while in women, in addition to adipocyte hypertrophy, there is also an increase in the number of cells. The regional accumulation is in a large extent due to the action of estrogens and the distribution of their receptors which are present in almost all cells, particularly in the endothelium, in smooth muscles, in adipocytes and in the attached extracellular matrix.

In the hypodermis, this matrix can be organized differently in the two sexes, thus highlighting a different aspect. Normally, the hypodermis has collagen fibers that delimit the septae, arranged both perpendicular and 45° to the skin plane (in the presence of a high quantity of estrogen, the conformation is predominantly perpendicular). With such a conformation, when the cells of the female adipose tissue which are already in greater numbers for the reasons we expressed above, become larger due to an incorrect diet, a thickening of the perpendicular septa occurs in order to oppose the hypodermic pressure. The thickened and longitudinally oriented septae are responsible for the characteristic "orange peel" appearance of the skin affected by cellulite.

The term *cellulite* is usually used to indicate a pathology of the subcutaneous connective tissue distinct from obesity and lipodystrophies. It is also defined as a progressive gangrenous infection of the subcutaneous tissue. It occurs in a localized or diffuse form, with skin thickening and "orange peel" or "mattress" integument, which characterize the various stages. It manifests itself with paraesthesia, tingling and blood circulation disorders (alterations in the microcirculation and impaired drainage of the lymphatic system), and sometimes with dermatalgia (or pain from contact).

However, in medicine, the term "cellulite" is incorrect, since it implies cellular inflammation that is not actually present. The correct term is EFSP (Edematous FibroSclerotic Panniculopathy) which indicates a degeneration of the adipose and connective panniculus, with the presence of edema, water retention and fibrotic indurations induced by the slowing of the circulation and metabolic exchanges, which determine a tissue compression and an incarceration of the fat nodules inside it, causing the classic orange peel appearance; in its most severe form it is defined as *sclerotic*, since it presents with thickening and incarceration of fat cells, and the skin becomes hollow like a mattress.

Under normal conditions, the adipose tissue is very well vascularized and the adipocytes are well represented, with the nuclei in a peripheral position; moreover, the blood vessels are adjacent to the surface of the adipocytes and allow a normal cell exchange. On the other hand, in sclerotic cellulite, inflammation is so high that it causes pain.

Four stages of EFSP have been characterized, from the mildest to the most severe. In the first stage, the *reversible edematous* one, edema is caused by the stagnation of liquids in the hypodermis and the accumulation of fat, and it is characterized by heaviness in the limbs and by the absence of the fovea sign. Interstitial edema creates a slight alteration of the blood vessels, thus causing vascular microectasias, with an increase in vascular permeability and a consequent extravasation of fluid; skin loses its elasticity, becomes very adherent to the underlying tissues and appears pasty.

In the second stage, the *fibrotic* one, fat cells are wrapped in a fine network of collagen fibers and edema induces the hypertrophy and hyperplasia of the fibers, with occlusion of the vessels, alteration of membrane exchanges and suffering of the skin and the subcutaneous tissue. It is characterized by a stagnation of toxic catabolites derived from cellular metabolism and the epidermis has a dull complexion, reddens when compressed and takes on the appearance of an orange peel; there is a presence of dilated capillaries (*telangiectasia*), which are also found in a branched form. These all represent symptoms of poor oxygenation, vessel fragility and difficulty in the disposing of fats.

In stage III, called the *sclerotic* stage, micronodules encapsulated by collagen fibers are created, microcirculation is compromised, metabolic exchanges and tissue oxygenation are severely limited; this produces sclerosis and hyperkeratosis.

Finally, stage IV, called the *scarring* stage, is the completely irreversible one, in which macronodules, a classic mattress aspect and a complete sclerosis of the adipose connective tissue are formed. There are no suitable therapies to restore the normal functioning of the adipose tissue in the stage IV, during which it is possible to act only with surgery or with esthetic medicine treatments.

To counteract this skin imperfection, it is necessary to act on several fronts, such as the facilitation of the purifying action of the liver, regularization of the gastrointestinal tract, hormonal modulation, postural rebalancing, a dietary regime aimed at oxidizing as much fat as possible, an adequate physical activity, an intake of a lot of water, infusions, decoctions and cold macerates, to promote diuresis and anti-inflammation. Herbal teas based on Java tea (orthosiphon), containing potassium salts, which stimulate diuresis, and saponins, which counteract inflammation, are useful for this purpose; birch extract, containing birch, to drain and for its anti-inflammatory effect; the infusion of apple and cinnamon, which contain functional substances; and finally, draining massages also represent an important adjuvant.

In order to implement a food strategy, supported by a specific supplementation that is capable of assisting the processes that leads to certain pathophysiological conditions, it is necessary to know the foods (both solid and liquid) that can help.

First of all, **Java tea** (*Orthosiphon stamineus*), which boasts exceptional diuretic properties and is one of the best natural remedies for cellulite and swelling. Coming from Southeast Asia and the island of Java, from which it takes its name, it is rich in phenolic compounds, especially flavonoids. It is used in India and Indonesia as a remedy for kidney and bladder problems.

Preparations based on orthosiphon are indicated in the forms of arterial hypertension, heart failure and in all cases of water retention for which it is considered appropriate to intervene with substances that have a diuretic activity.

Among the numerous studies conducted, one in particular collected information on the pharmacological properties through a systematic investigation aimed at certifying the curative efficacy of this plant for some human diseases.

What emerged from the carried out observations is that it boasts numerous properties: it is a remedy for kidney stones and gout because, thanks to its diuretic action, it favors the increase in the volume of fluid that passes into the kidneys, helping to dissolve the stones, facilitating their release and avoiding other deposits; it is also an antipyretic remedy, as it lowers the hyperthermia within 4 hours of administration; it is an anti-inflammatory and analgesic, favoring the reduction of edema and swelling 3-5 hours after administration, in addition to the reduction of the associated pain; it acts as a hepatoprotective agent thanks to its antioxidant properties, as it reduces the concentration of bilirubin, bringing it to physiological levels; it is a hypoglycemic agent, since it reduces the concentration of glucose in the blood of diabetic subjects, with a consequent reduction of triglyceride levels and an increase of HDL cholesterol; it is an antiangiogenic agent, as it blocks the growth of neovascularization; it balances the levels of nitric oxide in macrophages which are stimulated by the inflammatory endotoxins, reducing one of the harmful effects of inflammation.

The gastrointestinal mucosa is constantly exposed to oxidizing agents that come from ingested foods, consequently it is subject to a prolonged oxidative stress from reactive oxygen species (ROS) generated during the aerobic metabolism. Therefore, there is a close relationship between ROS and the inflammatory process of the mucosa. The activation of the transcription of nuclear factor-kappa B (NF-κB) by means of pro-oxidant molecules (stress, diet, infections, obesity, etc.) leads to an expression of the genes that control the inflammatory phase responses, with the production of TNF cytokines and interleukins (pro-inflammatory). In this regard, polyphenols play a beneficial role, thanks to their antioxidant activity, as they prove to be useful in lowering the inflammation of the gastrointestinal tract.

Among the foods that are important for their anti-inflammatory properties we will mention the apple, which consists of 87% water and has a high concentration of potassium. This fruit has an effective diuretic and anti-inflammatory effect thanks to the high amounts of polyphenols.

A recent study focused on defining the content of polyphenols extracted from dried apple peels, determined their antioxidant and anti-inflammatory potential in the intestine. In this regard, cell lines were used to study the role of the preventive actions of these polyphenols against oxidative stress and inflammation.

Oxidative stress causes an increase in malondialdehyde, a depletion of omega-3 polyunsaturated fatty acids (omega-3 PUFA) and alterations in the activity of endogenous antioxidants (superoxide dismutase, glutathione peroxidase and glutathione reductase). The results of this study showed that polyphenols prevented peroxidation and counteracted inflammation, as demonstrated by the reduction of cytokines (TNF-α and IL-6) and prostaglandin E2, which trigger the inflammatory cascade; in addition, the mechanisms of action initiated by the polyphenols also induced a reduction in the regulation of COX2 and NF-kB. These results provide enough evidence for the ability of polyphenols to reduce the oxidative stress and inflammation, two central processes involved in inflammatory bowel diseases.

Another food that promotes diuresis and anti-inflammation is **cinnamon**, whose phytotherapeutic properties derive from its active ingredients: polyphenols, tannins, terpenes. The most valuable variety is *Cinnamon zeylanicum*, whose stem is used to obtain cinnamon in the form of sticks. It has antiseptic, neuroprotective and antioxidant properties which counteract cellular aging and help strengthen the immune system; it is an excellent natural remedy for blood sugar control and weight control.

Cinnamon was the subject of an in-depth study, in which the oxidizing activity of its extract was evaluated through a series of chemical reactions. Its results showed that the methanolic extract of cinnamon contains a number of antioxidant compounds that can effectively neutralize ROS, including hydroxyl radicals and other free radicals *in vitro*. Their ability to neutralize free radicals and inhibit the lipid peroxidation is of a considerable interest. Furthermore, it is possible to increase the effectiveness of the antioxidant barrier, which can be evaluated through specific tests such as the d-ROM (diacron Reactive Oxygen Metabolites) test, with substances such as vitamin E, vitamin C, carotenoids, polyphenols and anthocyanins by including kiwis, pomegranates, avocados, carrots, tomatoes, oranges, mangosteen, guava, garlic, extra virgin olive oil, onions and fish in our food plan.

The oxidation of fats at the level of a localized region can be prevented by improving the microcirculation. It is therefore advisable to stimulate the microcirculation by adopting good behavioral rules, by avoiding too high heels, tight clothes, postures with crossed legs, smoking; instead, you must consume foods that contain functional substances, such as: **berries** (currants, blackberries, blueberries and raspberries), which contain anthocyanidins and antioxidant polyphenols that improve the capillary tonus; **black grapes**, which contain resveratrol, with a vasorelaxing activity and capable of promoting an increase in vascular elasticity; **plums**, which contain polyphenols and quercetin, which thin the blood; **red chicory**, which contains anthocyanins; **Venere rice**, which contains more anthocyanidins than berries.

There was a study carried out particularly for **cranberries**, known for their great antioxidant and anti-inflammatory properties as they are rich in anthocyanins (flavonoids) and resveratrol (stilbene), which demonstrated a reduction in oxidative stress and in the inflammatory processes in the members of the Canadian national rowing team. A series of parameters were evaluated, such as TNF-α, ferritin, iron, IL-6, myoglobin, sTFR, hepcidin, TIBC and UIBC, but the greatest effects were obtained on TAC (Total Antioxidant Capacity). The results of the study show that blueberry extract contributes to an increase in the antioxidant potential of subjects exposed to intense aerobic exercise, who have an abnormal consumption of oxygen which, with the metabolization process of beta-oxidation, leads to the production of ROS. Therefore, athletes who have taken the supplement have significantly higher TAC levels.

Further studies investigated the effect of anthocyanins (which are present in the previously mentioned foods) on the *endothelial system*. The latter, which lines the internal surface of the blood vessels, modulates the vascular tone and controls the functionality of the arteries. Its dysfunction and the consequent oxidative stress represent the main mechanisms of various pathologies and cardiovascular diseases. Its normal functions are mediated by nitric oxide (NO), which is a powerful vasodilator agent. Therefore, it is necessary to stimulate its production not from macrophages, but from the endothelial tissue itself.

ROS compromise the endothelial functions resulting in less nitric oxide availability. Factors that can protect the endothelial system or neutralize ROS have potential beneficial effects on cardiovascular diseases, and the decrease in the incidence and risk of cardiovascular disease is associated with the consumption of fruits and vegetables that are rich in these compounds.

Recent evidence shows that plant-derived anthocyanins may have a strong potential as cardioprotective agents. *Anthocyanins* are water-soluble polyphenolic compounds that make up the red, blue and purple pigments of fruits. They have numerous benefits, including antioxidant, anti-inflammatory, antiviral, antidiabetic, cardioprotective properties, as well as vasoactive and vasoprotective effects on coronary arteries.

We find anthocyanins above all in aronia (*Aronia melanocarpa*), bilberry (*Vaccinium myrtillus*) and elderberry (*Sambucus nigra*). There is evidence showing that the extracts are directly vasoactive, directly modify the endothelium-dependent and endothelium-independent responses mediated by NO (nitric oxide) and protect coronary arteries from oxidative lesions. A study showed that the anthocyanin extracts from aronia and blueberry produced a dose-dependent relaxation of the coronary arteries (where the aronia recorded the highest relaxation value).

Low concentrations of these extracts do not affect the vascular tone of the coronaries but protect them from ROS. These results suggest that some components of aronia and blueberry extracts may have vasodilatory properties; consequently, these extracts can have significant beneficial effects in vascular diseases, thus also being useful for supporting the health of the microcirculation.

For the stimulation of the microcirculation it is possible to use preparations based on:

- **horse chestnut**, which contains *aescin*, capable of reducing the capillary permeability (which instead increases when blood vessels are compressed, as in the second stage of EFSP, with a consequent leakage of fluid and the formation of edema); it also improves the resistance of the vascular walls;
- **butcher's broom**, which contains ruscogenins and flavonoids that determine an increased vascular tone and diuresis;
- **sweet clover**;
- **witch hazel**, which contains flavonoids and tannins that protect the vessel walls;
- **centella asiatica** (or Gotu Kola).

On the other hand, there are also some ready-made supplements based on:

- *oligomeric proanthocyanidins* (OPC), or grape seed extract;
- *pycnogenol*, extracted from maritime pine, which preserves the collagen of the blood capillaries from the damaging action of the elastase enzyme;
- *oxerutin*;
- *butcher's broom*, extract from Butcher's broom rhizome;
- *beta-alanine*, capable of buffering lactic acid in the muscle;

- *vitamin B12* and *folic acid*, which promote erythropoiesis and consequently improve the transport of oxygen. In fact, the increase in the supply of oxygen levels in compromised tissues where there is sclerosis, hypoxia and a decrease in pH is a positive factor.

A supplementation that includes fatty acids of the omega series, on the other hand, improves the fluidity of cell membranes, as well as that of red blood cell membranes. This results in a greater fluidity of the erythrocytes, which are able to reach even the tissues with narrower capillaries, thus guaranteeing a higher oxygenation.

The complex of the listed molecules gives tone, elasticity and resistance to the capillaries and contributes to the metabolism of red blood cells and many other processes that are important for the vascular and circulatory health.

The reorganization of the microcirculation starting from the diet cannot be separated from a specific physical activity that takes into account biochemistry, biomechanics and energy metabolisms and in this regard, a training plan is structured on an annual basis, based on the body re-composition of the hypolipolytic woman.

For the first months, the program includes a training in the weight room for the regional capillarization, which consists in implementing a series of exercises with a low load that train body regions in sequences which are at the greatest possible distance from each other. There is an execution of the movements with a range of repetitions between 12 and 20 for the low body training which is followed, without a pause, by exercises for the upper body.

All this requires commitment from the cardiovascular system, which improves the drainage and redistribution of blood flow to and from the body areas located at different extremities. It is considered effective because it allows a rapid reflux from the lower body areas and prevents the excessive stagnation of lactic acid. To plan a sequence of training schedules for a woman, especially if the subject is initially out of shape and with alterations in the microcirculation, it is now well established that producing as little lactic acid as possible, while fundamental for muscle hypertrophy, is deleterious for an already compromised microcirculation. In fact, the increase of the levels of acid catabolites in the microcirculation beyond the norm can favor, through the local lowering of the pH, conformational changes in key plasma proteins, such as transferrin and ceruloplasmin. Therefore, there is a release, respectively, of iron and copper in their free states. These transition metals, on the other hand, through the so-called Fenton reaction, can catalyze the conversion of circulating hydroperoxides (deriving from the cellular oxidative stress) into highly harmful oxygen free radicals (alkoxyls and hydroperoxyls), resulting in endothelial dysfunction and oxidation of lipoproteins. Therefore, having to lay the foundations for weight loss aimed at critical areas, in the first months of training, the trainer's attention will be directed not to hypertrophy (which in this period will take second place), but to the vascularization and the reduction of the general inflammation state.

CHAPTER 27

Nutrition and physical activity for pregnant women

by Fabrizio D'Agostino

A woman's life passes through several crucial phases which are characterized by different nutritional needs, as physiological, pathological and hormonal changes occur. It is necessary for women to be aware of the basic rules of nutritional education, as they will feed their babies both during pregnancy and during weaning. In order for women to face pregnancy without causing future problems for the unborn children, linked to nutritional deficiencies, there is a series of preventive actions. The intake of folic acid prevents a malformation called "spina bifida" and usually must be carried out in the first 28 days of conception; in addition, calcium intake in children increases the bone mass peak, triggering a mechanism to prevent the possible onset of future diseases such as osteopenia and osteoporosis. Pregnancy is marked by two phases: the first phase, of an anabolic type, is characterized by an increase in maternal lipid deposits and of the sensitivity to insulin; the second phase, on the other hand, of a catabolic type, is characterized by the reduction of insulin sensitivity, with a consequent increase in the concentration of glucose and free fatty acids.

By analyzing the hormonal picture of the pregnant woman in detail, it is possible to observe the modification of the production of hormones, such as: gonadotropin, human placental lactogen hormone (HPL), cortisol, progesterone, prolactin and estrogen. In particular, HPL increases the insulin resistance, increasing the blood concentration of glucose in the mother (hyperglycemia and hyperinsulinemia, which is a physiological condition during pregnancy) which will be made available to the fetus, ensuring an appropriate amount of carbohydrates, fundamental for the energy production and development. HPL also induces the lipolysis of maternal reserve fat deposits, which will be used as a source of energy by the mother herself, as an alternative to glucose made more available to the fetus. Eventually, ketones, formed from fatty acids, will also pass through the placenta to be used by the fetus.

It is therefore important to reduce the intake of foods with high GI (glycemic index), since prolonged postprandial hyperglycemia favors the flow of nutrients from mother to fetus, with a trans-placental passage of glucose which will lead to fetal hyperglycemia. This will result in a compensatory hyperinsulinemia which, by accelerating the anabolic processes, can lead to fetal macrosomia, with a consequent hyperglycemia of the unborn child.

As for lipid metabolism, there is an increase in FFA (Free Fatty Acid), triglycerides, fatty acids, cholesterol, lipoproteins and circulating phospholipids, since the mother tends to use lipids as an energy source, saving glucose and amino acids in favor of the fetus. However, the excess of the circulating fatty acids contributes to fetal macrosomia (weight greater than 4.5 kg).

To avoid ketosis after an overnight fast, three main meals and three snacks are generally recommended, which are important for avoiding the glycemic fluctuations that would lead to a situation of hyperglycemia with all the related consequences, up to a full-blown gestational diabetes, as well as a condition of obesity or overweight, both maternal and fetal. In general, for the intake of macronutrients we usually follow the guidelines of the Mediterranean diet.

Nutritional requirements in non-pathological pregnancy

The pregnant woman's diet does not differ much from that of other women, although it must be commensurate with the maternal-fetal nutritional needs and must take into account the effect that some foods may have on the health of the unborn child. The chosen foods can be eaten according to what is reported in the food pyramid suggested by the Dietary Reference Values (DRVs).

The carbohydrate requirement, following the rules of the Mediterranean diet, oscillates between 45 and 60% (up to 40% in the case of gestational diabetes) of the total daily energy, paying attention to the index and glycemic load, while the intake of fiber is 30 g per day and the sucrose intake must be less than 10% of the total daily energy.

The increased demand for energy is associated with a greater need for some nutrients, in particular proteins as the need for amino acids by the fetus increases, both during the organogenesis phase and during the growth phase, but also for the construction and storage of the mother's tissues (adipose tissue, breast tissue, uterus), which occurs from the 1st to the 6th month. The protein requirement should provide about 20% of daily energy and a prevalent share of this intake should come from foods with high biological value proteins, or proteins of animal origin such as milk, meat and eggs. The indicative weekly protein frequencies include a protein intake from meat 2-3 times, fish 2-3 times, legumes at least 4 times, eggs 1-2 times, cheeses 1-2 times. It is important to avoid cold cuts and prefer safe fresh cheeses, not marbled or seasoned, in adequate quantities, and ricotta. The lipid requirement in pregnancy is no different from that of the non-pregnant woman and should provide about 25-30% (35% in the case of gestational diabetes, when the intake of carbohydrates is reduced) of the total daily calories. The distribution of the daily lipid content also remains unchanged: no more than 7-10% of the total calories should be provided by saturated lipids; up to 20% from monounsaturated lipids; the cholesterol intake is 300 mg/day and about 7% must derive from polyunsaturated lipids. Among the latter, about 1-2% of the total calories should be represented by omega-6 essential fatty acids and about 0.2-0.5% by omega-3 essential fatty acids, with an omega-6/omega ratio -3 of 5:1. The development of the fetal CNS requires an important supply of DHA, which is synthesized mainly in the liver and placenta, then it is carried directly to the fetus. Their blood levels in the fetus are affected by the maternal diet. DHA is detected on the membrane of the outer segments of the rods of the retina and in the brain, where it mediates the phenomenon of neurotransmission at different levels. Its maximum accumulation occurs during the intrauterine life, therefore a deficiency in this phase will affect the development and will cause disorders that affect the central nervous system and the visual apparatus (Danish National Birth Cohort; 2007).

The importance of DHA during gestation has also been recognized in Italy, and it became so important that a revision of the LARNs and the distinction between DHA and other omega-3s are necessary. The minimum level that is currently recommended by the SINU (Società Italiana di Nutrizione Umana) is 200 mg per day (obtainable for example with 100 g of grouper or trout). DHA is contained in high quantities in fish oil (salmon, sardine, herring and cod liver) and in fish (mackerel and salmon). High levels of DHA are associated with a lower risk of preterm birth and its adequate intake is associated with a cognitive and functional improvement of the baby. The requirement of essential fatty acids for pregnant women is not fundamentally different from that of other adult women. According to the LARN, in fact, the intake of EPA-DHA remains the same, that is, 250 mg/day, while DHA intake increases from 100 to 200 mg/day. Essential fatty acids are found not only in fish, but also in other different food sources, listed in the table below.

It is important to pay particular attention to folic acid, since the deficiency of this acid (or vitamin B9) represents a risk factor for the onset of congenital malformations of the central nervous system (spina bifida) and it is also a cause of megaloblastic ane-

Table 27.1 Dietary sources of omega-3 and omega-6

Omega-3 fatty acids	Food source
Alpha-linoleic acid (18:3 n-3, ALA)	Linseed oil and seeds, oils and vegetables in general, nuts, algae, avocado, green leaves, soy beans
Eicosapentaenoic acid (20:5 n-3, EPA) Docosahexaenoic acid (22:5 n-3, DHA)	Fish
Omega-6 fatty acids	**Food source**
Linoleic acid (18:2 n-6, LA)	Oily seeds and fruit, vegetable oils and margarines, whole grains and legumes
Arachidonic acid (20:4 n-6, AA)	Meat, eggs and fish

mia. The Mediterranean diet is rich in folic acid (legumes, green leafy vegetables and fruit), but supplementation of this vitamin is required in preparation for a pregnancy.

The development of the embryonic structures from which the brain and spinal cord of the fetus will form is completed just 28 days after conception, while often the woman still does not know she is pregnant. Therefore, if pregnancy is planned, folic acid supplementation must begin 3-4 weeks before conception. The minimum levels are reached with an intake of 200 µg/day through food and 400 µg/day through supplementation. Women who are "at risk" (previous pregnancy and/or family history of spina bifida, concomitant treatment with chemotherapy or anticonvulsant drugs) require a daily dose corresponding to 4-5 mg of folic acid. Supplementing with vitamin B9 seems to reduce the risk of other pregnancy complications: preeclampsia, intrauterine growth retardation, congenital malformations, in particular cardiovascular, and presumably the subsequent development of tumors of the nervous tissues. Folic acid is present in numerous foods, such as dehydrated yeast (useful for vegetarian diets), wheat germ, white beans, escarole, spinach, nuts, etc.

As for vitamin D, the contribution during pregnancy is essential for the correct absorption of calcium. Vitamin D can be found in many foods, such as cod liver oil, fish oil, anchovies, scampi, cheese, etc., and a proper nutrition throughout the week guarantees the right amount of it. The recommended intake of minerals, on the other hand, indicate an increase in the need for calcium and iron. If the calcium intake is insufficient, it does not always induce disorders in the fetus, but it can cause excessive bone demineralization in the mother, since the fetus takes calcium from the maternal deposits.

Calcium supplementation is recommended in particular cases, such as in women who do not consume calcium food sources (intolerant, vegan), women with pre-pregnancy obesity (generally associated with low levels of vitamin D), women with hypovitaminosis D and adolescents in full growth. To cover the calcium requirement (**1200 mg/day**) it is important to take into account that a small glass of skimmed milk and a jar of yogurt provide 150 mg each; 5 teaspoons or a portion of 25 g of grated Grana Padano PDO or Parmigiano Reggiano provide about 300 mg; a portion of anchovies eaten with the bone provide 150 mg; therefore, with the proper nutrition, food supplementation is not necessary.

Among the foods that are rich in calcium we find cheeses, anchovies, chocolate, dried fruits, almond milk, yogurt, milk, etc. For the phosphorus requirement, on the other hand, a balanced diet already provides the necessary quantities that are required for any physiological situation.

Iron is the nutrient that has a greater increase in the needs of the pregnant woman, due to the increased production of erythrocytes. In the fetus, it is required for the formation of molecules such as hemoglobin and myoglobin and for the hepatic deposit of iron (during neonatal life it compensates for the low concentration of this element in the breast milk). Among the foods which are rich in iron we find clams

Table 27.2 Factors pros and cons the iron absorption

Factors that favor the intestinal absorption of NON-HEME iron	Factors against the intestinal absorption of NON-HEME iron
Gastric acid	Some minerals: calcium and phosphorus
Citric acid	Chelating agents
Ascorbic acid	Dietary fibers
Physical activity	Tannic acid (chocolate, coffee, etc.)
Air rarefaction	Polyphenols
Iron deficiency	Gastric hypochloridia or achloridia
Pregnancy	
Amino acids	

and similar sources, such as dehydrated yeast, liver, legumes, dried fruits, cereals, lean meat, etc. The concomitance of various factors affects the intestinal absorption of iron and there are factors that favor intestinal absorption and others that counteract it, as shown in the following table.

Iodine requirements are not particularly high; in fact, according to the 2014 DRVs, the estimated requirement is 200/g/day. An iodine deficiency, however, causes serious problems for the fetus, especially for the CNS, resulting in severe intellectual deficits and in an inadequate synthesis of thyroid hormones. It is possible that these problems are widespread in areas where food and drinking water are particularly low in iodine and endemic goiter is present, but the simple use of iodized salt or whole sea salt is sufficient to prevent them. One of the consequences of iodine deficiency is hypothyroidism, whose effects on pregnancy are manifold: pregnancy hypertension, preeclampsia, low birth weight, intrauterine death, congenital malformations and *postpartum* hemorrhage. Hypothyroidism causes damage to the neurological and intellectual development of the newborn, which in its most severe form configures the clinical picture of the endemic cretinism. If the mother is hypothyroid during pregnancy, this involves a damage to the fetal nervous system due to a lack of the maternal thyroxine (first weeks of gestation, when the fetal thyroid has not yet begun to function, or later, if the fetal thyroid is also hypofunctional).

The daily iodine requirement of an adult is 150 µg; a maximum of 50-100 µg is introduced with the diet, in some areas of Italy even 30 µg; during pregnancy, its requirement increases up to 200 µg. The maximum tolerable dose of iodine during pregnancy and lactation is 600 µg per day (European Commission, September 26, 2002). An increase in the nutritional availability of iodine is therefore necessary for at least 3 months to avoid the onset of maternal (mostly subclinical), fetal and neonatal hypothyroidism, which can arise with an intake of less than 100 µg/day.

The strategy that is recommended by WHO, the Iodine Global Network and UNICEF for the eradication of iodine deficiency disorders is to use food salt as a vehicle, enriching it with adequate amounts of iodine. Bearing in mind that 1 g of iodized salt provides 30 µg of iodine, the use of iodized salt is not in contradiction with the WHO recommendations to reduce salt consumption (no more than 5 g per day in adults, 2-3 g in children over the first year of life) for the prevention of hypertension, cardiovascular diseases and other diseases due to excessive salt consumption. Sea fish is the richest food in iodine, as it contains about 50-100 µg/100 g, while other foods contain much lower quantities (the iodine content of meat, fruit, vegetables and cereals varies between 2 and 5 µg/100 g); however, the consumption of fish in western country is modest and the iodine we introduce in our diet comes mostly from milk, meat and vegetables.

Another important condition in pregnancy is the state of hydration; in fact, water is the essential constituent of the human body and it is essential for the performance of all physiological processes and biochemical reactions. The water requirement for non-pregnant women is 2 liters per day, while 2.3 liters of water per day are needed during pregnancy and 2.7 liters during breastfeeding. The need during pregnancy increases due to the increase in the volume and production of the amniotic fluid.

An adequate hydration is also effective in reducing the risk of constipation and the onset of urinary tract infections. It should also be considered that a certain amount of water (600-800 mL) comes from foods, which contain it in various concentrations, in particular: fruits, vegetables, greens and milk are made up of 85% of water; meat, fish, eggs, fresh cheeses contain 50-80%; bread and pizza are made up of 20-40% of water and cooked pasta and rice contain 60-65%.

Foods to be avoided during pregnancy

One of the first foods to avoid during pregnancy is certainly alcohol, on which numerous studies have been conducted that have shown negative effects on the development of the fetus; in particular, teratogenic effects have been found on the nervous system with the development of structural and cognitive damage, risk of spontaneous abortion and low birth weight. The teratogenic effect is able to cause fetal malformations and induce the fetal alcohol syndrome, which involves a low weight at birth, mental retardation and facial dysmorphism (cleft lip and palate). In addition, any alcohol intake affects the absorption, metabolism and excretion of zinc, magnesium, copper and iron.

Caffeine, on the other hand, is able to cross the placental barrier. In fact, there are studies that state that the children of women who consume more than 500 mg of caffeine per day are more likely to have high heart and respiratory rates and tremors. Consumption of caffeine during pregnancy should therefore be limited to 300 mg/day. However, there is insufficient evidence to confirm or deny the effectiveness of abstaining from caffeine in relation to birth weight or other pregnancy outcomes; some studies show an increased risk of spontaneous abortion or fetal death following the intake of high quantities of caffeine (>300 mg/day), especially when combined with smoking and alcohol, or following an excessive use of caffeine (>800 mg/day).

An important caffeine content is not only found in coffee, tea and similar beverages, but also in numerous foods, such as unsweetened cocoa powder and dark chocolate. The CREA (formerly INRAN) guidelines simply recommend reducing the consumption of foods such as coffee, tea and herbal teas, caffeinated beverages such as cola or energy drinks, coffee liqueur, chocolate and cocoa.

It is important to pay attention to all those drinks that contain quinine, such as bitter lemon and tonic water. The undesirable effects can be neurotoxic, particularly visual and gastrointestinal disturbances, they can affect the heart conduction system, decrease the blood pressure, induce hematological problems, hypersensitivity reactions of the skin, fever and bronchospasms.

Even the consumption of fish should be controlled, as there is a risk of the presence of methylmercury, which can damage the CNS of the fetus. Women should no longer eat fish 1-2 times a week and pregnancy and lactation are the most critical periods for methylmercury toxicity. This substance is able to overcome the blood-brain and placental barrier, causing damage to the CNS and in the development of the fetus; high doses, in fact, cause severe mental retardation of the unborn child; lower doses cause alterations in the psychomotor development. From an examination of the literature it is estimated that 90-99% of the mercury present in fish is in the form of methylmercury (toxic). In particular, predatory species, such as swordfish, tuna, shark and others (such as emery, blue shark and dogfish), may contain high levels of methylmercury (between 500 and 1500 µg/kg). Fish and crustaceans such as salmon, cod, sole and shrimp contain less. The European Commission, in a recent information note, advises women of childbearing age, pregnant or breastfeeding, and children, to avoid the intake of swordfish, shark and mackerel or, not to consume more than a small portion per week (less than 100 g).

During the pregnancy, among the increases in the needs of some micronutrients (calcium, phosphorus, iodine, folic acid, iron, vitamin C) there is also an increase in the need of vitamin A. In this regard, an additional intake of about 100 µg per day of RE (retinol equivalent) is required, but the daily dose should never exceed 6 mg per day (in the form of retinol). With a dose that is equal to, or higher than 6 mg per day, there are greater risks of congenital malformations, given the potential teratogenic effect on the body.

In addition to the foods to be avoided during pregnancy that are already mentioned, other foods which are not allowed are offal and uncooked eggs, as they can be a carrier for salmonella, and seafood, both cooked and raw, raw and smoked fish, raw unpasteurized milk, soft cheeses from raw milk, raw meat and raw sausages in general, and all those other foods that can be sources for main pathologies of food origin that can cause harm to the mother and the child.

Physical activity in pregnancy

The benefits of physical activity during pregnancy are many, both from a maternal and fetal point of view. Through training, first of all, it is possible to control weight gain; in addition, the risk of gestational diabetes is reduced, due to the increased expression of membrane glucotransporters that promote the glucose uptake, allowing for a better control of blood glucose levels. It has also been shown that sports help to improve posture and movements, both during and after childbirth; There is also a mood improvement, as physical activities release hormones such as endorphins or other hormones that are involved in numerous activities such as the appetite control, the sense of well-being and sleep regulation. As a result, exercising helps you rest better, eat regularly, relieve stress and feel fitter.

The peripheral vascularization is also improved, since training the leg muscles promotes a better venous return of blood to the heart and, therefore, improving the circulation and reducing the sense of heaviness and swelling which is typical for the state of pregnancy.

An additional benefit for the mother is the **prevention of lower back pain**, sciatica and back pain; in fact, it is important to train back and shoulders muscles to counteract the displacement of the center of gravity. Some studies have shown the benefits of the physical activity also on the fetus. In fact, it represents a preventive tool against obesity and against the development of metabolic diseases; moreover, it has been shown that it guarantees a bigger and more mature brain activity in children who are born to trained and sporting mothers and, finally, it is able to increase the placental surface, favoring an increase in the oxygen exchange between the mother and the fetus.

Regarding the time when it is appropriate to start the physical activity during pregnancy, the guidelines indicate that it is possible to start as early as the 12th week; in this regard, however, it is necessary to know what type of pregnancy it is, if it is a physiologically achieved pregnancy, if the embryo is well implanted or if there are any uterine contractions. In this case, it is advisable to rest up to the 15th week or have a light or reduced physical activity if the woman is sporty, obviously without overloading. Physical activity should be reduced and not interrupted, as it could be deleterious; obviously, before starting, it will be necessary to wait for the gynecological certificate.

The preferred physical activities are: aerobic activities, which are important for the weight control and for the cardiovascular system; water activities, which reduce the sense of heaviness caused by pregnancy; activities with a wide synergy of the various muscle groups; muscle conditioning activities with moderate overload and mobility, and stretching activities (not maximal).

The intensity of the exercise must be such that the expectant mother is able to speak without excessive breathlessness and it can be assessed through the talk test, which analyzes the ability to converse while performing physical activity. Ideal intensity percentages based on heart rate have also been defined, ranging from 65 to 85% of the maximum heart rate (HRmax): 65% of HRmax for untrained women, 85% of HRmax for trained or even competitive women and 75% of the HRmax for women who exercise at least three times a week. All this, therefore, implies that the woman must train while attached to the heart rate monitor or while having other devices that are capable of detecting the heart rate.

As for the exercises, multi-articular high synergy ones are to be preferred, in order to increase the energy expenditure, with continuous and repeated movements, light loads between 50 and 60% of the maximum load, high repetition exercises and *core* and balance exercises. After obtaining a correct and careful medical history of the pregnant woman, it will be necessary to organize the training program, which will be differentiated according to the term. The **first trimester** does not present evident esthetic changes and is characterized by hyperemesis gravidarum; even though it is advisable to abstain from training for at least the first 12 weeks, pregnant women who still want to practice physical activities will be given a training program based on the cardiovascular work, balance, *core*, on mobility work and on the pelvic floor. The **second trimester** is characterized by a hormonal phase that gives the pregnant woman more energy, but at the same time there is a weight gain, for which it will be necessary to practice a muscle training aimed at controlling the weight gain, working with circuits, which combine the anaerobic work with aerobic work. In the **last term**, on the other hand, there is a significant increase in the volume of the uterus, a greater tissue laxity due to the action of relaxin hormone and a greater breathing difficulty. Therefore, the training program will be structured by first reducing the time of the sessions to a maximum of 40 minutes and by preferring aerobic, proprioceptive and deep muscle work.

CHAPTER 28

Nutrition and circadian rhythms
by Ivan Martellato and Vittoria Troianiello

Introduction

In 1729, the French botanist Jean-Jacques Dortous de Mairan, through the observation of plants in relation to the rhythms of the day, noticed the possible existence of an internal biological clock which is independent of light stimulation. Thus, for the first time, he began to draw the distinction between two types of rhythms that are conceptually very similar, namely the diurnal rhythm and the circadian rhythm.

The term diurnal rhythm refers to any physiological behavior or biological rhythm that is repeated approximately every 24 hours, while the circadian rhythm means the ability of a specific organism to generate its own rhythm at an endogenous level, marked on the needs that the selective pressure exerted has generated on every single species by the force of natural selection, for thousands of years.

The importance of this distinction must be kept in mind, since in the term circadian rhythm the word "circadian", which has a Latin root (*circa* = around, *diem* = day), does not actually coincide perfectly with the etymology.

Living organisms with a circadian rhythm have what is more commonly called the biological clock, that is, that physiological mechanism of adaptation that allows homeostatic regulation based on external stimuli, such as light and temperature.

It is thought that the first living organisms to possess a biological clock were protocells, which had to protect their organelles from daytime ultraviolet waves. Cyanobacteria, the first bacteria that, through the production of oxygen, made life on earth possible, also had a diurnal rhythm, probably based on the presence of radiation.

To date, we know that the ability of every living being to modulate their homeostasis according to external conditions is the basis of evolution; in fact, each eukaryotic cell has an autonomous nictemeral clock that shows oscillations over the course of 24 hours. It is a proper intracellular clock, regulated by specific clock-genes. This clock, as mentioned above, also exists in bacteria, therefore in prokaryotic cells. To demonstrate the topicality of this argument and its relevance in the scientific landscape, the 2017 Nobel Prize in Physiology and Medicine was awarded to Hall, Rosbash and Young for the "discoveries of the molecular mechanisms that control the circadian rhythm" and in particular for the description of the functioning of *PER* genes, where *PER* stands for period.

Central clock and peripheral clock

On the other hand, the connection between the central clock and the peripheral clock deserves a more specific wording. The term central clock refers to a particular structure found in the hypothalamus, known as the suprachiasmatic nucleus (SCN), which is capable of picking up the diurnal variations and which, through the epiphysis and the HPA axis (hypothalamus-pituitary-adrenal), modulates the behavior of all other organs on the basis of specific external stimuli or *Zeitgeber*:

- light and dark cycle;
- temperature;
- changes in gravity during the lunar cycles;
- social contact;
- consumption of food;
- physical activity.

However, even though there are many factors involved in modulating the biological clock, as for the central clock, light and temperature remain the main ones.

The term peripheral clock, on the other hand, refers to all the other clocks. The musculoskeletal system, every organ of the digestive system, the immune system, every part of the brain, in short, every somatic and germ cell has its own clock in which gene expression, transcription and post-translational modifications are finely adjusted according to the type of organ/system. The peripheral clock operates both on the basis of the efferences derived from the master clock of the central nervous system and on the basis of all the other *Zeitgebers* (i.e. external stimuli).

Training, for example, is the main *Zeitgeber* for the musculoskeletal system, the same way as food intake is for the intestinal endocrine regulation systems, gastric, hepato-biliary and pancreatic (for the secretion of insulin, glucagon, ghrelin etc.). Unlike the central clock, the peripheral clock has an important plasticity that underlies the generation of what is familiar and comfortable. An example could be the habit of always training in the afternoon, as well as the need to feed on time at 12.30 pm or wake up 30 minutes before sunrise.

As for nutrition, the digestive peripheral clock is called the gastric FEO (Food Entrainable Oscillator) (a peripheral clock that serves to modulate the appetite based on our food timing); this mechanism explains the familiar phenomenon of having an appetite at times when we are usually used to eating. Bodybuilders, for example, by eating every 3 hours, will adapt the rhythms that are already epigenetically marked by the clock of the digestive organs to secrete insulin, to produce gastric juices, to modulate the behaviors of hunger and satiety, all reflex behaviors that are before consuming a meal.

Circadian misalignment

As mentioned above, daytime rhythms are driven both by the biological clock and by environmental factors such as light, sleep, physical activity and nutrition.

More and more evidence shows that, when environmental rhythms are misaligned with respect to the internal circadian rhythm, various metabolic physiological processes are altered. We will begin by describing the effects of incorrect exposure to light and then move on to sleep, nutrition and training.

Light is the main *Zeitgeber* of the central clock; the time, intensity and duration of exposure to light are connected with the metabolic well-being. Reducing exposure to light during the day from 5000 lux to 80 lux causes a reduction in the secretion and in the motility processes of the gastrointestinal organs, thus resulting in a slowing of the intestinal transit, a higher absorption of nutrients, hyperglycemia and hyperinsulinemia.

As for the effects on metabolism, scientific research shows that, regardless of the quality and quantity of food consumed, being exposed to lux intensities that are not in line with the internal clock timing, alters the insulin sensitivity. As a demonstration of this, in the researches in which the subjects ate breakfast and/or dinner with a light intensity not in line with the physiological expectations of the CNS, altered glycaemia and insulinemia were found more often when compared to the groups that respected the chronobiology.

It must be taken into consideration that the quantity and quality of sleep, at times, may not be enough. Sleeping in circadian misalignments leads to a lowering of the pain threshold, a lower thermoregulatory capacity and an altered glucose metabolism. As for the training, late in the evening the effects depend on the type of the desired performance, the state of fitness, genetics, the type of work. Those who practice power sports benefit greatly from training sessions that take place from 6 to 10 pm; on the contrary, untrained subjects should avoid training too close to bedtime, due to their inability to degrade the produced catecholamines.

The same is true for those who possess the low-functioning variant of the *COMT* gene. As for night workers (shift workers), training should be done just before bedtime due to its positive effect in inducing a physiological sleep.

As for energy expenditure, staying awake at night and sleeping during the day causes, compared to normal night rest, a reduction of about 16% in the energy metabolism at rest, with a consequent reduction of 5% of TDEE (Total Daily Energy Expenditure). If we add the lower energy metabolism to the altered insulin and glycemic response, it all leads to an unbalanced body re-composition in favor of fats.

Particular attention should also be paid to breakfast. Nutrient timing studies have reported notable differences in the morning glycemic curve based on the times of the last meal, showing that eating after 9 pm results in a lower responsiveness of pancreatic beta cells the following morning, when compared to eating dinner before 8 pm. It follows that having a hearty breakfast is preferable in order to have more energy during the day and less hunger at night.

Circadianity of the nutrition

Resetting the biological clock is a so widely recognized method in nutrition science and in functional medicine, that intermittent fasting practices are effectively used in order to re-educate the body in order to keep up with the natural and physiological circadian rhythms. In the practice of intermittent fasting, a limited time window is chosen during the day during which to feed, and then fast in the following hours. Currently, the best known and "in vogue" is 16:8, where 16 are the hours of fasting and 8 are the hours of the scheduled feeding.

However, the beneficial effects are also found after 12 and 10 hour fasts. Even though the positive effects of fasting are strongly recognized, there are still doubts in the literature as to what is actually responsible for the beneficial effects of this diet. Caloric restriction and ketogenesis, in fact, bring results that are comparable to those of fasting and very often the trials that study the effects of fasting are trials in which subjects are subjected for several days to a low-calorie diet with levels of ketone bodies varying from 2 to 4 mmol/L. But what does fasting have to do with circadianism? Can intermittent fasting work the same way while maintaining the same calories?

A very important study from 2018 shows how, for the same calories, subjects who had consumed meals in a restricted period ranging from 8 in the morning to 2 in the afternoon (6:18) were found to have lower levels of insulin, lower blood sugar levels and a low HOMA index. They also had higher adiponectin levels than subjects who consumed the same calories but in a period between 8 am and 8 pm.

Intermittent fasting did not involve a caloric restriction compared to the control group and no significant weight changes were found between the two groups, demonstrating how the improvement in insulin and in the glycemic parameters is probably limited to the improvement in muscle insulin sensitivity, which is dependent on the modulation of the *PER*, *CLOCK*, *CRY* and *BMAL* genes. The stabilization of the blood glucose in the study group can therefore be attributed to two events:

- the time span of 18 hours between meals, which allows for a greater depletion of glycogen and in hepatic and muscle triglyceride reserves, resulting in more space for the future meals;
- consuming food in a time window long before the nocturnal melatonin peak.

The second event is of fundamental importance, as it represents a connection point between the calorie balance and the food timing, almost definitively overcoming the historical conception of the daily calorie balance on the improvement of the anthropometric parameters. Studies show that eating long before the melatonin peak offers a very important metabolic advantage. It is so important that every other factor aimed at improving the body is overshadowed. Research shows that:

1. There is a significant association between the last snack before the melatonin peak and the lesser amount of sleep.
2. Those who eat closer to 4 hours of the peak, sleep less.
3. Overweight individuals, on average, eat later than lean individuals and have more body fat.
4. If a person sleeps too little, the next day they will be hungrier in order to recover the energy they spent while being awake; moreover, most of the food will be ingested in the evening, near the melatonin peak.
5. The dynamic-specific action of a meal consumed at 8.00 pm is 4% lower than that of the same meal consumed at 6.30 pm.
6. There is a risk of generating a vicious circle that leads to binge eating disorders.
7. Those who eat late are more exposed to higher light intensities which, by slowing down the gastric emptying due to the shift in melatonin levels, lead to a higher absorption, resulting in altered blood sugar levels in the next morning.

Studies on the effects of a variant of the *MTNR1B* gene (Melatonin Receptor 1B) confirm the importance of melatonin in the management of blood sugar and intestinal motility. The gene encodes a receptor located in pancreatic beta cells, whose role is the modulation of insulin secretion based on melatonin levels. Different allelic variants of the gene result in different abilities to use substrates based on the time of day, which means that having the CC variant in the *MTNR1B* gene (two alleles that present cytosine instead of guanine) involves an anticipated secretion of melatonin.

Since melatonin inhibits the insulin secretion and the gastric motility, if a subject with the CC allelic variant consumes a large carbohydrate meal late in the evening, their blood glucose and insulin levels worsen. 30% of the population has two guanines (GG) in place of cytosines in the *MTNR1B* gene. This variant results in an increase in the density of melatonin MT1 receptor in the membrane of pancreatic beta cells. Since the mutation is directly correlated with the senescence of beta cells, subjects with the GG variant should exclude the supplements of melatonin from their diet.

Compared to carriers of the CC variant, individuals with the GG variant experience a postponed melatonin peak. This shift results in less gastric motility and less insulin secretion in the morning. Given this inhibitory effect on the gastrointestinal tract caused by the high levels of melatonin, subjects with this variant should refrain from eating a breakfast with high amounts of carbohydrates. It should be considered that carriers of this variant are more at risk of metabolic diseases, linked to the malfunction of pancreatic beta cells.

As for the effects of intermittent fasting in circadian desynchronization, we can refer to the most recent review published in *Nature*, in 2019, which demonstrates the benefits of Ramadan towards LDL, HDL, triglycerides and HOMA indices. However, no important results were found regarding the waist/hip ratio, BMI and weight, especially when considering the female sex. However, even though the results are surprisingly positive, it should be borne in mind that the review, based mainly on observational studies, did not take into consideration a homogeneous population with regard to certain habits, such as smoking and the caloric intake anticipating the fasting. In fact, if we consider that during Ramadan smoking is prohibited and that smoking limitation brings significant positive effects regarding cholesterol and BMI, in order to confirm the effectiveness of fasting on health, they should take these important variables into consideration.

In fact, in this case it is not possible to determine whether the effect is given by the presence of intermittent fasting, by calorie restriction or by smoking cessation, or if the three factors work synergistically to produce a positive effect. Another factor that must be considered is that Ramadan means fasting during the day, while it is possible to consume food in the hours following the sunset, therefore in the evening hours, or in the time window in which there is the greatest melatonin peak. From the comparison of several studies that have analyzed the effect of day and night fasting, it is possible to say that, generally, both practices are beneficial for the health. Considering the effects of circadian misalignment on health, it is possible to say that daytime intermittent fasting is less positive than nocturnal fasting. One of the reasons why eating at night can create problems and increase inflammation and fat accumulation could depend on the effect of melatonin and growth hormone on the insulin secretion. Sleep is a period in which the body takes care of eliminating the wastes that are accumulated during the day. The up-regulation of liver enzymes and the release of liquids by the glymphatic system require a lot of energy, which mostly derives from the circulating glucose. It follows that maintaining a stable insulinemia and glycaemia is essential in order to allow these expensive processes. Returning to practice, if insulin is stimulated following the nocturnal intake of food, it produces critical effects on the body and on the management of sugars. Basically, the consumption of food at night could compromise the physiological inhibitory action of melatonin on insulin secretion and insulin sensitivity. **However, the individual differences between each subject must always be taken into consideration.** The fact that the results were less positive for women suggests that the biochemical, hormonal and metabolic differences that characterize each of us are important factors that should be taken into consideration in the context of a circadian reset. Women, who tend to be ginoid and hypolipolytic, are better off consuming food in the morning and fasting in the evening; this is because the higher levels of estrogen in women lead to an epigenetic modification that results in a minor synthesis and translocation of glucose transporters (GLUT4), with a consequent lower insulin sensitivity marked by the circadian rhythm. The effects of estradiol on cortisol levels depend on the presence, sensitivity and location of the ER-alpha and ER-beta receptors, which in turn are modulated by the management of circadian rhythms. The circadian misalignment strongly alters the expression of these two receptors, with a particular overexpression of ER-beta. Since ER-beta limits the insulin sensitivity, it can be confirmed that men and women must adhere to chronobiologically defined dietary principles. In fact, if we are taking the male gender into consideration, the situation changes. The android-hyperlipogenetic subject tends to have higher cortisol levels, especially in the early hours of the day, when glucocorticoid glucose and lipid mobilization is needed in order to prepare for immediate movements. The circadian rhythm leads to an elevation of cortisol from the morning until the early afternoon. To avoid having a too high blood sugar, in these subjects it is not recommended to consume excessive calories (particularly carbohydrates) in the early hours of the day. On the contrary, in this case it would be appropriate to take a large part of the calories (especially from carbohydrates) towards dinner. In addition to lowering the cortisol levels, this dietary decision favors the relaxing action induced by serotonin (precursor of melatonin), ensuring better sleep quality.

In conclusion, taking into consideration the different hormonal profiles between men and women, and the consequent chronobiological differences, it is advisable to choose the appropriate fasting practices based on one's morphofunctional characteristics.

Regarding the effects of fasting on sports performance, a study published in the *Iranian Journal of Basic Medical Sciences* (2012) described the effects of Ramadan on the aerobic and anaerobic performance, and on the lipid profile of 14 wrestlers between the ages of 18 and 22 years old.

With the advancement of the studies on circadianity, many approaches on periodized nutrition have been studied for the purpose of optimizing endurance sports performance. The manipulation of the availability of carbohydrates pre-, during and post-training is successfully applied in cyclists and marathoners who want to up-regulate the enzymes involved in lipid metabolism (beta-oxidation), in order to allow a mitochondrial biogenesis with a consequent increase in VO_{2max} and a lower lactate production. One of these methods, the "sleep-low" carb diet, involves carbohydrate restriction in the evening, preceded by an exhaustion workout, and a moderate workout in the morning on an empty stomach, followed by a carbohydrate-rich breakfast. The effectiveness of this method is based on the management of the insulin sensitivity based on the circadian rhythm.

Optimal supplementation and circadianity

Some chronobiotic supplements which are useful for promoting the circadian alignment are mentioned below.

Melatonin – The term "chronobiotic" defines a substance that is capable of determining the alignment of the internal biological clocks in order to reset the body in line with the circadian rhythms. Melatonin is the endogenous chronobiotic par excellence and one of the main substances to exert this action (neuroendocrine transducer of the light-dark cycle). The pineal gland, which is the site of its synthesis, is an organ that is characterized by an endocrine secretion. In adults, it has a weight of about 0.2 g and it is not covered by the blood brain barrier, therefore it secretes directly into the capillaries of the systemic circulation. It has been observed that the gland undergoes a calcified degeneration process with the advancement of age.

Effective dosages of exogenous melatonin may vary, based on factors such as genetics and the amount of the daily light exposure. Even though the recommended dosage (antiaging) is 1 mg, particular conditions such as intercontinental flights (jet lag), and the prevention and support of prostate or breast cancer may require 5 mg or more.

Tryptophan – The pinealocyte produces melatonin starting from serotonin (5-hydroxytryptamine, 5-HT) and the cycle of the biochemical reactions has the amino acid L-tryptophan (essential amino acid) as its precursor. Since tryptophan must undergo hydroxylation, decarboxylation and methylation before becoming melatonin, it is recommended to supplement the hydroxylated form known as 5-HTP at a dosage between 200 and 400 mg per day.

Magnesium and Vitamin B6 – Of all the minerals and vitamins, magnesium and vitamin B6 play an indispensable role in the circadian modulation. Magnesium, through the inhibition of NMDA receptors, allows for less excitability with the promotion of the state of relaxation that precedes the physiological sleep. Vitamin B6, in addition to supporting the absorption of magnesium, allows the decarboxylation of glutamate in order to generate GABA, an inhibitory neurotransmitter inversely related to anxiety.

S-Adenosyl-Methionine (SAM-e) – A coenzyme involved in the transfer of methyl groups, SAM-e allows the synthesis of melatonin in the last step inherent in its creation. In addition, through the COMT enzyme, it allows the degradation of catecholamines, which normally counteract the physiological sleep.

Nobyletin – It is a polymethoxylated flavone, found in the peel of some citrus fruits. In addition to having a chemopreventive and NMDA inhibitory role, nobyletin has the peculiarity of synchronizing the peripheral muscle clock with the central clock, allowing greater insulin sensitivity with possible positive effects on life expectancy.

Putrescine and spermidine – These are polyamines derived from the metabolism of ornithine. During the course of life, the enzymes responsible for their synthesis undergo a selective repression. It has been found that, in addition to undergoing a circadian oscillation, the lack of polyamines is associated with a greater length of the period that marks the circadian rhythms. The integration of spermidine, both in aging and in conditions in which there is a circadian misalignment, could be considered.

NAD⁺ – It is the cofactor of sirtuins, enzymes that modulate the cellular epigenetic balance. By supplementing it, it is possible to reset the biological clock.

Lithium – A mineral that is widely used in bipolar disorders, it inhibits a micro-RNA (mir-34A) which in turn inhibits the enzyme responsible for the regeneration of NAD⁺ (a key molecule for evaluating the cellular energy status).

Phosphatidylserine – Numerous scientific evidence support the use of this supplement for the modulation of cortisol production, which also improves the GH-cortisol ratio.

CHAPTER 29

Intermittent fasting

Although there are a large number of studies performed on mice with incredibly promising results related to intermittent fasting (IF), which have been shown to cause weight loss, improve the blood pressure, cholesterol and blood sugar, at the same time it must be remembered that these are mice. Human studies, in the vast majority of cases, have shown that intermittent fasting is safe and also very effective, but in reality, it is no more effective than any other diet. It is usually described as an abstinence from some or all foods and drinks for a certain period of time, usually longer than 12 hours. During fasting, the body experiences ketosis and undergoes a metabolic change in its fuel source, from stored glycogen to fatty acids.

The stimulus that allows sugar to enter our cells is given by insulin, a hormone produced in the pancreas upon stimulation from glucose and proteins, which, in case the glucose levels are in excess, promotes the lipogenesis.

Between meals, insulin levels decrease, so the fat cells can release the stored sugars, to be used as energy. In fact, you can lose weight if you let your insulin levels drop; it is not a coincidence, in fact, that the idea behind intermittent fasting is to allow insulin levels to drop enough in order to allow the use of fats for energy purposes.

While the long-term effects of intermittent fasting have not been fully established, some studies suggest that certain benefits of fasting could be linked to the optimization of the mitochondrial function, leading to better energy production and improved general health. Mitochondria have a number of functions, from the generation of reactive oxygen species (ROS) to the synthesis of ATP, and their proper functioning can affect the health of the body as a whole. Mitochondria are dynamic organelles subjected to continuous cycles of fusion and fission. While excessive fission, or division, has been associated with mitochondrial functional defects that can lead to multiple disease states, a recent study on nematode worms has suggested that fasting could increase their overall lifespan, promoting a balance between the fusion/fission states and homeostasis in mitochondrial networks.

Mitochondrial biogenesis and function are mediated by several activators, regulators and transcription factors, such as PGC-1α and Nrf2. Research has suggested that fasting can enhance these mediators to promote mitochondrial biogenesis and optimize the mitochondrial function. For example, the co-activator of the gamma-1 peroxisome proliferator (PGC-1α) which is a fasting-induced transcriptional co-activator that mediates the mitochondrial biogenesis, is activated when the body receives a signal that it needs more cellular energy and increases its expression during fasting.

Erythroid nuclear transcription factor-2 (Nrf2) is a transcription factor that regulates the ROS production by mitochondria. Some studies suggest that Nrf2 is associated with mitochondrial biogenesis and may be involved in the control systems of the mitochondrial function. A 2019 study evaluated the impact of Ramadan's intermittent fasting on NRF2-mediated expression of antioxidant genes, and the results suggested that fasting improved the expression of the genes that regulate the production of antioxidants.

Some of the potential benefits of intermittent fasting have mainly been established through research on animals, observational studies, and anecdotal evidence. Additionally, fasting is not optimal for all patients, especially for those who are pregnant, have eating disorders, or have type 1 diabetes.

The first human studies that compared fasting every other day with eating less every day showed that both had equal effects on weight loss, although people struggled much more on total fast days.

One aspect that is never considered is that, by now, a growing number of researches suggests that the timing of fasting is critical and can make the IF a more realistic, sustainable and effective approach to weight loss, as well as to diabetes prevention.

Not all intermittent fasting approaches are the same; some, in fact, are very reasonable, effective and sustainable, particularly when combined with a nutritious diet based above all, but not limited to, on vegetables. Now let's see what the various approaches to intermittent fasting are. The methods of intermittent fasting are different and each person will choose the one that suits them best, probably based on their biochemical individuality and their hormonal biorhythms.

Fast for 12 hours a day

The rules of this diet are simple, in fact it provides a fasting window of 12 hours every day.

This type of intermittent fasting plan can be a good option for beginners, since, given that the fasting window is relatively small, a big part of the fasting occurs during sleep and you can consume the same number of calories every day.

The simplest way to do the 12-hour fast is to include your sleep period in your fasting window. For example, a person might choose to fast between 7 pm and 7 am. He/she would have to finish dinner before 7 pm and wait until 7 am for breakfast, and most of the fasting time would be spent while sleeping.

Fast for 16 hours

Fasting for 16 hours a day, leaving an 8-hour eating window, is called the 16:8 method or the Leangains diet. It is the most practiced and most studied type of intermittent fasting. A fundamental requirement is that in the 16 hours of fasting you must not consume any nutrients: carbohydrates, fats or proteins, not even a sweetened coffee or amino acids. The goal is to trigger the production of ketone bodies, which favor the metabolic shift in favor of the use of fats for energy purposes.

This type of intermittent fasting can be useful for those who have already tried fasting for 12 hours but had no benefits. In this type of fasting, people usually finish their evening meal by 8 pm and then skip breakfast the next day, without eating again until noon, or they finish eating by 3 pm, skip dinner and have breakfast at 7. The choice is linked to a greater compliance with one or the other approach, which can be related, as we will see below, to specific individual hormonal rhythms. A study in mice found that limiting their feeding window to 8 hours protected them from obesity, inflammation, diabetes, and liver disease, even when they were given the same total number of calories as the mice that ate at any time they wished.

Fast for 2 days a week

People who follow the 5:2 scheme, also known as the rapid diet, eat standard amounts of healthy foods for 5 days a week and reduce their calorie intake on the other 2 days. During the 2 days of "fasting", men generally consume 600 calories and women 500 calories. Generally, the days of fasting are spread within the week. For example, you can fast on Mondays and Thursdays and eat normally on other days. At least 1 non-fasting day should be interposed between the days of fasting. Research on the 5:2 diet is limited; a study on 107 overweight or obese women found that calorie restriction twice a week and the continuous calorie restriction led to similar weight loss effects. The study also found that this diet reduced insulin levels and improved the insulin sensitivity among the participants. A small-scale study looked at the effects of this fasting style in 23 overweight women. Over the course of a menstrual cycle (about 28 days), women lost 4.8% of their body weight and 8.0% of their total body fat. However, these values returned to baseline in most women after 5 days of normal feeding.

Fasting every other day

According to some, alternate-day fasting (ADF) must involve a complete abstention from solid foods during fasting days, while for others it is allowed to take up to 25% of the calories that are normally consumed in a single meal. One study reported that alternate day fasting is effective for weight loss and for the heart health in healthy, overweight adults; the 32 participants lost an average of 5.2 kg over a 12-week period. In another study (Hoddy et al.), Comparing the results of fasting every other day (24 hours of normal nutrition/24 hours with 25% energy intake at lunchtime, which proved to be effective for weight loss, but had a poor tolerability) has shown that moving the only meal at dinner time or dividing it into smaller meals can improve the tolerability and it produces weight loss and cardio-protective effects that are similar to those obtained with the consumption of the single meal at lunchtime. This flexibility in meal times can increase the tolerability and the long-term adherence to ADF protocols.

Alternate day fasting is a rather extreme form of intermittent fasting and may not be suitable for beginners or people with certain medical conditions. Moreover, it can be difficult to maintain in the long term.

24-hour weekly fast

Complete fasting for 1 or 2 days a week, known as the eat-stop-eat diet, involves abstaining from food for 24 hours. Many people fast from breakfast to the next breakfast or from lunch to lunch. Those who follow this diet can consume water, tea, and other calorie-free beverages during the fasting period. On non-fasting days, you should return to your normal eating patterns. Eating in this way reduces the total calorie intake but does not limit the specific foods that the individual consumes. A 24-hour fast can be challenging and can cause fatigue, headaches, or irritability. Many people find that these effects become less extreme over time, as the body adjusts to this new eating pattern. Before moving on to 24-hour fasting, you can try fasting for 12 or 16 hours.

Skip the meal

This flexible approach to intermittent fasting, which involves occasionally skipping of one or more meals, can be helpful for beginners. People can decide which meals to skip based on their hunger level or temporal needs. However, it is important to eat healthy foods with every meal. Meal skipping is likely to be more successful when individuals monitor and respond to their body's hunger signals. Basically, people who use this style of intermittent fasting eat when they're hungry and skip meals when they don't. For some, this method may seem more natural than the other fasting methods.

The warrior's diet

The warrior's diet is a relatively extreme form of intermittent fasting, but which in reality could not really be defined as such because consuming very small amounts of food throughout the day is allowed. The warrior's diet involves eating very little, usually only a few portions of fruits, nuts and raw vegetables, during the day, then eating a large meal at dinner in a 4-hour eating window. Proponents of the warrior's diet claim that humans, during the Paleolithic, mainly hunted during the day, in the meantime eating what they found, some berries, roots or eggs, and then consuming the real meal on their return from hunting; the same goes for the warrior, who marched or fought during the day, only to refresh himself at the end of the day. Consequently, they claim that eating at night allows the body to obtain nutrients in line with its circadian rhythms.

It is easy to understand that this approach, which is not really in line with general circadian rhythms, works fine especially for those with adrenocortical prevalence, who have particularly high morning cortisol levels that rise the blood sugar, as cortisol is a hyperglycemic hormone. On the other hand, hunters and warriors certainly had to have a particular activation of the sympathetic system to produce cortisol and adrenaline (hormones that slow down the digestive processes), necessary to face the hunt or the battle, and then, once the hunt or battle is over, leave the field to the parasympathetic system which activates the vagus nerve, favoring the digestive systems.

During the 4-hour eating phase, you should make sure that you are consuming plenty of healthy vegetables, proteins and fats. However, some carbohydrates should also be included. While it is possible to eat certain foods during the fasting period, it can be difficult to stick to strict guidelines on when and what to eat in the long run. Additionally, some people find it difficult to eat such a large meal just before bed. There is also a risk that people who follow this diet will not get enough nutrients, such as fiber. This can increase the risk of cancer and have negative effects on the digestive and immune health. Furthermore, this approach is certainly contraindicated for those who have had a heart attack, as emerges from a study that was recently published in the *European Journal of Preventive Cardiology*, the official journal of the European Society of Cardiology (ESC), which found that people who skip breakfast and eat dinner just before bed have worse outcomes after a heart attack. This study found that people with these two eating habits are four to five times more likely to die or suffer from another heart attack or angina (chest pain) within 30 days from the hospital discharge from a heart attack. This study was the first to evaluate these unhealthy behaviors in patients with acute coronary syndromes. Skipping breakfast was observed in 58% of the cases, late night dinner in 51% and both behaviors in 41% of them.

Intermittent fasting and circadian rhythms

The human being has evolved to be in tune with the day/night cycle, developing a circadian rhythm. Our metabolism has adapted to consuming food during the day and sleeping at night. In fact, nighttime food consumption is associated with a higher risk of obesity and diabetes.

Based on this, researchers from the University of Alabama (Sutton et al.) conducted a study on a small group of obese men with prediabetes. They compared a form of intermittent fasting (IF) called "time-limited early feeding", in which all meals were placed in an 8-hour period during the day (7.00 am to 3.00 pm), i.e. with 16 hours of fasting, with another form of fasting in which meals were spread over 12 hours (between 7.00 am and 7.00 pm). Both groups maintained their weight, but after 5 weeks it was observed that the group who ate in an 8-hour time window had significantly reduced insulin levels and significantly improved sensitivity to it, as well as a significantly lower blood pressure. Furthermore, despite only 8 available hours to eat, the group experienced a significant reduction in appetite. Just changing the timing of meals, eating early in the day and extending the fasting during the night, greatly benefited the metabolism. In fact, the results of TRF (Time Restricted Feeding) in humans seem to depend on the time of day of the food window is placed (Gill and Panda, 2015, Tinsley et al., 2017).

Limiting the food intake to mid-day ("mid-day TRF", mTRF) reduced the body weight or the fat tissue, fasting glucose and insulin levels, insulin resistance, hyperlipidemia, and inflammation (Gill and Panda, 2015, Moro et al., 2016). However, restricting the food intake to late afternoon or evening (after 4 pm; "late TRF", lTRF) resulted in mostly nil results or worsened the postprandial glucose levels, beta cell reactivity, blood pressure and lipid levels (Tinsley et al., 2017).

The circadian system, or the internal biological clock, can explain why the effects of TRF seem to depend on the time of day. Glucose, lipids and energy metabolism are all regulated by the circadian system, which upregulates them at some times of the day and downregulates them at other times (Poggiogalle et al., 2018). For example, in humans, insulin sensitivity, beta cell reactivity, and the thermal effect of the food are all higher in the morning than in the afternoon or evening, suggesting that human metabolism is optimized for an intake of food in the morning (Morris et al., 2015).

In fact, human studies show that eating in line with the circadian rhythms of the metabolism, increasing food intake at breakfast and reducing it at dinner, improves the glycemic control, weight loss and lipid levels, and also reduces hunger (Jakubowicz et al., 2015, Ruiz-Lozano et al., 2016).

This suggests that the effectiveness of IF interventions is linked not only to weight loss, but also to the time of the food intake. Furthermore, these data from circadian

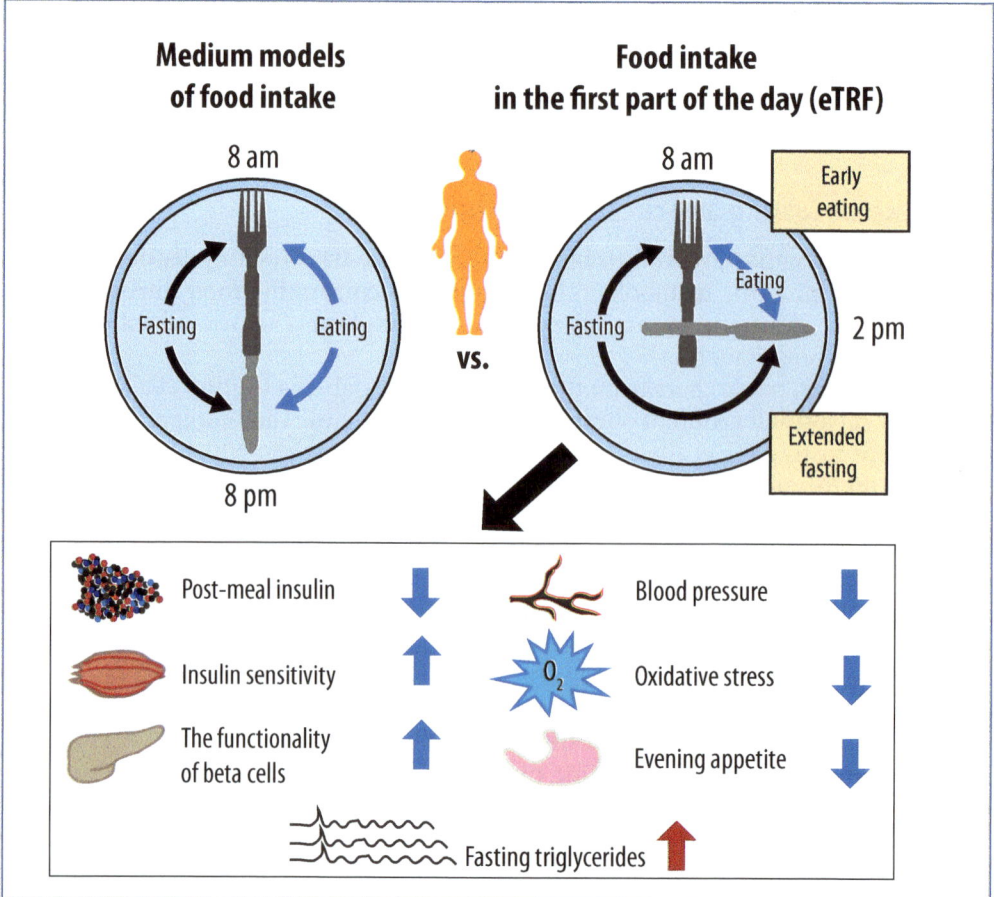

Figure 29.1 The comparison between normal food intake *vs.* early TRF (eTRF).

studies suggest that combining two different meal timing strategies (IF and eating in alignment with circadian rhythms) may be a particularly beneficial form of IF. This combined intervention is called "early TRF, eTRF" and it is defined as a subtype of TRF in which dinner is eaten in the mid-afternoon. This study tested eTRF in men with prediabetes – a population at a high risk of developing diabetes – and found that eTRF is an effective strategy for the treatment of both prediabetes and prehypertension. It can be hypothesized that eTRF, by virtue of the combination of the daily intermittent fasting and eating in line with the circadian rhythms of the metabolism, will prove to be a particularly effective form of IF. In light of these promising results, future research is needed to better elucidate the underlying mechanisms for both intermittent fasting and meal times, to determine which forms of IF and which meal times are effective, and then translate them into useful interventions for the general population. The limitation of this study, in my opinion, is not comparing the results of the eTRF group with a group in which the 16 hours of fasting were between 8.00 pm and 12.00 pm, which means, skipping breakfast. This would have further clarified the influence of the circadian rhythms compared with the duration of fasting. Personally, I believe that the effectiveness of the timing of one form of TRF rather than another is largely linked to the circadian rhythms of cortisol, which should be monitored before prescribing a personalized protocol.

Intermittent fasting and weight loss

Intermittent fasting lends itself above all to an approach aimed at weight loss. We have seen how it can be structured in different ways, for example fasting partially every other day or 2 days a week, or, the most practiced, 16 hours of fasting and 8 hours of eating window every day. This is easily achieved, for example, by starting from the last evening meal and taking advantage of the night fast, which normally consists of 8-10 hours, followed by skipping the breakfast, passing directly to lunch; or starting from breakfast, consuming a series of meals until 2.00-3.00 pm and, from that moment, fasting until the next day's breakfast.

The different ways of carrying out this diet depend on one's ability to adapt; for example, referring to the Chronomorphodiet, a hypercorticosadrenal android individual would be more likely to skip breakfast, as he/she already has high blood sugar in the morning.

In my opinion, this IF dietary approach works: there are studies that show a lowering of the blood sugar, a better insulin sensitivity, a higher lipolysis and an increase in adrenaline and GH, which are lipolytic hormones. Furthermore, there is a decrease in the levels of chronic inflammation, free radicals and toxins that derive from food. Last but not least, there is an effect that derives from autophagy, which removes the damaged cytoplasmic components and promotes apoptosis (programmed death) for the damaged cells, which can also be a prelude to tumoral pathologies.

In fact, there are contradictory studies on IF and weight loss and there has always been a lack of long-term randomized clinical trials to evaluate their real effectiveness. This until recently, because in 2017, a study carried out on 100 people and which lasted one year was published in the prestigious journal *JAMA International Medicine*. The study found that IF did not produce a higher weight loss or protection from cardiovascular disease than a simple calorie restriction. The researchers found that those who experienced IF had more difficulty following the diet and were more likely to quit the trial than those who followed the daily calorie restriction diet. The results showed that fasting every other day did not have superior results in weight loss, weight maintenance and cardiovascular risk indicators.

To conclude, there are some good pieces of scientific evidence which suggest that IF, when combined with a healthy diet and lifestyle, can be a particularly effective approach to weight loss, especially for people at risk of developing diabetes. However, other studies have also observed the negative effect of an increase in LDL (Low Density Lipoprotein), which is the so-called "bad" cholesterol. This could be attributable to the lowering of the thyroid metabolism following the fasting days. In my opinion, IF is a feasible diet only for limited periods of time, which may be good for some, but not for all. For example, I believe that this dietary method is not very suitable for a power athlete. However, if it is true that we are not all the same, we should not say that a balanced IF for a weightlifting athlete is not beneficial. There is no absolute rule in this regard, it is a practicable path but only for the subjects who really benefit from it. Even people with advanced diabetes or people who are taking diabetes medications, individuals with a history of eating disorders such as anorexia and bulimia, and pregnant or lactating women should not attempt IF unless they are kept under close medical monitoring.

Intermittent fasting and the physical performance

IF is a practice that has found a lot of followers in the fitness world, as an approach aimed at improving the body composition. In fact, almost all the studies on IF have been carried out on overweight individuals who did not train or otherwise not-trained individuals. The only study that takes into consideration trained bodybuilders is that of Moro et al. (2016), in which 37 athletes with at least 5 years of overload training experience were recruited and they trained 3 times a week with a split routine, training each muscle group once a week.

The study participants were divided into two groups and all followed a diet divided into three meals for 8 weeks, a diet that remained faithful to their usual caloric intake, which was measured before the start of the study. One group consumed their meals at 8.00 am, 1.00 pm and 8.00 pm (ND group), the other at 1.00 pm, 4.00 pm and 8.00 pm (TRF group), according to the concept of Time Restricted Feeding (TRF), a variation of IF. After 8 weeks, the TRF group had recorded a significant decrease in their fat mass (−16.4% *vs.* 2.8% in the ND group), while lean mass was maintained in both groups (+0.86 *vs.* + 0.64). Total testosterone, IGF-1 and T3 had dropped significantly in the TRF group and not in the ND group. The conclusions that can be drawn from this study may be that TRF is a practice that can promote a greater loss of body fat, even for the same consumption of calories (especially in a person who trains, given that other studies on untrained overweight people had shown the opposite) and that the decline in the anabolic hormones levels (T and IGF-1) does not lead to higher muscle catabolism. The latter evidence, which is the decline in the anabolic hormones, suggests that TRF is not a suitable practice for increasing the muscle mass. A recent systematic review by the Moro's group (2021) concluded that IF has potentially beneficial effects in combination with RT for reducing body mass and body fat relative to non-IF control diets, with similar preservation of fat-free mass.

In my opinion, in general, IF for muscle mass gain is an approach that has no practical, scientific or field basis. Even if IF can promote a decrease in body fat and perhaps even more in the body "weight", a decrease in the levels of glycated hemoglobin, insulin and insulin resistance, an increase in the levels of adrenaline, noradrenaline and glucagon, a decrease in the related inflammation and a promotion of autophagy at the cellular and mitochondrial level, it still does not promote an increase in the muscle mass.

This does not mean that with IF you cannot have results in terms of muscle mass gain, but only that it is not the best approach because, in addition to making the adequate nutrient timing more difficult, it does not induce the optimal hormonal conditions and does not allow you to make the most of the stimulus of protein synthesis. The latter occurs when we have an intake of a quantity of protein that contains all the essential amino acids together with at least 3 g of leucine, and it remains in these levels only for a few hours after the meal. It is no coincidence that bodybuilding champions often eat at least six meals a day and in some cases a protein shake at night is also recommended to counteract the slowdown in nocturnal protein synthesis, caused by prolonged fasting.

As far as nutrient timing is concerned, I think it is an added factor to consider; on the other hand, countless chronobiology studies show it, although I certainly don't consider it the most important factor in terms of muscle mass increase. I put the caloric quantity in the first place, as a possible caloric deficit does not allow a positive nitrogen balance, except in rare exceptions; the balance of macronutrients comes second, where proteins are king, because if there is a protein deficiency, muscle mass cannot be increased, while carbohydrates and fats are relatively interchangeable (within certain limits); after that come the micronutrients, because if there are sub-deficiencies of vitamins and minerals, which are enzymatic cofactors, the enzymatic processes of protein synthesis cannot take place in the best way possible, and in order to increase the muscle mass the body must maintain an optimal function.

Consequently, it is not certain that the muscle mass gain is not possible even in the IF regime, but in my opinion it is certainly not the best solution. If you really want to adopt an IF regime, you must make sure that the training is carried out during the food window or at the end of the fasting period, so that the catabolism is immediately interrupted in favor of anabolism. At this point, in order of importance, I would put the nutrient timing before the use of supplements, and you know how useful I think the use of supplements is; this means that I find nutrient timing particularly useful.

Finally, I obviously do not recommend training with anaerobic overloads for hypertrophic purposes during fasting conditions, as I believe that by doing so, catabolic conditions prevail, and even though they can be compensated later, it will not be optimal.

Another reason why I think it is not appropriate for a bodybuilding athlete to skip breakfast is that having breakfast helps to regulate the weight, as a certain amount of carbohydrates in the morning gives a signal for the production thyroid hormones, which are the most involved hormones in the regulation of metabolism; on the contrary, not taking food in the first 30-60 minutes after getting up would be a signal of "famine" to which the body would respond by reducing the lipolysis (the consumption of fat) and by promoting the production of cortisol, which has a catabolic effect.

At this point, we begin to have information that is of interest to us as a function of training. If, in a normal person, a little morning catabolism could be easily recovered with the subsequent meals, in an athlete who trains regularly this could be more difficult, especially if the training is carried out during catabolic conditions. In addition, we must take into consideration what type of training we are interested in, because in some cases even catabolism can be useful, depending on the goal.

For example, if the goal is endurance, training in the morning on an empty stomach favors the use of lipid catabolism for energy purposes, accustoming the body to the use of lipids for aerobic purposes; in addition, protein catabolism also predisposes the body to the ability of using amino acids for energy purposes. These metabolic adaptations will be very important during the moments of long-lasting competitions, when the body will be able to take advantage of the lipid and muscle tissue to obtain the necessary energy to complete the sports performance in the best possible way, without running the risk of depleting the muscle glycogen reserves, which would result in a decreased performance.

Another situation in which it may be a good reason to train on an empty stomach is when the goal is the weight loss. In fact, during steady state aerobic activities, i.e. at constant and moderate intensity, since blood sugar is lower, as well as the muscle glycogen levels, the trained body will mainly use fats for energy purposes, given the greater availability of their substrate and lower insulin levels due to fasting.

A recent published study by Moro et al. (2020) showed that a 8/16 TRE program decreased body fat, increased the ratio between peak power output and body weight, improved inflammation and immune conditions in elite cyclists.

In my opinion, in this case, we must consider the person's biotype: if the individual is hyperlipogenetic, which means, tendentially hypercorticoadrenal, with high cortisol and glycaemia levels in the morning, even an aerobic activity will not have the desired effects and, indeed, it could mainly lead to muscle loss; if you do not belong to this biotype, aerobics in the morning on an empty stomach can give excellent results for weight loss. In a 2007 study (Polak et al.) it was found that a lipid meal taken after an overnight fast inhibited the antilipolytic effect of alpha-2 receptors during low-intensity aerobic exercises.

The researchers suggest that lipid ingestion, by promoting an increase in plasma free fatty acids, modifies the lipolytic response which is dependent on the relationship between the activation of beta-2 receptors (stimulating lipolysis) and the inhibition of alpha-2 (inhibitors lipolysis), at the level of the adipocyte membrane. This should be taken into consideration especially in the case of stubborn localized fat deposits that respond poorly to the catecholaminergic stimulus induced by both training and diet, precisely because it has a higher concentration of alpha-2 antilipolytic receptors.

It is different if you train to gain muscle mass or strength. First of all, a natural activation of the neuromuscular system is also important for this type of training, which in the early morning struggles a little and needs time to maximize its abilities; this is one of the reasons that even though testosterone is high in the morning, strength is lower. Furthermore, if we train with weights for strength and mass, the training is necessarily anaerobic, so it can only use carbohydrates for energy purposes; if these are not there because we are fasting, the proteins (of the muscles) will be converted into glucose through gluconeogenesis and this is certainly not good.

There are now several studies that show that the most important meals to maximize the protein synthesis are the ones that are consumed pre- and post-workout. So, if for reasons of time you can only train with weights in the early morning and for obvious digestive problems you cannot have a full breakfast, it is good to take at least 20-30 g of whey protein, perhaps with a fruit juice or with some honey, in order to stop the catabolism and to have a little more energy; immediately after, please, have a hearty breakfast.

As for the aerobic activity in the morning for slimming purposes, I consider it the only possibility for a fasting workout (in addition to training aimed at metabolic efficiency in the use of fats, in view of extreme endurance sports) but not necessarily the best choice, for the reasons I have already explained in my book *The COM Diet & spot reduction*, of which I report an extract:

"Training on an empty stomach in the morning has often been commonplace in the fitness environment, in order to lose weight faster. However, recent studies suggest that it may not be the best solution. While it is certainly true that in this situation it is easier to deplete the glycogen stores because its levels are already lower after a night of fasting, it may not be true that more fats are consumed for energy purposes." From a physiological point of view, the rationale of doing aerobic activities in the morning on an empty stomach is sensible, since the glycogen is partly depleted, and in this condition the fat is more easily mobilized. However, recent studies seem to refute this theory. Researchers evaluated the effects of carbohydrate intake before exercise and during exercise, and the results showed that there is no evidence of a decreased fat oxidation associated with carbohydrate consumption, either before or during the exercise (B. Schoenfeld, *Strength and a Conditioning Journal*, February 2011). This may be due to the fact that fasting results in a slower basal metabolism and this is reflected in the ability to oxidize fats. In the end, this creates a sort of compensation between the decrease in the oxidative metabolism and the increased use of fat due to glycogen depletion. It would be interesting to see what happens differently between the administration of a protein meal (among other things, proteins have a greater thermodynamic effect) and the administration of carbohydrates. We know that proteins stimulate the GH, cortisol and glucagon, which all are lipolytic hormones, and instead carbohydrates stimulate insulin, which inhibits the lipolysis. The administration of a protein meal before training, compared to fasting, could make a difference. Another reason why training on an empty stomach may not be recommended is that in this situation there is a greater proteolytic effect that affects the loss of the muscle mass. Research has shown that twice as much nitrogen is lost (resulting from the protein catabolism) so you train in a glycogen-depleted state, compared to training with full glycogen stores (P.W. Lemon, *Journal of Applied Physiology*, 1980). Therefore, carrying out a cardiovascular activity in the morning, on an empty stomach, may not be useful for those who want to maintain or improve their muscle mass. We should also remember that decreasing the muscle mass means lowering your basal metabolism. In addition, training on an empty stomach promotes an increase in the cortisol levels, which, on the one hand, in the short term, stimulates fat loss, but on the long term increases the muscle catabolism. At this point, it seems legitimate to suggest a workout preceded by a small meal, which includes mainly proteins with a minimum intake of carbohydrates to buffer cortisol, accompanied by supplements such as BCAA, glutamine, phosphatidylserine, vitamin C, omega-3 and green tea, in order to stimulate the metabolism, prevent catabolism and buffer cortisol".

However, I believe that aerobic activity in the morning, even on an empty stomach or after taking protein and amino acid supplements (and in this case we can no longer talk about IF), is a useful strategy in promoting the consolidation of a habit or a lifestyle. After all, getting up early in the morning to do aerobics must involve going to bed early in the evening, and in this way we better synchronize our circadian rhythms, which favor the correct hormonal secretion of GH, melatonin and cortisol, in addition to the fact of having no excuse for not training due to work commitments. In doing so, we "take that daily physical activity home" every day and "without excuses".

CHAPTER 30

The ketogenic diet
by Antonio Paoli

Biochemical/physiological bases and applications

What is ketosis?

Ketosis is a perfectly preserved physiological mechanism that allows living species (especially mammals) to survive the periods of fasting that they periodically face. Without carbohydrates, our body cannot follow the metabolic pathways it usually uses to assimilate fats. After a few days of fasting or dieting with a drastic reduction in carbohydrates (less than 20-30 g per day), the body's reserve glucose becomes insufficient to allow for both normal oxidation of fats through the supply of oxaloacetatate in the Krebs cycle and the supply of glucose to the CNS (central nervous system). We recall that oxaloacetate is an intermediate of the Krebs cycle (Figure 30.1) which derives by dehydrogenation from malate and it is the acceptor of acetyls that derive from macronutrients.

Why does oxaloacetate need to be supplied externally starting from glucose? Oxaloacetate is relatively unstable at a normal body temperature and cannot be accumulated in the mitochondrial matrix. There is therefore a need to replenish the cycle of tricarboxylic acids with oxaloacetate through the "anaplerotic cycle", which leads precisely from glucose to oxaloacetate, through the ATP-dependent carboxylation of pyruvic acid by means of pyruvate-carboxylase (biotin-enzyme ATP -employee) (Figure 30.2). This mechanism, that is, the supply of oxaloacetate to the Krebs cycle, justifies the phrase "fats burn in the flame of carbohydrates".

As for the supply of glucose to the brain, it is well known that, not being able to use fats for energy purposes (since they cannot pass the blood brain barrier), the CNS normally uses glucose; therefore, after the first 3-4 days of absence of carbohydrates in the diet, the CNS is "forced" to find alternative sources of energy, as demonstrated by the now historical studies of the Cahill group. This alternative source of energy consists of ketone bodies (KB), produced from the excess of acetyl-CoA, which the CNS is able to use for energy purposes.

These ketone bodies, produced in particular metabolic conditions (prolonged fasting, diabetes, lipid overconsumption and very low carb diets) are, more precisely,

Chapter 30 ▸ The ketogenic diet

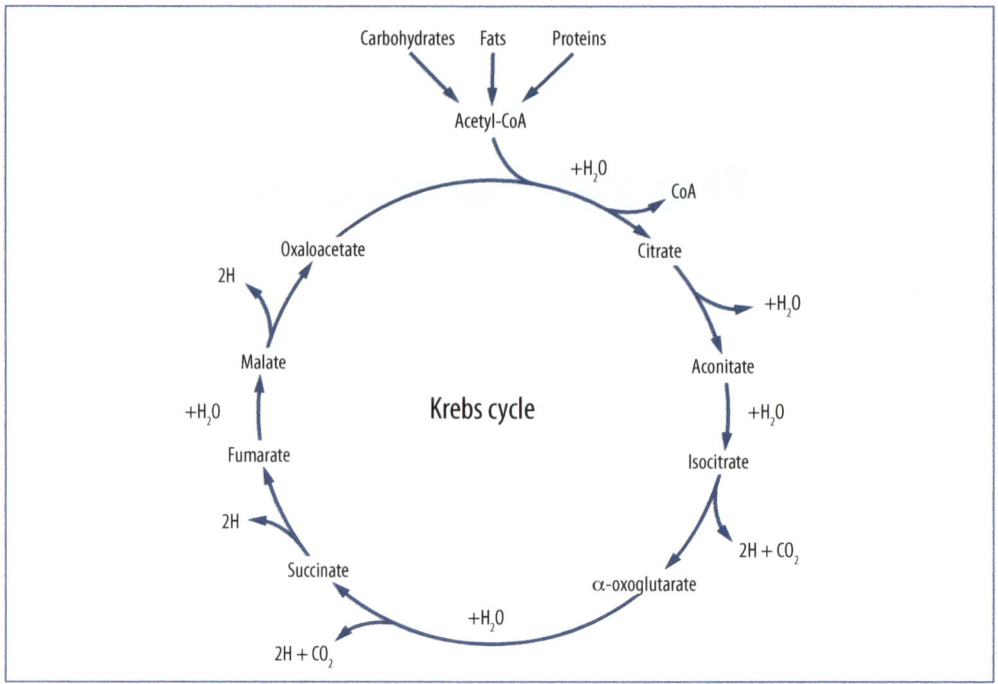

Figure 30.1 Krebs cycle or the tricarboxylic acid cycle.

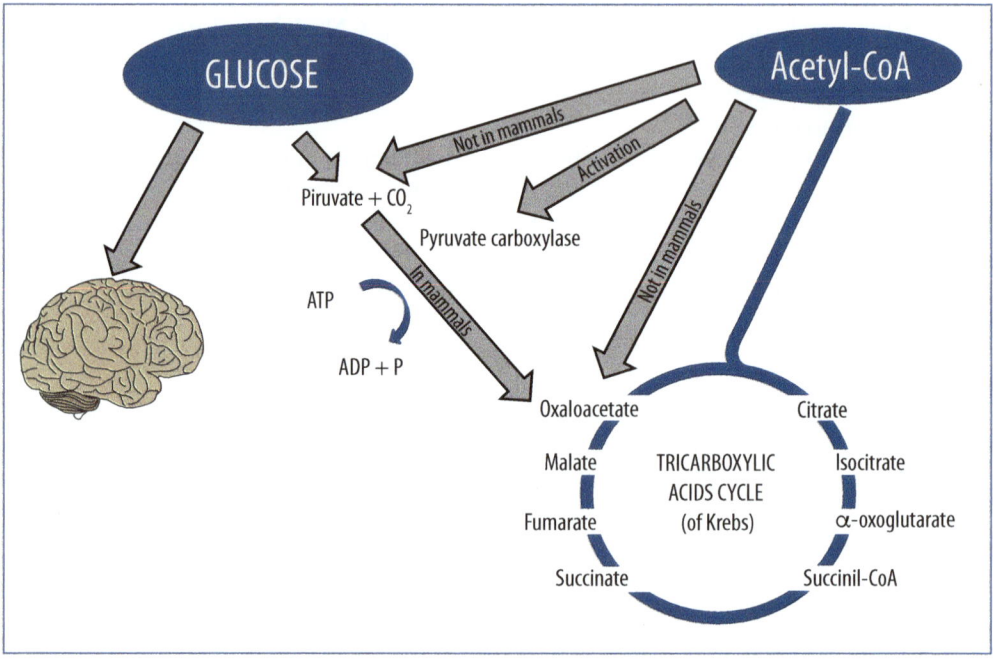

Figure 30.2 The replenishment system of oxaloacetate from glucose in mammals.

acetoacetic acid (AcAc), β-hydroxybutyric acid (3HB) and acetone. The production of ketone bodies is called ketogenesis and takes place particularly in the mitochondrial matrix of the liver.

We owe to Hans Krebs for the description of this process, together with the definition of "physiological ketosis", to differentiate it from pathological ketosis that we will see shortly. He described it in 1966, identifying the liver as the organ responsible for regulating ketones in the body. It was already understood that ketones did not represent a habitual intermediate in the breakdown of fatty acids, and that they could effectively serve as fuel for the respiration in animal tissues, playing an important role in what was called the "caloric homeostasis". When the level of glucose in the blood plasma is low, such as during fasting, with a low-carbohydrate diet, or when glucose is not usable, such as in diabetes, the concentration of free fatty acids in the plasma increases. This increase almost goes hand in hand with the increase in the concentration of ketone bodies, which represents a third source of energy. In other words, moderate ketosis that occurs in a variety of circumstances must be regarded as a normal physiological process that supplies the tissues with an easily usable fuel in the cellular respiration, when glucose is in a short supply. During the hepatic process of ketogenesis, all three ketone bodies are produced. The biosynthesis of ketone bodies begins with two acetyl-CoA molecules which join together to form acetoacetyl-CoA, in a reaction catalyzed by 3-ketothiolase. A second condensation follows with another acetyl-CoA molecule, catalyzed by hydroxymethylglutaryl-CoA synthetase, from which 3-hydroxy-3-methylglutaryl-CoA (HMG-CoA) is obtained, which is then cleaved to acetyl-CoA and acetoacetate. 3-hydroxybutyrate is formed from the reduction of acetate, according to a ratio which is dependent on the NADH/NAD⁺ ratio within the mitochondrion. Finally, the acetoacetate undergoes spontaneous decarboxylation to form acetone (Figure 30.3).

The main ketone body is acetoacetate, from which acetone is produced by spontaneous decarboxylation. Acetone is the cause of the characteristic and symptomatic

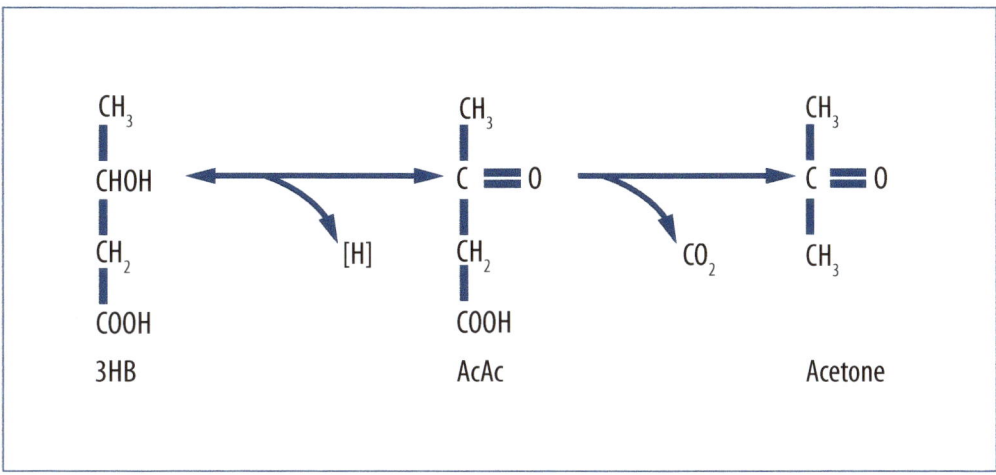

Figure 30.3 The ketone bodies: acetoacetic acid (AcAc), β-hydroxybutyric acid (3HB) and acetone.

"fruity breath" reported by internal medicine texts, thus assuming a certain importance from a clinical point of view. On the other hand, strictly speaking, 3-hydroxybutyrate is not a ketone body because the ketone part is reduced to a hydroxyl group. Under normal conditions the production of free acetoacetic acid is negligible and this compound, transported into the circulation, is easily metabolized in various tissues, particularly in the skeletal muscles and in the heart. In overproduction conditions, acetoacetic acid accumulates and a part of it is transformed into the other two ketone bodies. The presence of KBs in the circulation and their elimination in the urine cause ketonemia and ketonuria. The elimination of acetone, being a very volatile compound, occurs mainly with respiration. The pathway that leads to the formation of HMG-CoA (hydroxymethyl-glutaryl-coenzymeA) from acetyl-CoA is also present in the cytosol of hepatic cells, where it is instead used for the biosynthesis of cholesterol. KB therefore derives from a fat-bearing process that takes place in the liver. Under normal conditions, KBs are in very low concentrations (<0.1 mmol/L) compared to glucose (about 4 mmol/L). As the concentration of KBs increases, they begin to be transported across the blood brain barrier via the monocarboxylate transporter; this carrier is also up-regulated by the increase in the concentration of the KBs themselves. We would like to underline again that ketosis is a completely physiological mechanism that allowed our ancestors to survive and remain efficient even in the event of food deprivation. The physiological levels of ketone bodies are illustrated in Table 30.1 and demonstrate how the condition of physiological ketosis (fasting, ketogenic diet, etc.) is completely different from ketoacidosis, where KB levels reach up to 20 mmol/L (see Table 30.1).

During ketosis, it is possible to measure the blood concentration (in addition to the urinary concentration, which is simpler to detect but less indicative of the real state of ketosis) of acetoacetate and 3-hydroxybutyrate. However, 3-hydroxybutyrate

Table 30.1 Blood glucose, insulin, KB and pH values during a normal diet, a ketogenic diet and diabetic ketoacidosis

Blood values	Normal diet	Ketogenic diet	Diabetic ketoacidosis
Glucose (mg/dL)	80-120	65-80	>300
Insulin (µU/L)	6-23	6.6-9.4	~0
KB concentration (mmol/L)	0.1	7/8	>25
pH	7.4	7.4	<7.3

appears to be a better indicator than acetoacetate, and the KB ratio gives useful information for a metabolic evaluation. The normal 3HB/acetoacetate ratio is 3:1 but in ketosis you can find values of 6:1, and up to 12:1. In physiological ketosis (which is reached during fasting and VLCKD diets, Very Low Carbohydrate Ketogenic Diet, a ketogenic diet with a low carbohydrate content) ketonemia reaches maximum levels of 7-8 mmol/L with an unchanged pH, while in decompensated diabetes it reaches and exceeds 20 mmol/L with lowering of the pH (13, 14).

The blood values of KB do not exceed 8 mmol/L in the healthy individual, because the CNS, actually, efficiently uses these molecules for energy purposes to replace glucose.

Ketone bodies are used by tissues for energy purposes through a pathway that requires 3HB to be converted back to AcAc by D-β-hydroxybutyrate dehydrogenase. Subsequently the acetoaceate is transformed into acetoacetyl-CoA, thanks to the intervention of β-ketoacetylCoA transferase (with the donation of CoA from succinyl-CoA); finally, two acetyl-CoA molecules are formed from acetoacetyl-CoA, thanks to thiolase; these two molecules will then be used in the Krebs cycle (Figures 30.2 and 30.4).

It is interesting to note that the KB are able to produce more energy than glucose, in fact the high chemical potential of D-β-hydroxybutyrate leads to an increase in

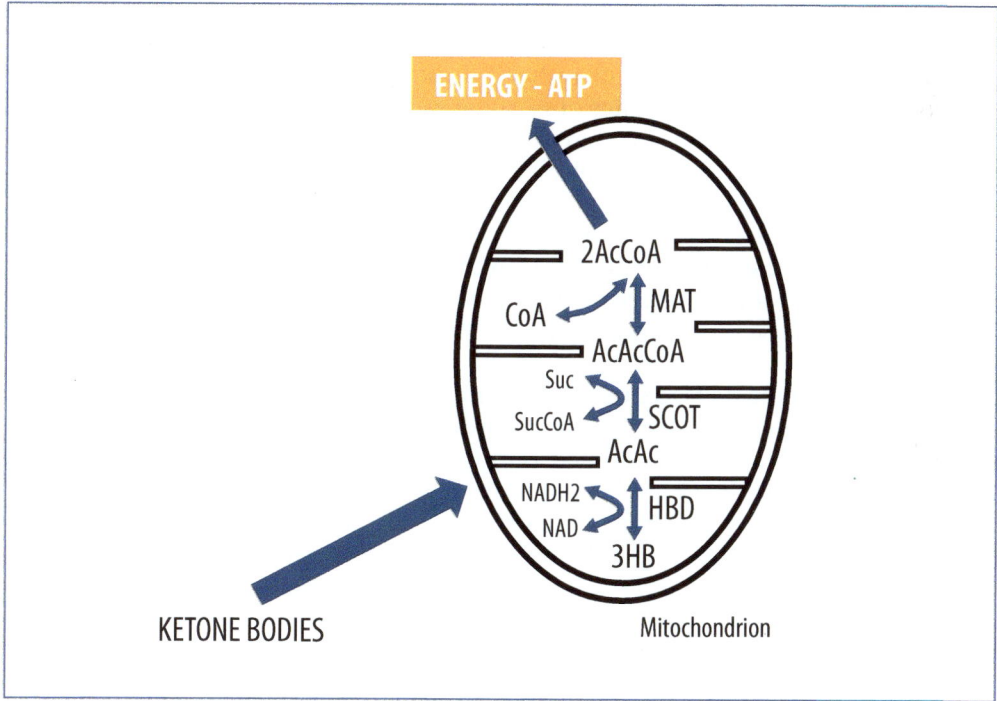

Figure 30.4 The utilization of ketone bodies in the mitochondrion (ketolysis).

ΔG_0 during the hydrolysis of ATP. It has been shown that KBs could increase the hydraulic efficiency of the heart by 28% and this effect cannot be explained only by the changes in the glycolytic pathway, but rather by the variations induced in the production of mitochondrial ATP by ketone bodies. Another point to underline, as shown in Table 30.1, is that the glycaemia, although being lower, remains at physiological levels. In fact, the glucose that is formed from the gluconeo-genetic amino acids and from the glycerol that is released by the lysis of triglycerides, is sufficient for the maintenance of euglycemia; the importance of the glucose produced through neoglucogenesis and of that produced from glycerol of triglycerides acquires, as the condition of ketosis is prolonged, an increasing importance. Glucose derived from glycerol can represent more than 16% of the glucose produced by the liver during a ketogenic diet, and about 60% during a complete fast.

What is a ketogenic diet?

The term ketogenic diet defines a diet based on a drastic reduction in the carbohydrate intake (less than 20-30 g per day), associated or not with a relative increase in the amount of proteins and fats. The metabolic state of ketogenic diets is attributable, in many ways, to fasting; even in fasting, in fact, there is an establishment of a particular metabolic state known under the name of ketosis. The first in-depth scientific studies on this metabolic condition were those conducted by the Cahill group in the 1960s, starting precisely from the "fasting" conditions.

Fasting, in fact, is a practice, or rather a technique, used for thousands of years in order to achieve particular states of spiritual well-being during religious rituals or practices. This practice is mentioned in the Old Testament, as well as in the Koran and in the Mahabharata. For example, we can find a reference to fasting in Matthew (17:14-21) where, in the episode of the healed epilepticus, it is said: "This race of demons cannot be cast out except by prayer and fasting"; and it is not a coincidence that we talk about fasting when it comes to epilepsy, as it has been known since the 1920s that ketosis (and therefore fasting) is able to improve some types of epilepsy. Obviously, one of the problems of fasting is the progressive depletion of the body's protein reserves.

Modern ketogenic diets, on the other hand, try to induce a state of ketosis while providing an adequate protein intake, in order to maintain the lean mass; in fact, they have often been called modified fasting diets or modified low-carbohydrate, protein-sparing diets. It should be emphasized that a classic ketogenic diet is not a high-protein diet but a hypoglucidic, normoproteic, possibly hyperlipidic diet. An excess of proteins, in the long term increases the gluconeogenesis, impairing the synthesis of ketone bodies; in fact, if it is true that in the first days of the ketogenic diet the main source of glucose to keep blood sugar stable is amino acid neoglucogenesis, with the passage of time the demand for amino acids decreases and glucose is synthesized starting from glycerol released from the hydrolysis of triglycerides. The protein content varies according to the conditions, whether there is a physical or a sporting activity, etc., but in any case, it is not higher than 1.2-1.5/kg/day.

These diets have known a great diffusion since 1972, with the publication a book by Dr. Atkins, who proposed a drastic reduction of carbohydrates for the purpose of rapid and effective weight loss. Since the publication of that book, studies on ketogenic diets have multiplied, but, despite the proven effectiveness in reducing the body weight, as well as reducing the markers of inflammation and the cardiovascular risk, this therapeutic weapon is often ignored or rejected by many nutrition field professionals. This a priori rejection is often motivated by a lack of knowledge on the mechanisms linked to ketosis.

The ketogenic diet and fat loss

There is a lot of research confirming that ketogenic diets are more effective than classic low calorie diets for fat loss, at least in the medium term. The mechanisms underlying this effect are not entirely clear, but a number of causes can be hypothesized: one of these is the suggestive hypothesis that there is a metabolic advantage that could explain the important effect of VLCKD on weight loss. The authors who embrace this line of thought hypothesize that the use of proteins, for energy purposes, in VLCKDs is an "expensive" process for the body and therefore it can lead to a "waste of calories". In a very low carbohydrate diet, in fact, our body needs in the first phase about 60-65 g of glucose per day, which is obtained in a minor part (16%) from glycerol and the major part is obtained from the gluconeogenesis of food or tissue proteins. The role of the energy expenditure for gluconeogenesis in VLCKD has been confirmed by several authors, and the cost of this process (starting from endogenous and dietary proteins) has been calculated to be about 400-600 Kcal/day. In fact, this hypothesis has been denied several times by the works of Kevin Hall, who demonstrated that there is no metabolic advantage (or rather, how this is reduced) during a ketogenic diet. Hall's position has been contested by other researchers (considering that Hall's model used the metabolic ward or the metabolic isolation of the subjects, which made the experimental setting not "natural" and that the small variations recorded by Hall, in the long term, could lead to substantial changes in body weight). Another factor to take into consideration is the dynamic-specific action of food, now called the thermogenic response to food. This parameter calculates the energy expenditure that our body must sustain to absorb and metabolize the nutrients. Taking an average of the literature, this energy expenditure amounts to 7, 2.5 and 27% of the calories supplied by, respectively, carbohydrates, fats and proteins. It is intuitive that, by changing the nutrient ratios, we will be able to act on this aspect of the daily calorie expenditure and the increase in the percentage of proteins inevitably leads to an increase in acute and chronic calorie expenditure. Another aspect that recently seems to have emerged is the minor influence that ketogenic diets seem to have on the mediators of hunger (ghrelin) and satiety (PYY, CCK etc.); in fact, it seems that low-calorie diets cause an increase in the hunger signals and a reduction in those of satiety, even months after the end of the diet, while ketogenic diets seem to have a minor influence on this scenario. Finally, it is now clear how ketogenic diets act on the metabolism by lowering the respiratory quotient (the ratio between exhaled CO_2 and consumed O_2), thus indicating a privileged use of fats over sugars.

To conclude, we can therefore state that the effect of VLCKD diets on weight loss seems to be caused by several factors:

1. A reduction of the appetite thanks to the action of proteins and ketone bodies.
2. Less influence on "signals" related to hunger and satiety compared to classic low-calorie diets.
3. A reduction of the liposynthesis mechanisms and an increase of the lipolytic mechanisms.
4. A decrease in the respiratory quotient at rest. The respiratory quotient (RQ) represents the ratio between the produced CO_2 and the consumed O_2 (CO_2/O_2); the QR of sugars is equal to 1, while for a mixture of fatty acids it is 0.7.

5. An increase in the metabolic expenditure caused by gluconeogenesis and the thermal action of proteins (even if the data are not definitive).

Regarding the so-called insulin hypothesis, i.e. the theory that high insulin levels stimulate the fat storage and weight gain, at the moment there are no data to confirm its existence and they rather suggest it has a possible marginal role.

Not just low insulin...

Ketone bodies have been thought for a long time to be of little physiological importance, if not frankly toxic. In reality, ketone bodies do not perform their function only as an energy source but, recently, several other functions for the body are emerging.

For example, it has been observed that beta-hydroxybutyrate exerts an epigenetic control on the genome: it acts as an endogenous inhibitor of class I histone deacetylase, increasing the expression of the *FOXO3A* and *MT2* genes (involved in the resistance to oxidative stress), reducing inflammation, reducing the production of cholesterol, having neuroprotective effects and stimulating the lipolysis. In addition, ketosis, mainly through β-hydroxybutyrate, acts by stimulating the AMPK. AMPK is the main regulator of the metabolic homeostasis and it can also exert its action directly. AMPK is affected by the AMP/ATP ratio and activates the processes that lead to the production of ATP, while inhibiting those that consume it. The modification in the intake of certain nutrients can affect these pathways: for example, the reduced availability of carbohydrates has been shown to be a stimulus for the activation of AMPK and SIRT-1, increasing the phosphorylation and deacetylation of PGC1α in the skeletal muscles (the transcription of genes involved in mitochondriogenesis, in the transport of fatty acids, in β-oxidation and oxidative phosphorylation is controlled by PGC1α, a co-regulator that is able to perceive the energy signals or the metabolic deficit and, consequently, it is able to activate mechanisms to modify the gene expression). After its activation, PGC1α translocates from the cytoplasm to the nucleus, which can occur through different pathways, including the phosphorylation by AMPK, CaM kinase and MAPK p38 and the deacetylation mediated by SIRT-1, without changing the total amount of AMPK, PGC1α or SIRT1. Surprisingly, carbohydrate restriction appears to be sufficient for the activation of these pathways in human muscle cells, even in the presence of excess caloric lipids, in line with the finding that AMPK is sensitive not only to the intracellular AMP/ATP ratio, but also to the glycogen reserves. In the same study, a low-calorie diet with a high carbohydrate/lipid ratio saw a reduced AMPK phosphorylation and PGC1α deacetylation. The effects of activating SIRT1 and AMPK also translate into better glucose homeostasis and an increase in insulin sensitivity.

AMKP also exerts an inhibitory action on mTOR, which in a dietary restriction of carbohydrates is accompanied by the effects of low insulin levels: mTOR, in fact, is a central regulator for the cell division and anabolism in response to signals mediated by nutrients and growth factors. The action on mTOR, together with the other effects mediated by AMPK via SIRT1, FOXO and PGC1α on oxidative stress and autophagy, could explain the role of the calorie restriction on longevity. Therefore, physiological ketosis opens up numerous interesting perspectives in health and even therapeutic fields.

The safety of ketogenic diets

If we *de facto* assume that ketogenic diets are diets with a high protein content, which it is not entirely correct, then the risks that are feared by critics of this type of dietary approach are essentially aimed at an alleged kidney damage due to an increased nitrogen excretion during the protein metabolism, which would cause an increase in the glomerular pressure and hyperfiltration. But the data in the literature do not agree: some authors support the possibility of kidney damage, especially on experimental models on mice and pigs, while others, still based on animal models but also on meta-analysis and human data, affirm that even an elevated protein intake does not alter the kidney function. In fact, although some authors have shown a positive influence on albuminuria, in the short term, by the reduction of the protein intake from 1.2 to 0.9 g/kg in subjects with type 2 diabetes, the same authors subsequently stated that a restriction of the protein intake is neither necessary nor useful in the long term.

Furthermore, it remains to underline that ketogenic diets are only relatively high in proteins and that, indeed, recent studies have shown that VLCKD can even reverse the diabetic nephropathy in mice. As for the possible risk of acidosis, since during VLCKD the concentration of ketone bodies never rises above 8 mmol/L, this risk is practically nil in subjects with an intact insulin function.

Another objection to the safety of the ketogenic diet is the excess of lipids in the diet, which is usually accused of being a risk factor for cardiovascular diseases.

In this regard, the studies are conflicting, also because ketogenic diets can be elaborated in very different ways, and often according to the habits and food resources of the territory in which the study is carried out.

Furthermore, many studies have been conducted on epileptic patients, whose proportion of dietary lipids is particularly high compared to the protocols that are used in other situations, and this could affect the results. However, what was most evident, even in these cases, is that although there is sometimes an increase in the blood lipid values, which can theoretically be interpreted as a pro-atherosclerotic profile, the cytokine structure that is determined is not in favor of the cardiovascular risks. Some studies seem to indicate that a possible increase in total cholesterol and LDL cholesterol is temporary and it is limited to the first period. Others show that the lipid profile tends to improve significantly. A meta-analysis published in 2012, analyzing the results of 23 studies conducted between 1966 and 2011, compared the long-term effects of low-carbohydrate versus low-fat diets on the metabolic risk in overweight or obese adults: the reduction in weight and waist circumference, as well as the overall improvement in the lipid profile, were roughly comparable, but in the low-carbohydrate groups, although the reduction in total cholesterol and LDL was slightly lower than the low-lipid groups, the reduction in triglycerides and the increase in HDL was more pronounced. The discrepancy identified between less significant changes in LDL reduction and more significant changes in triglyceride and HDL values, apparently in contrast, could be explained by the fact that low-carbohydrate diets, compared to low-fat diets, have demonstrated to increase the size and volume of LDLs and this would agree with the general improvement of the typical dyslipidemic picture of the metabolic syndrome, generated by the insulin resistance, in which low HDL, high triglycerides and LDL, increase the atherogenic potential. After all, there is a biochemical rationale behind the effects of the ketogenic diet on the synthesis of endogenous cholesterol: HMGCoA reductase, a key enzyme in the biosynthesis of cholesterol, is activated by insulin, which means that an increase in blood sugar and consequently an increase in insulin levels, will lead to an increase in the synthesis of endogenous cholesterol. On the contrary, a reduction in the dietary carbohydrates, together with a correct intake of exogenous cholesterol, will inhibit the biosynthesis of cholesterol.

This reflection has stimulated further research on the composition of fatty acids of the diet, as it is now established that these can influence the cardiovascular risk.

It cannot be excluded that many studies, especially the older ones, coming from the Anglo-Saxon world, were built on diets that were richer in long-chain saturated fatty acids.

The idea of verifying whether the lipid profile could have been further improved by shifting the percentages in favor of the unsaturated fatty acids, in a sort of hybrid between the ketogenic diet and the Mediterranean diet, came to a group of Spanish researchers, who created a protocol for obesity based on fish, fresh vegetables, olive oil and even red wine.

The extremely encouraging results were confirmed in patients with metabolic syndrome and in patients with NAFLD (Non-Alcoholic Fatty Liver Disease). In another study, instead, the effect of supplementation with omega-3 fatty acids (EPA and DHA) was tested by comparing it with a control group that was subjected only to a ketogenic diet: the results suggested that the supplementation with omega-3 does not alter the effects of a ketogenic diet on the reduction of the body weight and on the improvement of blood cholesterol values, but it rather increases even more the positive effects on the inflammatory markers, adiponectin, insulin and triglycerides. This type of supplementation can therefore optimize the positive effects of the ketogenic diet on some cardiovascular risk markers and on obesity, with chronic low-grade inflammation. A well-constructed ketogenic diet, with a particular attention to the quality of nutrients, does not currently seem to represent a potential danger for cardiovascular diseases, or for other metabolic problems, both because in most cases these are limited time protocols, and because by setting a normocaloric or even a hypocaloric regime, without sufficient glucose, the body is more driven to oxidize lipids to obtain energy than to accumulate them, and because the proinflammatory profile improves significantly. It certainly becomes necessary to carefully evaluate a family history of dyslipidemia.

There are still doubts for cases in which the ketogenic diet should be followed for life, as it happens in children with GLUT 1 deficiency, especially when the disease requires higher dietary restrictions on carbohydrates and proteins, with a share of lipids that reaches even 90%. These cases do not have a sufficient observation time yet, in order to understand the long-term effects of the diet. To date, however, the data are comforting, especially if adequate monitoring is put in place.

A rather common side effect during the diet is constipation. In order to counteract it, it is advisable that among the allowed foods, to include those with a greater laxative action, and above all to encourage the patients to drink adequate quantities of water, generally higher than usual. In ketogenic diets, in fact, on the one hand, the intake of water with food is significantly reduced, and on the other hand, the rather intense oxidative metabolism increases its consumption.

Generally, it is possible to carry out dietary protocols exclusively with common foods; However, in the cases of very restrictive protocols it is advisable to use some types of supplements.

The ketogenic diet remains contraindicated in a number of particular conditions:
- pregnancy and breastfeeding;
- kidney failure;
- liver failure;
- type 1 diabetes;
- porphyria, angina, recent myocardial infarction;
- alcoholism;
- mental disorders.

The ketogenic diet and sports

What are the applications of the ketogenic diet in sports? Basically, we can divide its applications into four main categories (Figure 30.5):
- Weight categories.
- Strength/power.
- Endurance.
- Muscle hypertrophy.

Weight categories

One of the recurring problems in sports that belong to the weight categories is the need for some athletes to "fall into a category" before a competition. Reiterating that the optimal option would be to reach the correct weight gradually, without losing weight too fast near the race, it is undeniable that the problem of falling into the weight categories remains constant for many athletes. The various procedures used to lose weight have various side effects that can reduce the performance and effectiveness, as well as being harmful to the athlete's health.

Unfortunately, the use of low-calorie diets, dehydration, saunas, etc. remains very widespread. These methods, in addition to being dangerous for the health of the athletes, disturb the normal physiological functions, affect the water and electrolyte balance, the glycogen stores and the lean mass and, in the case of the use of diuretics, they are also illegal and sanctioned by the sports code. A rarely considered option in these cases (except bodybuilding, where it has been known for years) is the ketogenic diet. The athletes' fear is that this type of diet can negatively affect their sports performance. In reality, there are very few studies on the ketogenic diet and the physical exercise. Kreider and collaborators (2011) studied the effects of an exercise program on overweight women with a normal diet or a ketogenic diet, demonstrating a benefit of combining the ketogenic diet with a circuit training with weights.

However, this work was based on health effects (weight loss and the maintenance of lean mass in sedentary women), while there are very few studies on its effects on the sports performance. We know that the ketogenic diet is effective in terms of fat loss in overweight/obese individuals, but how manageable this is in athletes is still unclear.

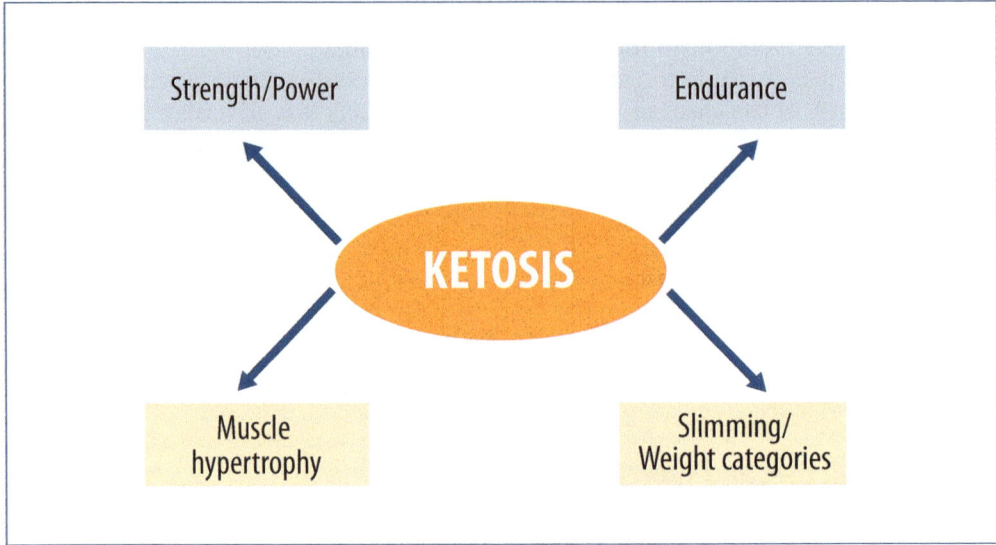

Figure 30.5 Areas of application of the ketogenic diet in sports.

Generally speaking, in trained individuals, weight-loss benefits of KDs were shown in ad libitum studies (Sawyer et al., 2013; Zinn et al., 2017). The BM and/or FM loss may likely be explained by a resultant calorie deficit created by the KD, as enhanced feelings of satiety and a reduction in overall food intake (Zinn et al., 2017). Indeed, when combining exercise with a KD, studies showed an increased efficacy of KDs in BM and FM loss, especially in ad libitum condition (Dostal et al., 2019; Gregory et al., 2017; Jabekk et al., 2010; McSwiney et al., 2018). Our group has shown that the ketogenic diet is able to reduce the percentage of body fat in high-level artistic gymnastics athletes (with already low levels of fat mass) without negatively affecting their performance (Paoli et al., 2012) and same results were obtained more recently by other groups in powerlifting and Olympic weightlifting athletes (Greene et al., 2018). It is clear that the management of the weight loss with the ketogenic diet must be prudent, foreseeing at least 7 days and considering that, in these 7 days, the greatest weight loss will be given by the decrease in muscle glycogen and the associated water. This loss will be compensated after the weight operations, in order to facilitate, at least partially, the recovery of the muscle glycogen.

The ketogenic diet and endurance performance

The effect of ketogenic diets on endurance performance has been a debated topic at least since the 1980s with the first, pioneering studies by Phinney's group. In their first study, Phinney and his collaborators followed a VLCKD diet for 6 weeks. The protein for this diet was derived from lean meat, fish and poultry, providing 1.2 g of protein per kg of body weight per day. In addition, supplements of sodium as broth (3 g) and 25 mEq (1 g) of potassium as bicarbonate were provided daily. The treadmill performance test included the determination of VO_{2max} after 2 weeks on the eucaloric diet and after 6 weeks on a ketogenic diet. The resistance time to exhaustion was quantified at 75% of VO_{2max}. The endurance test was repeated after 1 week and after 6 weeks since the beginning of the VLKD diet. To compensate for the fact that the subjects had lost an average of over 10 kg at the end of the diet, the final treadmill resistance test was carried out with a loaded backpack equal to the weight they lost. After 1 week on a ketogenic diet, the resistance time to exhaustion decreased, but instead, after 6 weeks a significant increase was reported. In a further study, Phynney used trained cyclists as subjects for a 5 week period. During the first week, the subjects consumed a (eucaloric) diet that derived 67% of its energy from carbohydrates. This diet was then followed by 4 weeks of VLCKD, which provided 83% of the energy from fats, 15% from proteins and less than 3% from carbohydrates. On average, subjects lost 0.7 kg in the first week of the VLKD diet, after which their weight remained stable until the end of the study. In this study, a test of resistance to exhaustion on the cycle ergometer was performed both at the end of the first week on an eucaloric diet, and at the end of the fourth week on the ketogenic diet. The test of resistance to exhaustion on the cycle ergometer was performed at 65% of VO_{2max}. The average continuous exercise time on the cycle ergometer until exhaustion at 65% of VO_{2max} was 147 minutes at the end of the eucaloric diet, and 151 minutes at the end of the VLKD diet. It should be noted that during the second test, a QR of 0.72 was measured, indicating a preferential use of fats for energy purposes. This historical work therefore suggests that a VLCKD can increase the time to exhaustion during an endurance performance. Actually, by analyzing the data obtained by individual subjects, we notice a factor that is constant in the various studies on the ketogenic diet and sports, that is the extreme variability of the individual response, which some authors have tried to explain in various ways, including the effect of the microbiota.

Subsequent studies disagree on the effects of the ketogenic diet on the performance; in fact, we have numerous studies that demonstrate an improvement in the oxidative capacity, but the effect on the performance remains controversial, if not downright negative. A very well conducted study that demonstrates its negative results is the one carried out by Burke's group in Australia (2017): they verified the effect of the ketogenic diet in a group of walkers during a retreat with important training loads. Researchers, in fact, found an improvement in the fat oxidation, accompanied by a worsening of the walking performance and a lower improvement (compared to the group that trained with a high carbohydrate diet) of the times of the performance after the training period.

Another observation should be made on the muscle glycogen: if it is true that it lowers to baseline, the data show that after a demanding performance there are no differences between subjects on a normal diet and those on a ketogenic diet; in other words, the glycogen levels after the performance were similar.

But how to explain the conflicting results of the different studies? There are three factors that can be taken into consideration to explain this contrast: 1) the time allowed for keto-adaptation; 2) the use of electrolytic supplements; 3) the amount of the consumed proteins. Regarding the first factor, studies that have generally shown a decline in the performance have not maintained the ketogenic diet for a sufficient period (at least 10 days). Whilst most studies investigating the effects of short ketogenic diet periods (less than 7 days), recently Shaw and colleagues (2019) showed that one month of KD was able to preserve submaximal exercise capacity in trained runners without confirming, on the other side, the high interindividual variability. Another interesting finding of this study is that exercise efficiency was maintained when exercising at an intensity <60% VO_{2max}.

These observations suggest that it takes 2 to 4 weeks to stimulate the so-called keto-adaptation. The second factor has to do with the adequate supplementation of minerals as long as the ketogenic state is maintained. During a ketogenic diet, an intake of about 3-5 g of sodium/day and 2-3 g of potassium/day is required in order to maintain an adequate performance and a balanced nitrogen balance. The third factor affecting the physical performance is an adequate protein intake. It is generally accepted that the preservation of the lean mass and the performance during any degree of energy restriction occurs when dietary protein is in the range of 1.2 to 1.7 g of protein per kg of body weight. Putting together anecdotal and scientific data, it could be suggested that when the performance is conducted at intensities lower than 65% of the VO_{2max}, for example in ultramarathones, the ketogenic diet may represent a viable option.

The ketogenic diet and strength performance

Regarding the strength performance, as mentioned above, our group demonstrated that 30 days of a ketogenic diet does not negatively affect the explosive strength capacity in highly skilled gymnasts. Eight highly qualified artistic gymnastics athletes were tested, who followed a Mediterranean diet for 30 days and a Mediterranean ketogenic diet with phytoextracts for an additional 30 days, in two overlapping competitive periods for training load modes. The athletes performed a variety of tests, such as folding at the bar (bringing straight legs at the bar), push-ups, parallel push-ups, pull-ups, squat jumps, countermovement jumps and 30 seconds of continuous jumps. The subjects reduced their fat mass significantly after 30 days of VLCKD, without affecting their performance in any way. In this case, the protein intake, also given the important training load, was much higher (2.2 g of protein per kg of body weight) than the normal indications of a ketogenic diet for weight loss. Other, more recent studies confirm how, by combining a resistance training and a ketogenic diet, body fat can be decreased without affecting the strength performance even in weight lifters.

The ketogenic diet and hypertrophy

Although, at the moment, there are no reliable published data on the ketogenic diet and muscle hypertrophy, the analysis of the molecular pathways linked to hypertrophy and the effects of the ketogenic diet on these pathways suggests that this type of diet, despite the high protein intake, is, at best, irrelevant for the purpose of increasing the muscle mass. The only one to speak out against that is in a work by Jacob Wilson's group, which demonstrated an increase in muscle mass after 10 weeks on a ketogenic diet, even higher than that of a normal diet; but this difference from the normal diet appeared only after a week from the reintroduction of carbohydrates (and therefore the replenishment of glycogen stores). If, on the other hand, we look at the common pathways between the ketogenic diet and hypertrophy, we realize

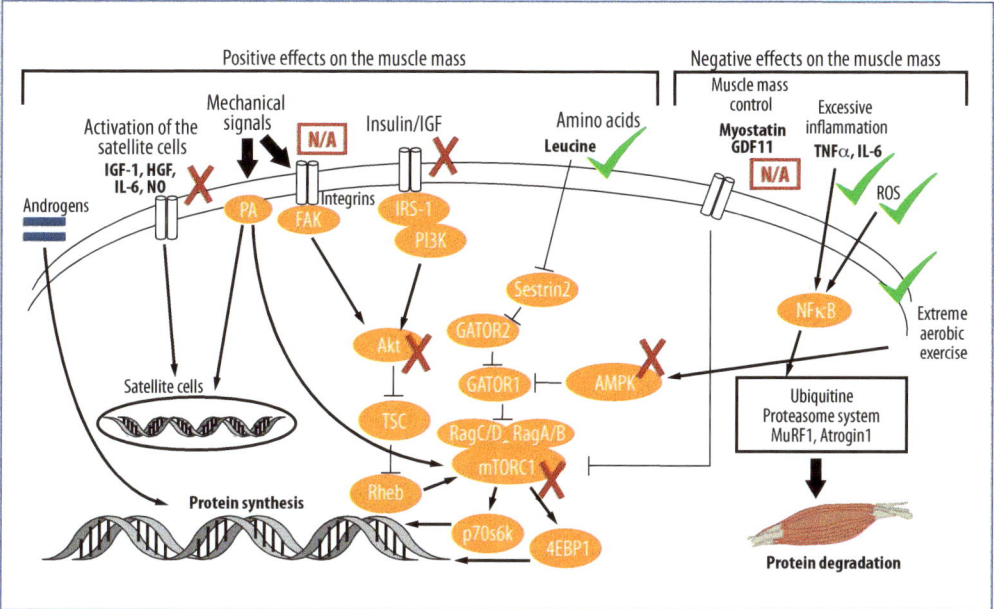

Figure 30.6 The molecular mechanisms of muscle hypertrophy and the sites of the probable action of the ketogenic diet.

(Figure 30.6) that there are some points in favor and others against. It is evident that the richness of leucine, the decrease in inflammation and the decrease in the production of free radicals are factors that favor the growth of the muscle mass while, at the same time, the lowering of the levels of IGF-1 and insulin, and the reduction mTOR activity, negatively affect the increase in muscle mass with a subsequent effect, in our opinion, in the balance. On the other hand, Thomsen et al. reported that BHB has potent anti-catabolic effects in muscle at the whole-body level; in muscle, reduction of MPB overrides inhibition of MPS (Thomsen et al., 2018), As a matter of fact, recently (Paoli et al., 2021), we demonstrated that a KD may maintain lean body mass and decrease fat body mass in competitive natural body builders, with the caution that hypertrophic muscle response could be blunted considering the smaller increase of muscle mass in KD group compared.

Conclusions

Ultimately, based on the data in the literature, it is possible to deduce that as long as it is conducted according to some criteria, with awareness and with the correct settings, the ketogenic diet can represent a useful tool for weight loss, for the treatment of some pathologies and also in sports, limited to athletes who need to return to their weight category in a relatively short time, without negatively influencing their explosive strength performance, and for athletes who undergo extreme endurance activities.

CHAPTER 31

Supplementation for strength

Strength supplementation must be suitable for maximizing the energy reserves to work in both alactacid and lactacid anaerobic conditions. During periods of strength (competitive and otherwise), it is of fundamental importance to promote the muscle recovery, increase its growth and preserve the integrity of structures, such as tendons, nerve membranes and bones. So, let's analyze the most important supplements related to increasing the strength.

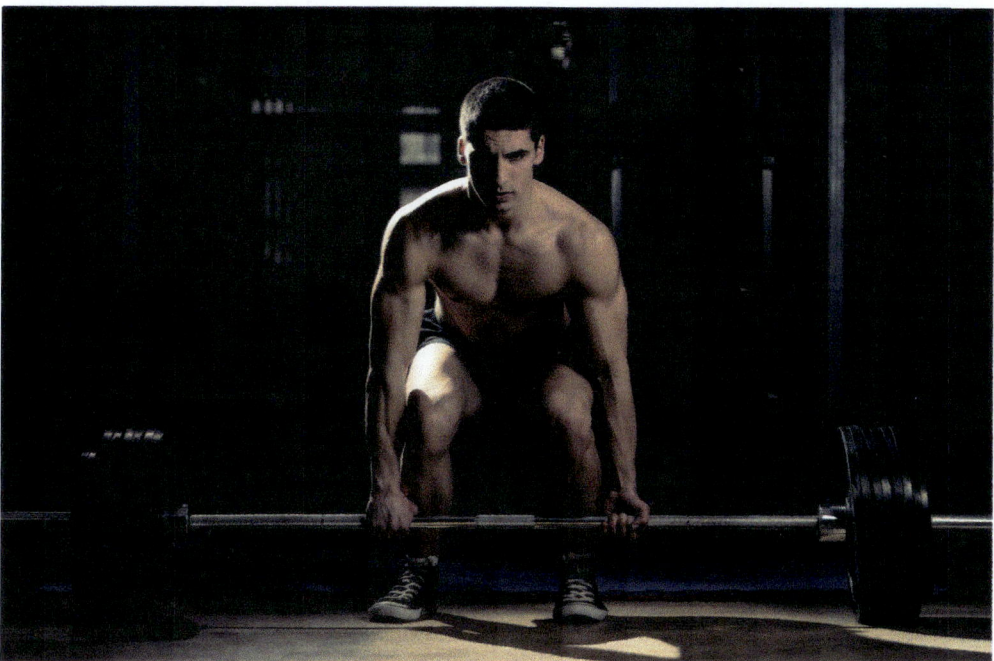

Figure 31.1

Creatine

It is undoubtedly the most important supplement for increasing the muscle strength and power. Creatine is a molecule composed of three amino acids (glycine, arginine and S-Adenosyl-Methionine), whose reserves in our body can vary from 120 g (for a 70 kg subject) up to 160 g. The amount of creatine stores varies according to our body mass; in fact, this molecule resides in our muscles. Its main function is to bind to the orthophosphate ion to form creatine phosphate or CP, and donate this phosphate group to an ADP molecule to form an ATP, which is our energy currency that will be used in the processes of muscle contraction. The Cr-CP system allows you to carry out high efforts for a very short time (five to ten seconds) and it is quite understandable how an increase in creatine can lead to an increase in the time of use for this energy system. In maximal efforts, a large amount of ATP is used and to work with these high loads it is necessary to increase the supply of the phosphate groups to the muscle. At this moment, creatine comes into play as a supplement that allows to increase the endogenous stocks by a variable fraction from 5 to 20% (Buford T.W., 2007). Several studies document that to achieve this increase in muscle creatine stores it is advisable to start with a "load" period with a dosage of at least 20 g for a week, and then take a maintenance dose (5-6 g) for at least three to four weeks. In this way, it is possible to benefit from creatine as a supplement to increase the maximum strength and promote the muscle recovery. The methods of administration during the "loading" include the fractional intake of creatine in two doses (possibly 10 hours apart from each other), or four doses (including it in the pre and post-workout), accompanied by a carbohydrate beverage and a good amount of water, in order to avoid creating accumulations of creatine salts in the intestine that could cause diarrhea, cramps and intestinal pain. The use of carbohydrate beverages allows creatine to be better conveyed into the muscles and increase its supplies.

Betaine

Being a methyl donor, it contributes to the synthesis of S-Adenosyl-Methionine which is a precursor of creatine. Furthermore, for the same reason, it promotes the synthesis of dopamine and adrenaline, which are fundamental neurotransmitters for performing a power exercise. These properties underlie the ability of betaine to increase the strength performance, as well as the fact that it is able to stimulate the production of IGF-1.

Proteins and amino acids

Proteins and amino acids are essential for maintaining and increasing the muscle mass and for promoting the muscle recovery. The doses and methods of intake are identical to the supplementation for muscle mass and in this case they are about 30 g of whey protein isolate, concentrate or hydrolyzed in the post-workout. They can also be associated with caseins, in order to reach the daily protein quota, in the snacks between the main meals (for those who do not want to take large quantities of meat or fish per day) and in the evening before bedtime; in the latter case, caseins should be preferred, to promote the muscle recovery and to reduce the nocturnal catabolic state, as they are absorbed more slowly and therefore have a more prolonged effect on aminoacidemia. As for amino acids, both branched ones and the essential ones are very useful for preventing energy losses and for reducing the muscle catabolism during the training. Branched amino acids can be taken before and during the training session, in dosages that must be calculated according the amount of 1 g for every 10 kg of body weight, while the essential amino acids (EAA) can be of valid help during the post-workout period as a replacement for proteins, along with 2 g of leucine. It is enough to say that around 20 g of essential amino acids offer the same anabolic effect as 45 g of whey protein.

Hormonal stimulators

As mentioned earlier, it is necessary to have good secretion of anabolic hormones to improve the strength. The substances that are the best stimulant in the sense of hormone secretion are ZMA, colostrum and arginine alpha-ketoglutarate (AKG). The first increases the free fraction of testosterone (which is the one that is actually active on the muscle tissue); colostrum, on the other hand, is a type of milk that is rich in growth factors such as IGF-1, and its supplementation allows a significant increase in the concentration of this hormone, which in the biological field is considered as the most powerful activator of anabolism. Furthermore, colostrum contains other growth factors which are useful for regenerating tendon and cartilage structures. As for AKG, various studies have shown its ability to improve the maximal strength performance, probably through a simultaneous stimulation of the nitric oxide production and an increase in IGF-1 levels.

Caffeine

It is very important to maintain the concentration, thus improving the contractile capacity and the blood flow to the tissues. Caffeine, by reducing the feeling of fatigue and by stimulating the release of adrenaline, allows you to be more concentrated and to have a faster nerve signal conduction speed, improving the coordination and the recruitment capacity of muscle fibers. In order to improve the explosive strength, it should be taken about 30-60 minutes before the training. By doing so, we can take advantage of its peak blood concentration to perform the most demanding performances; it is effective at a dosage of about 600 mg in subjects who are not regular users. Side effects such as tachycardia and muscle pain may occur at this dosage.

In a study by Dominguez et al. (2021) it has been found an achievement of a greater maximum power, average power, and a shorter time to reach these values in the Wingate test, as well as a lower RPE (Rate of Perceived Exertion), both on a muscular and general level with 6 mg/kg of caffeine *vs* a sugary placebo.

Supplementation for muscle mass

Bodybuilding is the sport in which nutrition and supplementation techniques are always at the forefront. In this sport, muscle development and a degree of definition are sought, and they involve great sacrifices both in terms of nutrition and training. Since it was born, bodybuilding has been characterized by two phases: mass gain phase, in which maximum muscle growth is sought even at the expense of the lean appearance, and the definition phase, in which there is an inevitable loss of a part of the muscle mass that was acquired in the previous step. The same principle has also been adopted in all those sports where it is important to increase the muscle mass for performance purposes.

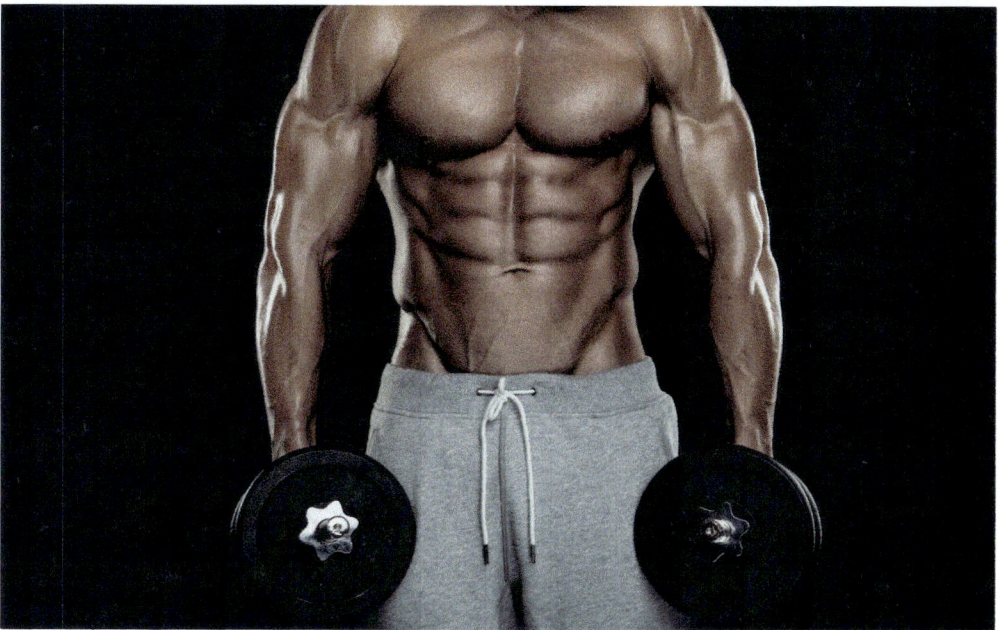

Figure 32.1

In the past, in order to increase the muscle mass, they tried to obtain a muscle development through the consumption of huge quantities of food (an unhealthy practice in many aspects, as the distinction between healthy and unhealthy foods was not well defined yet), with the side effect of an inevitable increase in the subcutaneous and visceral fat, the first with esthetic and performance repercussions, the second with long-term repercussions on health. However, today, even in the bulking phase, the athlete always feeds adequately, with healthy foods and a caloric surplus that allows him/her to train intensely, to grow the muscle mass and to control the body fat in order to facilitate the subsequent slimming phase.

The caloric surplus can be provided by concentrated **protein-caloric supplements** that can be easily eliminated during periods of low-calorie diets, without noticing the lack on a psychological and physical level. To achieve the required amount of protein, they use protein supplements whose calories and nutrient composition are known. These have the property of being easily digested and do not tire the digestive system, as opposed to what occurs by ingesting food, especially if it also contains a certain amount of fat (which, in the case of meats, is saturated fat, therefore an unhealthy one).

Of course, I am not saying to eliminate the traditional foods that are the basis of a healthy diet, but to adjust the quantities in order not to have excessive stomach dilations and a sense of bloating and heaviness (unsightly and harmful to health) due to the introduction of high amounts of food and/or because of the intestinal fermentation that occurs when too much food stays in the digestive system for a long time.

Let us now schematize the type of suitable proteins and indicate which protein supplement could be better in the bulking phase, listing their characteristics.

Let's start by talking about **whey protein**. Whey proteins are very useful in situations of increased protein requirements and for those who want to have a stimulus for increasing the muscle mass; in fact, thanks to their ability to quickly release amino acids into the bloodstream, they allow an acceleration of the protein synthesis. But, if it is true that whey proteins considerably raise the levels of amino acids in the blood, it is equally true that they are metabolized very quickly and that in a short time the level of the amino acids in the blood is drastically lowered. If we use only whey protein, eating every 3 hours may be insufficient and the number of snacks would have to be increased in order to maintain a stimulated state of protein synthesis. It is for this reason that they are preferred as a supplementation during the post-workout recovery, in which the muscle receptor capacity that is increased by the physical activity must be exploited as quickly as possible, and in which it is essential to supply the substances that allow the muscle to recover its energies and start the protein synthesis in the shortest possible time. As for the period of the major muscle building, protein supplements that contain a mix of calcium caseinate and whey proteins obtained by ion exchange are preferred to exploit the optimization of the protein synthesis that they produce by working in synergy. Whey proteins have strong anabolic characteristics thanks to their absorption speed and their amino acid release, while **calcium caseinate** has higher anti-catabolic properties (i.e. it spares the muscles) thanks to its slow amino acid release. Together, they allow a continuous and constant release of amino acids into the blood for a few hours. This mix of proteins is therefore useful as a snack, especially if it is accompanied by low glycemic index carbohydrates to make sure that the proteins are not used for energy purposes. In addition, it is also excellent as a snack before going to sleep if accompanied by a fruit, to avoid nocturnal catabolism. **Soy proteins** can also be added to this mix for their richness in arginine and antioxidants, for their easy digestibility, the cholesterol-lowering effect and the physiological modulation of the testosterone levels. In fact, although they are proteins of a vegetable origin, they contain protein quantities which are higher than 90% and they have very few fats and sodium; lactose is absent.

In a hypothetical maintenance phase, you can opt for the choice of a protein powder supplement that contains all three protein sources mentioned above, in order to benefit from their effects.

Some adjuvants to a diet which is rich in calories are those substances, such as **lipoic acid** and **hydroxycitric acid**, which do not directly promote muscle mass gain, but which allow excess carbohydrates to be stored in the form of glycogen instead of fat. Moreover, they help to maintain a more constant blood sugar level and they do not cause high blood sugar peaks, which are harmful to the body and they are the main cause of fattening.

Before training, it is useful to take a good **antioxidant complex (vitamins A, C, E, selenium**) to prevent the damage caused by the formation of free radicals and to reduce the post- workout DOMS (Delayed Onset Muscle Soreness), which may limit subsequent workouts. However, the use of antioxidants before the training is able to inhibit the catabolic inflammatory process that is the basis of the subsequent anabolic stimulus for the muscle reconstruction, therefore, in a mass program, it would be preferable to take them at a distance from the workout. After the training, if you are looking for a faster muscle recovery, it is useful to take a carbohydrate supplement, even with a medium-high glycemic index, and proteins dissolved in water which are easily assimilated. It may be better to take proteins immediately after the training to immediately stimulate the protein synthesis through the acute increase in the blood level of amino acids, and after that consume some carbohydrates to restore the muscle glycogen. A simultaneous intake would delay the digestion and the protein absorption, and the acceleration of the protein synthesis is what matters most when the goal is to increase the mass. To those who argue that carbohydrates are useful for insulin stimulation, which is necessary for the anabolic effect, we say that the insulin stimulation induced by whey proteins is more than sufficient and that an excess would only favor the liposynthesis. Another good supplement to be taken after the training in order to accelerate the recovery and the muscle growth is a mix of **creatine, leucine, HMB (hydroxy-methyl-butyrate), amino acids, glutamine, minerals and vitamins**; this mix is also very useful before a weight training because it allows you to "push" more and it counteracts the muscle catabolism, a pitfall for all competitive athletes. Among the amino acids, leucine and its metabolite, HMB, are those that have been shown to have the highest ability to stimulate the muscle growth and their use can be particularly useful close to training or, in the case of leucine, to enrich the meals in which this amino acid is deficient.

Betaine, or trimethylglycine, is an osmolyte which is normally present in the cytoplasm of the muscle cell that exerts a protective effect against dehydration and it has a catabolic effect on the muscle. Furthermore, since betaine is a methyl group donor, it increases the formation of creatine, acting in synergy with it in stimulating the hypertrophy.

As previously mentioned, before going to sleep, many athletes take milk caseins, a particular type of protein that is absorbed slowly and therefore has an anti-catabolic effect in the long sleeping period. During meals it is also preferable to take a complex of B vitamins which is essential for a good use of proteins and carbohydrates.

The use of supplements to stimulate the anabolic hormones in order to increase muscle mass can also be useful: **arginine, ornithine and fenugreek** to stimulate the GH, *Tribulus terrestris* and **ZMA** to stimulate the testosterone. Recent studies indicate that **phosphatidic acid** is a promising supplement to promote the increase of the muscle mass, thanks to its ability to stimulate mTOR through an insulin-independent pathway.

It is good to know that taking caffeine before training increases performance. Caffeine increases adrenaline levels, which helps to increase the intensity of the workout and this can also be functional for hypertrophy. However, researchers in Taiwan have shown that caffeine reduces GH levels after training by increasing the serum concentration of free fatty acids, which inhibits the release of growth hormone.

Beaven et al, in 2008, administered incremental doses of caffeine (from 0 up to 800 mg) and only the higher dose raised testosterone levels beyond what resistance training already did, but with concomitant elevation of cortisol as well such that they concluded: "Caffeine has some potential to maximize results through the anabolic effects of increased testosterone concentration, but this benefit could be counteracted by the catabolic effects of increased cortisol and subsequent decline in the testosterone:cortisol ratio".

For more in-depth details and to avoid unnecessary repetition, please refer to the specific chapters.

Don't forget water, the essential source of life. We are made up of 70% water and from this fact we should already deduce its importance for our health: water keeps our cells active, promotes the transport of nutrients and oxygen thus keeping our muscles healthy. A good hydration, through the effect of cell voluminization, promotes anabolic processes, while any situation of dehydration has a catabolic effect. Epigenetics has taught us that just as food is, water is a source of energy and information, so keeping us hydrated, taking quality water, can only improve the quality of our lives.

CHAPTER 33

Supplementation for endurance sports

In this part of the discussion, which concerns the supplementation and endurance sports, I will not dwell on the need for carbohydrate supplements, nor on the hydration and the use of hydrosaline drinks, as the topic has already been treated in the chapter concerning nutrition. Instead, I will analyze the supplements that can be useful to an athlete who faces, in a more or less intense way, an endurance sport discipline (cycling, marathon, cross-country skiing, etc.), considering which are the metabolisms involved in long-duration sports.

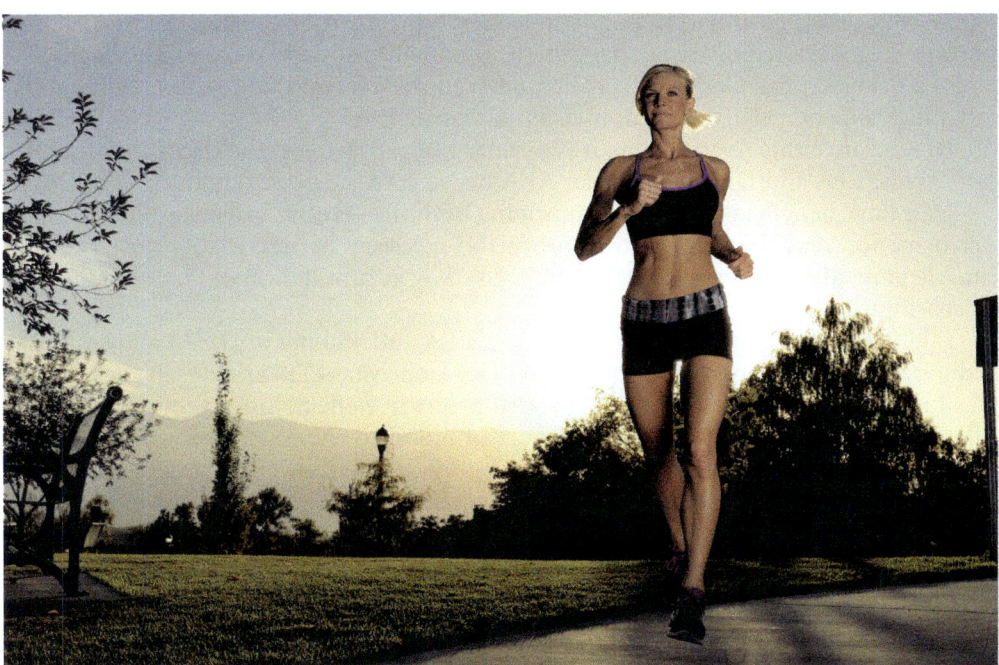

Figure 33.1

Omega-3 essential fatty acids
(DHA: docosahexaenoic acid; EPA: eicosapentaenoic acid)

Fatty acids of the omega-3 series are normally found in marine foods (especially salmon, mackerel, sardines) and some plants. The precursor fatty acid of the omega-3 series, most represented in the plant world and essential for humans is **alpha-linolenic acid (ALA)**. This must be transformed into **EPA** (eicosapentaenoic acid) and **DHA** (docosahexaenoic acid) to exert its biological effects, which, as we know today, are crucial for the correct functioning of some organs and systems such as the brain, retina and gonads. They also have protective effects against atherosclerosis and cardiovascular diseases. Furthermore, these fatty acids are present in various tissues and cells of our organism, where they contribute significantly to the fluidity of the cell membranes and they also modulate the production of some compounds with multiple biological activities: this explains the numerous physiological and pathophysiological roles of these compounds.

The production of these fatty acids (EPA and DHA) depends on the **enzymatic activity of the desaturases** (Δ-6 desaturases or D6D) and of the **elongases** on their precursor, that is, the essential alpha-linolenic fatty acid.

A stressed organism such as that of an athlete (especially competitive athletes) may face difficulties in implementing these biochemical reactions that lead to the transformation of alpha-linolenic acid into EPA and DHA; this is why supplementation can be very useful for those who play sports.

An imbalance between omega-3 and omega-6 (in favor of the latter) will create a greater formation of bad eicosanoids, which leads to the production of type 2 prostaglandins, with pro-inflammatory properties, which can be the basis of most of the chronic degenerative diseases that afflict humans in modern society. They can also cause a delayed post-workout recovery, delayed muscle pain, joint pain, etc. that often afflict the competitive and non-competitive athlete.

To rebalance this relationship, it is essential to supplement the diet with omega-3 fatty acids, EPA and DHA more than ALA because of the poor functioning of D6D.

They have beneficial effects on improving both the aerobic and anaerobic physical performance, and they can also improve the recovery by decreasing post-exercise muscle pain, also known as DOMS, not caused by accumulation of lactic acid but by micro-injuries in the muscles.

Taking 6 g of salmon oil daily (480 mg of EPA and 480 mg of DHA) allowed a net reduction of the lipid peroxidation marker (F2-isoprostane) in athletes. If the amount was lowered to 3 g daily, there was no such protective effect. Since they have a vasodilating effect, they improve the transport of blood to the muscles even during the contraction (the greater fluidity of the red blood cell membrane, thanks to the omega-3s, allows a greater deformation) and consequently determine a greater supply of oxygen and a better elimination of the toxins that are produced during the exercise.

They are essential because they inhibit the formation of bad eicosanoids and increase the formation of good ones, helping to maintain the balance of eicosanoids and thus improving the physiological processes.

They have a very important role in the cell membrane, as they are a structural part of it together with arachidonic acid, and they help in maintaining an excellent fluidity and permeability of the membrane itself, so that the passage of molecules from the outside to the inside of the cell (and vice versa) happens in the best way.

The required quantity of DHA+EPA for a healthy person can reach 2-2.5 g/day.

For a sportsperson, the need may increase based on the intensity and duration of the effort.

Magnesium

99% of the magnesium in our body is located within the cells, of which:
- 50% is concentrated in the bones;
- 24.5% in the muscles;
- 24.5% in the nervous system, myocardium, liver, kidneys and other organs that have a high metabolism.

Minerals make up only about 4% of the body's tissues, but they are vital for the body's functions:
- some minerals help strengthen the bones and teeth, others help regulate the activity of the muscles and nerves by affecting the permeability of cell membranes;
- other minerals serve as essential cofactors in enzyme catalysis;
- they also function as electrolytes, being really important in maintaining a balanced charge of the body's fluids.

Magnesium has all these functions and also serves to regulate the transmission of the nerve impulses; in fact, it is fundamental for the neuron and its deficiency causes a nervous hyper-excitability:
- it regulates the muscle contraction, interacting between the electrical stimulus of the nervous system and the mechanical response of the muscle fiber cell;
- it is a very important constituent of bone tissue;
- it participates in the DNA synthesis and in the energy metabolism;
- it is involved in the biosynthesis of proteins, fats and nucleic acids. It is part of the glycolysis which transforms glucose into energy;
- it promotes the transport and synthesis of proteins (30 g of proteins, in order to be assimilated, require about 200 mg of magnesium), improving the muscle building process, so it is indispensable for any athlete during the muscle building phase.

In recent years, studies on this precious element have intensified enormously and have shown how it is involved in a large number of biological reactions and how its deficiency, even in moderate levels, is the cause of numerous dysfunctions. Symptoms of magnesium deficiency include nausea, muscle weakness, irritability, and some mental disorders.

A loss of magnesium or a decrease in its availability can be caused by:
- intense and prolonged aerobic workouts;
- taking medicines such as diuretics, digitalis, tetracycline and corticoids;
- diets and the use of diuretics to lose weight;
- consumption of fast foods;

- excessive presence of phytates in the diet (plant components), as they negatively interfere with its absorption;
- alcohol consumption.

Magnesium deficiency in athletes produces:
- a decreased performance, with frequent cramps;
- an early increase in lactic acid levels;
- a reduced capacity of the heat resistance;
- a reduced capacity of the physical endurance;
- a reduced resilience;
- easy crises of "spasmophilia".

Some dietary factors that can decrease the amount of magnesium are the high consumption of fats, soft drinks (the ones that are rich in phosphates, which remove magnesium from the body) or an excess of vitamin D.

Acid rain takes the magnesium out of the soil; fluoridation eliminates it from the drinking water and the processing of grains and foods carried out by the food industry decreases the content of this mineral.

The endogenous causes that cause magnesium deficiency are various, but the main ones can be summarized as follows:
- asthenia and stress, which would lead to a displacement of magnesium from the intracellular to the extracellular space;
- some gastrointestinal diseases, which would cause a reduced absorption.

The normal requirement for an adult male is estimated to be 5 mg/kg of body weight, but in athletes this amount increases as a greater loss occurs through:
- perspiration;
- short and intense efforts due to the increase in lactic acid and adrenaline;
- prolonged efforts where magnesium is used for the combustion of fats.

For athletes, a daily intake of magnesium of about 500-1000 mg/day may be useful.

An essential amino acids pool

The physiology of sport tells us that the muscle needs a protein-amino acid replacement, not only to repair the damage caused by the training, but also to meet the inevitable caloric demands deriving from the physical activity. In fact, about 5-10% of the energy used during a purely aerobic performance (50% of VO_{2max}) is composed of protein structures.

Alongside this reality, there is a very strong need for recovery. The more the athlete practices trainings with high frequency and intensity sessions, the more marked the need for recovery. It is especially typical of competitive sports, but it can happen in amateur ones too, and the essential amino acids assist the recovery by facilitating the protein synthesis.

In addition to acting as building blocks for the protein synthesis, essential amino acids play a fundamental role in the physiological stimulation and in the constitution of important hormones such as growth hormone (GH), insulin and glucagon.

As for branched chain amino acids (BCAAs), in addition to their plastic/structural function (a common function of all essential amino acids), they can also perform an energetic function. BCAAs also help to mitigate the sense of fatigue in subjects who go through intense and prolonged physical exertions.

Phytonutrients and free radicals

It is now established that free radicals are an important risk factor that can no longer be ignored. The antioxidant system that each one of us is equipped with (superoxide dismutase, catalase, glutathione peroxidase) and the antioxidant substances that we take with our food (such as vitamin C, E, beta-carotene, polyphenols, minerals, deriving, for the most part, from fresh fruits and vegetables) allow the level of free radicals, which are continuously formed in a living being that is able to breathe, to remain at normal values. However, if the production of the free radicals increases in non-physiological quantities (the reasons can be many), our antioxidant system goes haywire and it becomes unable to counteract and keep the free radicals within a normal level, thus causing harmful oxidative stress. Oxidative stress leads, over time, to certain organic damage caused by the attack of free radicals on the structures of the cell membranes, consisting mainly of polyunsaturated fatty acids, phospholipids and proteins, with a compromise in the functionality of the cell. In these cases, it is necessary to intervene by modifying the diet and the lifestyle, and if it is necessary, by administering antioxidant agents.

Regarding the damage produced by the free radicals, athletes are a category at risk, especially those who are involved in long-term endurance disciplines, which lead to a significant production of ROS (Reactive Oxigen Species).

These athletes usually take care of themselves in all forms, from their nutrition to their social life, physical appearance, etc. However, they often neglect the prevention and the treatment of the oxidative damage, not out of laziness or because it requires more sacrifices, but because it is neither visible nor tangible, even if it causes disastrous consequences in the long term. The heart, brain, lungs and all the other organs and tissues of the athletes are more exposed to the threat of free radicals, as, during intense and/or prolonged exercises, there is an increase in the oxygen consumption, which is responsible for the overproduction of free radicals with a consequent oxidative cell damage. It determines a structural alteration of the cell itself and also of the DNA. According to a study conducted by Brooks and Fahey (Brooks GA, Fahey TD, Exercise Physiology. New York, John Wiley and Sons, 1984), during major efforts, an athlete can consume 12 to 20 times the volume of oxygen that is consumed by a sedentary person (imagine the free radical production and attack this could entail). It is known that training, followed by the right recovery, stimulates and strengthens the activity and the production of antioxidant enzymatic systems which, in partnership with vitamins C, E, beta-carotene, selenium and other anti-radical substances, can neutralize the produced free radicals. Despite this strengthening of the organic defenses, after an intense training session or after a competition, the athlete will always have significantly higher levels of the free radicals.

Other factors that contribute to an overproduction of the free radicals are the following:

- the decrease in the activity of cytochrome oxidase, which would cause an increase in the percentage of oxygen that escapes the normal metabolic pathway, that leads to the synthesis of free radicals;
- the oxidation of lactate in the muscle, through the enzyme lactate dehydrogenase (LDH), with a reduction of oxygen to the superoxide anion;
- hyperthermia, which favors the decoupling of the oxidative phosphorylation, with an oxygen deviation towards the production of free radicals;
- activation of intracellular adenylate cyclase, with a subsequent increase in AMP and hypoxanthine, which lead to the production of the superoxide anion through xanthine oxidase, with a mechanism that is similar to the one observed in the reperfusion syndrome.

To protect yourself from the production and the negative action of free radicals produced by intense physical activities, it is useful to take a food supplement based on fruit and vegetable concentrates, capable of providing the main phytonutrients that are naturally present in plants, which are useful in the daily nutrition and provide an antioxidant protection against the free radicals. If derived from "natural" and not synthetic origin, it seems to be absorbed and used better by the body.
This substance mix is also necessary for those who are not used to consuming fresh fruits and vegetables daily or for those who, due to logistics or lack of time, cannot carry them everywhere. It is certainly useful to also take antioxidants such as vitamin C, vitamin E and lipoic acid, which by acting in synergy can provide a 360 ° protection of the cell membrane against free radicals. If a sportsperson optimizes the functions of their organism, they have the possibility to make the best use of the energy resources during training and competitions. It also helps to speed up the recovery and the protein synthesis processes, and to minimize the damage caused to organic structures by the free radicals.

Carnitine

Carnitine is an amino acid responsible for transporting long-chain fatty acids within the mitochondria, where they are used for energy purposes. During aerobic exercises, especially prolonged ones, the use of fats for energy purposes can reach up to 80%, so the need for carnitine increases. Carnitine stimulates the activity of the pyruvate dehydrogenase complex, directing pyruvate towards the Krebs cycle and thus limiting the production of lactic acid, with the result of a reduction in fatigue and an improvement in the performance, even in aerobic sports where, given the intensity of the maximal effort, people often work above the anaerobic threshold, with the inevitable production of lactic acid (for example, cycling). Furthermore, since carnitine is a ketogenic substance, the simultaneous intake with ketogenic amino acids such as leucine and isoleucine could lead to a greater production of ketone bodies, inhibiting the catabolism at the level of structural proteins, saving the muscle glycogen and thus allowing a longer performance in endurance sports.

Taurine

This amino acid decreases the feeling of fatigue and has strong antioxidant and cytoprotective properties, demonstrated in different studies on animals and athletes. Taurine is destroyed during the training, and its deficiency brings a cell damage caused by an excess of peroxide (a harmful free radical), a classic situation in those who perform a lot of physical activities (especially aerobic).

Zhang et al. found an increase in VO_{2max}, in the time to exhaustion and in the ability to withstand a workload in those who took taurine supplements (*Amino Acids* 26: 203-207, 2004).

Taurine allows for a faster elimination of cholesterol and it is able to improve the insulin sensitivity with a consequent improvement in the use of carbohydrates in the muscles. Those who take taurine supplements have a higher production of nitric oxide than those who do not take it. Other research indicates its importance in the cellular hydration. The increase in the cell volume decreases the muscle catabolism and at the same time stimulates the protein synthesis (*Nutr Hosp* 2002 Nov-Dec; 17 (6): 262-270).

Among the possible benefits of taurine for athletes, there is an increase in the cardiac performance during exercise. Some scholars have evaluated the effects of an "energy drink" containing taurine (400 mg/100 mL) and caffeine (and other ingredients) on 13 athletes subjected to an intense and strenuous endurance workout. The drink increased the volume of the blood pumped by the heart during each beat by 21%, which was not the case with caffeine alone (*Amino Acids* 20: 75-82, 2001).

Inosine

Inosine is a natural substance that increases the body's ability to transport oxygen. It is also a molecule that allows you to support both aerobic and high intensity anaerobic exercises.

Inosine is able to cross the cell membrane of both cardiac and skeletal muscles. Once it gets in the cell, it promotes the production of ATP, which helps with the muscle contraction. In addition, it helps to carry more oxygen from the bloodstream to various tissues, including the muscles. It seems to be able to facilitate the hemoglobin/oxygen bond, given that much of the inosine is absorbed by red blood cells (in practice, its effect to CO would be the opposite of the smoke and pollution effect).

If we consider the heart as the most important muscle of the athlete (and not only), inosine is able to quickly recover the heart muscle after intense efforts.

Guarana

It can have a double effect on athletes, the ergogenic one and that of exerting a powerful antioxidant action to inhibit the effects of the free radicals.

However, a little known function of guarana, which is instead very useful both for sportspeople and for those who do not practice sports, is that it acts as an antiplatelet agent, preventing the formation of blood clots and probably also dissolving the ones that are already formed, thus exerting a protective effect at the cardiovascular system level.

Arginine

It is the amino acid precursor of nitric oxide.

Nitric oxide also allows (thanks to its vasodilating properties) a higher blood flow to the muscle, improving the transport of oxygen and other nutrients. An increase in the blood flow creates a greater pumping effect on the muscles, resulting in an increase in the muscle volume. The increase in the transport of nutrients creates favorable conditions for the formation of the new muscle tissue.

Nitric oxide (NO), by increasing the blood flow and the transport of nutrients, promotes a complete recovery after intense workouts. Having anti-inflammatory properties, it also decreases the post-workout muscle pain and promotes cell repair. Scientific studies indicate that L-arginine improves the muscle performance in aerobic exercise regimens through an increase in the NO production, and this confirms the already known role of this amino acid on the athletic performance.

Coenzyme Q10

Coenzyme Q10 is a lipid coenzyme, extremely widespread in nature, which plays a fundamental role in the production of energy, and it is synthesized in our cells in the mevalonate pathway. It is found in the mitochondria and in the innermost part of the membranes, and it is involved in the transfer of electrons in the respiratory chain, whose main function is the production of ATP. Thanks to its antioxidant properties, this coenzyme is widely used in the treatment of numerous pathologies, such as neurodegenerative disorders (including Parkinson's, Alzheimer's and encephalomyopathy), cardiovascular diseases, migraines and diabetes.

In 1997, Ylikosky studied the effects of CoQ10 supplementation on a group of 25 Finnish cross-country skiers. The results showed improvements in all physical performance indices (aerobic threshold, anaerobic threshold and VO_{2max}). Specifically, 94% of the athletes improved their times and their performance, while in the placebo group, only 33% achieved better results.

A study published by Dr. Bill Misner (Montana, USA) in 2005, examined 18 volunteer athletes (cyclists and triathletes), divided into two groups: to one group with ten athletes, was given coenzyme Q10; to another group, with eight athletes, was given a placebo. After 28 days, the concentration of coenzyme Q10 in the plasma was significantly increased in those who took the supplement, going from 0.91µg/mL to 1.97 µg/mL.

The anti-fatigue action of CoQ10 has recently been confirmed, with interesting implications both in duration and high intensity performances.

Lipoic acid

Alpha-lipoic acid naturally exists within the body's mitochondria and it is called a universal antioxidant because it is both water and fat-soluble.

Various studies have demonstrated its effectiveness in preventing death from heart damage dependent on the nerve function, typical of the diabetic patient, by inducing significant improvements in the heart function. The action of alpha-lipoic acid is also expressed directly in the management of type 2 diabetes, as it improves the body's ability to burn sugars and reduces the insulin resistance, (i.e. increasing the action of insulin itself on the peripheral tissues), both by increasing the production of

ATP. These last two characteristics are of a significant interest for those who practice physical activities.

Lipoic acid is an integral part of the oxidation process of the pyruvic acid, as it accepts the aldehyde groups created by thiaminapyrophosphate (TPP), an important substrate in the lipolytic cycles for the production of energy. It also prevents the protein glycation that occurs during the state of hyperglycemia. Alpha-lipoic acid, by increasing the uptake of glucose into cells, contributes to the prevention of the damage to collagen fibers due to glycation.

The high levels of glucose in the blood stimulate the production of insulin, facilitating the inflammation, which then leads to the glycation and the formation of very powerful free radicals called AGE (Advanced Glycation End-products).

ALA is important in many critical steps of the Krebs cycle, which produces free radicals. It regenerates many other antiradicals, such as vitamin C, vitamin E and coenzyme Q10. It is one of the few substances that increase the glutathione (tripeptide) levels. Alpha-lipoic acid, alone and in synergy with gamma-linolenic acid has an improving effect on the conduction of nerve stimuli.

According to a study (*Nat Med* 2004 Jun 13), lipoic acid has the following properties:

- it has a dose-dependent slimming effect;
- it may be able to increase the burned calories by 36-50%;
- it has no toxic effects;
- it reduces blood glucose and insulin levels;
- it reduces appetite;
- it is an essential cofactor for the enzymes of the mitochondria and consequently for the production of energy (ATP);
- it increases the function of uncoupled protein 1 (UCP-1) in the brown adipose tissue (higher energy expenditure).

Iron

The body of an adult subject contains about 5 g of iron; the majority of it is found in hemoglobin (a fundamental component of red blood cells), a good percentage is present in myoglobin (contained in the muscles) and a smaller amount is found in the form of deposits such as ferritin and hemosiderin, and as a cofactor of some enzymes. The iron in myoglobin and hemoglobin performs the function of transporting oxygen.

An iron deficiency can be created in the body due to insufficient food intake or by increased losses (micro- and macro-haemorrhages). In the athlete, the losses are higher than those who have sedentary lifestyles. The main causes are: profuse sweating, especially in those who train daily and in humid environments; microhemorrhages in the intestine and kidneys (with the presence of microhematuria, i.e. blood in the urine); greater exfoliation of the intestinal epithelium; increased hemolysis of red blood cells due to mechanical causes such as crushing the sole of the foot during running. Numerous studies document that athletes who practice endurance sports or who undergo intense and prolonged trainings are those who most easily undergo a reduction in the iron deposits. There are other mechanisms that cause an iron deficiency in athletes: intravascular hemolysis due to traumatic effects from an increased circulation speed; mechanical compression during the muscle contraction; acidosis; osmotic and mechanical erythrocyte alteration due to an increase in catecholamines; bladder trauma; lipoperoxidation of the erythrocyte membrane by an increased production of free radicals. Iron deficiency leads to iron deficiency anemia, which manifests itself with symptoms such as: weakness, paleness, chills, palpitations, difficulty concentrating. The effectiveness of iron supplements depends on their absorption and usage. Vitamin C, lysine, *Equisetum* and *Avena sativa* improve its bioavailability, as do some chelated forms such as ferroprotein succinate and iron bisglycinate.

Caffeine

The ergogenic effect of caffeine in endurance activities is expressed through the ability of this molecule to act as a competitive antagonist of adenosine receptors, reducing the feeling of fatigue and through its ability to stimulate the release of catecholamines (adrenaline and noradrenaline) by the medulla of the adrenal gland, with effects on muscle, adipose and vascular tissue and on the metabolic system, increasing lipolysis and sparing muscle glycogen, increasing coronary flow (increased blood supply to the heart), increasing cardiac output (increased blood supply to tissues) and increasing systolic blood pressure.

Water

Sweating is the main system for maintaining thermoregulation during endurance muscle activity. This physiological mechanism involves a significant evaporation of water from the skin by subtracting it from circulating fluids. The amount of fluids lost through perspiration, during physical activity, are significant and proportional to the amount of heat to be dispersed and the environmental temperature. It is suffice to say that in basal conditions of rest, the body transpires about 700mL/day of water. With physical activity, this value can reach even 25mL/min. Fluid losses are then conditioned by climatic conditions, humidity, wind, altitude, clothing and physical preparation of the athlete. With so many variables, it is difficult to accurately estimate the specific water needs of an athlete. Along with fluids, there are also significant losses of minerals. Indispensable are saline supplements to be reconstituted in the right proportions according to need. In case of lack, use 500 mL water, a lemon, half a teaspoon of salt and 1 sachet of fructose.

Those who practice endurance sports know their bodies and know how to perceive the first alarm bells that lead to a possible hydro-saline imbalance: thirst, a drop in concentration, muscular weakness, are all late symptoms that occur if replenishment has not been optimal during physical activity.

CHAPTER 34

Supplementation for slimming

There are many sports where it is necessary to fall into the right weight category and obviously it is better to achieve this by losing fat and not muscle. In bodybuilding, the maximum performance is achieved with a higher muscle mass combined with a lower fat mass, and most sports generally benefit from a better lean/fat mass ratio.

There are various types of supplements on the market that act in different ways, but always aimed at fat loss. In this chapter, we will mention the most common ones which are normally used for this purpose, without necessarily being dealt with exhaustively in the specific part of the book dedicated to supplements, as they go beyond the specific subject of the book itself and it could be the subject of another dedicated book.

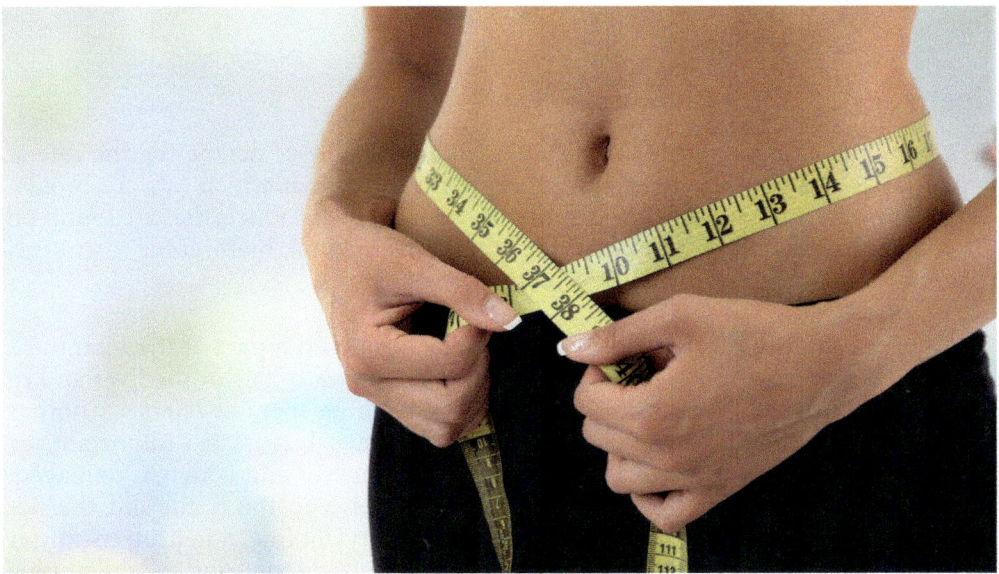

Figure 34.1

However, in general, the integrative approach in a weight loss phase could be summarized as described below. In the weight loss period, that is, the search for the minimum percentage of body fat, always preserving the health and the physical functionality, we switch to a low-calorie diet which therefore must contain supplements of the essential elements for the body, which are not sufficiently included in the diet due to their poor nutritional values.

First of all, you need to take a good multivitamin-multimineral supplement and omega-3 essential fatty acids to avoid a deficiency. Lipotropics help the liver to perform its functions concerning the fat metabolism, and without a well-functioning liver, an adequate weight loss cannot be obtained: this is the reason why a weight loss diet should always be preceded by a detoxification phase. To speed up the metabolism, you can take thermogenics containing synephrine and guarana, which increase the fat burning process and keep the muscles toned. They also have a slight effect at the central level, helping to maintain a higher concentration, thus avoiding the physiological mental decline that occurs in low calorie diets.

Before the training, to preserve the lean mass, you can use completely natural substances (phosphatidylserine, acetyl-L-carnitine), which are able to attenuate the secretion of the catabolic hormone par excellence (cortisol), associated with branched amino acids for their energetic and anti-catabolic effect. During this phase, you can also take substances that aid the weight loss, such as thermogenics and carnitine (the latter especially before aerobic activities).

After the training, the intake of branched amino acids, glutamine and small amounts of fructose will facilitate the energy and protein recovery and restoration, without compromising the lipolytic process (weight loss) that occurs in the period that follows the training session.

Before going to sleep, the intake of proteins and/or amino acids can facilitate the nocturnal release of growth hormone, resulting in a slimming and regenerating function.

Lipotropics

Let's start by talking about lipotropics, which are capable of decreasing the rate at which fat is stored in the liver and accelerating the rate at which fats are broken down into water, carbon dioxide and energy. Usually, the products that are found on the market are made up of associations of choline, inositol, methionine, carnitine, chromium.

Choline – Found in all living cells, choline is considered a part of the vitamin B complex. It works with inositol to prevent the formation of fats in the liver and to remove the fats that are present in the cells, by burning them as energy. Another function is that they help the body in using cholesterol. It is also important for the health of myelin, which forms the lining of the nerves and which, if damaged, would not allow a correct exchange of impulses between the brain and the periphery. It is a constituent part of lecithin and of acetylcholine, a neurotransmitter that is necessary for the muscle control, for proper muscle tone and for the muscle memory.

Inositol – This is also a B complex vitamin. Together with choline, it acts to prevent dangerous accumulations of fat in the arteries and keeps the liver, heart and kidneys healthy. It is involved in promoting the production of lecithin, a natural constituent of the cells and an emulsifier of cholesterol aggregates in micro-particles, preventing atherosclerosis.

Carnitine – This is a protein-type nutrient that shuttles the fats, transporting them to the mitochondria to be burned as energy. It improves the sports performance, as it makes fatty acids more available to be used as energy for the muscles; in this way it saves the muscle glycogen reserves and reduces the formation of lactic acid during the physical activity.

Chromium picolinate – It is a trace mineral essential for the metabolism of fats and carbohydrates. It helps to increase the insulin sensitivity, which means, the cell receptors for this hormone are activated and do their job by requiring smaller amounts of insulin. High-sugar diets and intense exercise regimes can create a chromium deficiency.

Methionine – It is an essential sulfuric amino acid. It helps to detox the liver from the fats present in it and participates in the formation of carnitine, trimethylglycine, choline, adrenaline, ergosterol and nucleic acids.

Thermogenics

Other effective "fat burners" are the thermogenics, which stimulate the basal metabolism. In this way, they increase the thermogenesis and the body's ability to burn more calories even at rest. Thermogenesis is a physiological process that takes place above all in the muscles and in the brown and beige adipose tissue, through a series of biochemical reactions intended to metabolize fats or their derivatives, releasing energy for the production of heat. Some molecules have the ability to interact with the beta3-adrenergic receptors of the adipose tissue and thus activate lipolysis.

Synephrine – It is a beta-agonist alkaloid with thermogenic properties but without side effects on the central nervous system and on the heart, unlike ephedrine, and it has the ability to keep the muscles toned, preserving them from the loss of the muscle mass, often associated with low calorie diets. It is present in the majority of these supplements.

Octopamine – It is a molecule chemically similar to synephrine and noradrenaline. It has a catecholamine-like effect, being able to stimulate the beta3 receptors present in the brown adipose tissue, by activating the lipolysis, increasing the metabolism and promoting the transport of glucose at the cellular level.

Guarana – With its content of gradually releasing caffeine and other xanthine derivatives (theophylline, theobromine, etc.), it allows to maintain high mental and physical abilities and it is able to stimulate the lipolysis.

Green tea – The main components of green tea are polyphenols and purine bases, mainly represented by theine, theophylline and theobromine. Catechins prevail among the numerous phenolic compounds, (the best known is epigallocatechin gallate). The presence of polyphenolic derivatives and theanine modulates the stimulating activity of green tea, making it milder and with more prolonged effects than theine alone. It should also be considered that the presence of polyphenols is essential in stimulating the production of a high level of norepinephrine through the inhibition of COMT (an enzyme that degrades norepinephrine), which is able to promote the lipolysis. In addition, some catechins have the ability to inhibit alpha-amylases (enzymes that are necessary for the digestion of starch) and with this mechanism, they can contribute to a significant reduction in the absorption of carbohydrates in the intestine, promoting the weight loss. Dosage: 100-200 mg, two to three times a day.

Guggul – This compound contains guggulsterones, which in addition to the well-known cholesterol-lowering and lipid-lowering properties have shown, in some studies, to stimulate the production of the thyroid hormones, responsible for an acceleration of the metabolism and therefore a greater consumption of iodine, a fundamental mineral for the proper functioning of the thyroid gland, the endocrine gland responsible for maintaining the basal metabolism and the vital processes.

Capsaicin – It is a capsainoid contained in chili, with a thermogenic effect, capable of increasing the caloric expenditure for a few hours by increasing the adrenaline levels. Most studies have shown that capsaicin increases the daily calorie consumption by 4 to 5% and it also increases the use of fats by 10 to 16%. In one study, the administration of 10 mg of capsainoid increased the adrenergic activity and the energy expenditure, with a greater use of fats in resting conditions, but not during exercise and during the recovery phase. Therefore, it is a supplement that can be useful for weight loss but should not be taken close to the training.

Coleus forskohlii

Coleus forskohlii is a plant that is used for centuries for the normalization of the blood pressure, unconsciously exploiting all the other properties that derive from a substance contained in it (forskolin), the ability to increase the intracellular concentration of cAMP (anti-platelet aggregation, vasodilation, reduction of inflammation, bronchodilation, contrasting action against glaucoma, positive inotropic effect on the heart muscle, etc.). This substance is able to activate adenylate cyclase, on which the cellular concentration of the second cellular messenger "cyclic adenosine monophosphate" (cAMP) is dependent on.

The exact mechanism governing this activation has not yet been well clarified; however, it seems that forskolin, interacting with the beta-adrenergic receptors, determines the release of noradrenaline from the endings of the sympathetic nervous system. The studies carried out on *Coleus* are now significant and concern various aspects of the organism.

The well-established properties that this plant possesses are: a positive inotropic effect, the reduction of inflammation, the reduction of blood pressure, bronchodilation, anti-platelet agglomeration, anti-glaucoma action.

It can help in the improvement of the insulin secretion (which can promote the transport of carbohydrates and amino acids into the muscle cells for their use for energy and recovery).

It has an antioxidant action aimed at the lipid peroxidation of the cell membrane of the red blood cells, caused by high glucose levels in the blood (*Cell Mol Biol* 45 (8): 1203-1207, 1999).

If you rely on certified and standardized extracts, studies have highlighted the following possible effects and results:

- an increase in lean body mass;
- the optimization of the release of fatty acids deposited in the adipose tissue;
- an increased thermogenesis;
- a stimulation of the activity of the T4 5-deiodinase enzyme, responsible for the formation of the thermogenetic thyroid hormone, T3. At the same time, the increased metabolic activity, dependent on beta-adrenergic receptors, causes an increase in the lean mass through the activation of phosphorylase in the skeletal muscles, a release of insulin and the synthesis of anabolic hormones;

  a mood modulating action, also useful for those who follow a restrictive diet for
- weight loss.

Lipoic acid

Another good product that has recently entered the field of slimming is the combination of lipoic acid and pyruvic acid. These two substances work synergistically, increasing the Krebs cycle's ability to burn nutrients for energy. They are also capable of increasing the flow of nutrients (especially fat metabolites) within the cycle itself. They are also useful for limiting the weight gain in high-calorie diets, as both substances have the ability to direct excess carbohydrates to the muscle cells rather than to fat cells, allowing the formation of a higher reserve of muscle glycogen. Lipoic acid is also an excellent antioxidant and an insulin mimetic, as it tends to maintain the blood glucose at physiological levels, allowing a better use by the cells, not causing high secretions of insulin that are harmful to the body and that can inhibit the weight loss.

Replacement meals

They help in reducing the calories while introducing the necessary macro- and micronutrients which come from the so-called replacement meals, thus avoiding a state of malnutrition which is characteristic of do-it-yourself diets or for diets that are extrapolated from magazines. They consist of powders and/or bars with a pleasant taste, which are easily consumable. They are excellent substitutes for the midday meals, healthier than the usual sandwich eaten in a hurry on the go. The most modern replacement meals also contain fibers and fructo-oligosaccharides (inulin, acacia fiber, etc.), useful for regulating the metabolism of fats and carbohydrates, but also for nourishing and balancing the intestinal bacterial flora, with positive repercussions on the whole body. It is not advisable to replace too many traditional meals with supplements, as the purpose of a correct diet is also to educate people to eat the correct foods. However, remember to divide your daily calories into at least five meals (three main meals plus two snacks), as they will allow you to maintain a constant level of energy and attention throughout the day, and they are also more effective for weight loss, since our body must consume energy to metabolize the foods that we consume each time.

Multivitamin-multiminerals

One thing that should never be lacking in low-calorie diets is a good multimineral and multivitamin supplement, as, due to a poor diet, we consume quantities that are lower than the real needs for vitamins and minerals, which are essential for cellular metabolism.

Water

A very important aspect when it comes to losing weight is hydration. Everyone will have heard that it is important to drink for their health, but few have any idea of how much water is actually needed to lose weight. A study has shown that drinking 500 mL of fresh water promotes an increase in metabolic rate of 30% through an increase in thermogenesis that is activated after 10 minutes and reaches its maximum after 40 minutes leading to a consumption of 25 Kcal. This means that by drinking 2 liters of water you consume about 100 Kcal more. Water is equally important for appetite control, it is not by chance that we often hear people say that when dieting it is necessary to drink more water in order to feel full for longer. The reason why this strategy is done is because in many cases what we perceive as hunger is actually thirst. Many sensations that tend to be associated with hunger, such as rumbling in the stomach, low energy levels and even mental fatigue, can actually be synonymous with dehydration. Several studies have shown that people who consume more water before and after meals are likely to consume smaller amounts of food and lose weight.

CHAPTER 35

Supplementation for concentration
by Marco Tullio Cau

The times (not very distant) when boxers, to "make" the weight, fasted and drank only ox blood, with the result of arriving in the ring drained and devoid of energy, seem to be over!

However, in addition to supplementation for, so to speak, "plastic" and pro-energetic purposes, there is a "third" that still appears to be neglected, and it is related to maximizing the concentration (or the mental clarity), which can assist the sportsperson, for example, in expressing their potential in a better way, making them able to carry out a more profitable workout: we could say that it allows you to make the most out the first two types of supplementation!

This could relate to a workout in the gym, but in reality every sport has its nuances: obviously, if we talk about concentration, we immediately think of shooting discs with a pistol, or even with a bow and arrow, all disciplines that require maximum attention and tranquility; here, in these cases, a supplement that is too "invasive" would create a state of excessive tension, which could turn out to be deleterious in the same way as a food that induces lethargy.

The same is true for any of the athletic throwing sports: competitive grit is required, but an extreme state of neural activation would affect the technical gesture, made up of precise body positions and rigorous timing. An excess of mental energy could distort these parameters, or eventually a good measure could be achieved without being able to remain inside the platform, with the result of doing a nice "null"!

Or, again, in a team sport, after half a game, the drop in the concentration could lead to an injury or a slight lackening of attention could cause a crash on a motorcycle: I remember a similar episode, which happened to a rider who was leading a race, during a time when I was following a group of professional motorcyclists.

Sports psychology - my first specialization - can certainly help, but why not further facilitate its intake with some *ad hoc* substances?

All this by always keeping in mind what is written in the chapter on nutrition: so to speak, we cannot fixate on the tree and lose sight of the forest!

Caffeine

It is almost a duty to start this review with caffeine (which until a few years ago was considered doping if taken in large quantities, while today it is present "only" in the monitoring list). This substance is certainly the best known ergogen and has been studied at 360 degrees for many years; just recently, in fact, I received an e-mail from Medscape in relation to a trial illustrating its beneficial effects against the recurrence of colon cancer.

Caffeine is a natural alkaloid substance (trimethylxanthine) contained in some plants and it is rapidly absorbed when consumed in drinks or capsules, since it appears in the blood within 5-15 minutes from the intake and peaks between 40 and 80 minutes. Returning to what is of interest to us here, most of the research concerned aerobic activities. However, anaerobic sports are also finding space recently, albeit to a much lesser extent.

A first interesting discriminant to take into consideration, is that relating to the quantities to be ingested in order to improve performance: Spriet (2014) carried out an excellent review on the subject (the chapter entitled "The changing landscape of caffeine research" alone would suffice), starting from the assumption that the most used doses in the studies were medium-high ones (5-13 mg/kg), which often provided good results, but also strong alterations of numerous biological parameters, such as increases in the heartbeat, gastrointestinal disturbances, nervousness, mental confusion, difficulty to focus, sleep disturbances and also (and here we enter another field) a doubling of the levels of catecholamines, higher values of lactate, free fatty acids and glycerol.

Some studies that have treated intermediate quantities (5-6 mg/kg) have still found a good efficacy, with a moderate reduction (but not elimination) of the physiological and side effects, while the few studies that have tested lower doses (<3 mg/kg, ~200 mg) always found a good efficacy and no change in the parameters described above, clearly indicating that the ergogenic power of caffeine passes through an interaction with the central nervous system.

To deepen this aspect, it is useful to consult the work of Nehlig (1992), which proposes three mechanisms through which caffeine acts: the mobilization of the intracellular calcium, the inhibition of specific phosphodiesterases (however, they occur with the highest dosages) and the mechanism that sees methylxanthines as adenosine antagonists, which is most likely to happen at medium-low quantities; the studies by Tarnopolsky et al. (2000), are also very interesting. They carried out a very technical analysis, whose results would support the hypothesis that "at least a part of the ergogenic effect of caffeine on endurance performance occurs directly at the muscle level". Kalmar et al. (1999), who after having administered the conventional 6 mg/kg implemented a complex protocol and, through electrodes, verified that "the mechanism is, at least partially, peripheral".

I will report only a recent research (2015) relating to the average quantities, which consisted on a pool of Brazilian and German researchers led by de Oliveira Cruz. As a subject, it had some well-trained cyclists who went through an exhaustion test after an administration of 6 mg/kg: the improvement was 22.7%.

However, given the aforementioned results obtained with higher doses, I believe that it is more useful to examine the researches that use moderate dosages (or "mixed" ones, where the lower quantities stand out), also by virtue of the fewer side effects: 200-300 mg of caffeine are equal to about two cups of coffee and can be used (almost) by everyone, possibly even in capsules.

The interest in caffeine as a potential ergogenic aid was sparked by Costill's studies in the late 1970s, which saw some professional cyclists improve their maximum pedaling time at 80% VO_{2max}, from 75 minutes in the placebo condition to 96 minutes following the ingestion of 330 mg of caffeine; it was an average dosage, about 5 mg/kg, unlike that adopted by a second study by the working group of the Ball State University (Indiana, USA), which had administered 500 mg of caffeine (divided into two doses, before and during the exercise) to another group of cyclists, who also made excellent progress, partly as a result of an increase of 31% in lipid oxidation, which likely provided the necessary substrate for the increase in the performance, as proof of the effects of higher doses of this substance that is loved so much in a major part of the world.

Continuing in the examination of the Spriet review, we find other studies: in one of them, some runners who received 3, 6 and 9 mg/kg of caffeine were compared, obtaining excellent results with the lower dosages, with a 22% increase in running at exhaustion (~ 85% VO_{2max}) when compared to placebo. In another study, caffeine was administered at intervals, before and during a trial with the "ordinary" cyclists (2.1, 3.2 or 4.5 mg/kg): the results sequentially decreased as the substance increased!

A different strategy was used in two experimental tests, one by the Australian Institute of Sport and the other one by Spriet himself: in the first one, some cyclists received a very low dose of caffeine (~ 1.9 mg/kg) after 80-120 minutes from the start of the race, showing a tangible improvement (without incurring appreciable changes in the various physiological parameters mentioned above, indicating the effects on the central nervous system), while in the second group, some triathletes underwent a tough protocol on the cycle ergometer (2 hours plus a click of about 30 minutes), receiving relatively moderate doses of caffeine (1.5-3 mg/kg) at 80 minutes from the start; the group that consumed 200 mg of caffeine had even more important results than the one that had consumed 100 mg. They were much faster than the placebo group, always without alterations in the blood values as seen previously, to once again comfort the opinion that we just expressed in relation to the CNS.

In another recent study by Jenkins (2008), in which some cyclists who received 1, 2 or 3 mg/kg of caffeine before a long warm-up and then went through a 15-minute sprint, the increase was 4 and of 3% with doses of 2-3 mg/kg, so the intermediate dose was the most effective, as opposed to the lower one... obviously there is a minimum threshold!

Irwin et al. (2011) tested a very interesting hypothesis: to find out if a medium-low dose of caffeine (3 mg/kg, 90 minutes before) has the same ergogenic effect in professional cyclists who regularly consume caffeine, after 4 days of constant use or abstinence: the results were almost the same, even with a slight advantage for those who had continued their usual routine, in contrast to the general beliefs and to many other studies (such as that of Ganio et al., 2009).

Van Soeren et al. (1998) wanted to test the hypothesis on the possible drop in the performance of subjects who were addicted to caffeine (as much as 761.3 mg/day), on a *normal* day or after a 2 and 4-day period of abstention: the parameter was the time to exhaustion on the cycle ergometer, pedaling at 80% of the VO_{2max} (previously tested). On the normal day, subjects taking (only) 6 mg/kg achieved 74.8 minutes *vs.* 59.0 of the placebo subjects, after 2 days of abstinence, 81.1 minutes *vs.* 59.5, and after 4 days the result was 81.5 vs. 63.6 minutes... excellent proof of the ergogenic potential of caffeine, also being in opposition to the general opinion, the same as the test that we mentioned above. Desbrow et al. (2012) compared some trained subjects who had received 3-6 mg/kg of caffeine 90 minutes before a cycle ergometer ride (75%, 60 minutes): the improvements were 4.2 and 2.9%, with a difference that is not extremely significant at a statistical level but sufficient to push the authors to advise against a higher dosage.

As Burke (2008) rightly points out, all these studies have been carried out in the laboratory, even if many have tried to reproduce as realistic as possible situations, in any case they stood far from the competitive climate: in ancient Greece, l'ἀγών (agon) was a challenge, a public event. An aseptic cycle ergometer in a sterile laboratory is just a pale imitation even if even field studies involve difficulties, given that the performance control is difficult to implement in climatic and competitive conditions that vary from one day to another (especially in team sports). However, let's not be discouraged, because the excellent review by Ganio et al. (2009) which, in addition to reiterating the concepts that we just expressed above, nonetheless confirms the validity of the results obtained from caffeine in field studies (3-4% on average, with peaks of 17%), with low to medium doses (3-6 mg/kg); however, the variability is higher than in laboratory studies, confirming the environmental and situational volatility of the former.

Durlac et al. (2002) carried out a "practical" trial, as can be seen from the title "A rapid effect of caffeinated beverages on two choice reaction time tasks", and administered 60 mg of caffeine to two groups, finding a marked improvement in the reaction times, which was always the same after different time intervals from the consumption, confirming the rapidity of the action: "the rapidity of the caffeine action on the psychomotor performance was of the order of a few minutes".

We now come to the researches that focus on the anaerobic activity, which are fewer in numbers, especially the ones relaed to medium-low dosages: you can get an overview by reading the review by Astorino et al. (2010), which shows that over 50% of the scrutinized studies (very selectively) show noteworthy results, but at the same time he complains about the discrepancy between the various exercise protocols; however, it is fundamental reading in order to know the state of research on caffeine and high intensity exercises, and it is also full of detailed explanatory tables. Very similar results were obtained by Davis and Green (2009), authors of a very thorough review, interesting and full of ideas... and criticisms, given that, according to them, the evaluation methods published up to that moment left much to be desired, not only regarding the uniformity but also the short duration of the sessions and the small number of exercises. However, the success rate is quite high, but with medium dosages, around 6 mg/kg. According to the two scholars, the ergogenic effect of caffeine at an anaerobic level is maximized in well-trained athletes, while tests on beginners have had much lower results; unfortunately, the reasons have not been spelled out.

Furthermore, Davis and Green also underline that in short efforts, the mechanism by which caffeine obtains good ergogenic results cannot be, as hypothesized by some, (only) the release of fatty acids and the consequent glycogen-saving effect, given the reduced operating times, an aspect that can be shareable and indeed shared by other authors.

Among the first ones to be interested in this aspect (and to detect excellent results) were some French scholars (Collomp et al.) who, in the relatively distant 1992, carried out two studies, both very convincing: in the first one, they compared two groups of swimmers, experts and beginners, with or without the aid of caffeine, however in low dosages (250 mg). The elite swimmers clearly improved their performance in the 100 m after taking caffeine, unlike the beginners, to confirm what we have seen above ("it would seem that some specific training is necessary to benefit from the metabolic adaptations of caffeine during the maximal exercises which require a high anaerobic capacity").

In the second study, the same team, directed this time by Anselme and again in the same year, tested a group of 14 subjects (250 mg of caffeine *vs.* placebo) to verify their maximum anaerobic power and obtained results that were almost as good as the previous ones.

Schneiker et al., In 2006, were interested in another type of physical activity, which involved intermittent sprints, in this case two "runs" of 36 minutes each, with 18 sprints of 4 seconds, interspersed with 2 minutes of active recovery: moderately trained subjects took 6 mg/kg of caffeine and achieved excellent results, 8.5% higher than a subsequent trial (without caffeine) for the first half, and an equally good 7.6% for the second half. In 2006, Beck et al., studied 37 trained subjects who underwent some tests after being given 201 mg (!) of caffeine or a placebo: only the 1MR on the bench press improved significantly, while the cycle ergometer and leg press had very little changes. Green et al. in 2007 tested 17 subjects, after ingesting the usual 6 mg/kg of caffeine or a placebo, "on the maximum lifting weight in the bench press and leg press": this time, only the leg press showed noteworthy increases (almost three more repetitions) without the perception of additional fatigue, and according to the authors, it means that "in high-intensity training, caffeine can mask the sensation of muscle pain with the result of shifting the perception of fatigue over time".

Timmins et al. (2014) tried to test the hypothesis that exercises that engage the largest muscle groups can respond better to the effects of caffeine; however, despite having obtained a good result compared to placebo in general, they concluded that "the influence of the muscle group remains uncertain". Warren et al. (2010) found consistent improvements but also stated that "caffeine appears to improve the relative strength of the maximal voluntary contraction mainly in the knee extensors". Duncan et al. (2014) tested only one movement for the knee extension and found that "muscle power production was significantly higher with caffeine than with the placebo". Instead, in 2008, Woolf et al. they administered 5 mg/kg of caffeine to 24 subjects, who achieved substantial improvements in bench press and in the peak power on the Wingate test (used for anaerobic power via cycle ergometer), but not on the leg press! In reality, judging the increase in the exercise of the upper part, I found it strange that the one for the legs has not improved, given the concomitant success of the cycle ergometer: I found that the complete study (and another study that criticizes it, which confuses the Wingate test with another one that is related to multidirectional sprints [Jones, 2011]) and in fact the procedures are not fully explained. The total times of performance are specified, but not the criteria with which the load percentages were chosen, then we talk about endurance related to anaerobic exercises, a bit of an oxymoron, even if we can imagine that it investigated the anaerobic lactacid mechanism; moreover, the volunteers had ingested, after caffeine, a breakfast that in our latitudes would be defined as lucullian and which certainly influenced the various blood parameters measured in different ways, even if we exclude cortisol, which is notoriously influenced by caffeine!

It is precisely these inaccuracies, verified in more than one study, which could constitute one of the problems to which the two authors of the reviews cited above refer (Astorino/Davis-Green), and which I have actually personally encountered in other fields, such as the one related to anabolic steroids to resistance training (weight training), but in the context of fighting sarcopenia or improving the brain performance; surely, the researchers were trained in their field but were not entirely experts in the field, which ended up in invalidating an otherwise valid research.

As I already stated, interest in the interrelation between caffeine and anaerobic activity has increased only recently and one of the studies on this subject is that of Glaister et al. (2015), which also takes into account the imperfection of many of the protocols used by the aforementioned reviewers: in the search for Wmax (maximal anaerobic power) many other scholars used a fixed load, while the group from Queen Mary's University, London, increased this parameter exponentially until reaching the maximum, from the sixth sprint onwards. The subjects, who were extensively trained, received 5 mg/kg of caffeine and ran numerous series of sprints of (only) 6 seconds (mind you, interspersed with 5 minute pauses), and in the end the Wmax of the treated group was higher when compared to that of the placebo group. Other researches, in addition to using, as mentioned, a fixed *wattage*, also required pauses of less than 60 seconds, which (especially after many sprints of 20 and more seconds) do not allow the maximum anaerobic expression due to the incomplete replenishment of the energy substrates; therefore, caffeine could not have brought a neural advantage anyway (as well studied by a team composed of Bishop and Girard, who in two 2011 studies analyzed the problem of the recovery times for repeated sprints, typical of many sports). Pontifex et al. (2010) carried out a trial that provided recoveries of as little as 20 seconds between sprints of 20 m: the group that had consumed caffeine managed to obtain significantly better results, both in total and in the fastest single sprint ($p < 0.05/p < 0.01$), but this is certainly not the best way to test the effect of a substance on the anaerobic parameters!

At this point, returning to the discourse of imperfect protocols (and researchers...), I was further intrigued, especially noting that another study by Glaister et al. (2012) was mentioned on a website among those that had not reported positive results: I found, with some difficulty, the original study, and I realized that even the team of scholars from across the Channel had used a fixed *wattage* of the recoveires in the previous trial, which was insufficient between the pre-test "warm-up" sprints and, finally, only one probative sprint, when we saw in 2015 that the improvement of the "under caffeine" group was progressive: a point in favor to the one that wrote the reviews on the subject, is the good highlighting of the pros and cons of the research on caffeine.

Continuing in the (brief) examination of some other studies, we come to a work by Trexler (2015), who compared 300 mg of caffeine, both in liquid formula and in capsules (obviously, also the placebos were administered in the same way): the results of some capsules proved better in this case, especially at the leg press (!), but both "forms" of caffeine were superior to the untreated group in five sprints of 10 seconds each; the only problem, so to speak, is that the dose was fixed and expressed based on the weight of the subjects, into a 3-5 mg/kg dose, from moderate to medium... singular, at least.

A different study is the one of Bliss et al. (2008), who compared some young practitioners of the shot put in order to see if a chewing gum with 100 mg of caffeine was able to make them throw farther and make them more responsive to specific tests when compared to the placebo; the test took place in the morning, a notoriously difficult moment for throwers, who in fact often fail to qualify for important competitions when the competition is carried out early: well, the athletes threw the tool farther away (especially in the first three throws) and they were more responsive.

The same Astorino et al. (2010b) performed a test to find out if 2 or 5 mg/kg/day were able to improve the performance of 15 well trained young individuals in leg extension/leg curl: only the medium-high dose had excellent results, with an increase between 5 and 8%. I will also report a study by Chen (2015), comparing men and women, in order to evaluate whether caffeine (6 mg/kg) exerts different effects in young elite athletes of both sexes: maximum voluntary isometric contraction improved on average by 5.9% and the submaximal one had an improvement (50%) of 15.5%, with good statistical significance compared to the placebo group and no difference between males and females, an often overlooked parameter.

I will also report an interesting work by Doherty and Smith (2005), which analyzed 109 studies that consisted in caffeine administration. The focus, this time, is on the Rating of Perceived Exertion (RPE), a score of the perceived exertion: the average perception of the subjective *improvement* was 5.6%, compared to the placebo group (with an increase of 11.2% in the objective performance).

The statistical variance (which identifies the sum of the squares of the rejects for the relative probabilities) indicates that the psychogenic intake of caffeine "weighs" for 29% of the final result: not bad! The same authors, a year earlier, had performed a very high intensity test on some cyclists, obtaining, with 5 mg/kg of caffeine, an important improvement compared to the placebo group.

By updating this chapter, I have noted with pleasure, how the interest in the relationships between caffeine and anaerobic exercise has increased and, in any case, how the attention towards this substance in general remains high, as it can be seen from the very recent review by Del Coso. et al. (2020), which counts over 200 new studies on Pubmed, although only a small part explicitly investigates the improvement in the performance.

In particular, "Caffeine and exercise, what next?" (Pickering and Grgic, 2019), a very interesting all-round study, deserves a reading, as well as "Caffeine supplementation for powerlifting competition: an evidence-based approach", again by Grgic et al. (2019), which discusses the ways in which to optimize the intake of caffeine, both in the form of gel and in the form of chewing gum, as well as the timing in relation to the duration of the races and more.

Venier et al. (2019), in this regard, report excellent results in numerous parameters with caffeine in the gel form (300 mg).

Again Grgic et al. (2019), in "Wake up and smell the coffee: caffeine supplementation and exercise performance – an umbrella review of 21 published meta-analyzes", collected a series of 21 studies concluding that "two cups of coffee, about 3 mg/kg, taken 60 minutes before the physical activity, should exert an ergogenic effect for most sports in almost all subjects".

Here, where a considerable controversy opens: to "The role of genetics in moderating the inter-individual differences in the ergogenicity of caffeine", he replies "Are there non-responders to the ergogenic effects of caffeine ingestion on exercise performance?", in which debates on how many are "immune" to the influences of this substance. To the question "Challenging the myth of non-response to the ergogenic effects of caffeine ingestion on exercise performance", he replies that this number is small.

A review from 2019 (Mielgo-Ayuso et al.) addresses the problem related to the importance of gender related to the results: if in the aerobic field men and women obtain practically the same results, at an anaerobic level it is the males who have the greatest benefits on an equal basis of quantities (incidentally, some of the analyzed studies have at least a "particular" evaluation of anaerobic exercises…). A recommended reading, for obvious reasons, is the "Administration of caffeine in alternate forms" by Wickham et al. (2018), as well as "Is coffee a useful source of caffeine pre-exercise?", by Pickering et al. (2019): in the latter, sent to me by one of the authors (a former level athlete), we analyze the differences between coffee as a drink and other forms of caffeine administration, between the ergogenicity of coffee and the influence of "decaf": the results are not univocal, but the authors also open an interesting range of in-depth proposals.

To conclude, another recent study (Jodra et al., 2020) confirms what is written a few lines higher: caffeine at a dose of 6 mg/kg has an ergogenic effect in both elite athletes and amateurs, but the former get the most consistent improvements.

Guarana

At this point, guarana or *Paullinia cupana* deserves a few lines. It is an evergreen climbing plant, native to South America, in particular to the Amazon region and the State of Bahia (the Guaraní used it to increase their vigor and resistance during long hunting trips, and its use in Brazil is still ubiquitous nowadays): it is often mistakenly assimilated to coffee, due to its caffeine content (up to 6-7% in the seeds), which in reality becomes very variable depending on the final preparations and in any case fails to explain the full spectrum of the produced effects (even though not everyone agrees, see Woods et al., 2012 and Smith and Atroch, 2007). In fact, the second review is particularly interesting, also because it traces a brief history of guarana, as evidenced by the captivating title: "Guarana's journey, from a regional tonic to an aphrodisiac and a global energy drink"; while noting the fundamental contribution of caffeine, the two authors correctly point out that, according to *The Encyclopedia of Psychoactive Plants* (Rätsch, 1998), "the stimulating effects of guarana last longer than coffee because *apparently* the caffeine in g. binds to the tannins".

Moreover, perhaps thanks to the cultural melting pot that springs from the nationalities of the two professors (one American, the other Brazilian, from an Amazonian university), we discover how this plant, once a miraculous tonic for various tribes, so important that the missionaries told that among the natives it was considered as precious as orosia, which became a carbonated soft drink in southern Brazil in 1909, finally transforms itself into a global energy drink, thanks to the exotic halo that has accompanied it for centuries; it is interesting how it is emphasized that most of these drinks contain the deleterious *fructose syrup derived from corn*, due to the bitterness of guarana, thus affecting their healthy characteristics!

However, during recent years this substance has attracted more and more attention of researchers, who are realizing the incisiveness of its other constituents, in addition to caffeine: we are talking about other methylxanthines (theophylline and theobromine), of saponins and also of polyphenols (including tannins, proanthocyanidins, catechins and epicatechins).

Schimpl et al. (2013), for example, underline how the only widely investigated constituent was caffeine, forgetting that guarana contains other potentially effective substances; the socio-economic appeal that the authors envisage when they wish for new research is detailed, given that a renewed interest in this phytoextract could represent a greater source of income for the indigenous Indians, who are among the major growers.

The study by Moustakas et al. (2015), in fact, examines the possibility that some other component besides caffeine is particularly active in guarana (in an animal model); it must be said that the researchers produced a very complicated series of experiments, some of which also included carbohydrates, to simulate the energy drinks. A complete technical examination goes beyond this space, but I will report some conclusions that go in the direction that we just outlined: "We were able to identify the presence of other stimulating substances in a guarana seed extract" and "The impression we got from this work is that g. offers an additional stimulation compared to caffeine". Weckerle et al. (2003) and Espinola et al. (1997) have dealt with this aspect. The latter, after having found notable ergogenic effects only with the lowest dose of guarana (0.3 mg/kg), point out how the other substances contained in guarana certainly have their own peculiar effect that is added and/or amalgamated with that of caffeine. One of the most convincing studies is that of Haskell et al. (2007), who frequently dealt with nootropic substances: in 2007 they compared some young people who took a placebo or different doses of guarana (37.5, 75, 150 and 300 mg). Well, only the first two doses produced significant cognitive effects, while containing only 4.5 and 9 mg of caffeine respectively; therefore, quoting the words of the authors, "It seems difficult that the effects we have seen can be attributed only to the amount of caffeine contained in guarana"! Incidentally, the higher doses only gave better results in mood and alertness. At this point, the Anglo-Saxon researchers suggest that "It is also possible that, at higher doses, the effects of higher levels of caffeine somehow mask the effects of other active substances. Herbal extracts can have a complex dose-effect relationship on the behavior and it is possible that, at lower doses, the components of guarana are able to exert a greater synergy". Very interesting!

A few years earlier, Haskell (with Kennedy as first author, 2003) had also compared guarana and ginseng, reporting excellent results with both substances, especially if taken together; however, given the dosage of 75 mg of guarana, the scholar was able to state that "These results provide the first demonstration of the psychoactive effects of guarana on humans, in its total [...] given that the low caffeine content (9 mg) of this dose of extract is not sufficient to explain these effects". More recently, in 2013, Haskell alone wrote an interesting review that includes many of the plants that contain caffeine and therefore deserves reading, since it acts as a *trait d'union* between the substances we are dealing with, as can be seen from some statements such as "A large number of research is now accumulating, showing that there is an independent effect for many of the phytochemicals that coexist with caffeine" and "This review highlights the need to implement more research aimed at understanding the effects of these compounds and, even more importantly, *the synergistic relationship they may have with caffeine*". Again in 2015, Veasey et al. administered a vitamin and a guarana complex to a group of volunteers: after a 30-minute run, the subjects reported a significant reduction in the subjective effort during the exercise, compared to the placebo group. They also reported a greater mnemonic accuracy and also an improved alertness, reflected in some computerized tests. A study by Campos et al. (2005), on the other hand, compared caffeine and guarana in a mouse model: the animals were very "stimulated" by both substances (given the dosages served, this is no wonder), but what catches our eye is how the researchers hypothesized different mechanisms of action compared to caffeine alone, writing that their conclusions "suggest that some mechanisms, other than the adenosinergic ones, must be present in the activity of guarana".

For sporting purposes, it turns out that the research by Miura et al. is particularly interesting (1998), since another effect would be added to the nootropic effects of guarana, that relating to an increase in the availability of glucose for the muscle activity, as reported by the Japanese team: "These results indicate that the suppression of hypoglycemia may derive from a better use of glycogen".

Two substantial reviews (both of 2018, by Marques et al. and Santana et al.) collect the state of the art on the subject, also insisting on the best extraction methods to guarantee a good product; moreover, in 2018, a research paper by Salomão-Oliveira et al. proved guarana to be useful because it also deals with some interactions with numerous drugs, which are quite numerous.

In 2019, a review by Konstantino and Heun, while confirming the potential of this substance, questions its synergy with caffeine, in contrast to other previous researches.

For space reasons, I will only mention another important potential of guarana: the induction of a moderate thermogenesis and the oxidation of fats: an agile study by Hursel et al. (2011) analyzes its scope and shows how the combination of catechins/caffeine is much more effective than caffeine alone (see also Lima et al., 2005), while Bérubé-Parent et al. (2005), while recognizing its thermogenic value, attribute it to the caffeine component; I will also mention its antioxidant and antiplatelet properties, two faculties that significantly broaden its range of action (Bydlowski et al., Basile et al. 2005-2012).

From the above, it is clear that the dosages must take into account the caffeine titration of the used product, considering the probable concomitant use of coffee, at least in our latitudes: however, they can vary from 500 mg to 3 g, depending (also) on the titration of caffeine.

Rhodiola rosea

A few years ago, a close friend of mine (one of the best bodybuilders of the 1980s and now an established photographer and filmmaker in the United States) started producing a line of sports supplements in California, where he has been residing for some time, and sent me a sample of a product containing (also) *Rhodiola rosea*: I found immediate benefits and, scrolling through the components, I realized that the effect had to depend on that ingredient that I had never tried, despite having heard of it, or rather from its combination with tyrosine, which we will discuss shortly, since the synergy of these two substances is truly remarkable. In fact, I had experienced a particular recharge: not that excessive – determined by some thermogenics that are now banned from sale, but a peculiar mental acuity, a focus that allowed me to train better, with a greater determination and without nervousness or tremors of any kind.

At this point I must emphasize that the other substances that we will discuss have not been studied as much as the previous two for sporting purposes: however, what interests us, is the nootropic effect that we can use to concentrate better during a mental task, but also to focus on a competition tactic, to complete a hard training or to keep a strong attention until the end of the competition. So let's see what, first of all, this plant product, also called the golden root/arctic root is: it is a perennial herbaceous plant native to the cold and mountainous areas of Siberia, Mongolia and Tibet, but also present in the highest mountains of Northern Europe and on the Alps. It can reach 70 cm in height and has yellow flowers with a typical rose scent; contains a myriad of different compounds that can be separated into different groups: flavonoids, phenylpropanoids, phenolic acids, triterpenes and monoterpenes; the most interesting constituents are salidroside and rosavins (rosavin, rosin, rodiosin). Its use is certainly not recent, if it is true that the Greek physician Dioscorides, already in 77 AD, spoke of it in the *De materia* (reputed to be the most important treatise on pharmaceutical botany of antiquity), as well as many centuries after him, it was mentioned by the famous Linnaeus (who changed its name to *rosea*, precisely because of the fragrance it gave off). In the following centuries *Rhodiola* continued to be used, but further east, especially in Siberia (where its name, *zoloty koren*, means "golden root"), and has been handed down from generation to generation as the ethno-botany tradition of those lands which later became the USSR; in fact, many of the studies carried out recently are in Slavic or Scandinavian languages (Strandberg, 1997; Aly, 1997) and without abstracts in English, which slowed down their diffusion in the West, especially until the fall of the Iron Curtain.

Rhodiola, for example, is considered an adaptogen (a natural agent capable of increasing the body's resistance and ability to adapt to internal and external stress factors). It was a Russian, Lazarev, who "invented" this term while carrying out research to find substances to improve the energy and the concentration of the soldiers in order to replace amphetamines and cocaine, which determined, according to the scholar, strong short-term effects but heavy relapses in terms of depression and low energy in the long term (!). The Soviet doctor was mainly interested in chemicals, while his student, Brekhman (who also wrote in English), in the 1960s, studied in depth four plants that were traditionally used in Asian medicine, including *Rhodiola*. So let's see how this substance is not "the latest arrival" not only in popular use, but also on a scientific level! Its mechanisms of action have not been fully clarified: five reviews by Panossian et al. (1999, 2007-2009, 2010-2014) try to shed light on some of these processes: "The effects of a multiple administration of adaptogens are associated with the hypothalamus-pituitary-adrenal axis" or "In the case of single dose, the effects are instead linked to another part of the stress-related system, the sympathetic-medullary system of the adrenal gland". They are extremely technical analyzes and their in-depth analysis would steal precious space for our discussion; however, to those who are particularly interested, we recommend reading it.

Fortunately, nowadays, studies have become more numerous, even if, as we will see, those carried out in the former Soviet Union are still predominant and not always easily accessible; they focus on the various indications for which this phytoextract is recommended, but we will limit ourselves to the aspects relating to the increase in the physical and mental performance, as they are linked to each other.

Research relating to *Rhodiola* has expanded, as mentioned, to many fields (too many for this site) and, furthermore, as Ishaque et al. (2012) in a long review, found that a large part use uncertain protocols or have methodological limitations; however, the researchers at Alberta University have in any case narrowed their interest to a few studies, illustrating them in the best possible way and highlighting lights and shadows: a recommended reading.

As mentioned above, many of the works come from the former Soviet Union and from the present-day Russia and, except for those of the forerunners of Lazarev's group, a large part comes from Tomsk State University, located in the town wtih the same name which is close, not coincidentally, to Siberia and Mongolia; some are contained in a review published by this university (Saratikov): in the first study, 52 men took 150 mg of *Rhodiola*, another phytoextract or a solution containing a psychotropic chemical substance similar to *Ritalin* or, again, a placebo, and after 30 minutes they performed a test on the cycle ergometer to establish a work base: after 5 minutes of rest, they started pedaling again to establish the maximum duration of work at a given intensity, fixed on the basis of the test that was just performed. All of them had better results than the control group, but the subjects who had taken *Rhodiola* clearly outperformed the others (+9% compared to the placebo) and also had a subsequent better recovery, measured by blood pressure and speed of the heartbeats recovery to the baseline. Furthermore, as already reported by the aforementioned Lazarev, the subjects who had taken the other drug complained of insomnia and irritability, unlike those who had tested *Rhodiola*: adaptogens differ precisely in this from other stimulants, as the increase in working capacity due to the stimulation of the central nervous system does not decay as massively as with synthetic products, which deplete the neurotransmitters, bringing them to lower values than normal.

Another work contained in this review involved 42 elite skiers engaged in a biathlon competition (20 km of Nordic skiing and target practice): compared to the placebo group, the subjects receiving *Rhodiola* demonstrated a higher overall efficiency, with a better coordination, less tremor of the arms and a more precise aim; also in this case, the return to the normal values of the vital signs was faster in the treated group. A laboratory study by Abidov turns out to be very interesting because, by comparing two different types of Rhodiola, it emphasizes the correct choice of the products: he compared three groups of rats were compared, to which he administered *Rhodiola rosea*, *Rhodiola crenulata* (50 mg/kg) or a placebo; the tank resistance and the ATP content in the mitochondria of the muscle cells were evaluated. Treatment with *R. rosea* extended the duration of the swim to exhaustion by up to 24.6% more than the other groups, and also activated the synthesis or resynthesis of ATP in the mitochondria, stimulating the recharge of the energy processes after the exercise.

In this regard, it is better to choose the supplements that contain *Rhodiola rosea* since, without entering the taxonomy (which is still quite controversial), only its extracts have been the subject of numerous tests (as can be seen from some tables that would be too long to be published here); however, 51% of the animal studies and 94% of those on humans have had *R. rosea* as their object. Furthermore, the content of the different species differs significantly and has not even received an adequate toxicological screening, at least in the majority of the cases (although, as we will see a little further on, the situation is changing and the use of other *Rhodiola* species is gaining momentum). Furthermore, the ratio between rosavins and salhidroses must be 3:1, as occurs in nature: while salidroside is present in all species of *Rhodiola*, only *R. rosea* contains rosavins; for the sake of truth, some studies overturn the importance of the two components, but the question is somewhat controversial, too much for these pages!

In 2007, Perfumi and Mattioli used variable quantities (10, 15 and 20 mg/kg), confirming that *R. rosea* "significantly induced antidepressant, adaptogenic, anxiolytic and stimulating effects in mice (not in a dose-dependent manner)"; in the same year, the same authors (but with reverse roles) tested again the adaptogenic potential of *Rhodiola*, always with good results.

Another interesting work is that of Kucinskaite et al. (2004), unfortunately in Lithuanian: luckily, at least the abstract is in English and in its few lines we can read that "these active components affect the central nervous system by increasing the concentration, as well as the physical and mental power"; the Baltic authors, who have not simply tested *Rhodiola*, but have thoroughly analyzed it, add tyrosol among the highly active components. The same team then wrote again on the subject, finally in English, unfortunately dealing more with the technical aspects of the extraction. Lee (2009), on the other hand, carried out an accurate test, again on mice, this time also collecting very useful biophysical parameters, since mice models cannot express their sensations! The poor animals were tested in a 90-minute session of continuous swimming and then on swimming to exhaustion with an overload of 5%. The measurements concerned numerous biomarkers of fatigue, the analysis of which showed an increase in the hepatic glycogen and in the enzymes related to the lipid metabolism. There was also an improvement of a whole typology of the body's defense mechanisms, including transaminases, as well as a marked dose-dependent increase in the time under exertion.

These results had already been cited by Tomsk State University scholars, such as Salnik, Adamchuk, Danbueva and Revina, almost 50 years ago: in 1970, the first one investigated the possibilities of *Rhodiola* to increase ATP/CP in the muscles and in the brains of rats, and obtained results that were similar to those seen above (dating back to 2004), including the increase in performance; the second (1969) reported similar conclusions regarding the energy mechanisms, also adding notes on the optimization of the protein and amino acid synthesis, as well as on the mitochondrial functionality; the third one, on the other hand, successfully investigated the improvements in the lipid metabolism (1968) and the fourth (1969) obtained an optimization of the brain energy parameters during an intense physical effort. We understand why we must regret that at the time Soviet magazines were not exactly easy to obtain!

Huang (2009), on the other hand, tested once again the effect of *Rhodiola* on rats, analyzing the results on the oxidative stress and noting that the effect on reactive oxygen metabolites, responsible for oxidation, was very high: the increase in performance was therefore combined with an effective antioxidant effect.

In 2008 Ryu et al. have implemented an extensive series of swimming experiments, always on mice models, administering *Rhodiola* with different temporal modalities and with different types of exercises, reporting that "it has an anti-fatigue effect and reduces the nervous stress induced by the physical effort, also thanks to the positive influence on the lactate metabolism": a different mechanism of action from those usually mentioned. Recently (2015) Kang et al. reported a valid action of *Rhodiola* in increasing the time under exertion and also the improvement of some blood parameters. Returning to the human studies, in 2004 de Bock et al. carried out a comparison of young volunteers on different parameters, subjecting them to various physical tests after taking an acute dose of 200 mg of *Rhodiola*, the same dosage for 4 weeks or a placebo: subjects who had taken the phytoextract had a fair progress in resistance compared to the control group, together with the improvement of some physiological values, with both methods of administration. Another interesting study is that of Noreen et al. (2013), in which slight progress was found in a performance on the bicycle ergometer, with a lower heart rate, together with a much higher score on a test that measured the perceived exertion, mood and cognitive functions. It was so significant that the authors suggested that the better mood was able to make you feel less fatigued, allowing not only an aerobic improvement but also a better energy condition at the end of the test. Spasov (2000), on the other hand, measured the physical and the mental performance of some students through objective and subjective observations: the most notable improvements were found in the physical fitness, mental fatigue and neuromotor tests, but their subjective evaluation was also improved significantly in the *verum* group.

Shevtsov (2003), on the other hand, compared 161 cadets, with a variant: apart from the placebo and the "physiological" group, there were two other categories of subjects, treated with different quantities of *Rhodiola* (strong, of a very high titration of salidroside), 370 mg or 555 mg (1.5 times higher than the former).

The results showed a pronounced anti-fatigue effect, evaluated according to the AFI (Anti Fatigue Index) for the subjects that were given *Rhodiola* compared to the others (significance even $p < 0.001$): the author suggests that the minimum dosage may be preferable, as reported by other scholars who, in fact, have observed paradoxical effects with too high dosages, an aspect that deserves more space.

Regarding *R. crenulata*, I partially contradict myself by reporting a trial by Den et al. (published after the first edition, at the end of 2017), as the product used is extracted from a large Chinese company that seems to guarantee a more constant titration and the results, in addition to being excellent, show a synergy between *Rhodiola* and the aerobic exercise, and not only, as can be seen from the title: "Exercise combined with *Rhodiola sacra* supplementation improves exercise capacity and ameliorates exhaustive exercise-induced muscle damage through enhancement of mitochondrial quality control".

In 2018 Anghelescu et al. wrote a review that positively evaluates the effects of *Rhodiola* and in the same year Jòwko et al. carried out various tests on male students, obtaining good results in terms of mental alertness (and also at the antioxidant level), but only modest results in terms of physical endurance, although reading the research thoroughly, it was not as insignificant as this group of Polish scholars stated.

A couple of other works from 2017 reaffirm the proven efficacy of *R. rosea* in fatigued subjects, underlining its adaptogenic value.

In a very recent study (Ballmann et al., 2019) a dosage of 1500 mg/day of *R. rosea* plus 500 mg before a Wingate test allowed to obtain excellent results (with more than discrete statistical significance) in college students. Precisely because it is an adaptogenic substance, particularly stressed subjects *may* have to take high dosages, as in some cases described above, but the standard dosage ranges from 100 to 400 mg/day, even in several stages, the last of which it is advisable to take place towards lunch time, so as not to run the risk of disturbing their sleep.

Tyrosine

Tyrosine is a precursor amino acid of dopamine, adrenaline and noradrenaline that is used to improve mental alertness: Salter, in 1989, experimented with some young cadets, being aware of the potential of tyrosine in times of stress, and demonstrated how his use reduced the norepinephrine deficiencies (decreased due to physical-mental tension), while improving the performance, and he recommended it for military use. Moreover, even Owasoyo et al., in 1992, wrote an agile review on the potential of this semi-essential amino acid in relation to particularly long and stressful military operations, suggesting its use in situations of prolonged stress, in this case in battle or during particularly hard military trainings. This is exactly what Deijen did, who in 1999 gave a group of soldiers 2 g of tyrosine contained in a protein drink five times a day and compared them to another group that took the same number of drinks (isocaloric but only with carbohydrates): the "protein" group was superior in various attention tests, while the blood pressure values were decreasing. Reading these results, two things stand out: the first, that the researchers magnified the "tonic" effect of tyrosine by inserting it in a protein drink vs. one of carbohydrates only, since we have seen the different influences that these two macronutrients have on the central nervous system. The second is the fact that this amino acid is less "exciting" when compared to common substances that used to energize, also considering the decrease in the blood pressure (at least in this trial, despite the fact that it raises the dopamine levels). Deijen himself had obtained similar results in 1994 in another study. In fact, supplementation with tyrosine was initially studied in conditions of preventive stress, which depletes the reserves of dopamine and noradrenaline: there are numerous researches that foresee its intake after the exposure to temperatures below normal (with excellent results) but we will not report them here. A study by Thomas (1999), on the other hand, administered tyrosine in high doses (150 mg/kg) in "normal" conditions: the subjects of the *verum* group demonstrated a higher alertness and concentration than the placebo: stress, in this case, was not preceding, but the effect was still good. A review by Jongkees et al. (2015) extensively illustrates the various uses for which this amino acid has been tested, many of which are also related to psychiatric pathologies (with no consistency of results), and a passage relating to its role as depletion reverser is very interesting: when a significant brain activity reduces dopamine and norepinephrine, with a consequent performance decay, the administration of tyrosine can reverse the process. In our case, it could be an athlete stressed by a long preparation for a competition, subjected to a low-calorie diet in the middle of a particularly demanding and heavy leg workout, or a "differently young" subject who continues to train at an advanced age, given that the dopamine metabolism loses its bumps with the passage of time, which may therefore need a greater supplementation of tyrosine (Carfagna et al., 1985).

Furthermore, researchers belonging to three different Dutch universities insist on what is expressed in another review ("People are different: tyrosine's modulating effect on cognitive control in healthy humans may depend on individual differences related to dopamine function", 2014), in which, in addition to recognizing the potential of tyrosine as "a product capable of improving the concentration", they list a long series of "measurements, tests and factors that can have an effect on its supplementation, since each individual will have its own particular response" and underline how the influence of genetics, with its various polymorphisms, should not be underestimated. Here we return to the initial discussion of the subjectivity of the results, to remember that there is not a single recipe for everyone, but that each step must be customized. A review by Baker et al. (2014) examined what was alrady published on tyrosine, stressing once again that most of the research started with physical and mental stressful states (exposure to cold and very high temperatures, sleep deprivation, high altitude, relationship stress) and how many studies on animals are finally overlapping with those on humans; after having listed a series of works that have been largely successful, he concludes by hoping for a greater number of investigations in relation to the (possible) effects on the sporting activity, as already demonstrated by Tumilty et al. in 2011, in a trial in which some cyclists obtained excellent results (with significance of $p < 0.01$) in a test carried out at 30° C and with a 60% humidity.

Unfortunately, studies on sportspeople continue to be scarce, but what is stated by me in another chapter, and also by other authors in this book, regarding the various types of nutrients and neurotransmitters, it is certainly an excellent reason to experiment with macro- and micronutrients, also for the purpose of the physical performance.

Neri et al. (1995), on the other hand, subjected a group of people who did night work to a battery of tests of performance tasks and moods: 150 mg of tyrosine significantly reduced (up to 3 hours) the drop in the performance which, instead, occurred in the control group. Dr. Paul has compiled an agile flyer (not quoted) in which she briefly lists the potential of tyrosine, also underlining its excellent synergy with *Rho-*

diola, as I had previously written: an interesting idea for a galenic preparation, since I believe that their combination can maximize the results.

We now come to two studies by Colzato et al. (2013, 2015) (often a co-author of the Dutch researchers): in the first one, subjects who had taken 2 g of tyrosine responded markedly better ($p < 0.05$) to the more complex part of an *n*-back test (after a sequence of stimuli, we need to indicate whether the current stimulus is the same as that displayed *n* times before) without the results to a mood questionnaire, and heart rate and systolic and diastolic pressure measurements being dissimilar from the baseline, indicating, as the authors suggest, that a connection of the results with the physiological or mood changes can be excluded. The researchers then conclude that the maxim of the philosopher Feuerbach "Der Mensch ist, was er ißt" (man is what he eats) has a further meaning: food really influences our mind, in this case, by acting as a cognitive facilitator, without having the side effects of popular drugs such as *Ritalin*, which in some cases could eventually be replaced by tyrosine. The same working group led by Colzato (2014) proposed a work with the explanatory title, "Food for creativity: tyrosine promotes deep thinking", in which once again the results obtained underline how the effects of tyrosine are more evident in the resolution of complex tasks.

In 2015 Haze et al. confirmed the efficacy of tyrosine in acute doses and also highlighted how behavioral changes take place after a longer period, hoping for studies on long-term effects; just what Kuhn et al. did, in 2017, which examined the use of tyrosine over a long period of time, analyzing the diet of nearly 2000 subjects and relating it to performance in various cognitive tests; the conclusions are decidedly positive: "to a much higher extent than the previous studies".

A recent study by Frings et al. (2019) reported modest benefits on attention, but the dosage was 2 g: the average one for athletes is around 500-2000 mg, but many of the papers have used much higher quantities, in a range that is around about 100-150 mg/kg: probably an intermediate dose, taken gradually, could be the most profitable way.

DMAE

DMAE (dimethylaminoethanol), known in Europe as deanol, is an element naturally present in low concentrations in the brain and also in salmon, sardines and other similar fish. DMAE is a precursor of acetylcholine, at least according to most studies (Pfeiffer et al., Haubric et al., 1975-78; Millington et al., 1978, London et al., 1978, Jope et al., 1979), while others go in the opposite direction (Zahniser et al.); however, this substance seems to be involved in the metabolism of choline, which is important, both for the brain functions and for the muscle contractions, so it is obvious that its optimization may be of interest to us.

A review compiled by Dean et al. (1993) lists its potential, underlining how DMAE produces a mild stimulating effect that occurs over a period of several weeks, an aspect also underlined by other authors, who highlight the difference compared to other nootropics, with a faster effect. A further benefit for elderly people (whom, however, have decreased values of acetylcholine with the passing of the years) is its effect – so to speak – rejuvenating at the dermal level (since it slows down the deterioration of the cell membranes and decreases the excess of arachidonic acid, which can cause wrinkles and skin aging) and its powerful antioxidant action, as recently highlighted by Malanga et al. (2012).

In fact, DMAE had some success in the 1960s and 1970s, when it was marketed under the name of *Deanol*: at some point the American FDA changed its pharmacological status and required more studies to continue its sale, and the manufacturing company withdrew it from the market because the cost/benefit ratio had become unsustainable.

Acetylcholine and its precursor choline have difficulty in passing the blood brain barrier, while DMAE, thanks to a similar but not the same chemical structure, succeeds better and therefore can express a greater nootropic action, as evidenced by Ceder et al. (1981). Some studies have checked the effectiveness of DMAE through the use of the electroencephalogram, verifying tangible results for the substance in question but not for choline (Goldstein et al., 1960). Also Dimpfel et al. (2003) used the electroencephalogram to verify the effect of DMAE, this time coupled with some tests on the mood: the subjects who had taken the substance detected brain wave values such as to prove a better state of alertness and the volunteers "were manifestly more active and felt better"; moreover, the results of the questionnaires were also clearly superior, "in full agreement with the laboratory tests". A very interesting piece of work is that of Coleman et al. (1976), who managed to highlight the potential of DMAE on a sample of hyperkinetic young people, on whom, at a dose of 500 mg/day, it exerted a balancing effect, showing how the substance truly optimizes brain levels of neurotransmitters at 360 degrees, whether starting from a "normal" state or from a hyperactive one. Also a French study (Caille, 1986) showed (with a rather high dosage, 1200 mg) that patients who had taken DMAE showed "a significant and progressive synchronization of the two hemispheres [...] which was correlated with better neuromotor control and better results in behavioral tasks " on the electroencephalogram. An investigation by Kapoor et al., in 2009, tested the effectiveness of DMAE with regard to memory, learning and brain function, as did Oettinger (1977), but this time in pediatric subjects: there was found an increase in attention and in concentration without any kind of overexcitement or nervousness; Kugel et al. (1963), on the other hand, unlike many scholars, did not report relevant results in minors to whom he had administered 100 mg of the substance in question; moreover, in a couple of reviews it can be read that they would have achieved significant improvements in depression and chronic fatigue states… probably the habit of writing "*ad usum Delphini*" has not been lost. The analysis of Lewis and Young (1975) is also relevant in minors, who used 500 mg of DMAE or 40 mg of the "usual" *Ritalin*: both substances, albeit with different nuances, have improved the reaction times and the results from a series of psychometric tests of 79 patients. Danysz et al. (1967) reaffirm the cholinergic properties of the substance in question and recommend it for the "mental and physical efficiency in man"; in 1974, Re compiled a review listing the positive effects of DMAE on the concentration, finding better results than *Ritalin* on 124 students. Geller (1960) also reported positive results on the intellectual functioning and alertness of 75 young people, with a dosage of only 100 mg/day, as did Pfeiffer (1957), who achieved cognitive improvements in two thirds of boys and three quarters of girls whom he had examined (sample of over 100 subjects).

Pfeiffer himself, in 1959, found that DMAE was able to relieve chronic fatigue through its effects "on physical energy and motivation" in 100 patients, without creating addiction, unlike some chemical preparations. Pieralisi et al. (1991) added ginseng to DMAE and administered the compound to some physical education teachers: both the final result on the treadmill (carried out with progressive increases in resistance) and various biological parameters were better in the treated group, especially in the less trained subjects. Finally, Ray Shaelian, a physician-nutritionist (author of books covering the entire spectrum of supplements, which have sold over a million copies), strongly recommends DMAE. In fact, he has included it in his mixes of nootropic substances, also reporting a personal experience, shared by other experts: over 350 mg the substance can cause muscle tension in the neck and shoulders. DMAE dosages range from 100 to 600 mg, although some studies have used higher amounts; however, also considering what is written a few lines above, it is still advisable to start from the minimum quantities and, probably, stop at 200 mg: Pfeiffer himself, a true pioneer of DMAE, had noted in an old study (1963, not cited.) how the individual response, also in this case, was quite varied.

It should also be remembered that the substance can interact with different categories of drugs, so it is recommended not to take it on your own initiative.

Vinpocetine

Vinpocetine is obtained from the lesser periwinkle (*Vinca minor*), a rather widespread herbaceous perennial vine, typical of the undergrowth, where it forms extensive evergreen carpets, but also common along the roadsides. In fact, vinpocetine is a semi-synthetic derivative of an alkaloid derived from periwinkle, vincamine, widely used in Eastern Europe for the prevention of epilepsy, cognitive decline and for the recovery from strokes. The product, while being effective, showed relative liver toxicity that made vinpocetine preferable, a more tolerable substitute, synthesized in 1975 in Hungary, where it has been sold as a "drug" for over 40 years (*Cavinton*). A number of studies support its use for the diseases listed above, which interest us for the benefits deriving from the increased cerebral blood flow: mental focus and efficiency. Subhan and Hindmarch (1985), for example, administered 10, 20, 40 mg of vinpocetine or a placebo for two days to a group of subjects who, on the third day, completed a battery of psychological tests: significant results were obtained with the higher dosage, especially regarding the memory and the mental alertness. In fact, a research by Valikovics (2007) shows how this substance can improve the cerebrovascular flow on "post-stroke" patients or patients who are suffering from senile dementia, who had taken it for 12 weeks: the "mechanical" measurements with transcranial Doppler (TCD) were clearly superior for the verum group, as were the results of the cognitive tests that were administered in parallel; incidentally, also an instrumental investigation by Bönöczk et al. (2002) had already demonstrated the excellent ability of vinpocetine to increase the cerebral blood circulation, thanks to the use of TCD and Near Infrared Spectroscopy (NIRS), able to highlight what other more common methods of investigation had failed to show. A few years later, Valikovics et al. (2012) examined some patients with chronic cerebral hypoperfusion, this time for 18 months: the increased blood flow had led to a massive improvement in the various psychometric tests assigned to the subjects. The foregoing had already been examined by a review by Horváth, who in 2001 had dealt with the argument relating to how the positive effects of vinpocetine extended to patients who presented brain problems "regardless of the type of disease that had caused the hypoperfusion". Two other reviews, edited by Patyar (2011) and Szapáry (2012), substantially confirm the potential of vinpocetine, underlining that it is not easy to trace all the modes of action of this substance, one of which, certainly, is the inhibitor of type 1 phosphodiesterase, resulting in the relaxation of the cerebral vessels and in a better blood flow, mainly in the brain. Another interesting study is that of Balestrieri et al. (1987), in which two groups of 42 subjects took a placebo or 10 mg of vinpocetine, three times a day for 30 days and then 5 mg, three times a day for 60 days: the results, established through a large battery of cognitive tests, were clearly superior in those who had taken the product. The list is still long, but it should be added that vinpocetine also has an excellent antioxidant and anti-inflammatory effect; in addition, the facilitation of blood flow allows for a greater supply of oxygen and nutrients that also improve the synthesis of ATP in the brain, which certainly promotes mental alertness; worthy of interest is its positive influence on the values of the brain neurotransmitters.

In 2017 Zhang et al. wrote "An update on vinpocetine: new discoveries and clinical implications" and, in addition to re-listing the potential of the substance at a cognitive and mnemonic level, they add "anti-inflammation, antagonizing injury-induced vascular remodeling and high-fat-diet-induced atherosclerosis, as well as attenuating pathological cardiac remodeling"; in 2019, Lourengo-Gonzales et al. inserted an analgesic effect, precisely in relation to the anti-inflammatory effect mentioned above.

A study by Ali et al. (2019), "Physical and mental activities enhance the neuroprotective effect of vinpocetine and coenzyme Q10", as the title suggests, studied its effects together with CoQ10, while another study by Svab et al. (end of 2019) investigated the mechanisms through which the substance operates, identifying several mechanisms at the mitochondrial level. Average dosages start from 5 mg and gradually reach 30 mg; in this regard Ding et al. (2017) and Golob (2016) tackle some new methods of administration that manage to improve the absorption of the substance through the use of polymeric micelles, associated with borneol and a form of co-crystallization, continuing a fairly abundant theory of studies on the subject, indicating both the not-excellent bioavailability of vinpocetine and the interest in it.

Ginkgo biloba

We also briefly mention *Ginkgo biloba*, also frequently used in the treatment of erectile deficits, which has a field of use that is similar to that of vinpocetine, thanks to the fact that it also promotes the cerebral blood circulation. It is the oldest seed plant in the world: in fact, it is the only survivor of the *Ginkgoaceae* family, which was already present on Earth over 250 million years ago. It is so old, that Darwin considered it a living fossil; extinct in the Old Continent and in America, it was found by a German botanist only in the 18th century in Japan, although it was later discovered that the monks had cultivated it for millennia in China; it is very resistant (it lives up to 1000 years) and some specimens have even survived the radiation of Hiroshima! For reasons of space and the similarity of the effects with vinpocetine lead us to cite only a few studies in this regard. To frame the topic quickly but comprehensively, some reviews may be useful, such as those of DeFeudis (2000) and Diamonds (2000-2013), which show how this plant is used for the improvement of cognitive memory abilities, for senile dementia and other pathologies, while its mechanisms of action include a marked increase in the cerebral blood flow and a strong antioxidant, anti-inflammatory and antiplatelet effect. The review by Clostre (1999) is also very stimulating, starting from the first lines: "At the dawn of the third millennium (the sixth for *Ginkgo biloba*), we envision the state of the art with respect to this substance"! The author begins by underlining the wide spectrum of pharmacological activities that allows *Ginkgo* to be used for the numerous haemodynamic, haemorheological and metabolic pathologies that can occur in cerebral, retinal, cochleo-vestibular, cardiac or peripheral ischemias, and continues by listing the effects at the neural, molecular and cellular level; the French researcher does not fail to point out the high antioxidant and antiplatelet power of this phytoextract, as well as its ability to improve the cerebral ATP value and the state of the endothelium; he continues by stating that, on the basis of the works passed under review, *Ginkgo* can allow an improvement in the signs and symptoms of cognitive functions, especially attention, alertness, arousal state, memory and mental fluidity. The review by Yang et al. (2016) who, after evaluating all the published research on the subject, narrowed their screening to 21 studies that had examined 2068 patients: in general, the conclusions regarding memory and alertness are positive, but the authors, due to the uneven methodological quality and the sometimes reduced number of patients, rightly recommend a greater number of investigations in order to be able to express a more definitive opinion. Kaschel (2009) also calls for new observations (correctly designed), and in any case reports that "there is consistent evidence that its chronic administration improves the selective attention, some behavioral processes and the long-term memory for verbal and non-verbal materials". Moving on to clinical studies, we again find Subhan and Hindmarch (1985), who tested some volunteers with the same protocol as the aforementioned research for vinpocetine, this time with 120, 240, 600 mg of *Ginkgo biloba* or a placebo: also in this case, there was a significant improvement only for short-term memory and reasoning, and always with the highest dosage. Another interesting work is that of Kennedy et al. (2000), in which 20 volunteers were subjected to a computerized battery of specific tests for the evaluation of drugs that can improve the cognitive faculties, Cognitive Drug Research (CDR). After receiving a single dose of *Ginkgo* (120 mg, 240 mg and 360 mg), to test its effectiveness after an "acute" administration compared to the placebo group, the subjects who had taken 240 mg and 360 mg obtained excellent results (for over 6 hours after ingestion), especially in the speed of attention. Other factors were also improved, so much so as to push the authors to declare: "We can conclude that the acute administration of *Ginkgo biloba* is capable of producing a consistent and lasting improvement in the attention capacity". The same group directed by Kennedy, a few years later, carried out another study by coupling *Ginkgo* this time with also ginseng, and the synergy between the substances improved the already good results obtained by the two substances taken alone. Elsabagh et al. (2005) subjected two groups of young volunteers to psychometric tests: 120 mg of *Ginkgo* allowed a clear improvement in the memory and in the attentional capacity, while the same dosage for 6 weeks did not bring detectable benefits, demonstrating that, probably, a cyclization of the substance is indicated. At the end of the paragraph relating to this ancient plant, also celebrated by Goethe, it should be noted that the extract of *Ginkgo biloba* is made up of different constituents, and a series of researches (one by Ahlemeyer, 2003, and three by Chandrasekaran et al., 2001, 2002, 2003) has shown how the various components of this plant exert different actions: in this case, even the non-flavonic part of the substance demonstrates a strong neuroprotective action, as it was possible to observe thanks to a series of experiments conducted by these researchers.

A review by Suliman et al. (2016) delves into the molecular mechanisms of the functioning of *Ginkgo biloba* and also Gorby et al. (2010) confirm its potential: "The strongest evidence suggests specific effects of *Ginkgo biloba* on certain aspects of mood and on attention"; similar comments can be found in a more recent review (O'Connor et al., 2019). The average dosages used in the studies range from 80 to 720 mg/day, while in sports practice, it is used in dosages from 200 to 600 mg: the usual *caveat* is applied starting from the bottom, to reach around 300 mg.

There are obviously other nootropic substances, one of all the *Panax ginseng*, but it is not possible to treat all of them here.

I would like to conclude by recalling how supplements must remain such: you cannot make up for any errors made in terms of macronutrients with one or two phytoextracts, but these substances, if combined with a correct diet, can make the difference!

CHAPTER 36

Supplementation for the immune system

The immune system is a complex network for regulating the homeostasis of our organism, mainly in charge of defending us from the aggression of internal or external elements that can alter the state of functionality of our organism. The immune system is the one that destroys cancer cells as soon as they form and that attacks bacteria and viruses when they enter our body.

Competitive athletes are generally more exposed to the risk of infections, as they are subjected to physiological, psychological and environmental stresses that cause immunosuppression, and also to pathogenic microorganisms due, for example, to open mouth breathing, skin abrasions and using the changing rooms.

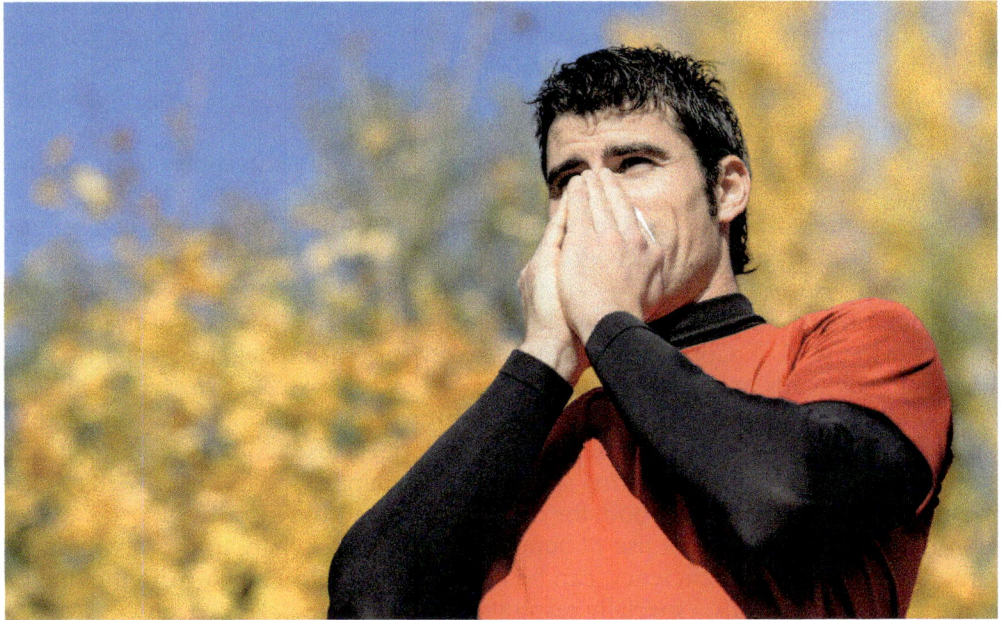

Figure 36.1

Physical activity itself has a modulating effect on the immune system and, while moderate activity has an empowering effect, intense and prolonged activity, as in endurance sports, causes numerous changes in the immune system and body parts, increasing the risk of URTIs (Upper Respiratory Tract Infections). Intense physical activities cause physiological stress and transient but significant changes in the immune system; the main parameters involved are cortisol, adrenaline and pro- or anti-inflammatory cytokines.

The stress hormones (adrenaline and cortisol) produced during intense exercises probably contribute by decreasing and lowering the functional capacity of circulating leukocytes, as well as by decreasing **glutamine** levels (an essential amino acid for leukocytes); in addition, intense physical training causes the production of inflammatory cytokines that can be superimposed to infection and trauma. Finally, during intense physical exercise there is an increase in the production of ROS (Reactive Oxygen Species) and we know that some functions of the immune cells can be compromised by excess free radicals. In light of the multiple effects of intense and prolonged training on the immune system, it has been concluded that there is an immune "susceptibility" phase (which can last from 3 to 72 hours), during which viruses and bacteria can get the better of the immune defenses, therefore the risk of clinical and subclinical infections increases.

There is therefore a sort of a J-curve in which there is an increased risk of upper respiratory tract infections, both in sedentary people and in those who train at high intensity, while there is a notable decrease in those who perform moderate exercise. The exact frequency, duration, type and intensity of the physical exercise required to lower the risk of infection or, conversely, to increase it, remain to be determined. Obviously, the diet is important for the immune function and it must provide an adequate amount of calories, proteins, fats, carbohydrates, vitamins and minerals. An inadequate protein and energy intake, or the lack of some micronutrients (such as zinc, iron, magnesium, manganese, selenium, copper and vitamins A, C, E, B6, B12 and folic acid) lower the immune defenses against pathogens, causing an increased susceptibility to infections.

Many minerals and vitamins have been associated with the ability to boost the immune system.

Zinc has numerous studies to its credit, which show that its deficiency can lead to immune system dysfunctions. A zinc deficiency, as demonstrated in a study carried out by Emily Ho of the State University of Oregon (USA), promotes inflammation through an impaired activation of immune cells and a dysregulation of the inflammatory cytokine IL-6. Competitive athletes easily suffer from deficient states of zinc, which already tends to be low in our diet.

Selenium, a key nutrient for the immune function, is also an antioxidant that helps strengthen the body's defenses against bacteria, viruses and cancer cells. It can be particularly useful for protecting against some strains of the influenza virus. Selenium is easily obtained from food, for example by consuming Brazil nuts.

Vitamin A: a short-term use of supplementation, especially in those who have a moderate vitamin A deficiency, can be extremely useful in supporting the body's ability to fight infections, especially respiratory pathogens.

Vitamin D has also recently been recognized for having an important role in regulating the immunity and an inverse correlation has been seen between the number of upper respiratory tract infections and low vitamin D levels. A study published in the Journal of Sports Sciences examined the effects of vitamin D3 supplementation with 5000 IU per day for 14 weeks, in athletes who trained intensely during the winter months. The results showed that vitamin D3 supplementation significantly increased the levels of antimicrobial proteins and peptides, both of which are critical for the immune system.

If fat fisches, egg yolk and dairy product are not taken daily, then the use of supplement must be considered. Athletes with a monotonous nutrition (rice and chicken for bodybuilders), vegetarian athletes and even more so vegans, athletes who often eat junk food, poor in nutrients, and athletes who are subjected to "weight loss" and take drastic diets (combat sports) to fall into the right weight category, must be particularly careful in order to avoid such deficiencies.

Some supplements can actually increase the immune functions and reduce the risk of infection in immunocompromised individuals, but there is little scientific evidence regarding their effectiveness in preventing the exercise-induced depression of the immune system. We will now see what can really help and what scientific evidence exists.

Several placebo-controlled studies in runners and cyclists have shown that the intake of **a carbohydrate-based beverage** during prolonged exercise is effective in decreasing the negative effects on the immune function.

In a series of studies, it has been shown that the intake of a sports beverage with 6% carbohydrates (1 liter/hour) during intense and prolonged exercise attenuates the increase in neutrophil and leukocyte count in the blood, and also the increase of stress hormones and inflammatory cytokines, but it has little effect on the decrease in salivary IgA immunoglobulins and T lymphocytes.

Thus, the ingestion of carbohydrates during the physical activity seems to be an effective, albeit partial countermeasure to the immune dysfunction, with favorable effects on changing stress hormones and inflammation. Some recent evidence suggests that regular intake of relatively high doses of **antioxidant vitamins** can reduce the cortisol responses during prolonged exercises, and these studies have been successful with both 500 mg of vitamin C + 400 IU of vitamin E. Only vitamin C supplementation can reduce the risk of URTI in ultramarathon runners.

A good balanced diet should theoretically promote the necessary amounts of **vitamin C**, but if fresh and organic fruits and vegetables are not available then the use of supplements must be considered. Vitamin C can help to prevent infections, including those caused by bacteria and viruses. A goob balanced diet should theoretically promote the necessary amounts of vitamin C,but if fresh and organic fruits and vegetables are not available then the use of supplements must be considered. A regular administration of vitamin C has been shown to shorten the duration of the common cold, and higher doses of vitamin C during an illness can also act as a natural antihistamine and anti-inflammatory agent. In fact, excessive antioxidant supplementation cannot be recommended because there is little evidence of the real benefits. It is also known that excess supplementation with antioxidants can reduce the formation of the natural endogenous antioxidant defense systems and it can also decrease the adaptation response to training.

Quercetin belongs to the category of flavonoids, which are substances generally endowed with antioxidant, anti-inflammatory, cardio-protective, anti-tumoral properties and contained in high quantities in onions, apples, blueberries, kale, chili pepper, tea and broccoli. The intake of flavonoids with the diet (with quercetin accounting for about 75% of them) varies from 13 to 64 mg/day. In a double-blind placebo-controlled study, it was shown that the intake of 1000 mg of quercetin per day by male cyclists significantly increased plasma levels of this substance and it also reduced the incidence of URTI during the two weeks following a three-day period of an intense exercise. The immune function, inflammation and oxidative stress in this study were not worsened, suggesting that quercetin may exert a direct antiviral effect.

Sulforaphans and acetylcysteine. Sulforaphans are sulfur compounds found in brassicaceae and particularly in broccoli. Sulforaphans and also acetylcysteine (both donors of thiol-SH groups) are able to increase the endogenous production of glutathione (GSH), which is a potent endogenous antioxidant. Recent studies suggest that the redox balance (oxidoreductive) of dendritic cells is a key factor in maintaining cytotoxic immunity and that its alteration may contribute to immunosenescence, decreasing the Th1 response, which is precisely against viruses and bacteria. The administration of sulforaphane and acetylcysteine (the latter decreases the pro-inflammatory cytokines IL-6, IL-1 and TNF-alpha) can restore this response by bringing the redox system back into balance. In one study, taking a smoothie of broccoli sprouts for a few days was found to protect against infection. Sprouts contain 20 times more sulforaphans than regular broccoli, and refrigeration increases the content. Suggested dose: 600 to 1,200 mg per day of broccoli sprout extract titrated to 10%.

Astragalus roots contain triterpene saponins, flavonoids, pyogenic amines and polysaccharides. In particular, polysaccharides stimulate the immune system, strengthening the body's natural defense mechanisms against infections.

This plant has immuno-stimulant and antiviral properties against viruses that cause the most common upper respiratory tract infections (common cold, cough), but it also protects against viruses that are responsible for more serious diseases, such as avian flu.

Astragalus, in fact, is able to favor the trophism of organs such as the spleen, thymus and the intestinal lymph nodes and it also improves the phagocytic capacity and the maturation of T lymphocytes.

Echinacea is a very popular supplement among athletes and numerous experiments have shown that echinacea extracts actually show immuno-stimulating activities; however, there are limited studies in terms of the numbers of participants and the methodological quality and, even if there is a basis of cultural traditions in the use of echinacea as a medicinal remedy, it is not yet known whether echinacea is effective in modifying the immunosuppression induced by physical exercise. It is to be used with caution in individuals with autoimmune diseases, as it can boost the autoimmune response.

Elderberry extract/syrup: elderberry can be useful in reducing the duration and the severity of the flu. It has been shown to help prevent the influenza virus infection, and it also has powerful antiviral properties that can help reduce the duration and symptoms of the flu. Doctors believe that the anthocyanins in elderberry prevent the virus from infecting our cells and are even more effective in slowing the spread of the virus once the cell is already infected. Elderberry inhibits the early stages of infection by blocking the viral proteins that attack and penetrate the host cell. In addition, elderberries stimulate some cytokines that positively activate the immune response against pathogenic microorganisms. Elderberries also need to be used with caution in some people with autoimmune diseases, due to the mechanism by which it stimulates the immune system.

The immuno-stimulating action of **eleutherococcus** is confirmed by numerous pharmacological studies and clinical trials. *In vitro* and *in vivo* studies show an increase in the number of leukocytes, cytotoxic T lymphocytes, T-helper lymphocytes, and B and T cell counts in the peripheral circulation.

In addition, an increase in phagocytosis was found in the activity of Natural Killer cells and T 18,19 lymphocytes. In vivo, it has also been seen that eleutherococcus stimulates the phagocytosis and the inactivation of pathogenic fungi (such as *Candida albicans*) by granulocytes and monocytes, with a 30-45% increase in phagocytosed cells compared to healthy control subjects. Furthermore, the mobility of the granulocytes and, therefore, their ability to migrate and reach the site of infection is increased by 45%. The therapeutic efficacy of eleutherococcus was confirmed in a double-blind clinical trial in 36 healthy volunteers. The subjects were treated with an eleutherococcus extract or placebo, three times a day for four weeks. In the treated group, a significant increase in the number of immunocompetent cells and a particularly evident effect on T "helper/inducer" lymphocytes was observed, but also on cytotoxic lymphocytes and on Natural Killer cells.

The immuno-stimulating activity of eleutherococcus, in addition to eleutherosides, is probably also due to its polysaccharide fraction (as in the case of other plants that act at the level of the immune system), especially regarding the prevention of common colds (sinusitis, flu, etc.) and other infections. The stimulating activity of the phytocomplex on the immune system was confirmed by an interesting study that involved a population of 3,000 healthy subjects, forced to work in adverse weather conditions. These were mainly workers from a city in Northern Russia, who worked at an average temperature of –5° C. Over the course of a year, there was a 40% reduction in the number of lost working days and a 50% reduction in the subjective findings of malaise. The preventive action of eleutherococcus has also been documented against acute and chronic respiratory diseases. Another study reports that the administration of the substance in 1000 workers (miners and foundry workers) for two winter months, reduced the incidence of acute respiratory diseases by two to four times compared to the control group.

Some studies indicate that **cysteine and/or theanine** supplementation can increase the immune efficiency of athletes exposed to prolonged periods of intense exercise. 700 mg per day of cysteine and 200 mg per day of theanine (an amino acid contained in green tea extracts) were administered in a study that was carried out in long distance runners, and it was found that the inflammatory response caused by exercise was attenuated, as evidenced by a lower increase in C-reactive protein levels and in the number of neutrophils. There was also a better immune adaptation, as evidenced by the lack of the decreasing number of lymphocytes. The researchers concluded that the intake of cysteine and theanine helped to decrease the exercise induced stress on the immune system, preventing a decline in its function, and it also hindered the infections during the continuous period of intense exercise.

Honey: honey is a good emollient (it relieves the burning sensation and the inflammation of the mucous membranes), it has antioxidant properties and some antimicrobial effects. It is useful for coughs and sore throats and can be added to hot tea.

Garlic: garlic contains a variety of compounds that can affect the immunity. Studies have shown that both fresh garlic, aged garlic extract and some other garlic-based supplements can reduce the severity of the upper respiratory tract viral infections and they also help in the prevention of viral infections that can cause colds.

Beetroot: beetroot juice is particularly rich in nitrates which promote the production of nitric oxide (NO). Additionally, supplementation with beet juice has been shown to provide a strong prevention of stress-associated cold symptoms, as well as being beneficial for asthma patients.

Probiotics are live microorganisms that, when administered in adequate quantities, modify the intestinal microbiota so that the number of beneficial bacteria increases and that of harmful microorganisms (pathogenic bacteria and fungi such as *Candida albicans*) decreases. Probiotics, in addition to providing a series of benefits for the intestine, exert a positive effect by modulating the immune function thanks to their interaction with the intestine associated lymphoid tissue. Some placebo-controlled studies have indicated that the daily intake of probiotics coincided with fewer overall days of respiratory tract diseases and with a decrease in URTI symptoms.

During recent years, countless studies have been published on intestinal microbiota and probiotics, but few studies have examined the effectiveness of taking probiotics for the immune system of athletes.

In a placebo-controlled study, 20 male long-distance runners took a *Lactobacillus fermentum* VRI003 probiotic for four months; during this time, athletes taking the probiotic experienced fewer sick days and experienced a reduction in the severity of symptoms when they became ill. Further large-scale studies are needed to confirm that taking probiotics can reduce the number of lost training days due to illness and to determine which probiotics are the most effective and whether their effects are strain-specific. However, the assumptions are good. Some mushrooms such as **reishi**, **maitake**, **cordyceps** and **shiitake**, given their content in terpenoids and beta-glucans, exert an antimicrobial action by attacking and eliminating only the pathogenic bacterial flora and also provide fibers that perform a prebiotic function, i.e. nourishment for probiotics. This mechanism underlies their ability to boost the immune system.

Beta-glucan: in a double-blind placebo-controlled study (*Journal of Sports Science and Medicine* – 2009 – 8, 509-515), beta-glucan was shown to be effective in preventing upper respiratory tract infection (URTI) infections and mood state.

75 marathon runners (35 men, 40 women) aged 18-53 years, took placebo, 250 mg or 500 mg of BETA 1,3/1,6 GLUCAN for 4 weeks after a marathon.

Over the course of the 4-week study, subjects in the beta-glucan groups (250 mg and 500 mg of beta-glucan daily) reported significantly fewer URTI symptoms, improved overall health and decreased confusion, fatigue, tension and anger, and increased vigor on the POMS (Profile Of Mood State) survey compared to placebo.

CHAPTER 37

Pre- and post-workout supplements in the gym

Pre-workout

For about 35 years, I have been going to the USA every summer, both to spend the holidays and for refresher courses and internships concerning fitness, nutrition, and also functional and anti-aging medicine. One thing that has always fascinated me about the USA is the widespread use of food supplements. Entire departments of supermarkets are dedicated to them; you can find specific shops on every street corner and inside each shopping center. For me, a person that has always been a big "fan" of food supplementation, it is a kind of "funfair" where I find myself wandering for hours and hours, if not for whole days. Obviously, the supplement market also follows trends, partly on the basis of commercial pressures and partly following the most recent scientific discoveries. Well, lately I have been impressed by the large space dedicated to the so-called "pre-workout", especially in advertisements and articles in the magazines of the supplement sector. But what do these "pre-workouts" consist of? Basically, they consist on the usage of some supplements before training, in order to improve the athletic performance. It is something that has always been common among athletes, especially those that participate in endurance sports, but also among gym-goers. Obviously, in the past, pre-workout among endurance athletes was aimed at increasing the duration of the performance and was mainly based on powdered carbohydrates, mineral salts and possibly amino acids. As for gym-goers, the pre-workout was often limited to amino acids to counteract the catabolism, and thermogenics in order to have more "grit" during training and possibly burn more fat. However, during recent years, the number of the scientific works regarding supplements that can improve performance in the gym has been so high, that it even creates uncertainty among consumers, who cannot decide which one to choose. They also don't want to use too many of them for both economic and practical reasons. At this point, the supplement companies, contravening a consolidated marketing rule that suggests diversifying into more products to increase the sales, have decided, perhaps also considering the economic crisis, to meet the demands of the average consumer, formulating a new supplement that contains various active ingredients in a single administration: the pre-workout. Obviously, each company, in order to differentiate the choice, has used certain formulations; but let's see from a theoretical-scientific and practical point of view what the perfect pre-workout should contain. First of all, while the post-workout must be focused on muscle recovery and growth, the pre-workout must increase the strength, concentration, energy and endurance, and perhaps it can also improve the muscle "pumping".

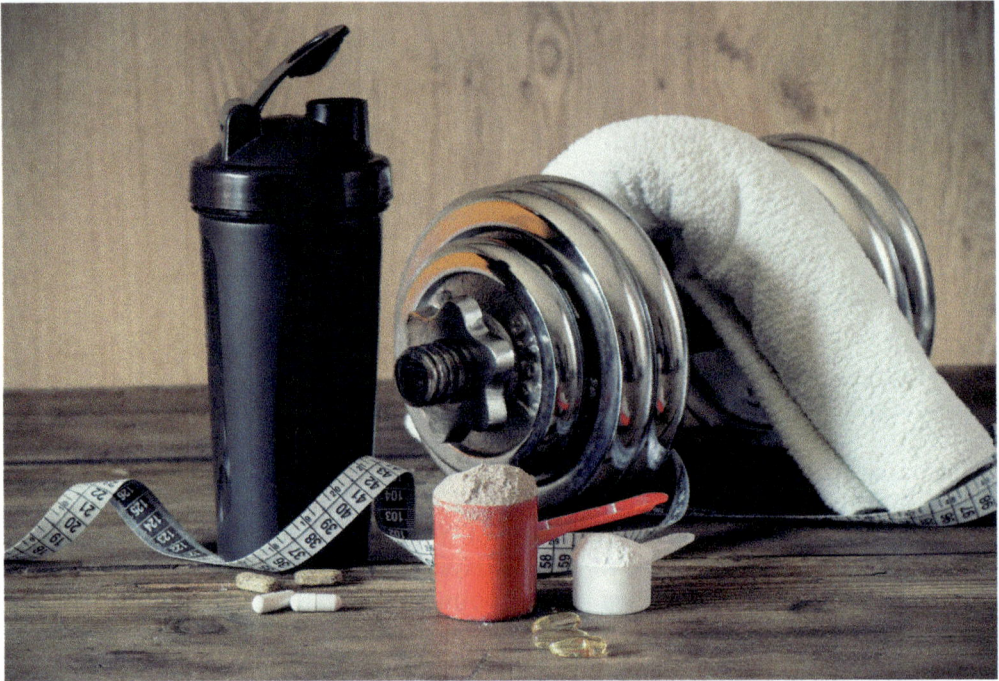

Figure 37.1

Creatine

It is the second best-selling supplement, after protein powders, and it also comes second in the number of studies. Creatine, from the functional biochemistry point of view, serves above all to build up the creatine phosphate reserves in the muscle. Creatine phosphate is an indirect energy reserve source for ATP and it is basically used in physical exercises of an alactic anaerobic nature, where the energy substrates consist on ATP itself and on creatine phosphate. These exercises include explosive strength and power exercises, which are normally performed over a 10-20″ time range. In reality, creatine exerts a buffering effect against cellular acidosis during the exercise and therefore, it should also be able to improve the resistant strength by delaying fatigue. A study by Jonathan Little et al. of the University of Saskatchewan in Canada, showed that taking creatine monohydrate and creatine monohydrate plus arginine alpha-ketoglutarate before training increased peak strength during repeated push tests on a static bicycle.

Beta-alanine

Beta-alanine is the supplement that has found a lot of space in scientific conferences in recent years. Beta-alanine is the amino acid that limits the formation of carnosine, a lactic acid buffer substance. This buffer effect allows you to perform longer and more intense sets, and consequently a greater training volume. It is mainly indicated for sports that exploit the anaerobic lactacid metabolism such as soccer, 400 meters, bodybuilding, and it is naturally complementary to creatine. Beta-alanine has a molecular structure that is very similar to taurine, as they both use the same membrane transporters (kind of "shuttles" that carry a molecule from the outside to the inside of the cells) and thus a competition is created that favors the prevalent molecule. Therefore, it is preferable that beta-alanine supplementation is accompanied by taurine supplementation, not so much with the intention of enhancing the absorption of beta-alanine, as they compete at the same carrier level, but to allow a sufficient entry of taurine in the muscle cell, which is an important antioxidant. However, there appears to be no significant difference in carnosine concentration when combining taurine with beta-alanine.

BCAA

Branched chain amino acids are an all-Italian discovery; I remember when, 30 years ago, I went to train at Gold's Gym in Venice, Los Angeles (the Mecca of bodybuilders) and, comparing myself with the local champions, I realized that they didn't even know what they were. It took more than 20 years to make sure that branched chain amino acids found their place on the supplement counter in that country, and I think it is one of those very rare cases, together with the widespread use of mobile phones, in which Italy preceded the USA (actually the same thing happened with lipoic acid: when I began to propose it in Italy at higher dosages as a normoglycemic agent and as an activator of lipolysis, in the USA it was still marketed only at dosages of 50 mg per capsule, and it was given as an antioxidant). There are three branched amino acids, leucine-valine-isoleucine, which have a selective metabolism in the muscles by practically bypassing the liver and, for this reason, they are also used in therapies for patients with liver diseases (when my patients nowadays still repeat to me that the general practitioner advised them against the intake of amino acids because "they are bad for the liver", I want to laugh, in order not to cry!). The ability of branched chain amino acids to limit the protein catabolism, through the neoglucogenetic function, and also to stimulate the anabolic hormones, such as testosterone and GH, is now widely demonstrated. In addition, the branched chain amino acids taken before training, thanks to the serum BCAA/tryptophan ratio, reduce the production of serotonin in the brain, thus delaying the feeling of fatigue. From this point of view, a 1-1-1 formulation with reduced leucine would be better, as there is a competition mechanism between the same branched amino acids, and the one that competes more with tryptophan is valine, while the one that performs the best energetic function is isoleucine.

Taurine

It is essential for the cellular health, as it is a powerful antioxidant and it preserves the mitochondrial function. Furthermore, this amino acid stimulates the metabolism by helping with the fat burn and it acts as a neurotransmitter, working against depression and also on the muscle contractility. In studies conducted on rats, it has been seen that taurine is able to stimulate testosterone.

Nitric oxide (NO) stimulators

In recent years, nitric oxide has become a very popular supplement among gym goers. NO has multiple functions, but the most recognized is the ability to increase the blood flow through vasodilation that occurs through a relaxation induced at the level of the smooth muscle of the arterial walls. It allows a greater influx of nutrients and oxygen, simultaneously facilitating the elimination of waste substances, which promotes a better muscle performance as well as greater ability to burn fat. Since NO is synthesized from the amino acid **arginine**, logic would have it that it is the first choice supplement to increase the NO production. However, arginine is oxidized in the intestine and is above all rapidly degraded in the liver; it is better to use **citrulline**, which is more easily absorbed in the intestine, avoids degradation in the liver and it is rapidly converted into arginine by our organism. Indeed, in a study by Osawska et al. it has been shown that the intake of citrulline allows a greater increase in the level of arginine in the blood and muscles, than the intake of arginine itself. Citrulline, in addition to promoting the "pumping" through the vasodilating capacity of NO, is also able to directly stimulate the protein synthesis by activating the mTOR enzyme, which promotes the muscle growth. In one study (Perez-Grisado et al.), 41 men performed 8 sets of horizontal bench presses with 80% of the maximum weight (weight that allows you to do only one repetition). Half of the subjects were given 8 g of citrulline, while the others were given a placebo. The group that received citrulline were able to perform more reps in all eight sets and, in addition, reported less muscle pain. **Arginine alpha-ketoglutarate** can be equally useful, as it follows a preferential path for the synthesis of NO.

Caffeine

The fact that caffeine is a powerful energizer is nothing new, and for several years it has been on the WADA doping list for the IOC, and it is currently banned in the NCAA. Caffeine promotes weight loss by increasing the consumption of fats for energy purposes (*Nutrition and Metabolic Insights* 4: 65-72, 2011). There are many studies that demonstrate the energetic properties of caffeine, I will mention only one: according to a study by Coventry University UK (Duncan MJ et al., 2010), caffeine-based drinks reduce the perception of effort during weight-training, they increase the number of repetitions to exhaustion and also increase the ability to train. The test subjects consumed an energy drink containing 179 mg of caffeine and a placebo (without caffeine) 60 minutes before training. They performed four different exercises (bench press, deadlift, barbell row, squat) to exhaustion, with 60% 1MR (1 maximum repetition) and the experimental conditions (caffeine or placebo) were repeated after (at least) 48 hours. The subjects that consumed caffeine completed significantly more reps in each exercise, and the mental predisposition for physical exertion was also increased. The results of this and other studies have confirmed that caffeine improves the performance in endurance and power sports, and it also improves the psychological approach to training (*Journal Strength Conditioning Research* 2612859, 2865,

2012). We all know the effect of caffeine on the central nervous system and on increasing the consumption of fat for energy purposes, but some recent studies show that caffeine is able to increase the release of calcium from the muscles, thus increasing the strength of the muscle contraction, and this may be another reason for its ergogenic effect (*Journal International Society of Sport Nutrition* 9:21, 2012).

Post-workout

I've been training with weights for over 45 years now. In the past, my main goal was to increase strength and muscle mass; however, my current target is to maintain the muscle mass and keep the body fat percentage low. I understood from the beginning how important biochemistry and nutrition were in order to obtain what I set out to be, and it was for this reason that I dedicated myself to the studies of Medicine and Food Science, which led me to deepen, in particular, the studies on hormonal modulation induced by foods and supplements, as a function of training. Recent scientific research has shown that the most important moment of the intake of macro- and micronutrients in the anabolic function is close to training, and specifically after training. However, the total amount of macronutrients is certainly more important than timing; for example, it is more important to reach the necessary amount of protein to better promote the increase of muscle mass, rather than worrying about taking them close to the training. However, there exists a so-called anabolic window of about 2 hours during which the assimilation of nutrients is aimed at the muscle anabolic purpose. Therefore, their accumulation in the form of glycogen and contractile and sarcoplasmic proteins in the muscle is more privileged than the transformation into triglycerides in the adipose tissue. In other words, after the training you can afford to eat more without gaining weight and, indeed, the meal consumed after the training is functional to muscle growth or, at the very least, to the recovery of glycogen and to the regeneration of the damaged muscle. On the other hand, if one fasts for more than 2 hours after the training, muscle catabolism will be more favored.

The best way to take advantage of this anabolic window is to consume a liquid meal consisting of proteins and carbohydrates in powder and various supplements (quickly absorbed and assimilated) immediately after the training. If your training is aimed at hypertrophy, it is better to consume the proteins first and then, after 30 minutes, the carbohydrates (thus favoring the acceleration of protein synthesis which is induced by a faster absorption of the proteins when they taken alone), followed then, within an hour, by a solid meal that is possibly easily digestible so as not to slow down the absorption. This meal must therefore contain lean proteins, low saturated fats and carbohydrates in the appropriate quantities in relation to the performed workout. For example, 80-100 g of rice or pasta; 150-200 g of chicken or fish; large quantities of vegetables dressed with olive oil; some dried fruits and a fresh fruit. After all, a simple healthy meal should be halfway between the Mediterranean diet and the Zone Diet. If, on the other hand, the goal is weight loss, both the pre-workout and post-workout meals must follow the concepts of the Chronormorphodiet, or COM Diet. Therefore, the android type subjects, i.e. hyperlipogenetics, must take a pre-workout meal that is low in carbohydrates, workout in the afternoon, and the following dinner should be richer in carbohydrates to better modulate cortisol and leptin, and thus promote weight loss. On the other hand, ginoid or hypolipolytic individuals will have to consume a lunch that is rich in carbohydrates to stimulate the thyroid metabolism, carry out an evening workout and take a subsequent protein-rich dinner to stimulate the nocturnal secretion of GH (Massimo Spattini, *The COM Diet & spot reduction*). In this chapter, I would like to focus on post-workout supplementation, the one to be consumed in the half hour following the workout.

The characteristics that a post-workout must have are listed below:

1. It must promote the recovery of muscle glycogen, which is depleted by the training.
2. It must stimulate the anabolism by optimizing the protein synthesis.
3. It must reduce cortisol, which, if present in high quantities, causes catabolism, i.e. muscle loss.
4. It must exert a volumizing and hydrating effect at the intracellular level, in order to favor the repair processes.
5. It must promote the disposal of toxic substances produced by training.

So let's see what the main ingredients must be.

Powdered carbohydrates

Carbohydrates are essential in the post-workout, in order to promote the restoration of muscle glycogen, limit the production of cortisol, hindering the catabolism, and to stimulate the protein synthesis, synergistically with proteins (this is not valid for the middle-aged athletes, who do not require post-workout carbohydrates and, by having a reduced insulin sensitivity, they do not benefit from it, and it has only negative aspects: which are, the possible increase in fat tissue and a further worsening of the insulin sensitivity). The "after workout" is perhaps the only moment in which carbohydrates with a high glycemic index find their place, i.e. with a rapid absorption and consequent high insulin stimulation. This is because after the training, there is a significant increase in the insulin sensitivity in the muscles, so the carbohydrates will selectively go into the muscle and not into the adipose tissue. Maltodextrin and glucose are fine for this purpose, but Vitargo® (patented polysaccharide derived from processing starch) is the most effective in restoring glycogen reserves, thanks to its hypotonicity, which allows it to be absorbed more quickly than glucose, and its glycemic index is comparable to that of glucose and higher than that of maltodextrins. The recommended dosage of carbohydrates is 0.5-1 g per kg of body weight.

Powdered proteins

Taking proteins immediately after the training seems to be the most important thing to stimulate the protein synthesis. Milk proteins are better than soy proteins, whey proteins are better than caseins, hydrolyzed proteins are better than isolated proteins, and differentiated absorption protein blends are able to prolong the activation of the protein synthesis, and therefore they are more preferable if the next meal is more than an hour apart. However, the most important thing is to take about 30 g of protein in an aqueous solution immediately after the training.

Creatine

Creatine is an excellent supplement which is also useful for endurance sports, but, especially if taken after training, it is particularly useful for increasing muscle strength and mass. Creatine works for various reasons: it increases creatine phosphate levels, stimulates muscle satellite cells, exerts a buffering effect, has a volumizing effect at the cellular level, increases dihydrotestosterone and so on. It was found that giving bodybuilders 5 g of creatine after weight training, five times a week for a month, produced a significant change in the body composition: a decrease in fat mass and an increase in strength, compared to its intake before the training. There are various forms of creatine in addition to the classic creatine monohydrate, for example the creatine ester, the buffered creatine, the PEC (polyethylene glycosylated creatine); the only advantage of the latter, apart from the individual tolerability, is the ability to load the muscle cells with creatine even with a reduced daily intake (3-5 g of creatine monohydrate for a month compared to 1.5-2.5 other creatines); however, this advantage is canceled out by the higher cost.

Leucine

Recently, the traditional 2-1-1 formula (2 of leucine, 1 of valine, 1 of isoleucine) of branched chain amino acids has been changed by several supplement companies (from 4-1-1 up to 12-1-1), as it has been discovered that leucine, above all other amino acids, plays an important role in stimulating the protein synthesis through the direct activation of the mTOR enzymatic pathway. Another reason why it would be better to take leucine rather than isoleucine and valine after the training, is that isoleucine favors the influx of glucose into the muscle and its conversion into energy, and therefore it would be better take it before the training, while leucine facilitates the accumulation of glucose in the form of glycogen and this is particularly useful in the recovery phase.

While valine is the major antagonist of tryptophan (precursor of serotonin) at the blood brain barrier level, leucine antagonizes dopamine, and since the sensation of fatigue during the training is actually conditioned by the relationship between these two neurotransmitters, it is better to avoid or in any case limit your leucine intake before the training. After a workout, although leucine represents only a modest percentage of the amino acids making up the body's proteins, its levels drop by about 30% and restoring its optimal levels as soon as possible is essential for protein synthesis. The recommended dose of leucine to compensate for the decrease caused by training is 500 mg for every 10 kg of weight. Obviously, for the protein synthesis to take place, the presence of all essential amino acids and indispensable cofactors such as magnesium, vitamin B6, zinc, niacin and others is necessary.

HMB

HMB is a leucine metabolite that promotes the muscle growth especially by attenuating the catabolism rather than stimulating the protein synthesis, as leucine does. HMB produces this effect by decreasing the production of a catabolic enzyme for the muscle, called atrogine-1. In one study, it was found that 3000 mg of HMB weakly stimulated the protein synthesis and that it was also able to decrease the protein catabolism by 57%. It is clear that by combining leucine and HMB we can obtain the anabolic effect of one and the catabolic effect of the other, thus favoring a significant increase in muscle mass. A study by Mobley et al. of 2014 demonstrated how a mixture containing leucine, calcium-HMB and creatine monohydrate is able to reverse the atrophy induced by myostatin in isolated muscle cells, by preventing the inhibition of the formation of new muscle fibers.

Betaine

Betaine increases the cellular hydration through an osmotic mechanism, thus reducing the negative impact of dehydration on the cellular anabolism. The cell volumization effect stimulates the protein synthesis and decreases the catabolism through mechanisms that are not yet well known. However, they seem to be linked to a restructuring signal that makes the muscle cell adapt to new dimensions. The ability of betaine to donate a methyl group promotes the synthesis of creatine and also its greater uptake within the muscle cell. Furthermore, its ability to act as a methyl group donor helps to keep homocysteine levels low, a molecule that decreases the insulin sensitivity; therefore, this positive effect on the insulin sensitivity further contributes to the insulin-dependent entry of creatine into the muscle cell.

Glutamine

Glutamine is a neoglucogenic amino acid, therefore it promotes the resynthesis of glycogen. Being the most represented amino acid at the level of the cytoplasm, that is, the non-contractile part of muscle cells, it exerts, like creatine, a volumizing effect and, consequently, by promoting hydration it also favors the anabolism. Its association with leucine is important because leucine enters the cell through a glutamine-dependent transporter. Glutamine is also essential for the immune system, as it is the nutrient of choice for lymphocytes, and intense training can depress the immune system, favoring infections, especially the ones that affect the upper respiratory tract. Glutamine peptide is better as a supplement, since simple glutamine is largely consumed by the intestinal mucosal cells that are greedy for it. The recommended dosage of glutamine is 5-10 g.

Arginine alpha-ketoglutarate

It is the most functional form of arginine as a precursor of nitric oxide. Arginine, taken after training, in addition to promoting the stimulation of GH, with lipolytic and anabolic effects, induces the production of nitric oxide, causing a vasodilation that increases the blood flow and favors the supply of nutrients to the muscle cells, improving their trophism. The recommended dosage is 3 g. Citrulline has been shown to be an effective supplement, working on the increase of plasma arginine, increasing the production of nitric oxide and it can be more effective than arginine, as it has a higher absorption rate and is therefore able to restore the nitric oxide production more quickly.

All these ingredients must be "shaken" in at least 500 mL of water, perhaps even with a sachet of mineral salts, and to be consumed immediately after the workout, making sure that all this "mash" will go into the muscles!

CHAPTER 38

Supplementation and stress

Well-being passes through the constant practice of a proper physical activity, an adequate nutrition and stress management. Stress generates cortisol, which, if produced acutely, can help in the athletic performance, but when it is produced in a chronic continuous manner, for example in overtraining conditions or during hectic everyday life, it takes on a negative value as it has a catabolic effect on the muscle, favors the increase of fat especially in the abdominal area and it is also deleterious for the memory and for other brain faculties. If the excessive cortisol produced by overtraining can be limited by decreasing the training, limiting the cortisol that is produced due to the rhythms of modern life is much more difficult; stress is due to the kind of life that we all lead by now, where time is scarce and excessive technology, instead of being a useful support, ends up becoming a sort of master for our lives, for which we must remain continually available. Obviously, the anti-stress techniques are many and they are based on breathing exercises, meditation, autogenic training, yoga, music therapy, massage therapy, etc.; all this, however, does not fall within the specific area of this book, so I will deal with the topic from the nutrition point of view and, above all, with supplements. As for nutrition, the advice is the usual: it is advisable to spread multiple meals 3-4hours apart, possibly always at the same time and they should not be too abundant. They should be balanced in the various macronutrients in order to keep blood sugar stable, with a good supply of foods rich in fiber, such as fruits and vegetables.

An excess of carbohydrates, especially with high glycemic index ones, raises blood sugar too much, leading to a hyperstimulation of insulin with a subsequent hypoglycemia which activates the production of cortisol, the main stress-related hormone. It has a hyperglycemic and catabolic effect on both muscular and cerebral levels. However, it is also not advisable to take too many proteins, because they directly stimulate the production of cortisol, which is involved in their transformation into glucose through the activation of neoglucogenesis.

If you have a disturbed sleep, perhaps also due to the habit of exercising late in the evening, or if you are very nervous and perhaps belong to the hyperlipogenetic category of the Chronormorphodiet (with accumulation of fat in the abdominal area), you can have benefits by consuming fewer carbohydrates during lunch and more at dinner. This habit allows an increase in the production of serotonin, which promotes better physiological sleep with a lower production of cortisol, which instead increases when sleep is reduced or irregular. It is also essential to take into account not only what and when you eat, but also how you eat. You have to do it in a conscious way, being focused on your food and its flavors, chewing slowly, possibly maintaining a good posture and avoiding being distracted by mobile phones, etc. The visual aspect is also important, so the dish should be as colorful as possible thanks to the varied choice of foods, not only to ensure that a large number of phytonutrients are automatically included, but because the colors have a relaxing effect, especially blue and green. So, only rice cakes, chicken breast and egg whites are not good for the body or the brain!

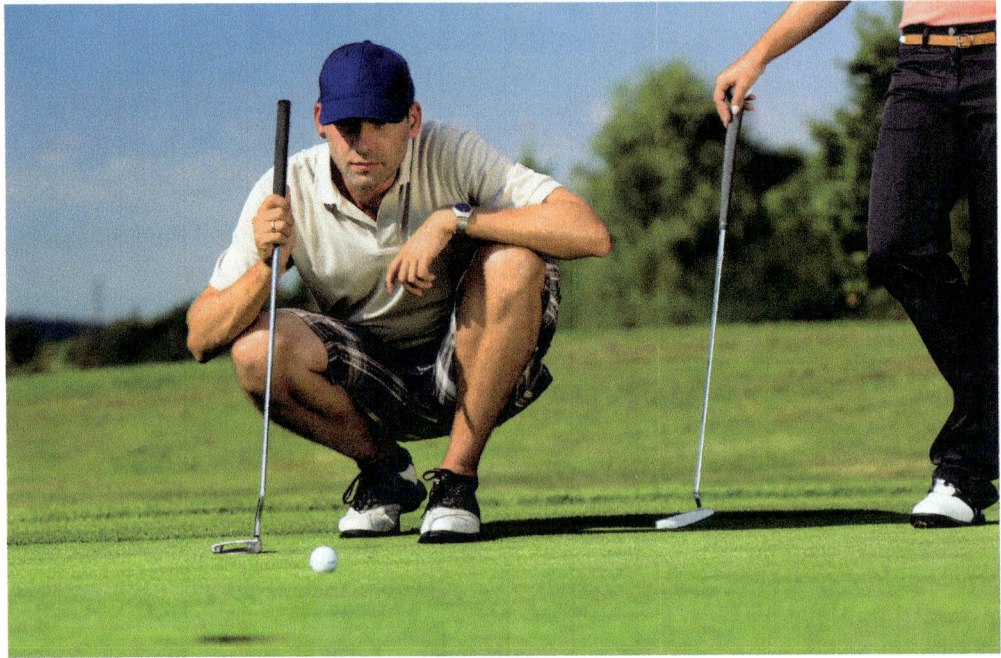

Figure 38.1

It also makes sense to eliminate coffee in the morning and opt for green tea. In fact, a study conducted by Duke University concluded that the effects of coffee in the morning can enhance the body's responses to stress and raise the cortisol levels throughout the day until late in the evening. Conversely, the theanine present in green tea promotes non-sleepy relaxation by stimulating the production of the neurotransmitter GABA in the brain, which counteracts the stimulating effects of theine.

But, in addition to nutrition, is there a magic pill to defeat this excess of cortisol? Well, there are some drugs that block its production, but in reality this is not a good strategy because cortisol is a life-saving hormone, so it is essential for our body; except in very rare cases of pathologies in which the production of cortisol is overexpressed, these drugs are absolutely not to be used. On the other hand, there are supplements or herbal products that are able to limit and modulate the production of cortisol during stressful situations.

Supplements in hypercortisolism

Phosphatidylserine (PS) is a phospholipid that constitutes the cellular matrix of all cell membranes. Numerous studies show that PS plays an important role in the synthesis of the neurotransmitter acetylcholine; it also decreases the secretion of ACTH by the pituitary gland during stressful workouts. ACTH is the hormone that stimulates the adrenals to produce various hormones, including cortisol, and in this way the PS reduces blood cortisol levels during and after strenuous exercises.

Tyrosine is the precursor of dopamine, adrenaline and noradrenaline: the latter two are very important for the process of adaptation to intense and sudden psychophysical stress. They have been tested on soldiers subjected to training in conditions of high stress and they have shown their abilities to increase the tolerance of physical and mental fatigue.

Rodhiola rosea has adaptogenic properties, which means, it actually creates a small stressful situation for the body which helps to adapt and better tolerate the most severe stressful situations. It is able to increase the level of betaendorfins and it also decreases the release of corticotropin releasing hormone (CRH), which is responsible for the hypothalamic stimulation that leads to the release of ACTH. It is particularly useful for athletes to shorten the recovery time after a long and intense workout.

Holy basil is another medicinal herb which is capable of reducing cortisol levels; it also improves the glycemic balance and insulin sensitivity when stress is the key factor.

Withania somnifera or **Indian ginseng** is another adaptogenic plant which is useful in states of anxiety and insomnia and it is also able to reduce the production of cortisol.

Magnolia bark, obtained from *Magnolia officinalis*, has an anxiolytic activity similar to benzodiazepines, it interacts with the GABA receptor (relaxing effect) and controls cortisol levels.

Ganoderma lucidum or **reishi** is an adaptogenic mushroom that has an anti-inflammatory and antioxidant effect. It regulates the blood pressure and blood sugar levels, lowers cortisol and improves the quality and duration of deep sleep.

Theanine, found mainly in green tea, promotes non-sleepy relaxation by stimulating the production of the neurotransmitter GABA in the brain, counteracting the stimulating effects of caffeine.

Betasitosterol, derived from wheat germ oil, balances the cortisol/DHEA ratio (DHEA is a sex adrenal hormone), which increases especially as a result of exercise-induced stress.

BCAAs are inhibitors of cortisol production. They work both by increasing the synthesis of glutamine in the muscles, and by preventing its release under the influence of cortisol.

DHA (docosahexaenoic acid) is a fatty acid from the omega-3 family that is able to improve the response to stress. A study that included 41 students, evaluated the effectiveness of a DHA-based treatment of 1.5 g per day in the 3 months before exams. The control group that had taken soybean oil, at the end of the study, when the students were under examination stress, showed a 58% increase in the expressed hostility, while the treated group showed a 14% reduction in the same indices. A study under similar conditions showed that DHA significantly reduced (-31%) adrenaline levels.

Magnesium helps regulate cortisol levels while being stressed. Low magnesium levels can cause headaches and fatigue, increasing the effects of stress.

Vitamin C reduces cortisol: in a study, it was found that 3000 mg of vitamin C given before a stressful workout can bring cortisol levels back to normal faster.

In recent years, the use of **probiotics** in the modulation of the stress response has been examined. By improving the synthesis of neurotransmitters (in the intestine) such as serotonin, melatonin, GABA, histamine and acetylcholine, the microbiota improves the response to stress by modulating the activity of hormones such as ACTH and cortisol. The administration of *Lactobacillus rhamnosus* for 28 days in laboratory animals led to a significant decrease in corticosterone levels and it also reduced the depressive states (Bravo et al., 2011). A possible mechanism of modulation of the stress response by probiotics is related to the metabolism of serotonin. When administered to mice, *Bifidus infantis* 35824 raised the levels of tryptophan, the precursor of serotonin (5-HT) (Desbonet et al., 2008). The concentration of serotonin in the central nervous system is closely related to the ability of the peripheral enzyme systems (intestine and enteric nervous system) to capture tryptophan and convert it into 5-HT (Ruddik et al., 2006).

If the problem of high cortisol is linked to situations of acute stress or to the early stages of chronic stress, when the stress has persisted for a long time, for months or years, it can lead to an adaptation situation in which you will find yourself with low cortisol levels, and then other supplements will be useful.

Supplements in hypocortisolism

Certain "adaptogenic" substances are particularly suitable for situations of hypocortisolism. These are defined as "compounds that increase the ability of an organism to adapt to environmental factors and to avoid damage from such factors".

In situations of hypocortisolism, these substances can improve the state of the subject, as they create an up-regulation of the (in this case) poor response to stress and maintain the adaptation state of the homeostasis; in addition, many of them contain polysaccharides which have been shown to produce an improvement in the immune response.

Used in single doses, these compounds are effective in situations that require a rapid response and the effects are associated with the sympathetic-adrenergic system, by increasing the levels of catecholamines, neuropeptides, ATP, nitric oxide, eicosaenoids.

If taken in repeated doses, the positive effect on stress is similar to that of the physical exercise, with a consequent increase in the endurance and duration. They do not inhibit the stress response, but rather act as agonists to induce an adaptive response to stress.

They are particularly useful in sports medicine, as they increase the physical endurance and promote a faster recovery.

The main adaptogenic substances to be used in the case of hypocortisolism are illustrated below.

Turmeric has been thoroughly studied for its strong anti-inflammatory properties. It improves the sensitivity of the cortisol receptors. A prolonged use increases cortisol blood levels. Turmeric reverses the effects of chronic stress on the behavior and on the HPA axis.

In animals subjected to chronic stress for 20 days, there was an increase in the thickness of the cortex and a decrease in cortisol receptors. The use of turmeric reversed the process (dosage 5-10 mg/kg). Probably the anti-inflammatory and pain-relieving effect of turmeric is due to this modulating action of the cortisol receptors.

Panax ginseng has a toning capacity attributed to a class of molecules called ginsenoids. It is defined as a "psychotonic" for its stimulating and tonic activities at the central nervous system. Not only does it improve the body from a physical point of view, but, by positively influencing the depressive states, it also improves the performance and concentration.

Low doses of **licorice** extracts, **glycyrrhizic** and **glycyrrhetic** acid inhibit the 11β-HSD enzyme. This inhibition leads to an increase in cortisol levels and a reduction in the activity of aldosterone, which no longer acts as a powerful mineralocorticoid, supplanted in this role by cortisol (glucocorticoid).

Maca (*Lepidium meyenii*) is a typical plant of the Andes that grows at more than 3000 m of altitude. It is also known as the Peruvian ginseng and it has important energizing properties.

The part that we use is its root, rich in essential amino acids, fibers, vitamins and minerals, including iron, phosphorus, calcium, potassium, zinc and manganese. Its function is manifested in the reduction of chronic fatigue and in athletes use it for the ability to increase the physical endurance and to strengthen the muscle mass. Maca implements glycogenesis and for this reason it increases the available energy.

Rhodiola rosea is a perennial herbaceous succulent plant, typical of the cold climates of the northern hemisphere. Among all the species of *Rhodiola*, the *rosea* is the one that has strong adaptogenic properties. This compound is exceptionally effective in increasing the production of serotonin in the brain (up to 30%), inhibiting the activity of COMTs and promoting the transport of serotonin across the blood brain barrier. It has antidepressant and anxiolytic properties, improves the concentration and the mood, and it also and reduces the feeling of fatigue by increasing the concentration of important neurotransmitters such as dopamine, adrenaline and noradrenaline.

Cordyceps sinensis is a native plant of China to which numerous properties are attributed. It is used in sports for its strong ergogenic effect in increasing the endurance and reducing the sense of fatigue, preventing overtraining in professional athletes. Its properties include an increase in the capacity of the immune system and a possible tranquilizing effect on the central nervous system.

Eleuterococcus or **Siberian ginseng** is a plant used in herbal medicine for its remarkable tonic properties. Eleutherococcus extract binds strongly to glucocorticoid and mineralocorticoid receptors (Pearce et al., 1982). *In vitro* tests have shown an increase in ACTH and LH levels after administration of the eleutherococcus extract (Wagner, 1995). The strong tropism towards the adrenals would explain the strong influence on the resistance to heat, cold, infections, physical stress in general, radiation and also the effects of weightlessness in space. Athletes demonstrated an increase in endurance of up to 9%.

Astragalus is a plant that belongs to the legume family. In traditional Chinese medicine, it is used to strengthen the immune system, and recent studies have shown that it also reduces the toxic effects of chemotherapy. It is hypothesized that the polysaccharides contained in this plant strengthen the immune defenses and improve the resistance to fatigue, by increasing the energy. It is also used to counteract the loss of appetite, chronic fatigue and excess sweating.

Schisandra is an adaptogenic plant rich in lignans, which is useful against stress and it also stimulates the heart and the nervous system. In addition to increasing the resistance to stress, it stimulates the central nervous system by improving the reflexes, endurance and the working capacity; it also performs an antioxidant activity and determines an increase in the immune activity.

In addition to adaptogenic substances, various vitamins are useful in case of hypocortisolism:

- **thiamine (B1):** has been shown to protect the adrenal gland from functional exhaustion after surgical stress;
- **pantothenic acid (B5):** induces the hypersecretion of cortisol following the down-
- regulation due to stress. It also optimizes the function of the cortical zone of the adrenal gland;
- **niacin (B3):** increases the quality and duration of sleep;
- **methylcobalamin (B12):** implements the circadian cycle and moves the cortisol peak to the morning;
- **pyridoxal phosphate (B6):** important cofactor for the synthesis of sedative neurotransmitters (GABA, serotonin);
- **vitamin C:** essential for the production of cortisol at the adrenal level.

In addition to these supplements with a direct effect on cortisol, both in situations of hypercortisolism and, at lower doses, of hypocortisolism, I would also add lipoic acid and chromium, which have a normoglycemic effect, in order to avoid the changes in blood sugar that cause cortisol differences and the phenomenon of "carb craving" (compulsive hunger for sweet things that occurs in situations of stress and an inability to manage the hypoglycemia).

CHAPTER 39

Supplementation and joints

There is no doubt that those who train against resistance with weights, despite using considerable quantities of loads, are fundamentally less subjected to trauma and injuries, especially compared to other sports, such as football, rugby and basketball, where in addition to the dynamism of the sport itself, there is also a physical contact with the opponent. This is particularly true if the execution of the exercises respects the correct form and if the individual performs exercises that are less dangerous from a biomechanical point of view. But it is also true that over the years – these are statistical data, as well as my personal opinion - almost all weightlifters have joint pathologies, especially at the shoulder level (it is so often that we talk about the "bodybuilder's shoulder"), knees, elbows and spine. Most of these conditions result in arthritis.

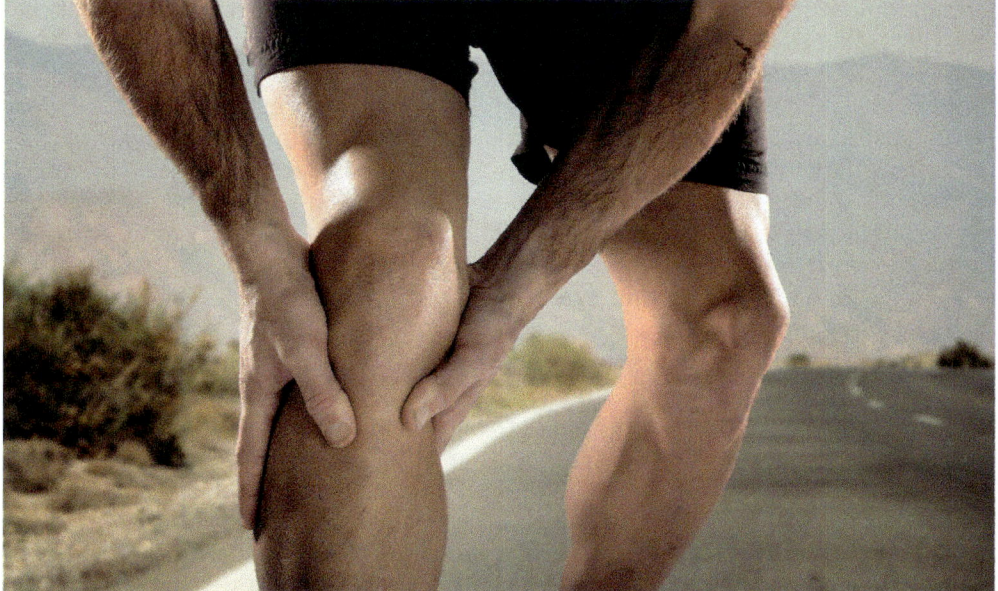

Figure 39.1

Arthritis literally means "inflammation of a joint" and it is characterized by pain, swelling, stiffness and redness. The term "arthritis" does not indicate a single disorder, but a joint disease that has many causes. Arthritis can affect one or more joints that can have different degrees of severity, from mild pain and stiffness to intense pain and, subsequently, joint deformity. Although arthritis has been divided by rheumatologists into about 10 categories, the most common ones can be grouped into three broad classes: osteoarthritis or arthrosis, inflammatory arthritis and extra-articular diseases. Although only one of these categories is defined as "inflammatory", in all of them you can find inflammation that involves the joints and the tissues surrounding the joints. Symptomatic therapy usually involves the use of anti-inflammatories such as acetylsalicylic acid and ibuprofen, if not cortisone. But these drugs have severe side effects in the long run. Isn't there any natural supplement that can help?

Certainly yes, but first let's understand this disease. Osteoarthritis, better known as arthrosis or degenerative arthropathy, is the most common type of arthropathy. Caused by the wear and tear of the articular cartilages, it usually develops in middle aged individuals and mainly affects the elderly. Rheumatoid arthritis is the most serious type of the inflammatory joint diseases. It is an autoimmune form in which the body's immune system reacts against the joints and the surrounding soft tissues, by damaging them. It affects women two to three times more frequently than men. Another inflammatory arthritis is the ankylosing spondylitis, which usually begins during adolescence and in young adults with a pain and stiffness in the lower back that gets worse in the morning, then improves during the day with a hot shower and moderate physical activity. After about 10 years or more, the spine may stiffen in a curved position, especially if the person suffering from it does not pay attention to doing the right exercises and maintaining the correct posture.

Among the extra-articular diseases, we include tendinitis and bursitis. Rotator cuff tendonitis, in which the tendons that help keep the shoulders in the correct position are inflamed, is one of the most frequent causes of the "painful shoulder" due to an overuse of the arms and is typical of bodybuilders. Tennis elbow, golfer's elbow, jumper's knee, sprinter's Achilles tendon are all common forms of tendonitis due to overuse, as is carpal tunnel syndrome, probably the most familiar of all extra-articular types of arthritis. The carpal tunnel is a narrow passage inside the wrist where nerves and tendons pass; if one of the tendons becomes inflamed and, by swelling, presses on the nerves, it causes pain and tingling. Wrist tendons can become inflamed if forced to work too hard in a forced position, such as at the computer keyboard, but also as a result of repeated flexion-extension of the wrists with heavy loads, as occurs in weightlifters and crossfitters.

Bones, ligaments, cartilages and tendons are all made up of connective tissue structured in different shapes. Connective tissue is made up of cells that produce fibers and proteoglycans that come out of the cells and become part of the connective matrix. These fibers include collagen, reticular fibers and elastin. Proteoglycans are molecules of various shapes and sizes and interact with fibers to help maintain the health and strength of the connective tissue. Proteoglycans are complex molecules formed by a central nucleus consisting of a protein and long branched chains sugars bound to it. **Glucosamine** is one of the major constituents of these sugars.

It has been shown (Drovanti) that the oral administration of glucosamine (500 mg three times a day) for at least 3 months, decreases the painful symptoms of osteoarthritis, perhaps because it stimulates the synthesis of proteoglycans. While glucosamine alone is effective, it is even more so when associated with chondroitin sulfate.

Chondroitin sulfate is a glucosaminoglycan and it is synthesized by fibroblasts that stimulates the chondrocytes, i.e. cartilage cells, to produce collagen and proteoglycans, and it also inhibits the enzymes that degrade the latter. In a 1991 study, 200 elderly patients received 1200 mg of glucosaminaglycans formed from chondroitin sulfate, and there was a significant improvement in pain without any side effects. Obviously, it is unthinkable that glucosamine and chondroitin sulfate alone are able to counteract a degenerative disease such as osteoarthritis. The dietary approach is also fundamental, and it must provide a diet rich in fruits and vegetables in order to obtain the right quantities of the antioxidants with protective properties.

In order to enhance collagen in the joints, supplementation with **type II collagen** (a particular type of collagen present in gelatin) was also considered. In a study conducted at Harvard Medical School, purified type II collagen was administered for 3 months to arthritic patients resulting in minor joint swelling and pain. It is believed that supplementation with type II collagen can prevent joint degeneration that occurs with weight training. **Collagen peptides** are made by breaking down whole collagen proteins into smaller pieces. When taken by mouth seem to build up in the skin and cartilage. This might help improve some skin and joint conditions. Numerous scientific studies have shown that collagen peptides can help improve joint health by protecting cartilage from deterioration and helping to reduce inflammation around joints.

Pycnogenol, a pine bark extract, was able to decrease joint pain and stiffness by 55% in patients suffering from arthritis who took it for 3 months. Pycnogenol is both an antioxidant and an anti-inflammatory.

A fundamental prerequisite for joint health is the optimal presence of sulfur. **MSM (methylsulfonylmethane)** is a compound with a high sulfur content that has proven to be particularly effective in the fight against osteoarthritis and joint pain. The proteoglycan molecules are linked together in disulfide bond chains that make the cartilage firmer and more resistant.

Silicon is necessary for the synthesis of elastin and collagen and is important for the health of tendons, bones, connective tissues, cartilage and joints. Collagen acts as a scaffold that provides support for tissues, while elastin provides elasticity.

Turmeric is a spice with numerous beneficial effects, including an anti-inflammatory effect. Turmeric owes its anti-inflammatory effect to its curcuminoid content and specifically to curcumin, which is able to inhibit the enzymes COX1, COX2 and lipoxygenase, responsible for the inflammation. In addition, curcumin increases the receptors for cortisol and also its half-life, thus exerting an enhancement of the anti-inflammatory effect of the same. In one study, subjects suffering from arthritis were administered a mixture of curcumin and ginger (another spice with anti-inflammatory properties) or indomethacin (an NSAID), and the results after 14 and 28 days were practically comparable. Obviously, it goes without saying that these spices are free from the side effects that NSAIDs have.

Among the many properties of **ginger**, there is that of decreasing soreness after intense training with eccentric weights, which is what normally causes more DOMS, that is, delayed muscle pain. It is also able to reduce inflammation after an intense endurance workout, as demonstrated by research carried out by Patrick Wilson at the University of Nebraska (USA).

In Scotland, Jill Bed conducted a study involving 49 subjects with rheumatoid arthritis: these subjects were taking **onagra oil and fish oils**, both of which were rich in essential fatty acids. The aim of the research was to find out the anti-inflammatory effect of polyunsaturated fatty acids that tend to increase the production of type 1 and 3 prostaglandins, as opposed to saturated fats which increase type 2 prostaglandins (with a proinflammatory effect). After 12 months, there was a significant subjective improvement.

Dr. McAlindon of Boston University Medical Center, in a retrospective analysis of 640 subjects, found that low to high **vitamin C** intake inhibits the progression of knee osteoarthritis. Vitamin C exerts this protective effect to a greater extent compared to beta-carotene and vitamin E, because, by being water-soluble, it acts better in the intra-articular aqueous environment. McAlindon and colleagues also found that patients who did not take enough **vitamin D** had a threefold chance of worsening their osteoarthritis. In 1963, Barton & Elliott from England, found low levels of **pantothenic acid (vitamin B5) i**n the blood of 66 people with rheumatoid arthritis. After 7 days of pantothenic acid supplementation and after its levels were normalized, the arthritic symptoms had decreased. Another British researcher (Ammand, 1963) began treating his osteoarthritis patients with a pantothenic acid supplement. Within 14 days from the beginning of the supplementation, 20 out of 25 patients showed a significant improvement. When the supplementation was suspended, the symptoms reappeared, only to improve again when the vitamin was resumed.

It seems that pantothenic acid, being the precursor of coenzyme A, essential for the production of adrenal hormones, favors the production of endogenous "cortisone" with an anti-inflammatory effect. The dosages that proved useful are 1 g per day.

CHAPTER 40

Supplementation and inflammation

by Giovanni Montagna

Let's start by saying that the body's natural healing response is inflammation. Acute inflammation is the trigger of a cascade of biochemical events that follows the repair of a wound or trauma.

Usually, the first action to take is to use non-steroidal anti-inflammatory drugs (NSAIDs) and cortisone, which are effective in relieving pain but carry the risk of a delayed healing.

Anti-inflammatory drugs inhibit the release of prostaglandins, which are responsible for dilating the blood vessels (vasodilation). As a result, the soft tissue healing process is delayed and / or inhibited.

The type of inflammation to fight is the chronic, low-grade and silent one that acts in the long term, while the acute one is to be encouraged.

Which are the main substances that control inflammation?

Eicosanoids, also called "super-hormones", are the first hormones that the body produces; they are biological agents that govern the synthesis of all other hormones in the body, control the immune system, the brain and the heart. They are synthesized from fatty acids and are also modulated through insulin, so they can be controlled through nutrition (omega-3 and omega-6), by regulating the ratio between insulin and glucagon. There are two types of eicosanoids, proinflammatory and anti-inflammatory, which must be kept in balance if you are to live healthily and avoid chronic diseases. An imbalance of eicosanoids, i.e. an increased production of proinflammatory ones, is responsible for chronic inflammation, which is the cause of many diseases: allergies, asthma, arthritis, heart attack, stroke, high blood pressure, cancer, depression, chronic infections, Alzheimer's etc.

Chronic inflammation became known to the general public thanks to an article (advertised on the cover of the magazine) published in *Time Magazine* on February 23, 2004 and the main causes of what has also been dubbed the "silent killer" are our Western lifestyle, sedentary, with a higher ingestion of "junk food" or otherwise foods that are poor in nutrients and rich in calories (mainly carbohydrates with a high glycemic index and industrial fats), and pollution associated with a constant increase in proinflammatory biochemical substances in our body.

What supplements can help us to keep the chronic inflammation under control?

In terms of supplements we also include spice concentrates and foods with a high concentration of nutrients that exert an anti-inflammatory effect.

Alpha-lipoic acid is a molecule comparable to a fatty acid and it is produced by our body. It plays a key role in the energy and antioxidant metabolism, in which it performs the function of protecting the cells from free radical damage, by regenerating the levels of other antioxidants, especially vitamins C and E.

Alpha-lipoic acid also helps in the **reduction of inflammation** linked in particular to insulin resistance, cancer, liver problems, heart disorders and other diseases. Furthermore, it is able to reduce the levels of inflammation markers detected in the blood, such as IL-6 and ICAM-1. **Recommended dosage:** 300-600 mg per day. No problems were found in subjects who took 600 mg of alpha-lipoic acid continuously, for more than 7 months.

Curcumin is a component of turmeric. It provides several benefits for the health of our body. It can decrease inflammation in diabetes, heart disease, inflammatory bowel disease and cancer, to name just a few diseases. Curcumin is also very useful for reducing inflammation and for improving the symptoms of osteoarthritis and rheumatoid arthritis.

A randomized controlled trial found that people with metabolic syndrome who took curcumin, had significantly reduced the levels of CRP and MDA inflammation indicators compared to others who received a placebo. In another study, when 80 people with cancer were given 150 mg of curcumin per day, most of their inflammatory markers decreased much more than in the control group. Their quality of life score also increased significantly.

Curcumin is poorly absorbed when taken alone and as it is, but its absorption can increase up to 2000% if it is taken together with piperine (contained in black pepper). Some supplements also contain a compound called BioPerine®, which works just like piperine and increases curcumin absorption. If it is bound to phospholipids (in the form of liposomal turmeric), absorption increases further. **Recommended dosage:** 100-500 mg per day, when taken with piperine. Dosages of up to 10g per day have been studied and are considered safe, but they can cause digestive side effects.

Fish oil rich in omega-3s. Fish oil supplements contain **omega-3** fatty acids, which are vital for good health. They can decrease the inflammation associated with diabetes, heart disease, cancer and many other conditions.

Two particularly useful types of omega-3s are eicosapentaenoic acid (EPA) and docosahexaenoic acid (DHA). DHA, in particular, has been shown to have anti-inflammatory effects that reduce cytokine levels and promote the intestinal health.

It can also reduce the inflammation and the muscle damage that occur after exercise.

In one study, levels of the inflammation marker IL-6 were found to be 32% lower in people who took 2 g of DHA, compared to a control group. In another study, adding DHA to the daily diet allowed to significantly reduce inflammatory markers such as

TNFα and IL-6 after vigorous exercise. However, some studies on healthy people and people with atrial fibrillation have shown no benefit from adding fish oil to their diets. **Recommended dosage:** 1-1.5 g of omega-3s from EPA and DHA per day. Fish oil supplements with molecularly distilled, undetectable mercury content should be preferred.

Ginger root is usually ground into a powder and added to sweet and savory dishes. It is also commonly used to treat indigestion and nausea. Two components of ginger, gingerol and zingerone, can reduce inflammation linked to colitis, kidney damage, diabetes and breast cancer.

In subjects with diabetes, the administration of 1600 mg of ginger per day allows to obtain lower levels of CRP, insulin and HbA1c, compared to the control group. Another study found that women with breast cancer who took ginger supplements, had lower levels of CRP and IL-6, especially if the intake was associated with exercise. There is also evidence to suggest that ginger supplements can decrease the inflammation and muscle pain after the exercise. **Recommended dosage:** 1 g per day, but up to 2 g is considered safe.

Resveratrol is an antioxidant contained in grapes, blueberries and other fruits with purple skin. It is also present in red wine and peanuts. Resveratrol supplements can reduce the inflammation in individuals with heart disease, insulin resistance, gastritis, ulcerative colitis and other pathological conditions. In one study, people with ulcerative colitis were given 500 mg of resveratrol per day. Their symptoms improved and there was also a reduction in the inflammatory markers CRP, TNF, and NF-κB.

In another study, supplementation with resveratrol was shown to lower the inflammatory markers, triglycerides and blood sugar in people with obesity. The resveratrol contained in red wine can also have beneficial health effects, but the amount present in it is not as high as many think. In fact, red wine contains less than 13 mg of resveratrol per liter, while most studies analyzing the benefits of this substance have used 150 mg or more per day. To get an equivalent amount of resveratrol, you should drink at least 11 liters of wine a day, which is definitely not recommended. **Recommended dosage:** 150-500 mg per day.

Spirulina is a type of blue-green seaweed with strong antioxidant effects. Studies have shown that it reduces inflammation, leads to a healthier aging and it can also strengthen the immune system.

Although most of the research carried out so far has investigated the effects of spirulina on animals, studies on elderly men and women have shown that it can improve the inflammatory markers, anemia and the immune system.

When diabetic people were given 8 g of spirulina per day for 12 weeks, their levels of the inflammation marker MDA decreased. In addition, their levels of adiponectin, a hormone involved in the regulation of blood sugar and fat metabolism that can exert an anti-inflammatory action, was increased. **Recommended dosage:** 1-8 g per day; based on current studies, this dose of spirulina is considered safe.

Astaxanthin has shown its potential as an antioxidant and anti-inflammatory therapeutic agent in cardiovascular disease models.

At least eight clinical studies were conducted on over 180 people using astaxanthin to assess its safety, bioavailability and clinical aspects relevant to oxidative stress, inflammation and its effect on the cardiovascular system. No negative results were reported.

Studies have shown a high capacity in reducing markers of oxidative stress and inflammation, and also an improvement in blood rheology. An increasing number of experimental studies using astaxanthin have been conducted. In particular, animal studies using a reperfusion myocardial ischaemia model have shown protective effects from previous administration of both intravenous and oral astaxanthin.

Future clinical studies will allow to determine the effectiveness of antioxidants such as astaxanthin on the vascular structure, and their functionality on oxidative stress and inflammation, in a variety of patients at risk or with cardiovascular disease.
Recommended dosage: the recommended dosage of astaxanthin in order to obtain an antioxidant effect is 2-4 mg per day; the same dosage is indicated for the protection of the cardiovascular and immune systems. Those who intend to use it as a sports supplement and to promote the health of the nervous system should take dosages of 4-8 mg per day. Its supplementation is also recommended for those who suffer from rheumatoid arthritis, tendonitis, carpal tunnel syndrome, etc. In this case, the recommended dosages are 4-12 mg per day.

Vitamin D. Vitamin D3, a steroid hormone, is a modulator of the immune system that reduces inflammatory cytokines, promotes cell maturation and increases macrophage function. maturing cells and increases macrophage function. **Recommended dosage:** 2000-3000 IU per day.

Vitamin A. Retinoids induce the migration of T cells into the bloodstream, where they are needed, and direct the production of anti-inflammatory type macrophages by inhibiting the production of interleukin-6 thus exerting a modulation of inflammatory cytokines. **Recommended dosage:** 10,000 IU per day.

Acetylcysteine is a donor of thiol-SH groups and is able to increase endogenous production of glutathione (GSH), which is a potent endogenous antioxidant. Acetylcysteine decreases the pro-inflammatory cytokines IL-6, IL-1, and TNF-alpha. **Recommended dosage:** 600 mg per day.

CHAPTER 41

Supplementation for the sexual performance

by Marco Tullio Cau

Humanity has always looked for ways to improve the (male) sexual performance: the testimonies are lost in the mists of time, but this is not the right place to deal with such a vast topic.

The decision to write this chapter arises from the fact that some of the supplements that were mentioned elsewhere in the volume, also have a significant effect on problems of a sexual nature: in fact, the erection of the penis or clitoris is mainly a vascular event. Obviously, there are many other factors involved in both sexual function and dysfunction (neurological, iatrogenic, hormonal, traumatic), but here we will mainly deal with circulatory and hormonal ones.

Furthermore, the sporting lifestyle and a consequent substantially correct diet that those who read this book are probably following, are the best viaticum to optimally preserve not only the muscles, but also the brain, the circulatory system and the sexual functionality.

I have written more extensively on this topic in other books, always edited by Massimo Spattini. However, I did not go into too much detail in the aspect related to supplements.

A good introduction to this topic can be found in "A review on plants used for improvement of sexual performance and virility", by Chauhan et al. (2014), where, in addition to the Ayurvedic vision of the matter, we can find a discussion of numerous herbs that are useful for the problem in question; in the Asia alternative medicine has never lost its importance. Ho and Tan also published a notable review, as did Drewes et al. Not less interesting, and closer to the products that are found in Europe, is the complete review written by Borrelli and a team of Italian researchers ("Herbal dietary supplements for erectile dysfunction: a systematic review and meta-analysis", 2018), the reading of which is certainly recommended.

The analysis of the products sold online by Balasubramian et al. (2019) is very recent and the two parts of "Plant-derived supplements for sexual health and problems", by Rowland et al. (always 2019) are also well thought: one of the authors of this last article, McNabney, sent me the complete copies before finishing this chapter and I think it is useful to read them both, because most of the studies I cited below are dealt with in these books, but in a more in-depth way, thanks to the greater availability of space, which allows a better understanding of the various nuances of the operating modes of a fair number of herbs.

We can divide the various substances into two sectors, albeit broadly: those that aim at an improvement of the hormonal means and those that improve the blood circulation and increase the levels of nitric oxide. Some substances can even fall into both fields.

In this volume, we will talk about supplements that improve the hormonal levels (*Tribulus, Cordyceps*, ZMA) and we will therefore consider only some specific studies, not failing to mention a review from Gunnels and Bloomer which is specific on the subject and it explains the possibilities of herbal extracts in general.

Nitric oxide

It is essential for the erection of the penis (Toda et al., 2005, among many others) and for the swelling of the clitoris: for this specific reason, phosphodiesterase V inhibitors (the famous "blue pills" and similar ones) work precisely on a series of mechanisms that maximize the levels of this ubiquitous substance. Furthermore, let's not forget that NO best expresses its action when testosterone is available on good levels (Zvara et al., 1995), so there is an evident interrelation between the two areas, beyond what is usually highlighted.

Tribulus terrestris

Using 250 mg of the substance (standardized in 112 mg of saponins), Kamenov et al. (2017) obtained excellent results depending on the fields of investigation on *Tribulus terrestris*. So did Zhang et al., but they used mouse models. Meanwhile, Santos et al. (2014), even with a higher dosage, did not find an advantage compared to the placebo group: this reminds us of the importance of standardizing the content and titration of herbal products.

"Pro-sexual and androgen enhancing effects of tribulus terrestris: fact or fiction" by Neychev et al. (2016) was really interesting. The authors, while recognizing the validity of the substance, formulated new hypotheses on the reasons of its effectiveness, probably due to an improvement in the endothelial function and the release of NO.

Excellent results were also obtained by Gamal El Din et al., in a study on 87 hypogonadal patients, with a significance, in some of the evaluated parameters, even of $p < 0.001$, while Roaiah et al. obtained evident increases in testosterone in 30 subjects (always hypogonadal). Zhang et al., in 2019, also highlighted important improvements, but on mouse models, confirming the results of Gauthaman et al. (2003). Spivak et al. (2018) documented the benefits of *Tribulus* on 173 patients while Stasiak et al. wrote an interesting article in 2016, confirming its potential. The studies by Palacios et al., De Souza et al., Vale et al. and Akhtari et al. have a particular importance. The average dosage was around 800 mg.

Cordyceps sinensis

Regarding *Cordyceps sinensis*, Hsu et al. (2003) were able to obtain significant increases in testosterone in laboratory mice, both in vitro and in vivo, and Huang et al., at the turn of the 2000s, also found good results in a number of studies.

Rossi et al. (2014) found significant increases in testosterone in a group of cyclists, using *Cordyceps* in conjunction with another fungus, *Ganoderma lucidum*.

The standard dosage was around 1-1.5 g.

There is also a long list relating to the influence on the sexual behavior of laboratory mice, all with positive results.

Ginkgo biloba

Ginkgo biloba, also recommended for its influence on blood circulation, had good results in a fair amount of studies that evaluated the effect of its administration on mice, but the benefits have been ascribed to neurotransmitter factors: this is plausible, also in relation to what has been seen in the chapter on concentration and a study by Oshio et al. (2015), which did not show great results on testosterone levels, unlike Wu et al.; another hypothesized potential factor is related to an increase in the blood flow.

Two studies report decidedly positive effects, on men and women, on sexual problems due to the use of certain antidepressants, known for some of their side effects (Cohen et al., Wheatley et al.). However, Ashton et al. used 300 mg in both sexes with modest outcomes, as did Kang et al., who found a moderate improvement even in the placebo group, which prompts them to emphasize the power of the mind!

Sohn and Sikora, who in a 1991 study (online in 2015) by administering 240 mg of the substance, reported both objective and objective improvements, which is important in this type of disorders that also greatly affect the psychological sphere of those who suffer from it. Yeh has shown great benefits on rats in three of his studies.

The recommended dosage is between 100 and 600 mg (the average dose is probably already sufficient), with a type of standardized extract that has a content of flavonoids and terpene derivatives of 22-27% and 5-7% respectively. We will also mention here the importance of the quality of herbal products... so be careful! I also cite a couple of studies by Palacios et al. and one by Ito et al., since they administered some products with various contents (ginseng, ginkgo, arginine etc.) and they obtained noteworthy results in female subjects (the half of the universe which is very neglected in these kinds of studies).

DHEA

DHEA (which requires a prescription in Italy, while it is free for sale in the USA) is a hormone that begins to decline from the third decade of life and whose decline is associated with a whole series of degenerative diseases related to aging: its role in nitric oxide metabolism and the related effects on smooth muscle and endothelium may suggest its potential use for the erectile dysfunction (ED), especially when its blood levels are low.

El Sakka, in 2018, described all the aspects in detail, in a review whose reading is certainly recommended, given the fact that it analyzes both the pros and cons; moreover, since it is recent, a large part of the published studies can be found there, such as that of Reiter et al., which obtained good results with a supplement of 50 mg; Lee et al., on the other hand, used female animal models, again with interesting results.

Liu et al. observed significant increases in testosterone with 50 mg supplements, even without specifically investigating the disorders of the sexual sphere. We recall that DHEA drops drastically after the fourth decade: its role in the hormonal orchestra is complex, and the discussion is not possible here. The dosages that are often used in these studies are around 50 mg, but a prescription is required.

Citrulline and arginine

When we look at the supplements that could increase the NO levels, citrulline and arginine immediately catch our eye: the second is the one that received the most attention first, thanks to the fact that it is directly involved in the synthesis of this ubiquitous gas, the discovery of which brought a Nobel Prize to three researchers who, at different times, made a decisive contribution to its exact definition.

A study carried out in Italy by Barassi et al. shows us the importance of these two amino acids ("Low levels of these nitric oxide synthase substrates might increase the erectile dysfunction risk by reducing the concentration of nitric oxide"), but it goes far beyond this fact. Those who have an arteriogenic erectile dysfunction are found to have the lowest levels, differentiating from those who have a psychological etiology, who obviously find the reason for their problem elsewhere.

This is a concept that would have been revolutionary only half a century ago, when the erectile deficit was largely ascribed to psychological problems!

As already specified, arginine has had more attention under the spotlight, but not only because of its direct function: some companies have produced compounds that (also) contain this amino acid.

In fact, we often find clinical trials that see this substance coupled to the **pycnogenol**: Lamm, Ledda and Stanislavov have obtained significant results by administering this commercial product, like Aoki, which has an independent combination of these two substances.

Is this synergy beneficial? Definitely, since the polyphenol extracted from the *Pinus pinaster* is very effective.

A very recent review by Rhim et al. comes to our aid. (2019), in which we can see how arginine alone is able to produce good results, even if the dosages vary from 1.5 to 5 g per day. Others, such as Klotz et al., found no benefit with the 1.5 g dosage, unlike Chen et al. who obtained positive results only with the highest dosage, as did Mozaffari et al., again with 5 g.

Zorgniotti and Lizza, had already tested successfully dosages of around 3 g in 1997. So did Moody et al., but on rats of advanced age.

Also, the review by Koolwal et al., also from 2019, confirms the above, including the wish to have a greater number of studies, with a better uniformity of parameters.

Some studies have not shown significant results; according to Bode-Böger et al., and the reason is that in the absence of certain pathological conditions, a surplus of arginine does not improve the synthesis of NO, certainly because arginine, although directly involved in the NO release mechanism, has the problem to be partially deactivated at two different pre-systemic levels before being able to carry out its precious functions.

It precursor, citrulline, comes into play at this exact moment. It has the advantage of undergoing the partial intestinal and hepatic deactivation to a lesser extent than arginine; however, unfortunately there are fewer studies, at least in this specific field of investigation.

Ochiai et al., albeit indirectly, have demonstrated the contribution that this substance can offer to solve some sexual problems, given the excellent results obtained with 5.6 g dosage (!) on the arterial stiffness, an important circulatory parameter, obviously, not only in the field we are dealing with. Tsuboi et al. have shown how citrulline not only reduces, but also reverses the endothelial senescence.

Some of the Japanese authors cited above (with Ignarro in addition) have also demonstrated the efficacy of citrulline on the endothelium-dependent vasodilation, on the intensity of the blood flow, a very consistent regression of atheromatous lesions and also a reduction of the superoxide that causes damage to the endothelium. A study by Cormio et al. reports substantial improvements with only 1.5 g of citrulline.

On the other hand, Shiota et al. obtained excellent results on mouse models, not only at the level of NO but also on parameters such as the smooth muscle/collagen *ratio*. The same results were found by Hotta et al., this time on castrated rats.

However, the excellent results obtained at the level of the maximization of the blood flow (often in the formula coupled with **malic acid**), are also excellent "references" and, moreover, as suggested by De Tejada, providing the precursors of NO can also improve the pharmacological effects of phosphodiesterase V inhibitors ("blue pills" and similar drugs) in subjects who do not obtain the expected benefits (30-40%).

Pycnogenol

I mentioned pycnogenol earlier, which is a flavonoid-rich substance capable of increasing (also) the endothelium-dependent vasodilation, extracted from the bark of a certain species of pine from southern France. The history of its discovery is special, but too long for this site; studies abound, again thanks to the fact that a company has registered the patent.

Since I have experienced it in various circumstances, I can say that, for once, its potential is not only a result of the marketing: for example, it is particularly effective in decreasing the swelling and stagnation that occur during long-haul air travel.

Research relating to sexual problems was partially mentioned previously, in conjunction with arginine. About its administration alone, Duračková et al. have highlighted the advantages on erectile deficit and on LDL cholesterol levels at a dose of 120 mg/day, while Enseleit et al., describe general effects, on the correlated endothelial function.

There is a myriad of research on the effects at the endothelial level, therefore related to sexual disorders, but since they are not specific, they will not be mentioned.

The recommended dosage is 60-180 mg, but unfortunately, the fact that pycnogenol has been patented has made its cost quite high.

Yohimbine

Among the herbal products we will also mention yohimbine, banned in many countries including Italy, but "tolerated" in the USA, at least in low doses. The problem is that it is often included without mentioning it in many products, in unspecified dosages, as evidenced by a 2015 study carried out at a US Army base and one at Harvard Medical School.

This substance, which is extracted from the tree from which it takes its name, can also cause pressure changes and heart rate increases and, given the uncertainty about the actual dosages, its use by those with cardiovascular problems is not recommended.

In fact, yohimbine exerts an antagonistic effect on a_2-adrenergic receptors, which are important in regulating the release of neurotransmitters from nerve endings, followed by an increase in the noradrenergic activity which allows an increase in blood flow and nerve impulses to the genital organs. However, the fact that it does not imply this function on the same receptors in other parts of the body explains the high probability of causing the aforementioned side effects, even minor ones, such as headaches, strong agitation and insomnia; moreover, it fights the side effects of some anti-depressant drugs that affect sexual activity.

The first study to be mentioned is that of Akhondzadeh et al., which used yohimbine in conjunction with the aforementioned arginine, on subjects with a moderate degree of ED who had a "significant difference" compared to the placebo group after 4 weeks; the same combination (6-7 mg yohimbine + 6 g arginine) and the same results were obtained by Lebret et al. and Kernohan et al. (the latter also evaluated the hypotensive effects in the co-use with nitroglycerin, a practice that instead proves problematic with phosphodiesterase V inhibitors). The clinical trial by Guay et al. reports good results, again in subjects with modest/medium degree ED, with different doses, 15/30 mg three times a day, with the highest dose having the most consistent improvements.

Discrete results were obtained by Vogl et al. with 30 mg dosages, while a review by Carey, analyzing various studies, highlighted "a trend towards a moderate improvement in erectile function".

Pittler also found moderate improvements, while Sonda et al. report a 38% partial satisfaction, coming to the hypothesis that the effect is dose-dependent (15/20 mg were administered) and also adding that this hypothesis should be tested (certainly, I add, given the possibility of side effects!).

A work by Tam et al. tackles the topic very thoroughly and combines the good results with the potential negative effects of the highest dosages, assuming that the synergy with certain NO precursors is the winning way.

Susset et al. reached up to 42 mg, not experiencing significant side effects and finding 34% positive results, between total and partial.

Pushkar et al. described results as from fair to excellent, depending on the severity of the disease, always with 15/20 mg dosages.

Morales is very interesting, who in various works defines yohimbine as "an orphan drug": as it is not patentable, the large pharmaceutical companies are not interested in studying it further. Yet, the author continues, there are years of scientific insights that could and should be exploited (also) to test alternative routes of administration; but probably "we will never know", given its status as an "outlaw". Lebret et al. combined 6 mg of yohimbine with 6 g of arginine glutamate, obtaining noteworthy results that prompted them to declare that this could be a very promising combination, to be investigated further.

However, 30 mg dosages divided into three different times of the day can be considered sufficient, **with all the limitations**.

Furthermore, many authors question the real content of the various products, more than in other cases.

Ginseng

For ginseng, a psycho-tonic capable of acting also at the endothelial level, good results were obtained from a review by Jang et al. (2008) (although hoping for a greater number of insights), as well as from a study by Choi et al. (1995) on 90 patients (fair statistical significance, $p < 0.05$) and one by De Andrade et al. (2007) on 60 subjects (from $p < 0.001$ to 0.05, depending on the parameters); equally valid results were obtained in animal models in 2013 by Lin et al. and Kim et al., and in 2014 by Li et al.

Tode et al. and Wiklund et al. studied the effects of ginseng on postmenopausal women, with more than a moderate success.

A substantial bibliography can be obtained from Lee et al., In "Ginseng for erectile dysfunction" (2018); the average dosage is around 600-800 mg of extract.

Icariin

Icariin is another interesting phytoextract, which is extracted from plants of the *Epimedium* genus and which improves the blood flow and exerts an activity similar to phosphodiesterase V inhibitors: in the USA, the plant from which it is extracted is known as the horny goat weed, from a legend about the effect that this herb would have on goats...

The potential related to the inhibition of PDE5 and NO-cGMP are confirmed by numerous trials: dell'Agli et al., Jiang et al., Ning et al., Zing et al., Xu et al... a plebiscite! Liu et al. carried out two studies on laboratory mice, finding hemodynamic improvements, an improved integrity of the smooth muscles and the endothelium, as well as, as expected, the ability to inhibit PDE5, while Shindel et al. also reported a neurotrophic effect.

Tian et al. praise its qualities in relation to the improvement of the erectile function, while Makarova et al. used an oily extract of epimedium and found an increase in the sexual activity of the mouse models.

The dosages extrapolated from the studies on guinea pigs reach up to 200 mg/kg of a 40% extract (80 mg/kg of icariin) or 10 mg/kg, based on the trials that used lower quotas: given that the substance is not legal in Italy and that excessive ingestion is not free from various risks and interactions, what has just been written is to be considered only at a level of hypothesis (in the USA, however, it is a substance of a freely commercially available and the dosages are quite high, but however, it is necessary to check the percentage of icariin: a capsule of 1500 g at 10% makes an impression only on the label...).

To complete its discussion, Zhang et al. also highlighted an increase in blood testosterone levels.

Peruvian maca

Another phytoextract is the Peruvian maca, which is extracted from *Lepidium meyenii*, which has been used for centuries in Central and South America to improve sexual function.

Zenico et al. achieved good results in subjects with a moderate degree of ED while Shin et al. reported fair results, but pointed them to the limited number of studies. A trial by Gonzales et al. reported an increase in sexual desire starting from the fourth week, with dosages of 1.5 or 3 g. Dording et al. carried out a double-blind study on post-menopausal female subjects, noting how maca (3 g) alleviated the sexual disorders due (also) to the use of antidepressants.

Brooks et al. used a sample of the same type, confirming the results that we mentioned above (with 3.5 g) and adding that the benefits are not derived from estrogenic or androgenic differences; similar results are found in Lee et al. and Meissner et al.

Zhenh et al. and Cicero et al., in two studies, reported excellent results in the sexual behavior of laboratory mice.

Dosages vary from 1.5 to 3 g, always trusting in the quality of the product and therefore in its content.

Other substances

Pomegranate extract, rich in antioxidants and with an estrogen modulating effect, has also shown promise, as reported by Azadzoi et al. in a study that explains the importance of this substance at the vascular health level and therefore, also (but not only) on the sexual level (see also Forest et al. and Kroeger). It is also confirmed by Ignarro, one of the scholars awarded the Nobel Prize for discoveries related to nitric oxide, who also wrote a study with De Nigris.

Another substance, **D-acetyl-glucosamine** (KP2647), obtained from chitosan, has been the subject of some promising studies and has been tested, together with Tribulus and a seaweed, by a team of researchers led by Dr. Iacono, demonstrating some influence on nitric oxide.

Even zinc (especially **ZMA**) has its importance, but it is more about the optimization of nutrition: I am not talking about a diet because, otherwise, we would have to refer more specifically to the original term, the Greek *diaita*, δίαιτα (lifestyle), which rightly includes physical activity, rest, etc.

A few lines should be added in relation to antioxidants, a term that embraces a vast array of substances, usually ingested for a similarly ample umbrella of pathologies.

I can mention, for example, *Glutathione levels in patients with erectile dysfunction, with or without diabetes mellitus* (Tagliabosco et al., 2005) where one can read that "Antioxidant defenses are reduced in men with ED [...] reduced levels of glutathione (GSH), an important intracellular antioxidant, men with and without diabetes had significant decreases of GSH if they also had ED".

Oral glutathione is not absorbed very well, unless taken in a special formulation, not readily accessible everywhere and to everyone, so one can turn up to acetylcysteine, actually a glutathione precursor (a minireview on N-acetylcysteine… Dhouib et al., 2016), a much cheaper and obtainable product.

Alternatively, in *A Dietary flavonoid intake and incidence of erectile dysfunction* (Cassidy et al., 2016), the authors write that "in analyses stratified by age, a higher intake of flavanones, anthocyanins, and flavones was significantly associated with a reduction in risk of ED in men [...] because a higher intake of several flavonoids reduces diabetes and cardio-vascular disease risk".

The list of antioxidants is too long for this particular chapter, but their use shouldn't be forgotten or underestimated.

Some folates and other B vitamins can help people that suffer from an excess of homocysteine, known for its adverse effects on cardiovascular endothelium and smooth muscle cells and therefore the insurgence of ED (Giovannone et al., 2015).

I would like also to underline the importance of oral health, in general, but also in relation to ED, as an ample evidence strongly supports the fact that periodontal disease is a major risk factor for various systemic diseases namely cardio-vascular disease, diabetes mellitus and, actually, ED.

One last mention for D vitamin: dozens of researches are in agreement with the theory that Vitamin D deficiency is independently associated with greater prevalence of erectile dysfunction (Farag et al., 2016), which is another role for this polyhedric substance.

The list is still long, as said, too much for these pages, and let's not forget that swallowing a few pills, cannot make up for essentially a bad diet!

Conclusions

We have mentioned how the use of some substances can favor the action of PDE5 inhibitors, providing a more efficient substrate, and in some cases, such as pomegranates- the efficiency was even too high, as highlighted by Senthilkumaran et al. in "Priapism, pomegranate juice, and sildenafil: Is there a connection?" and also reiterated by Lee et al.

As mentioned at the beginning, a lifestyle that includes the right relationship between the physical activity and the recovery phase, and a diet that is rich in the right nutrients, without excessive calories, is the best way to go for the longest possible but healthy life; the use of some nutritional precautions is part of this picture, as we can see, for example in "The andrologist's contribution to a better life for aging men: part 2" by Comhaire and Mahmoud.

As a reference to some books, written by well-known authors in the field, Meldrum and Gambone, in the evocative *Survival of the firmest*, they advise to exercise, not to eat too much (especially some foods), to use **omega-3**, **arginine/citrulline**, **folates**, **antioxidants**, not to smoke... in short, what we said above.

The same authors have a website where you can find a lot of information on erectile function and they have also written numerous scientific articles on the subject which are very interesting and complete, together with Prof. Ignarro, such as "A multifaceted approach to maximize erectile function and vascular health". In this article, they propose very stimulating concepts, such as the phylogenetic reasons for the redundancy of NO secretion and the importance of a multifactorial approach.

Two other milestones in this sector, with perfectly fitting titles, also by the same team, are *The link between erectile and cardiovascular health: the canary in the coal mine*, a true classic, and *Erectile hydraulics: maximizing inflow while minimizing outflow*. The latter has also the contribution of Dorey and Esposito, two equally famous specialists.

Another expert in the field, Steven Lamm, in *The hardness factor*, confirms what has just been written, adding pycnogenol and icariin.

Dr. Moyad (in the volume titled *Oral pharmacotherapy for male sexual dysfunction: a guide to clinical management*, edited by Gregory A. Broderick) wrote a chapter dealing with lifestyle modifications and nutritional supplements entitled "What works and what is worthless", in which he more or less inserts supplements and lifestyle changes, adding androstenedione and DHEA.

Androstenedione, on the other hand, has not given noteworthy results in the specific field and is in any case illegal even in the US.

Dr. Moyad pointed out that research must also develop towards experimenting with the joint use of PDE5 inhibitors and the supplements we have covered, given that the synergy appears to be promising, as we have seen, and that non-responders to the former could benefit from their synergy.

However, in other books, including *Male sexual function: a guide to clinical management*, edited by Mulcahy, there are only five lines dedicated to the subject, out of nearly 500 pages; however, the supplements - *briefly mentioned* - are more or less the same.

In conclusion, the use of some of the substances that we mentioned - and many not mentioned but highly publicized - is still poorly supported by sufficient scientific evidence, while others are better accepted by the scientific community. One thing remains clear: even the most effective ones must still be a small part of a larger design, one that focuses on a **balanced diet and the right amount of movement**.

Supplementation for the heart
by Paolo Conforti

Treating the heart is quite complex due to the metabolic implications of this organ and its function of support for all other organs and systems. The heart is composed of a contractile structure that mediates its pump action (which works perpetually and with certain metabolic characteristics) and a nerve stimulation tissue that mediates the transformation of the electrical impulse in mechanical work. The myocyte (the heart cell) has intermediate characteristics between smooth muscles and striated muscles (cells with smaller nuclei like the smooth muscle, but organized in sarcomeres like the striated muscle). Myocytes are communicating with each other and, when the stimulus arrives, they behave like a single large cell contracting almost in unison (syncytium type). Being an always active muscle, it has a purely aerobic metabolism and, to support this continuous production of energy and the cytoplasm of these cells, they are very rich in mitochondria (which make up about a third of the organ). For these reasons, the extraction of oxygen is very high at the level of this organ and the blood that carries it is conveyed by a network of vessels and capillaries that is considerably extended (much more than other muscles). These characteristics make the heart extremely dependent on oxygen for its pump activity, with a preferential fuel given by fats (we will see how important its mitochondrial transporter carnitine will be) and, subsequently, glucose and lactate. During physical effort a large part of the lactate produced by the muscles and put into circulation is metabolized by the heart, but always aerobically. Cardiac function therefore depends on vascularization, the supply of substrates and oxygen, cardiac metabolism understood as transporters, enzymes, complexes of the mitochondrial respiratory chain, etc. The force of contraction (inotropism) depends on the energy level of the cell and the correct entry and extrusion of calcium into the cytoplasm, which describes the cardiac cycle. The heart is inextricably linked with the peripheral muscles by a compensatory mechanism. If we are inactive and the peripheral skeletal muscles extract oxygen in an inefficient manner, the heart will have to beat more to compensate for this fact. If, on the other hand, our periphery is performing well, fewer beats will be enough to ensure a correct perfusion (one of the reasons why those who do aerobic sports have a lowering of the heart rate). Therefore, the heart is a particular muscle and understanding its physiology allows us to understand the possible areas of intervention, especially with a view to prevention.

Cardiovascular health has always been the health goal of all industrialized countries. People still die a lot from heart problems. Heart attacks are a silent killer that often does not give signs and, when it does, if you are lucky enough to survive, it often radically changes people's lives. Cardiovascular diseases remain the leading cause of death in the world and are mostly treated with a pharmacological approach aimed at minimizing the contribution of the main risk factors for heart diseases. Thus, in primary prevention (i.e. before there is a full-blown pathology), we often end up treating hypertension with an ACE inhibitor, cholesterol with a statin, diabetes with an oral hypoglycemic agent and so on. If there was a drug that cancels the effects of smoking, I am sure it would be very popular (of course, instead of quitting smoking). The fact that there is a tendency to do few blood chemistry tests for cost reasons, does not allow in itself for problems to be intercepted in time. Often, one realizes how much neglected one has been over the years, only in the course of evaluations made for other reasons (serendipity). However, not that this reflection of mine is not the usual ban on drugs. When there are important problems such as heart problems, medicines must be taken but it is true that they are often given by specialists and are not re-evaluated for years, until during a hospitalization, maybe a geriatrician takes the trouble to identify at what point the situation is at and to prescribe something. Drugs can be modulated, in some cases up to weaning (mainly in primary prevention, but something can also be modulated in a secondary prevention, i.e. after a cardiovascular event).

However, a whole series of precautions can be taken to avoid taking them or to delay their intake as much as possible. Over the years, supplements have become increasingly popular due to their preventive-therapeutic values, but they have also been used as adjuvants for pharmacological therapies at various levels. The scientific debate on heart supplements is still very heated and controversial, with major scientific societies of cardiology often distancing themselves from the use of vitamins and supplements. So, let's see what are the supplements that may have some indication in this area.

Vitamins

In Sweden, where fruit and vegetable consumption is low, a case-control study on the relationship between vitamin supplements and myocardial infarction (MI) showed an inverse association between a low intake of multivitamins and the incidence of MI. In contrast, in 2011, a large multi-ethnic study of 182,099 participants showed no significant association between taking multivitamins for more than 10 years and the risk of heart diseases. For multivitamins, evidence on the prevention of heart disease is still scarce, probably due to the different dosages, different reference populations and different methods of intake in the various studies. The only vitamin that seems to have strong correlations with the evidence on prevention is vitamin D. Low levels of vitamin D are associated with an increase in insulin resistance, hyperlipidemia and hypertension (all risk factors for heart disease). Many studies associate vitamin D deficiency with the severity and progression of the atheromatous disease (see below), while proper production would lead to the formation of life-saving collateral circulation in the heart. It therefore seems that most recent studies support the direct association between vitamin D deficiency and heart disease.

Coenzyme Q10 (CoQ10)

According to some publications, CoQ10 supplementation improves the cardiovascular conditions in several ways. Some authors have reported that CoQ10 supplementation improves the myocardial contractility, increasing the ejection fraction on heart failure patients, while others have shown how its intake could affect the endothelial function (coronary artery tone and peripheral perfusion are controlled by the endothelium, see below). A 2002 study (Landmesser et al.) showed that CoQ10 attenuates the production of the free radicals of oxygen (ROS) for low density lipoproteins, decreasing them (OX-LDL, cardio-cardiovascular risk factor). The protective effect of CoQ10 against lipid peroxidation was studied in patients with atherosclerosis in 2012. Lee et al. have shown that the supplementation of 150 mg/day of CoQ10 in 43 patients with coronary artery disease is associated with a lower oxidative stress and a lower production of the proinflammatory interleukin IL-6. Furthermore, administering Q10 in the context of a Mediterranean diet, especially in the elderly, reduces the expression of genes related to inflammation and stress. We know how hypercholesterolemia has correlations with heart disease in the literature, which is why statins are prescribed to lower it. The synthesis of cholesterol and CoQ10 depends on the activity of the 3-hydroxy-3-methylglutaryl coenzyme A (HMG-CoA) reductase. Statins inhibit HMG-CoA reductase, also blocking the production of CoQ10. The deficiency of CoQ10 and its consequences on the mitochondrial functions (it is part of the respiratory chain complexes) partly explains the incidence of myopathies induced by the use of statins in patients with a genetic susceptibility. Therefore, the supplementation of CoQ10 should even be encouraged in those who take statins. However, it seems that this is still not entirely clear, given that there is no unanimous consensus on the improvement of myopathies with the use of CoQ10.

Omega 3

We know how cardiac pathology largely depends on the atheromatous pathology, with the formation of lipid plaques in the arterial vessels which tend to stenate or occlude the lumen of these vessels when they become fixed. Atheromasia is caused by an inflammatory state of the vessel, which degenerates by infiltrating lipids and inflammatory cells with the production of oxygen free radicals (ROS), fibrin by fibroblasts, etc. Not all the plaques are the same and they are divided into stable and unstable, according to their predisposition to ulcerate. The ulceration of the plaque produces an activation of the coagulation factors which leads to complete occlusion of the vessel and an ischemia of the downstream tissues. The omega-3s would stabilize the unstable plaques, following a prompt absorption by them. As we know, omega-3s (EPA and DHA) have important functions in our body, including the anti-inflammatory role and maintaining the membrane fluidity. It is also true that modern diets (in particular the low consumption of fish), on the other hand, produce an increase in pro-inflammatory omega-6s. It seems that the increase in the omega-3/6 ratio over the decades has been accompanied by the increase in the organic inflammatory state (Low Grade Inflammation, LGI), which would be the common denominator of many frequent diseases (for example, all hypokinetic pathologies). Unfortunately, supplementation is often necessary, especially in subjects who do not consume fish, because the conversion of the plant precursors of omega-3 into EPA and DHA, is in fact frequently complicated by many factors (stress, excess of omega-6, old age, alcohol consumption, enzyme deficiencies, etc.). The American Heart Association recommends eating fatty fish (salmon, mackerel, herring, anchovies, sardines) at least twice a week (other studies indicate at least three), preferably small in size to avoid contamination by heavy metals and endocrine disruptors in general. Some European guidelines suggest supplementing omega-3s at dosages of 2-4 g/day to lower hypertriglyceridemia (which predisposes to cardiovascular diseases, as well as pancreatitis). Here, the mechanism would seem to be attributed to a decrease in lipogenesis and an increase in lipolysis. Lipidomics is emerging as a promising test for cardiovascular risk assessment. It assumes a measurement of the composition of the erythrocyte membrane and its components – arachidonic acid (AA), EPA, DHA, monounsaturated and polyunsaturated – with a gas chromatograph. The ratios of particular interest to the therapist are the omega-3 index (omega-3 ratio on total fatty acids), the AA/EPA ratio (arachidonic/EPA), the SFA/MUFA ratio (saturated/monounsaturated), the activity of desaturases (enzymes that convert omega-3 precursors into EPA and DHA) etc.

In particular, if the omega-3 index is <4% there would be a marked risk of heart disease, while the minimum safe value would be an omega-3 index> 8% (Harris et al., 2008).

Beetroot juice and "NO-boosters" (arginine and citrulline)

Beetroot juice is used because it can act as a precursor to nitric oxide (NO). It is believed that the mechanism of NO synthesis is due to the catabolism of arginine by the enzyme NO synthase (NOS). In fact, it has been shown that supplementing arginine or citrulline increases the NO levels. An alternative mechanism of the NO genesis is mediated by the inorganic nitrate found in beet juice, the high amount of which is able to increase the levels of NO in the body.

In the mouth, about 25% of the dietary nitrate is reduced to nitrites by a reductase produced by resident microorganisms, which are then reduced to NO through the subsequent action of the gastric acid. Nitrates are a significant component of our diets, mostly coming from green leafy vegetables. In the past, an excess of these molecules and the nitrite pool in particular, alarmed the scientific community for its association with carcinogenesis. The discovery of a metabolic pathway in mammals where nitrate is reduced to nitrite and NO, has justified a re-examination of the physiological role of this small molecule, which has consistently been shown to offer protection against obesity, type II diabetes and metabolic diseases. NO has numerous physiological functions at an organic level, which include hemodynamic and metabolic aspects. NO has an effect on smooth muscle fibers and causes blood vessels to dilate. This vasodilation effect increases the blood flow to the muscles, favoring the gas exchange and also inducing an improvement in biogenesis and mitochondrial efficiency, and all these aspects together can favor the cellular energy level. At the cardiac level, NO production must be carefully supported and for this action, there are three different ways of NO production at the cardiomyocyte level. The subcellular compartmentalization of these enzymatic isoforms imposes a specific signaling pathway for each of them, in response to specific physical stimuli (an example is the stretching of the heart chambers) or through a receptor. Gene suppression and overexpression experiments helped to characterize the respective role of each isoform in the normal and diseased heart. Endothelial NOS (e-NOS) and neurogenic-derived NOS (n-NOS) both help support the normal coupling between nervous excitation and myocardial contraction. The e-NOS form is more localized in the cytoplasm, while the n-NOS form is found in the mitochondria. They also inhibit the adrenergic stimuli mediated by β1 and β2 receptors (which would increase the heart rate and the contraction under stress), while strengthening vagal control (pre- and post-synaptic), thus protecting the heart from excessive stimulation by catecholamines. In the ischemic and non-functioning myocardium, the expression of another inducible isoform (i-NOS) increases, which further contributes to attenuating the effect of catecholamines. Many drugs that are currently used for the treatment of ischemic heart diseases directly or indirectly activate and/or increase the production of e-NOS in the myocardium, mediating a kind of cardioprotection. I allow myself a parenthesis on exercise: numerous researches have found that beet juice supplementation increases the performance, involving resistance exercises (aerobic metabolism), but a meta-analysis from 2018 (Domínguez et al.) concluded that beetroot juice supplementation reduces the muscle fatigue also associated with power exercises. Since phosphocreatine resynthesis requires an oxidative metabolism, beet juice could help restore the phosphocreatine reserves and thus also improve the alactacid anaerobic metabolism. In parallel, supplementation would limit the accumulation of metabolites such as ADP and inorganic phosphates, which are known to induce muscle fatigue. Beetroot juice was also shown to improve the release and reabsorption of calcium in the sarcoplasmic reticulum. This would facilitate the energy production associated with improvements in the muscle shortening speed. This brief examination of the role of beet juice on the skeletal muscle metabolism underlines why an improvement in the peripheral muscle function (as appears from the evidence gathered so far) always invariably leads to an indirect improvement in the heart level (in particular a decrease in heart rate). Arginine, citrulline and beetroot juice would therefore seem to have a positive effect on the cardiac performance, both directly and indirectly, an effect that would have the production of NO as its fulcrum.

Taurine

This amino acid is considered semi-essential for humans but it has strategic importance in many diseases, including heart disease. In Japan, taurine supplementation is used successfully in people with congestive heart failure (in whom it was seen that treating its deficiency improved the outcome of heart failure [Jeejeebhoyet et al., 2002]). This effective treatment subsequently spurred research into other possible uses of taurine and the discoveries were particularly interesting. A noteworthy study was conducted by the World Health Organization (WHO), which involved 50 population groups in 25 different countries of the world, and reports how a high consumption of taurine in the diet is associated with a reduced risk of hypertension and hypercholesterolemia (Sagara et al., 2015). Taurine supplementation is also linked to the reduction of the body mass index (Yamori et al., 2010) and to the reduction of the levels of inflammation markers in obese women (Rosa et al., 2014). The commonality of these researches, but also of many others, seems to be what is called the cytoprotective effect of taurine. First of all, taurine has an anti-inflammatory and antioxidant effect: anti-inflammatory because it directly neutralizes the products of activated macrophages (particularly hypochlorous acid) and antioxidant because it stimulates the activity of complex I of the respiratory chain (which has a very little effect in conditions of low taurine availability). If the mitochondrial respiratory chain is inefficient, there will be a decrease in the production of ATP and therefore a decrease of energy for the cell. There will also be an increase of the free radicals at the mitochondrial level, with membrane damage and mitochondrial DNA leakage at the cytosol level. Therefore, it brings a mitochondrial dysfunction that can worsen the function of the remaining mitochondria (further increase in ROS) and of the cell as a whole, with a subsequent apoptosis. On the other hand, supplementation with taurine would seem to block this vicious circle. On an energy level, a dysfunction of the respiratory chain leads to a decrease in the oxidation of fatty acids and a blockage of the citric acid cycle (related to the deficiency of taurine which would down-regulate the PPARα pathway). PPARα regulates several proteins and enzymes involved in the metabolism of fatty acids, the most important of which is the acetylcarnitine transport complex, which is essential for transporting fatty acids into the mitochondrion. Another cytoprotection mechanism is the blockade of oxidative stress at the endoplasmic reticulum level. When the endoplasmic reticulum is subjected to an excessive level of free radicals, the relationship between the production of proteins and their disposal is impaired, with an accumulation of the latter at the cellular level. Taurine would improve the control at this level by stimulating the intracellular autophagy. A further mechanism is the one related to the control of the intracytoplasmic calcium pool, in which taurine indirectly regulates the activity of the sarcoplasmic reticulum Ca^{2+} ATPase, which mediates the removal of calcium ions from the cytosol (Ramila et al., 2015). Last but not least in the cardiology field, like all the previous ones, is the diuretic and natriuretic effect of taurine on the kidney. Taurine exerts a mild positive inotropic effect on the hypokinetic heart and promotes natriuresis and diuresis. One of the main therapeutic effects of chronic administration of taurine seems to involve a reduction in the tone of noradrenaline and angiotensin II (known to reduce the performance of the myocardium – drugs such as beta-blockers and ACE-Is are used for a reason in this case). Although recent studies have shown that taurine therapy improves the exercise capacity of patients with heart failure (Ahmadian et al., 2017), it remains to be established whether taurine supplementation also reduces the risk of developing heart failure in the general population. However, there is reason to believe that taurine can prolong the life span of patients with heart failure, because it increases the availability of ATP in myocardiocytes. Taurine also appears to have an effect on hypertension. In 2016 a study (Sun et al.) investigated the vasodilatory effects of taurine on some patients with pre-hypertension (i.e. when the systolic is between 130 and 139 mmHg and the diastolic between 85 and 89 mmHg). The study was a single-center, double-blind, randomized, placebo-controlled study of 120 pre-hypertensive subjects, aged 18 to 75 years. After the administration of taurine (1.6 g/day) for 12 weeks, the subjects' systolic blood pressure was reduced by 7.2 mmHg and the diastolic blood pressure by 4.7 mmHg, while the placebo-treated subjects showed no sign of decreased blood pressure in the same treatment period. Administration of taurine resulted in a 1.5-fold increase in the plasma concentration of this substance. The study concluded that the reduction in blood pressure mediated by taurine was due to a better dilation mediated by NO. This would confirm a study of the same year (Katakawa et al., 2016) which reached the same conclusions and an old study (Ogawa et al., 1985) which observed that the plasma taurine pool was very low in subjects with essential hypertension. Atherosclerosis itself would benefit from taurine supplementation. The WHO-CARDIAC epidemiological study has shown that the intake of taurine in the diet is related to a reduced mortality of patients with ischemic heart disease (Yamori et al., 2001). In support, other studies have found that taurine increases the beneficial effects of omega-3 fatty acid supplementation on total cholesterol, LDL cholesterol, and triglycerides. Recently, Katakawa et al. (2016) noted a reduced risk of atherogenesis with a nutritional intervention (a diet supplemented with taurine and magnesium) which led to a reduction in the oxidative stress and an improvement in the endothelial function. Therefore, the multitude of the studies concerning the effects of taurine on cardiovascular well-being seems to be really conspicuous. I will conclude the discussion on taurine by emphasizing how mitochondrial dysfunction is also fundamental in the pathogenesis of diabetes (cardiological risk factor) and how treating it with taurine can improve the body's oxidative glycemic picture (also here, direct and indirect effects).

Carnitine

Carnitine is an amino acid, responsible for the transport of long-chain fatty acids within the mitochondria, where they will be used for energy purposes (beta-oxidation). It can be synthesized within the human body in the liver and partly in the kidney and brain.

Carnitine levels are much higher in the heart than in plasma (an extraction against a concentration gradient of about 60 times), since this transporter is essential for organs such as the heart, which use purely fats for their metabolism. Older people may suffer from a relative carnitine deficiency. Serum levels of carnitine tend to be stable up to about 70 years, while subsequently they undergo a decrease for reasons that are still unclear, probably due to the poor digestion of foods of animal origin that these subjects often suffer from (carnitine, in fact, tends to be in short supply even in vegans).

Carnitine, in the form of propionyl-L-carnitine (PLC), has been shown to improve the symptoms and the exercise capacity in patients with peripheral arterial disease (a form of occluding atheroma in the lower limbs that is usually concomitant with the cardiac atheroma). Acetylcarnitine, on the other hand, appears to have a sensitizing effect on the peripheral testosterone receptors (a hormone with a cardioprotective effect). A multicenter study (CEDIM Trial) conducted on 500 patients with severe myocardial infarction, performed intravenous carnitine treatment within 24 hours of a heart attack at a dose of 6-9 g/day, for one year, showing a significant improvement in the recovery of the impaired left ventricular functioning. It is known that a reduced availability of ATP is one of the main reasons that can lead to the decline in left ventricular function (due to a decrease in the activity of the respiratory chain). It has also been shown that the transition from aerobic ATP-producing metabolism to glycolytic metabolism participates in left ventricular dilation and subsequent heart failure. A meta-analysis revealed that early treatment with L-carnitine in patients with extensive myocardial infarction led to a reduction in serum levels of brain natriuretic peptides (BNP) and N-terminal natriuretic peptides (NT-proBNP). These natriuretic peptides are used for assessing the severity of the heart failure, which can be a complication of a massive infarction. Quantitative data showed a 50-60% reduction in the serum concentrations of BNP and NT-proBNP, following an oral administration of L-carnitine.

Probiotics

Last but not least, given the relevance of assuming in the medical literature, there is a relationship between gut microbiota and cardiovascular health. There is a growing number of studies that have verified how changes in the intestinal microbiota (dysbiosis) lead to systemic dysfunctions of organs and systems that seem disconnected from each other but which, in practice, are not at all. An interesting review in 2019 (Vasquez et al.) illustrates the mechanisms underlying these upheavals, with a particular focus on the cardiovascular aspect. Let's start with hypertension, which, as mentioned several times, is a risk factor for many heart and kidney diseases, and also for premature death. The classic therapy is pharmacological, but adjuvant protocols that involve a change in the diet with fermented foods and the use of probiotics can be set up. A large part of the immune system resides in the intestine and communicates through specialized cells with the intestinal lumen, where the mucous barrier and intestinal microbiota lodge. The various bacterial species of the microbiota must be quantitatively well expressed and in balance with each other. This balance is called biodiversity. An intestine is as healthy as it is "biodiverse" (this is a well established thing in the study of the microbiota). However, it is very common that this biodiversity is lacking for a whole series of conditions (caesarean section, stress, use of antibiotics, excessive and prolonged physical exertion, improper diets, infections, micronutrient deficiencies, etc.). In these cases, the bacterial strains decrease in number, the relationships between them are imbalanced and pathogenic strains easily take over. Frequently, there is concomitant damage to the intestinal barrier that produces systemic endotoxemia. The immune system reads these changes and prepares to react by eliciting proinflammatory cytokines to mediate violent immune responses, even for minimal noxious stimuli. This inflammation is also read by the autonomic system, with a consequent increased orthosympathetic tone and cortisol secretion (which in turn worsens the damage to the mucous barrier). An eubiotic stimulus, on the other hand, would produce an increase in T-reg lymphocytes, an anti-inflammatory pathway with IL-10 secretion. We have known for years that the brain influences the intestine (stress produces intestinal symptoms, while vagal stimuli such as meditation mediate anti-inflammatory effects) but now we know that the relationship is mediated by a bidirectional axis. The National Heart, Lung, and Blood Institute recently put pen to paper on possible future indications for the treatment and prevention of hypertension through the use of probiotics or functional foods such as kefir. Several clinical trials on humans have demonstrated the ability of probiotics to reduce high blood pressure levels. For example, in an old study from 1995 a Lactobacillus casei extract was shown to induce a reduction in systolic / diastolic BP and heart rate in hypertensive patients. In 2002, an interesting study showed that dietary supplementation with *Lactobacillus plantarum* produced a significant reduction in systolic BP in heavy smokers. In another study in prediabetic patients, there was a significant tendency to reduce hypertension in those taking a broad-spectrum probiotic. In 2014, a meta-analysis found that the effects of probiotics on the BP were all the more marked, the higher the starting levels were. The authors also concluded that different species of probiotics used together provided synergistic effects and that the duration of the intervention should be at least ≥8 weeks, with probiotics that ensure a daily intake of ≥1011 colony-forming units. Obviously, the meta-analyzes also describes studies in which the results were more disappointing, but this variability could depend on the different mechanisms of development of hypertension in the evaluated subjects, the choice of different bacterial strains, the different types of patients and the initial state of their microbiota. All these factors can be decisive in terms of satisfactory results for BP reduction.

The endothelial dysfunction, like hypertension, is a recognized and early risk factor for heart disease. This is characterized by a decrease in the activity of the endothelial enzyme NO synthase (e-NOS), with a reduction in the bioavailability of NO (a factor that promotes hypertension, among other things). It seems that oxidative stress contributes largely to the development of the endothelial dysfunction and we know how a state of dysbiosis favors an imbalance of the pro-oxidative sense of the redox balance. Human studies have shown an improvement in endothelial function in conjunction with a probiotic treatment. The 6-week supplementation with *Lactobacillus plantarum* in men with stable coronary artery disease improved the endothelial function, increasing the bioavailability of NO (measured by dilating the flow of the brachial artery) and simultaneously reducing the systemic inflammation. These results suggest that the intestinal microbiota is inextricably linked to the systemic inflammation and to the vascular endothelial function.

Another clinical study showed that a broad-spectrum probiotic improved the functional and biochemical parameters of the endothelial dysfunction, including systolic BP, vascular endothelial growth factor, interleukin-6 (IL-6), and tumor necrosis alpha (TNF-α) in obese postmenopausal women. In general, human clinical studies suggest that supplementation with different types of probiotics contributes to an improved endothelial function through various mechanisms.

Although more research is needed, the role of probiotic supplementation in correcting the endothelial dysfunction appears to be a promising field for future studies.

Patients with heart failure, due to ventricular dysfunction, undergo some changes in the gut microbiota. Some studies describe increased levels of pathogenic flora, which could potentially have deleterious effects on the heart function. This phenomenon could be explained by the reduced pump function of the heart and an intestinal congestion in patients with a decompensated heart failure (vascular damage). This would favor the bacterial translocation by increasing the release of endotoxins (LPS) into the circulation, which cause inflammation. Kummen et al. (2018) reported how the intestinal microbiota in patients with heart failure correlated with persistent activation of T cells (T, LT lymphocytes). The removal of Gram-negative intestinal bacteria by particular antibiotics would reduce the expression of LT, together with endotoxins and cytokines, with an improvement in the average intestinal blood supply. The use of antibiotics, however, must be reserved for special cases (removal phase) and implemented by specialists who insert it in a correct process of restoring the microbiota (re-inoculation phase). In all other cases it must be carefully evaluated. The contribution of the intestinal microbiota to the pathogenesis of heart disease is also supported by the discovery of toxic metabolites in the intestine, which have a negative impact on the cardiovascular system. Specifically, it is the increase of trimethylamine-N-oxide (TMAO), recognized as an important factor contributing to cardiovascular and kidney diseases. There is only one human study for heart failure and the use of probiotics. In this pilot study, patients with class II or III heart failure and ejection fraction <50% were randomized and treated with Saccharomyces boulardii or placebo for 3 months in a double-blind manner. Patients treated with the probiotic showed a significant reduction in the left atrial diameter (sign of pump deficiency), uric acid, CRP (C-reactive protein, sign of inflammation) and creatinine levels (useful for evaluating the kidney function). The treatment was safe and well tolerated, with no reports of side effects or adverse events.

From the above, it is clear that the world of food supplements is rich in evidence on the interaction between them and the cardiovascular system. This area, however, both in terms of primary prevention and in terms of secondary prevention, has for years foreseen a heavy pharmacological medicalization deriving from massive clinical trials on very large populations, that consequently leaves little room for adjuvant therapies. However, drug therapies are not free from side effects, which are often treated with other drugs. The hope is that the now abundant literature on lifestyles, proper nutrition, physical exercise and nutritional supplementation (as personalized as possible), will allow us one day, to leave room for a less demanding approach from a pharmacological point of view, perhaps more oriented towards those small synergistic metabolic changes, in which food supplements (always admitting a good quality of the product) find a proper application. The goal is that they can assist, help wean or delay the pharmacological intervention.

Nutrition and supplementation for American football

by Antonio Squillante

American football is an explosive, intermittent sport with short bouts of intense effort spread across 15-minute quarters. Despite the length of an average game, the ball is in play on the field for an average of 11 minutes with individual offensive and/or defensive play lasting anywhere between 1.87 to 12.88 seconds in length. The standard work to rest ratio for American football is 1:5 with an average number of series per game of about 14.4 and 4.6 plays per series. The average American football player spends 6 minutes per game on the field either running, blocking, passing or tackling. According to research, up to 90% of the energy production during a football game is provided by the ATP-CP energy system. Nevertheless, the repetitiveness of

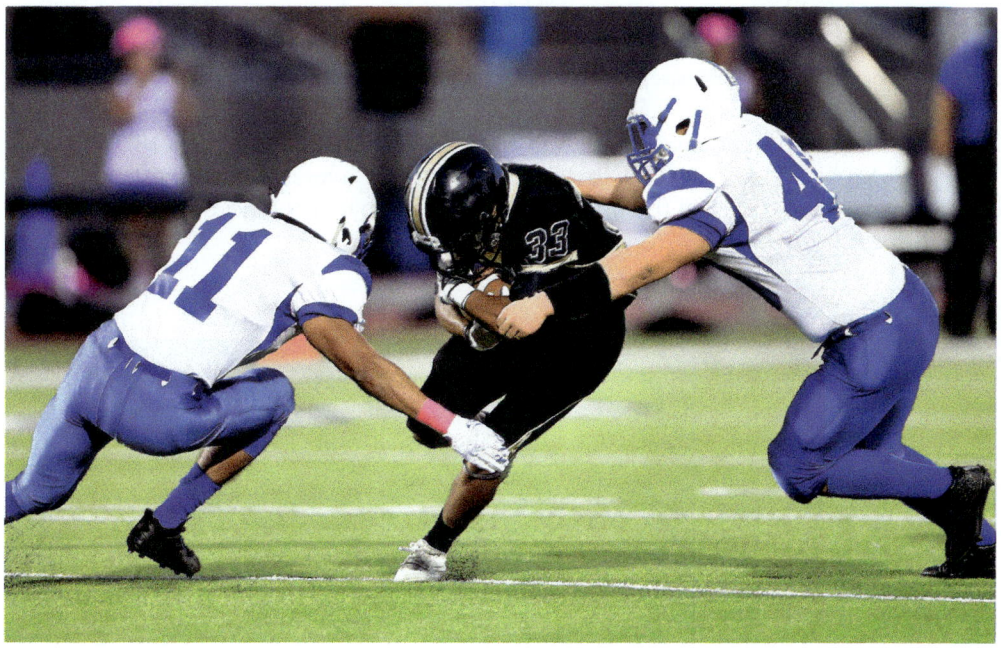

short bursts of acceleration, and deceleration places remarkable stress on the aerobic system as well.

The average VO_{2max} in American football has been measured at 53.1 mL kg^{-1} min^{-1} although results might vary quite broadly between positions. Offensive linemen and defensive linemen tend to have lower aerobic capacity than skill players with an average VO_{2max} of 50.9 +/- 6.4 mL kg^{-1} min^{-1} compared to 55.3 +/- 3.2 mL kg^{-1} min^{-1}. There is, indeed, quite a significant difference in body mass and body composition between linemen and skill players. Offensive and defensive linemen weigh in at 140.9 +/- 6.1 kg (310.6 +/- 13.4 lbs) and 132.9 +/- 14.7 kg (293.0 +/- 32.4 lbs) respectively. On average, offensive linemen have been measured at 28.8 +/- 3.7% body fat whereas defensive linemen have been measured at 25.2 +/- 7.6% body fat.

Table 43.1 Body Composition: Offensive Lineman/Defensive Lineman

Body Composition	Offensive Lineman	Defensive Lineman
Height cm/inch	192 ± 4.1 75.9 ± 1.6	190.9 ± 2.9 75.2 ± 1.1
Body Mass kg/lbs	140.9 ± 6.1 310.6 ± 13.4	132.9 ± 14.7 293.0 ± 32.4
Body Fat % body mass	28.8 ± 3.7	25.2 ± 7.6
Lean Mass kg/lbs	96.5 ± 4.5 212.7 ± 9.9	95.2 ± 5.5 209.9 ± 12.1
Fat Mass kg/lbs	39.3 ± 6.0 86.6 ± 13.2	33.3 ± 12.3 73.4 ± 27.1

Retrieved from: Dengel, D. R., T.A. Bosch, T.P. Burruss, K.A. Fielding, B.E. Engel, N.L. Weir, and T.D. Weston (2013). Body composition and bone mineral density of National Football League players. J. Strength Cond. Res. 28:1-6.

Running backs and linebackers weigh in at 105.4 +/- 8.5 kg (232.4 +/- 18.7 lbs) and 109.9 +/- 4.6 kg (242.3 +/- 10.1 lbs) respectively. On average, running backs have been measured at 16.0 +/- 4.0% body fat whereas linebackers have been measured at 17.4 +/- 3.2% body fat.

Table 43.2 Body Composition: Running Back/Linebacker

Body Composition	Running Back	Linebacker
Height cm/inch	181.5 ± 4.1 71.5 ± 1.6	186.7 ± 3.9 73.5 ± 1.5
Body Mass kg/lbs	105.4 ± 8.5 232.4 ± 18.7	109.9 ± 4.6 242.3 ± 10.1
Body Fat % body mass	16.0 ± 4.0	17.0 ± 3.2

Continues

Continued

Body Composition	Running Back	Linebacker
Lean Mass	84.5 ± 4.9	87.3 ± 3.5
kg/lbs	186.3 ± 10.8	192.5 ± 7.7
Fat Mass	16.3 ± 5.3	17.9 ± 3.8
kg/lbs	35.9 ± 11.7	39.5 ± 8.4

Retrieved from: Dengel, D. R., T.A. Bosch, T.P. Burruss, K.A. Fielding, B.E. Engel, N.L. Weir, and T.D. Weston (2013). Body composition and bone mineral density of National Football League players. *J. Strength Cond.* Res. 28:1-6.

Wide receivers and defensive backs weigh in at 94.0 +/- 6.0 kg (207.2 +/- 13.2 lbs) and 90.8 +/- 6.1 kg (200.2 +/- 13.4 lbs) respectively. On average, wide receivers have been measured at 12.5 +/- 3.1% body fat whereas defensive backs have been measured at 12.1 +/- 3.3% body fat.

Table 43.3 Body Composition: Wide Receiver/Defensive Back

Body Composition	Wide Receiver	Defensive Back
Height	185.7 ± 3.9	182.2 ± 3.1
cm/inch	73.1 ± 1.5	71.7 ± 1.2
Body Mass	94.0 ± 6.0	90.8 ± 6.1
kg/lbs	207.2 ± 13.2	200.2 ± 13.4
Body Fat % body mass	12.5 ± 3.1	12.1 ± 3.3
Lean Mass	78.3 ± 4.3	76.1 ± 4.2
kg/lbs	172.6 ± 9.5	167.8 ± 9.3
Fat Mass	11.3 ± 3.4	10.6 ± 3.5
kg/lbs	24.9 ± 7.7	23.4 ± 7.7

Retrieved from: Dengel, D. R., T.A. Bosch, T.P. Burruss, K.A. Fielding, B.E. Engel, N.L. Weir, and T.D. Weston (2013). Body composition and bone mineral density of National Football League players. *J. Strength Cond.* Res. 28:1-6.

Normative data refer to professional American football players in the United States and may vary from country to country as shown by Vitale et al. (2016).

Body composition changes quite significantly throughout the year, as the energy demand of the season is far greater than the average energy demand of the off-season. In-season, practice takes place once a day, five days a week. The average caloric expenditure during practice is in the order of 8 METs (1 MET = 3.5 mLO$_2$/kg/min). For an average lineman this figure equals to 1,150 Kcal during a 2-hour practice. For an average skill player, this figure is somewhat lower, in the order of 850 Kcal. Practice may last anywhere between 90 minutes and 2.5 hours. In-season training also includes an average number of 2-4 training sessions a week in the weight room, 45-60 minutes each in length. Intensity is moderate and counts for an additional 300-400 Kcal (3-6 METs). In-season, the recommended caloric intake for adult American football players is 50 Kcal/kg. This figure corresponds to 6,800 Kcal/day for linemen and 5,000 Kcal/day for skill players. Hardly such a high number of calories can be consumed daily. An average of 5,500-6,000 Kcal/day for a lineman and 4,000-4,700 Kcal/day for a skill player suffice to preserve adequate levels of daily energy availability. It is of paramount importance to preserve adequate levels of energy availability (EA), in the order of 35-40 Kcal/LBM. Low energy availability has been associated with a number of possible hormonal and metabolic factors associated with overtraining, energy deficiency, and compromised immune function.

$$EA = (EI - EEE)/LBM$$

EI: energy intake (Kcal)
EEE: exercise energy expenditure (Kcal)
LBM: lean body mass (kg)

IN-SEASON WEEKLY AVERAGE ENERGY AVAILABILITY Lineman					
	Monday	Tuesday	Wednesday	Thursday	Friday
EI	6,200	5,900	6,100	5,200	5,400
EEE Field	1,750	1,950	1,450	1,850	1,250
EEE Weight Room	450	0	450	300	0
EA	41	40	43	31	45

Average body weight: 136 kg. LBM: 96.5 kg. Average EA: 40 Kcal/kgLBM

IN-SEASON WEEKLY AVERAGE ENERGY AVAILABILITY Skill Player					
	Monday	Tuesday	Wednesday	Thursday	Friday
EI	4,500	4.300	4,700	4,500	4,100
EEE Field	1,050	850	1,150	950	650
EEE Weight Room	300	0	350	300	0
EA	38	41	38	39	42

Average body weight: 100 kg. LBM: 83.5 kg. Average EA: 40 Kcal/kgLBM

In-season, the recommended caloric intake for adult American football players is 50 Kcal/kg. Off-season the average caloric intake for an American football player might decrease substantially, down to 35-40 Kcal/kg of 1.4-1.8 times the basal metabolic rate (BMR). For a lineman this figure corresponds, roughly, to 4,300-5,000 Kcal depending on the physical activity level. For a skill player this figure corresponds, roughly, to 3,500-3,800 Kcal depending on the physical activity level. Physical activity has a big influence on the total energy expenditure (TEE). According to Brinkley et al (2015) Division I football players can lose up to 1.3 kg (1.2%) of body mass with a decrease in lean mass equal to or greater than 1.4 kg (1.6%) over the course of a 4-month season. Absolute fat mass tends to say approximately the same. Bodyweight does not seem to increase during the off-season; however, lean mass can increase by up to 2.2 kg (2.6%), and absolute fat mass decreased by 1.4 kg (6.7%) over the course of an 8-month off-season. These data are representative of collegiate athletes aged 18-21. Nevertheless, professional players might display a similar trend.

BMR: 88.362 + (13.397 × weight in kg) + (4.799 × height in cm) − (5.677 × age in years)[1]

Lineman

- Bodyweight: 136 kg
- Height: 191cm
- Age: 25

BMR:
- 88.362 + (13.397 × 136) + (4.799 × 191) − (5.677 × 25)
- 88.362 + 1822 + 916 − 142 = 2,684 Kcal

Estimated Energy Requirement (EER)
Approach 1:
Min: 2,684 × 1.4 = 3,759 Kcal
Max: 2,684 × 1.8 = 4,830 Kcal
Avg: 4,300 Kcal

Approach 2:
Min: 136 × 35 = 4,760 Kcal
Max: 136 × 40 = 5,400 Kcal
Avg: 5,000 Kcal

Skill Position

- Bodyweight: 100 kg
- Height: 184 cm
- Age: 25

---

1 Retrieved from; Roza, A. M., & Shizgal, H. M. (1984). The Harris Benedict equation reevaluated: resting energy requirements and the body cell mass. *The American journal of clinical nutrition*, 40(1), 168-182.

BMR:
- 88.362 + (13.397 × 100) + (4.799 × 184) – (5.677 × 25)
- 88.362 + 1340 + 883 – 142 = 2,170 Kcal

Estimated Energy Requirement (EER)
Approach 1:
Min: 2,170 × 1.4 = 3,100 Kcal
Max: 2,170 × 1.8 = 3,900 Kcal
Avg: 3,500 Kcal

Approach 2:
Min: 100 × 35= 3,500 Kcal
Max: 100 × 40= 4,000 Kcal
Avg: 3,750 Kcal

This figure corresponds to an average caloric intake of season of 3,900-4,400 Kcal, 2,300 Kcal shy of the average daily caloric intake in season. Off-season EER might vary quite widely based on activity level and/or any need to support additional muscle growth or fat loss. With an average of 3-4 training sessions a week, predominantly resistance training, the lower end of the range suffices. With an average of 4-5 training sessions a week and a combination of resistance training and endurance training, the higher end of the range suffices. An additional 500 Kcal/die can be added when the goal is to increase muscle mass or subtracted when the goal is to decrease body fat. During the season, carbohydrates make up 60% of the total caloric intake, a figure that corresponds to 6-7 g of carbohydrates per kilogram of bodyweight. For an average lineman, 800-950 g of carbohydrates a day – 3,200-3,800 Kcal or 50-55% of the daily caloric intake – suffice to preserve muscle glycogen and provide energy during training. For an average skill player, 500-600 g of carbohydrates a day – 2,000-2,400 Kcal or 50-55% of the daily caloric intake – suffice. On average, 0.5 g of carbohydrates per minute should be consumed during practice sessions lasting 90 minutes or longer. During practice, amylose or other low GI carbohydrates provide an advantage over glucose and high GI carbohydrates. The daily carbohydrate intake might decrease during the off-season down to 4-5 g/kg. Protein intake averages at 1.5-1.8 g/ kg or 15-20% of the daily caloric intake. For an average lineman, 200-250 g of protein a day – 800-1,000 Kcal or 15-20% of the daily caloric intake – suffice to preserve adequate levels of strength and muscle mass. For an average skill player, 160-180 g of protein a day – 650-750 Kcal or 15-20% of the daily caloric intake – suffice. Fat counts for 30% of the daily caloric intake. American football players should strive to consume a relatively higher percentage of saturated fats equal to 10% of the total caloric intake, with the remaining 10-20% of the total caloric intake equally distributed between monounsaturated and polyunsaturated fats.

Lineman
- Bodyweight: 136 kg
- Height: 191 cm
- Age: 25

BMR: 2,684 Kcal
- Off-Season Estimated Energy Requirement (EER) = BW*37.5 = 136*50 = 5,100 Kcal
- In-Season Estimated Energy Requirement (EER) = BW*50 = 136*50 = 6,800 Kcal

Macronutrients:
- **Off-Season:**
  CHO: 4-5 g/kg = 540-680 = 2,160-2,720 Kcal
  CHO_{avg}: 610 g = 2,440 Kcal
  PRO: 1.5-1.8 g/kg = 205-244g = 820-975 Kcal
  PRO_{avg}: 225 g = 890 Kcal
  FAT: 35% EER = 1,785 Kcal = 200 g

- **In-Season:**
  CHO: 6-7 g/kg = 810-950g = 3,240-3,800 Kcal
  CHO_{avg}: 880 g = 3,500 Kcal
  PRO: 1.5-1.8 g/kg = 205-244g = 820-975 Kcal
  PRO_{avg}: 225 g = 890 Kcal
  FAT: 30% EER = 2,000 Kcal = 225 g

Skill Position

- Bodyweight: 100 kg
- Height: 184 cm
- Age: 25

BMR: 2,170 Kcal
- Off-Season Estimated Energy Requirement (EER) = BW*37.5 = 136*50 = 3,750 Kcal
- In-Season Estimated Energy Requirement (EER) = BW*50 = 5,000 Kcal

Macronutrients:
- **Off-Season:**
  CHO: 4-5 g/kg = 400-500 g = 1,600-2,000 Kcal
  CHO_{avg}: 450 g = 1,800 Kcal
  PRO: 1.5-1.8 g/kg = 150-180 g = 600-720 Kcal
  PRO_{avg}: 165 g = 660 Kcal
  FAT: 35% EER = 1,300 Kcal = 145 g

- **In-Season:**
  CHO: 6-7 g/kg = 600-700 g = 2,400-2,800 Kcal
  CHO_{avg}: 650 g = 2,600 Kcal
  PRO: 1.5-1.8 g/kg = 150-180 g = 600-720 Kcal
  PRO_{avg}: 165 g = 660 Kcal
  FAT: 30% EER = 1,500 Kcal = 165 g

Nutritional supplements such as maltodextrins and whey proteins might help consuming adequate nutrients during periods of intense training. Moreover, the use of creatine monohydrate, beta-alanine, carnitine, and caffeine can help improve performance. Evidence shows the benefit of supplementing with 0.03 g of creatine monohydrate daily. This equals 4 g for a lineman, 3 g for a skill player. Creatine monohydrate can increase muscle creatine content and phosphocreatine content by 20-40%. Total muscle creatine levels up to or above 140 mmol/kg (dry weight) have shown to improve strength and power, anaerobic and aerobic endurance, promoting muscle growth and supporting protein synthesis. Supplementation with creatine monohydrate post-work out in combination with carbohydrates (1 g/kg) and protein (0.2 g/kg) has shown to further increase total muscle creatine content up to 155 mmol/kg (dry weight) potentially enhancing the ergogenic effects. Supplementing with beta-alanine helps preserve adequate levels of carnosine, a potent intramuscular buffer for hydrogen ions. Greater carnosine level can improve anaerobic endurance, mitigating the effect of fatigue during repeated bouts of high-intensity effort. The contribution of muscle carnosine to total intracellular muscle buffering capacity has been suggested to be approximately 7% under normal conditions but this may be increased to 15% following dietary supplementation with beta-alanine. On average, 3-6 g of beta-alanine per day have shown to increase carnosine levels by 50%, thus improving performance. Supplementing in 3-4 doses of 1-1.5 g each might help mitigate some of the collateral effects associated with beta-alanine supplementation such as gastrointestinal discomfort and tingling. Beta-alanine might be used in combination with sodium bicarbonate. Sodium bicarbonate too is a potent intracellular buffer. On average 300 mg of sodium bicarbonate per kg of bodyweight 1-2 hour before practice can improve performance, lowering the energy cost (VO_2) associated with short, repeated bouts of intense effort. For a lineman, 40 g of sodium bicarbonate should be consumed over a period of 2 hours with ample water and, if needed, food to decrease the likelihood of gastrointestinal distress. For a skill player, 30 g suffice. Evidence has shown the benefit of supplanting with carnitine as well. L-carnitine helps increase fatty acid oxidation during periods of intense training, sparing intramuscular glycogen and increasing time to exhaustion during short bouts of intense training. Moreover, recent studies support the use of L-carnitine supplementation to decrease muscle soreness and attenuate hypoxia-related tissue damage commonly associated with prolonged periods of anaerobic work. Supplementing with 3-4 g of acetyl-L-carnitine (ALCAR) per day in 3-4 doses or 1 g each suffice to increase intramuscular carnitine concentration. Caffeine can also have an ergogenic effect. Recent studies have shown how consuming 3-6 milligrams of caffeine per kilogram of body weight 45-60 minutes before a training session can improve strength and peak power output. The use of caffeine can mitigate the onset of fatigue, preventing the loss of muscle function normally reported during high intensity training sessions lasting longer than 60 minutes.

CHAPTER 44

Supplements, from A to Z

To facilitate the understanding and the choice of using one supplement rather than another, at the end of each discussion I decided to insert a table in which I assign a sort of score that distinguishes the specificity of the supplement. I preferred to adopt this system, instead of dividing the supplements according to their characteristics at the outset, as many of them would have fallen into multiple categories. The score is assigned by me based on evidence from scientific literature, but also on personal observations and feedback from the practical use in the world of sport and fitness. This choice is due to the fact that, as far as scientific studies are concerned, there is such a variety of elements to be taken into consideration – dosages, number of subjects involved in the study, starting conditions of the subjects themselves, confounding factors (smoking, alcohol, drugs, hormones, etc.), different diets, different genetic characteristics, use of different methods of statistical analysis, the company that sponsors the study – so it is normal to find apparently similar studies that demonstrate the opposite of each other. Obviously, the meta-analysis, that is the analysis of the various studies in this regard, becomes fundamental, but sometimes even this can be manipulated by excluding certain studies and inserting others, and by using subjective criteria that can influence the final result. For these reasons, in addition to my personal experiences, I believe that it is necessary to take into consideration also the experiences that come from the field. It is not the first time, and it will not be the last, that a supplement has been launched and placed on the market based on scientific research and then rejected by the sports community. The supplements that really work resist over time and are hardly affected by passing trends.

The indicated specificities are: strength, resistant strength, mass, endurance, weight loss, concentration and recovery. By strength we mean the maximal or submaximal explosive strength that still uses the anaerobic alactacid metabolism. By resistant strength, we mean the muscular endurance or in any case the short-term resistant strength (35"-2'), but also exercises of greater duration with intervals, which mainly use the aerobic lactacid metabolism. By mass we mean those adaptations of the muscle that lead to the phenomenon of hypertrophy and/or hyperplasia, stimulated by workouts that use the anaerobic alactacid metabolism and, above all, the lactacid metabolism. By endurance we mean the stamina and duration that mainly uses the aerobic energy metabolism, but which also benefits from a base of resistant strength and the ability to bear an effort. By weight loss we mean all those metabolic and biochemical processes that promote the loss of body fat, either through hormonal modifications, by increasing thermogenesis or through the best use of fats for energy purposes. By concentration we mean the ability to maintain the attention, determination, calmness, clarity and mental energy, especially during the athletic performance, and also outside of it. By recovery we mean the athlete's ability to restore their energy levels in the muscles, their hormonal balances, the facilitation of the sleep induction, the activation of detoxification mechanisms and the elimination of training-induced metabolic wastes and the ability to repeat the performance in the shortest possible time. Scores are assigned in the table at the end of each supplement. The sign – indicates no efficacy; the + sign indicates minimal effectiveness; the ++ sign indicates a fair efficacy; the +++ sign indicates good efficacy; the sign ++++ indicates an excellent effectiveness.

Having to opt for a supplement in order to obtain an improvement in a specific capacity, I recommend choosing supplements marked with the +++ or ++++ sign; however, also considering the overall effect of a supplement on the various capacities, it is also possible to opt for those supplements whose overall score reaches ++.

ACETYL CARNITINE (ALC)

Description
Acetyl-L-carnitine, also known as ALCAR, is a carnitine molecule linked to an acetyl group. From a chemical point of view, acetyl-L-carnitine (ALC) is the acetylated derivative of the amino acid L-carnitine and its endogenous production occurs starting from L-carnitine and acetyl-CoA, deriving from the fatty acids beta-oxidation process, thanks to the intervention of the carnitine-acetyltransferase enzyme, which is present in the mitochondrial matrix. Exercise naturally increases our levels of acetyl-L-carnitine; however, if you are obese, over 30, or if you have health problems, it will probably be necessary to take supplements of this molecule.

Properties
Acetyl-L-carnitine is considered a version of carnitine with a higher neurological efficacy. In chronic fatigue, for example, ALCAR can reduce the mental fatigue. Supplementation with acetyl-L-carnitine can attenuate the decline in the potential of the mitochondrial membrane and the reduction of cardiolipin (a constituent of the membrane), associated with age (and also with overfeeding). Cardiolipin is a fatty acid, exclusive to mitochondria, with numerous vital roles in the mitochondrion, such as the optimal maintenance of the structure of the electron transport chain and its enzymes. It has been hypothesized that acetyl-L-carnitine plays an important role in aging, as ALCAR is a part of the mechanisms aimed at restoring and/or maintaining cardiolipin levels and it also slows the decline of the mitochondrial function.

From a physiological point of view, acetyl-L-carnitine plays roles that are very similar to those of L-carnitine, with the notable difference of being able to add to the effects of L-carnitine, which you will find listed in the chapter dedicated to this supplement, those directly related to **its acetyl structure** and **its greater bioavailability**.

Because of these effects, several authors believe that it may play a role in the acetylcholine synthesis processes, which is a known neurotransmitter. Furthermore, speaking of the bioavailability, it is interesting to consider the data that seem to suggest a **more efficient absorption** of the acetylated form.

The possible applications of acetyl-L-carnitine are therefore multiple and they cover many areas, since it is effective not only for sportspeople but also in the field of pathology, as shown by medical research applied to the therapy of Alzheimer's disease, diabetic neuropathies, to ischemia and cerebral reperfusion, as well as to the improvement of cognitive faculties and degenerative neuropathies, such as those that follow chronic alcoholism.

A supplementation with acetyl-L-carnitine can have the following effects:
- an improvement of the cognitive abilities of human beings in good health (attention, visual coordination, reflexes, speed of execution of intellectual tasks);
- an improvement of the cognitive functions, emotional state and social behavior of patients that are affected by mnemonic deficiency associated with aging;
- a reduction of depression symptoms and an improvement in the perception of the quality of life;
- a delayed cognitive impairment in patients with Alzheimer's disease;
- an improvement of the symptoms of senility;
- an improvement of the cerebral circulation in patients affected by cerebral vascular insufficiency;
- a reduction of the formation of lipofuscin (the cellular "debris" which constitutes the "old age spots") and a decrease in lipofuscin deposits, a sign of brain aging.

The ergogenic aspect of acetyl-L-carnitine is exerted through:
- a direct increase in the activity of enzymes that participate in the cellular respiration;
- a reduction of muscle pain following strenuous exercise;
- a reduction of the increase in heartbeats during the moment of maximum intensity of the effort;
- an increase in the stamina of athletes during prolonged efforts;
- a decrease in the formation of free radicals during exercise;
- an increase in the metabolic efficiency of using high-energy molecules;
- an increase in the possibility of burning fat during the physical activity;
- an increase in the efficiency with which sugars are burned;
- a decrease in the lactate/pyruvate ratio with relative increase in the energy availability at the cellular level;
- an improvement of the CoA uptake in the mitochondrion during the fatty acids beta-oxidation process;
- an increase in the production of acetylcholine and a possible colino-mimetic action;
a stimulation of the synthesis of membrane phospholipids.

Evidence

When we are going through particularly stressful periods or if we are overtraining, we feel tired and lazy, positive hormones such as testosterone and growth hormone are lowered and stress hormones such as cortisol are increased, which, if they reach too high quantities, become harmful for our body. In this case, ALC can exert a positive effect by mitigating the negative impact of overtraining on the testosterone production. A study by Dr. Bill Kraemer showed how supplementation with 2 g of ALC favors the increase of androgen receptors in conjunction with weight training. In this study, it was noted that immediately after training, testosterone levels dropped even more, indicating that a greater amount of testosterone was being captured at the cellular level. The author of this study also claimed that this momentary drop in testosterone sends a signal in the brain to produce more endogenous testosterone. Studies on animals subjected to chronic stress have shown that ALC is able to **directly stimulate or prevent factors that decrease the release of gonadotropins (the pituitary hormones that stimulate the production of testosterone in the gonads)**. The modulating effect on the cortisol production is linked to the ability of ALC to increase the sensitivity of cortisol receptors and this means that, thanks to the feedback mechanism at the pituitary level, through a lower production of ACTH (the pituitary hormone that stimulates the production of cortisol at the adrenal level), it decreases the production of cortisol.

Therefore, these two effects on the hormonal level can only help us with a physical improvement, both through more effective muscle building and through a reduction in the muscle catabolism. When combined with glutamine and branched chain amino acids, it is effective in counteracting the action of cortisol during the immediate post-workout period. In a study by Ferreira et al. in 2017 who wanted to study the role and the neuroprotection played by L-carnitine and acetyl-L-carnitine during brain development. In recent years, there has been considerable interest in the therapeutic neuroprotection potential of L-carnitine and its acetylated acetyl-L-carnitine derivative in a number of disorders, including hypoxia-ischemia, head trauma, Alzheimer's, and in conditions that lead to the damage of the central or peripheral nervous system. There is compelling evidence from preclinical studies that L-carnitine and ALC can improve the energy status, reduce oxidative stress and prevent the subsequent cell death in adult, neonatal and pediatric brain injury models. ALC can provide an acetyl part that can be oxidized in order to produce energy, to be used as a precursor of acetylcholine or to be incorporated in glutamate, glutamine and GABA, or in lipids for myelination and cell growth. The administration of ALC after the brain injury in rat pups improved the long-term functional outcomes, including memory. Further studies are needed to better explore the potential of L-carnitine and ALC in protecting the brain development, as there is an urgent need for therapies that can improve the outcomes after neonatal or pediatric brain injuries.

Acetyl-L-carnitine, in addition to helping brain cells to have more readily available energy at their disposal, also acts as a **powerful antioxidant and helps to increase the level of an important molecular messenger, acetylcholine**. The availability of energy is particularly important for brain cells. Acetyl-L-carnitine is also able to decrease the loss of the cell receptors that normally occurs with the advancing age, precisely because of its ability to increase the vitality and energy in the brain. The intake of acetyl-L-carnitine is also indicated in the treatment of depression, especially in the cases where depression appears in old age.

In some scientific researches, acetyl-L-carnitine has been shown to be able to:

- increase the level of NGF (Nerve Growth Factor), which plays an important role in maintaining the functionality of neurons. The action of acetyl-L-carnitine manifests itself by improving the sensitivity of neurons towards this factor;
- keep the myelin sheath covering the nerves healthy and efficient (important for maintaining the health and functionality of the nerves themselves);
- help brain cells to use alternative energy sources, such as ketone bodies;
- help our brain cells adapt to lower blood glucose levels, such as those that can occur between meals. In this way, the brain is guaranteed a constant and an adequate supply of energy.

Scientific research has shown that giving acetyl-L-carnitine to people affected by a stroke allows for a faster recovery than placebo.

It can also be a valid support for low-calorie diets, in fact **it favors the entry of fats into the mitochondria**, and this allows, in addition to losing weight, also having more energy during the day.

Some observational studies have found a remarkable action of acetylcarnitine on the improvement of fatigue, angina pectoris attacks, aerobic endurance and mood, with doses of 0.5-1.5 g per day, taken with plenty of water in order to reduce the mild burning that this molecule can cause.

These observational studies, which lasted for long periods, demonstrated the following results, obtained through supplementation with ALC:

- an increase in optimism and good humor, associated with a general state of well-being, vitality and "grit", and a greater ability to deal with the difficulties of the daily life;
- an improvement of the depressive syndromes and "mental concentration", with a strong action also in female subjects, both young and geriatric ages;
- a reduction of rheumatic and muscular pains, such as lumbosciatica, arthritis, etc.;

- a greater endurance of "sporting" fatigue and an increased ability to "react" to acute stressful events, which are very different from routine daily stress. A faster post-workout recovery.

To understand the effects mediated by this molecule, it is necessary to understand the endogenous biosynthetic pathway that leads to the formation of carnitine, noting that it has an important molecule as a precursor: S-Adenosyl-Methionine (SAM-e).

The latter is formed in the liver from simple methionine and ATP, which is degraded to transfer adenine to methionine in order to form SAM-e. A formed SAM-e molecule has "consumed" an ATP molecule for its synthesis. Understanding this is fundamental, since the SAM-e sparing process by carnitine administration can help explain the **psychic** and physical **benefits** that we already mentioned, as SAM-e is fundamental for the synthesis of numerous brain neurotransmitters.

Clinical studies have found an improvement in sports and in the intellectual performance, an aid for the memory, the immune system and for the maintenance of intellectual faculties, against depression, against chronic fatigue syndrome, etc. These studies also indicate that appreciable cognitive benefits occur after a few months of additional administration and highlight the neuroprotective role of ALC on the cholinergic system. Carnitine and ALC should not be used in people with bipolar disease (manic depression) and epilepsy, unless recommended by the attending physician.

Dosages

The average dosage is 500-1000 mg/day, although in the presence of slimming regimes and intense physical activity, it can reach 1500-2000 mg per day.

It is interesting to note that ALCAR in daily quantities equal to 2 g, in combination with alpha-lipoic acid, can potentially reduce the hypertension thanks to its antioxidant and pro-energetic action, as well as improve the insulin resistance and glucose tolerance in people with compromised heart health.

Effectiveness

Strength	Resistant strength	Mass	Endurance	Slimming	Concentration	Recovery
+	+	++	+++	++	++	++

ACETYLCYSTEINE (NAC)

Description

N-acetylcysteine (NAC) is a precursor of L-cysteine, a non-essential but important sulfur amino acid for the hepatic metabolism and also for the metabolism of homocysteine and the antioxidant glutathione (GSH). In nature, it is found in plants of the *Allium* species, in particular in onion (*Allium cepa*, 45 mg NAC/kg). It is a donor molecule of thiol groups (the sulfhydryl-SH group) which, within the NAC molecule, directly eliminate reactive oxygen species (ROS) and modulate the redox state of NMDA and AMPA receptors (involved in transmission at the central nervous system level), and it also inhibits NF-κB (a transcription factor for inflammatory processes).

GSH, together with SOD (superoxide dismutase) and catalase, are the most potent organic endogenous antioxidant. The level of free radicals to which the cell is subjected is indicated by the GHS/GSSG ratio (reduced glutathione/oxidized glutathione). It is known that in athletes, the administration of exogenous antioxidants must be evaluated very scrupulously. The free radicals produced during the training must be managed primarily by the cell's endogenous antioxidant defenses. Nature has foreseen a hormetic adaptation of these defenses, which tend to improve the following sessions of physical activity with an intensive training (different from subject to subject). This happens, above all, if the correct recoveries are respected, which depend on the type of sport, intensity, duration, frequency, volume, etc. Muscle adaptation to exercise is also mediated by the hormetic stimulus of free radicals (increase in protein synthesis, mitochondrial biogenesis, recovery capacity), so much so that many studies suggest a worsening of the muscle adaptation and performance in subjects taking chronic and/or supraphysiological doses of antioxidants (typically vitamins C and E). With this in mind, encouraging the intake of thiols such as NAC could increase the body's anti-radical defenses without creating an exogenous abatement by downregulating the hormetic stimulus given by the training. In addition, NAC stabilizes HIF (Hipoxia-Inducible Factor), which is responsible for activating the erythropoietin transcription gene (EPO), which increases its production. EPO is a protein hormone produced mainly in the kidneys which increases in situations of poor tissue oxygenation and stimulates the erythropoiesis by increasing the production of red blood cells, which act as oxygen transporters for the tissues.

Properties

NAC is used as an antidote for paracetamol overdose in order to prevent acute liver failure. Another dated pharmacological use (from 1963) is that which sees it as a mucolytic (used as an aerosol or by mouth). In fact, it has also been used to combat the action of some substances that produce free radicals, such as carbon monoxide (CO) and some contrast fluids used in radiology. It is used both parenterally (intravenously) and by mouth. In the literature, in 2002, a single case of anaphylactic reaction from NAC was described at a dosage of 150 mg/kg in an asthmatic 40-year-old woman. When taken by mouth, however, side effects are very rare and the areas in which this molecule has been used vary from non-alcoholic steatohepatitis to COPD (chronic obstructive pulmonary disease), substance abuse, ovarian polycystosis, diabetic retinopathy, cataracts, for a total of 300 clinical studies. However, many studies focus on the preventive use of NAC in diseases such as Alzheimer's disease, irritable bowel, obesity, insulin resistance, cardiovascular diseases, heavy metal toxicity, diabetic retinopathy etc. Some studies on invertebrates and mammals have also reported an increase in the lifespan, with a substantially antiaging effect (yet to be confirmed in humans).

Evidence

NAC has also attracted considerable attention as a sports supplement for reducing the muscle fatigue, improving athletic performance and promoting muscle recovery.

However, there is a great variability of results in sports studies, also due to very heterogeneous methodologies. Some studies have shown very significant increases (over 50%) in athletic performance, particularly in single workouts consisting of interval exercises, performed under the use of NAC. These results were found in particular in subjects who, characteristically, had an enormous production of free radicals during a single workout.

In a 1994 study, it was found that the use of NAC was particularly useful for inhibiting the muscle fatigue especially in long-lasting sports (endurance), probably for its **effectiveness in countering free radicals** and oxidative processes, which cause fatigue once they're produced.

The main disputes regarding the use of NAC as a sports supplement are related to the dosages and the times of administration, which are not standardized. For example, the daily dose of NAC in the studies included by Rhodes and Brakhuis ranged from 1.2 to 20 g and the supplementation period varied from a few minutes to eight days before performing the exercises. In various studies, the heterogeneous effects of NAC reflect the fact that there is an optimal state of the redox balance in various tissues, which is, however, difficult to assess. In these conditions, an incorrect dosage of an antioxidant (too much or too little) can lead to a significant reduction in the performance. A 2018 study (Paschalis et al.) took into consideration three categories of athletes, 100 subjects divided according to their basic glutathione level (low, medium, high). These athletes were supplemented with NAC at a dose of 600 mg twice a day, for 30 days, and their redox balance and performance were assessed on the Windgate test (an exhaustion test that examines the subject's anaerobic capacity). The group starting with a lower GSH level reported a significant improvement in both post-NAC redox balance and in the performance level during the Windgate test, while there was little improvement in the groups that had medium to high baseline GSH concentrations. Other studies on rugby players (Rodi et al., 2019) and volleyball players (de Jesus Pires de Moraes et al., 2018) have found that supplementation with NAC gave better results particularly in acute cases, after an intense training session. According to the meta-analysis by Rhodes and Brakhuis, NAC doses >5 g have a greater potential to cause side effects. Although these side effects are generally mild and limited to gastrointestinal disorders, they can hinder the athletic performance and therefore affect the purpose of the supplement itself. However, the evidence of these side effects is limited and in many studies included in the meta-analysis of Rhodes and Brakhuis, they were not reported despite the generous doses of NAC.

In one study, 1200 mg of NAC were administered to well-trained athletes for eight days and, in addition to an increase in glutathione, they also found **an increase in EPO**. In another study by Momeni et al. it has been shown that with a single dose of 600 mg of NAC, there was an EPO increase of 20-30% during the 24 hours following the administration. The single dose, of course, did not produce an increase in the red blood cell production, as verified by a measurement made two weeks after the experiment. Conversely, the dose of 1200 mg for eight days significantly raised glutathione levels (+33%), EPO (+26%) and hematocrit (+9%), confirming the validity of NAC as a supplement for aerobic sports.

As mentioned, there is also evidence relating to pathologies that are characteristic of the elderly, such as in the prevention of neurovegetative pathologies, neuropathic pain, mild cognitive disorders and immune system disorders. However, some studies have considered administering hydrolyzed keratin as a thiol donor to build up GSH reserves, and both mouse and human studies have shown promising results. For humans, using hydrolyzed keratin dosages of 10-40 g per day have shown an increase in endogenous taurine (another sulfur metabolite that participates in the GSH cycle).

Dosages
Dosages are 600 mg once a day, preferably in the evening as an antioxidant and 1200 mg to improve the endurance. Other studies use dosages of 40-70 mg/kg of body weight.

Effectiveness

Strength	Resistant strength	Mass	Endurance	Slimming	Concentration	Recovery
+	++	+	+++	+	−	+++

AGMATINE

Description
Agmatine is a biogenic amine produced through the decarboxylation (elimination of a carboxyl group) of L-arginine, a non-essential basic amino acid in adults, produced in physiologically sufficient quantities through the urea cycle.

The main function of this amino acid is to represent the main precursor in the metabolism of nitric oxide.

Although agmatine can influence the metabolism of nitric oxide, it does not represent its metabolic precursor, which is carried out by L-arginine, but it represents an intermediate of "polyamines", cell growth factors capable of stimulating the proliferation especially in fast-growing cells such as cancer cells.

One of the possible agmantine metabolic pathways is represented by the formation of 4-guanide butyrate by the enzyme diamine oxidase (DAO), and by hydrolysis into urea and putrescine (polyamine) by the enzyme agmatinase1.

Although agmatine represents an intermediate in the synthesis of polyamines, it seems to have an inhibitory effect on the bioactivity of polyamines by reducing their intracellular quantity.

Like other biogenic amines (putrescine, tyramine, cadaverine, serotonin, histamine), agmatine can represent a by-product of bacterial fermentation, including that of the intestinal flora. In this regard, it seems that some bacteria are able to produce ATP and therefore energy, starting from substrates such as arginine and agmatine.

In the past, it was identified as "the substance capable of displacing clonidine", a drug classified as a selective agonist of α_2-adrenergic receptors, that acts predominantly as an antidepressant.

Agmatine accumulates in various parts of the body, although the highest levels are found in the stomach, small intestine and adrenal glands. Lower levels are found in smooth muscles, endothelial cells, heart, spleen and brain, where it is found particularly in areas where neuron terminals form excitatory synapses with pyramidal neurons.

Properties
Also known as 4-aminobutyl-guanidine, agmatine is stored in neurons at the level of synaptic vesicles (synaptosomes), from which it is released during the neuronal activity, and for this reason it is often considered a real neurotransmitter and neuromodulator.

Some research suggests that this amino acid may have potential in the treatment of neuropathic pain and in the context of drug addiction. These potentials work in synergy with the work done by painkillers such as morphine and other opiates, thus increasing pain tolerance. Studies conducted on guinea pigs have shown that taking agmatine sulfate significantly improves the insulin sensitivity, and it also promotes the release of anabolic hormones, such as the growth hormone-GH and the luteinizing hormone-LH, which stimulate the release of testosterone. Agmatine exerts its effects through various mechanisms; we will list the most interesting ones below:

- it can inhibit the N-methyl-D-aspartate receptor (NMDA) of glutamate (a very important neurotransmitter involved in neuronal plasticity and long-term memory consolidation), which, if excessively excited, causes excitotoxicity with induced neuronal death. Agmatine, by inhibiting this receptor, appears to improve the cognitive abilities and memory, resulting in a significant neuroprotective effect;
- it can act by activating the receptors of imidazolines, synthetic substances used as drugs in hypertensive states, or in the modulation of pain. A study has shown that the activation of

- imidazoline receptors by agmatine significantly improves the insulin sensitivity by reducing blood sugar levels in diabetic rats;
- agmatine is able to inhibit the calcium channels of some serotonin receptors, in particular the 5-HT1a type receptors with an antidepressant action;
- agmatine, by inhibiting the nitric oxide synthase enzyme, helps regulate nitric oxide levels. Despite this, it still seems to have vasodilatory and hypotensive effects;
- there is an interesting study that demonstrates the improving effect on the integrity of the vascular endothelium, as a consequence of supplementation with agmatine sulfate in the presence of damage to the vascular endothelium induced by the intake of nicotine;
- agmatine appears to improve the lipid profile, among other things, achieving a reduction in serum LDL cholesterol levels and an increase in HDL cholesterol levels. It should be noted that these improvements were observed only in conjunction with damage caused by the intake of nicotine;
- agmatine is able to influence a number of metabolic functions, however the mechanism by which they occur is not yet fully understood. A study done on laboratory animals with obesity induced by a high-fat diet suggests that the intake of high doses of agmatine is able, over time, to significantly improve the metabolism of these subjects. Agmatine appears to lead to a better expression of the genes that regulate thermogenesis, to a better gluconeogenesis and higher systemic levels of carnitine and acetylcarnitine, therefore a better activation of the beta oxidation of fatty acids. These metabolic changes are associated with a weight reduction and a reduction in metabolic and hormonal alterations;
- agmatine is known to inhibit nitric oxide synthase (NOS); this activity is carried out by modulating the inhibitory action, especially related to (inducible) iNOS which is its main objective, while the inhibitory action is mild on eNOS (endothelial). Remember that iNOS seems to contribute to an excess of nitric oxide production with harmful consequences, while eNOS appears to be protective through vasodilation;
- some studies have highlighted an involvement of nitric oxide production in the aging process; Specifically, it seems that a dysregulation occurs with increases in the levels of NOS and a sharp decrease in agmatine levels in certain areas of the brain. This dysregulation seems to be the cause of age-related behavioral disorders. Injections of agmatine in elderly rats seem to restore the NOS activity by correcting these disorders.

Evidence

In the sports field, the use of agmatine is fairly recent, especially because even if there are no visible side effects, there is still a lack of data that would make it safe in the long term. The use of this polyamine as a supplement stems from a shared thought; since agmatine represents the product of arginine catabolism (true proponent of stimulation in the production of NO), a surplus of agmatine would slow down this conversion process regulated by "arginine decarboxylase". At most, agmatine could be **considered a modulator of NO** and not a stimulator of its production.

However, even in sports, the use of agmatine cannot be limited to the sole vision of an "arginine saver".

Some probable or potential effects resulting from the use of this polyamine are listed below:
- it improves the insulin sensitivity and therefore the anabolic effect of this hormone in the post-exercise phase;
- it stimulates the production of the growth hormone GH by the pituitary gland and therefore, it amplifies its anabolic effects;
- not only does it relieve pain, but it also increases mental well-being by reducing the production of cortisol, which is released during intense physical exercise; this avoids muscle catabolism.

However, until there are further studies carried out on athletes in training, the possible ergogenic properties of agmatine cannot be confirmed.

Dosages
Agmatine, once absorbed after oral ingestion, is rapidly distributed in various tissues, also reaching the brain. In the systemic circulation agmatine appears to have a half-life of less than 10 minutes, however it remains in the brain for up to 12 hours. The passage through the cell membrane cannot take place in a passive way, but requires an active transporter; moreover, its absorption is shared with putrescine, which, if in high concentrations, can inhibit the absorption of agmatine. Even though there is insufficient research to determine an official recommended dose, dosages between 1300 and 2600 mg per day appear to be effective and well tolerated.

However, experience indicates that in order to have significant benefits, it is sometimes necessary to increase the dosage. Some studies indicate that dosages of 6 to 40 mg/kg of body weight are required to have benefits like increasing the mental concentration or an anxiolytic effect. Other studies indicate that the effects of agmatine are not dose-dependent and that it follows a "bell-shaped" trend. Taking it orally is recommended on an empty stomach or with a small non-protein meal, as agmatine competes with some carriers used by amino acids.

Effectiveness

Strength	Resistant strength	Mass	Endurance	Slimming	Concentration	Recovery
+	+	+	+	++	+++	+

ALPHA-GLYCERILPHOSPHORYLCHOLINE

Description
Alpha-glycerylphosphorylcholine (α-GPC) is a precursor of the neurotransmitter acetylcholine and a natural metabolite of phospholipids derived from soy lecithin. It improves the memory abilities and all brain functions in general. α-GPC is indicated to strengthen the release of GHRH (Growth Hormone Releasing Hormone), which in turn stimulates the secretion of growth hormone (GH, Growth Hormone) in young and elderly individuals.

Properties
The stimulation of acetylcholine and the consequent natural release of growth hormone are the result of the stimulation of neurotransmitters on the cholinergic system, however other modulations and biochemical-related systems may also be involved. α-GPC, in particular, **increases the synthesis and release of an important neurotransmitter called acetylcholine, which allows the growth hormone levels to increase even after physical exercises**.

Recent studies have also suggested that α-GPC may be an effective ergogenic aid.

Evidence
A recent study examined the GH release in endurance athletes after supplementation with α-GPC. In athletes supplemented with α-GPC, GH levels rose 68% more than those who took the placebo. In particular, the peak strength on the bench press in the athletes who had used the α-GPC was 14% higher than the controls.

Similar results were found in another study involving both young and elderly men. In younger subjects (30-34 years), α-GPC showed a 40% increase in the GH release compared to non-α-GPC group. In older subjects (80-82 years) taking α-GPC increased the GH secretion up to 140% more than in non-α-GPC.

The researchers suggest that α-GPC could amplify GHRH-induced GH release through two mechanisms. According to the first hypothesis, supplementation with α-GPC would lead to an increase in brain levels of acetylcholine, which, in turn, would increase the pituitary sensitivity and amplify the release of GH. The second hypothesized mechanism foresees that the increase of the growth hormone secretion is determined by the increase in the fluidity and permeability of the pituitary membranes, i.e. by a greater ease of signal transmission.

Lena Marcus et al., In 2017, designed a study to evaluate the effectiveness of two doses of α-GPC compared to placebo and caffeine for increasing the jumping performance, the isometric strength and the psychomotor function.

Forty-eight healthy college-age males volunteered for the study and underwent baseline jumping assessment, mid-thigh isometric pull (IMTP), upper body isometric strength test (UBIST), and psychomotor alertness (PVT). Following this evaluation, participants were randomly assigned to groups taking 500 mg of α-GPC, 250 mg of α-GPC, 200 mg of caffeine or placebo daily. Blood samples were collected 1 hour and 2 hours after the initial dose to quantify the free choline and the thyroid stimulating hormone.

Serum TSH was found to be significantly depressed in the 500 mg α-GPC group compared to other treatments ($p < 0.04$). Group differences were observed for maximum speed and mechanical power on jumping ($p < 0.05$) and the 250 mg α-GPC group demonstrated the greatest improvements in outcome. In conclusion, on the basis of these tests, α-GPC could be considered an efficient ergogenic supplement.

Another interesting aspect concerns the mitochondria. It has been hypothesized that α-glycerylphosphorylcholine (α-GPC) can influence the mitochondrial respiratory activity and, in this way, it can exert protective effects on the tissues. Rat liver mitochondria were examined with high-resolution respirometry to analyze the effects of α-GPC on the electron transport chain in normal oxygen conditions and in the absence of oxygen. The activities of reduced glutathione (GSH) and oxidized glutathione (GSSG), tissue myeloperoxidase, xanthine oxidoreductase and NADPH oxidase were measured.

The formation of tissue malondialdehyde and nitrite/nitrate was evaluated, together with the production of superoxide and hydrogen peroxide in the blood. It was observed that, following the cell damage and the oxidative stress, the administration of α-GPC reduced the inflammatory activation and also the inflammatory markers. In conclusion, α-GPC, by preserving the respiration of the mitochondrial complex, reduced the biochemical signs of oxidative stress. This suggests that α-GPC is a compound that also targets mitochondria and that it is able to indirectly suppress the activity of the main intracellular proximity enzymes.

Dosages

The normal use of α-GPC, in quantities ranging from 100 to 1000 mg per day, contributed to a significant improvement in the endogenous secretion of GH and to the stimulation of the enzymatic synthesis of phosphatidylcholine, especially in nerve and muscle cells. Small doses of 150-400 mg also appear to be effective.

Effectiveness

Strength	Resistant strength	Mass	Endurance	Slimming	Concentration	Recovery
+	+	+	++	+++	++++	−

ANTIOXIDANTS

Description
Free radicals are particularly reactive substances that have atoms with unpaired electrons, in excess or in defect, thus unbalancing their electromagnetic charge. In this situation, the atom is unstable and tries to equalize its electromagnetic charge by stealing an electron from another atom, and so on, triggering a chain reaction. If atoms that belong to cellular structure molecules are involved in this reaction, a damage occurs at the cellular level, which seems to be the cause of aging, degenerative diseases and tumors. The production of free radicals in the body is a physiological event and normally occurs in cellular biochemical reactions, especially in those that use oxygen for energy production. However, the body has a number of defenses, called antioxidants, which are able to neutralize these free radicals.

Properties
Exercise increases the production of free radicals, increasing the use of oxygen; among other things, the free radicals produced during exercise can cause direct damage to the muscle cell. It is equally true that training also improves the body's antioxidant capacity, so well-trained athletes are able to counteract these free radicals, but in the untrained individual and in overtraining conditions, the production of free radicals exceeds the defense capacity of the organism. It is obvious, at this point, that the athlete, together with the smoker (it has been shown that smokers have a lower level of antioxidants and a greater production of free radicals), are the major candidates for taking antioxidants as supplements, precisely with the intention of protecting themselves from the damage induced by the physical activity itself and also for the reasonable possibility of a better athletic performance over time. Among other things, many correlations have recently been noted between deficiencies of the immune system and the production of free radicals, and we all know that athletes are an easier subject to immunosuppression.

In the recent years, studies have shown that the category of antioxidants is wider than it was thought: there are dozens or even hundreds of substances, each of which with a specific function, but they must be synergistic with the function of the others: an excess or a deficiency could be harmful, so it is incorrect to emphasize a single substance, but you should have them all in the right amount. Just as there are dozens of antioxidants, there are also several types of free radicals. The chain reaction caused by free radicals can alter the cellular biochemistry so profoundly, that cells die.

For example, damage to the cell membrane inhibits the flow of nutrients inside the cell and the flow of toxins outwards, so at the same time, the cell does not receive nutrition and becomes intoxicated. The formation of free radicals is the basis of the aging processes and is also caused by numerous environmental events. Ultraviolet radiation from sunlight causes free radical damage. The same is achieved with the oxidation induced by the atmospheric pollution. Each breath is "toxic" due to the considerable variety of free radicals that are formed. Exercise can simply increase this damage. To counteract the harmful effect of free radicals, the human body produces endogenous antioxidants, mainly **superoxide dismutase**, **catalase** and **glutathione**.

These antioxidants "block" free radicals by receiving or donating an electron. This action converts the antioxidant itself into a free radical. However, a chain of antioxidants is activated in our organism, and they are capable of rebalancing the system. This chain of events, in practice, is interrupted with the formation of waste products that are harmless to our body, such as water and carbon dioxide, which can be excreted through urine, sweat and breath. Exercise generates a higher amount of these waste substances. Panting and wheezing during an exercise is because we require a greater effort to get rid of the excess carbon dioxide, rather than a higher need for oxygen. This is the reason why the most attentive athletes focus more on the exhalation activities, without paying much attention to the inhalation activities. Endogenous antioxidants alone do not always seem to be able to protect athletes. If we make calculations by looking at the pure and simple volume of oxygen used during the exercise, we see that the production of antioxidants by our organism cannot always be adequate, and in this case, the most important antioxidants must come to the aid. We know that exercise releases a significant number of free radicals in the protective membrane that surrounds each muscle fiber. These radicals include singlet oxygen, hydrogen peroxide, and superoxide anions. They oxidize some fats contained in the membranes, a form of damage known as *lipid peroxidation*. Oxidized fats continue the chain of damage in the form of peroxyl radicals. In a few days, inflammatory phenomena develop and damaged cells often die. Peroxyl radicals are often the main cause why muscles hurt more on the second day rather than the first day after intense physical exertion. **Vitamin E** is a fat-soluble antioxidant capable of blocking the peroxidation of lipids. In doing so, it becomes a pro-oxidant, producing *tocopherol* and *tocopheroxyl radicals*. At this point, **vitamin C** intervenes in blocking these radicals and by regenerating vitamin E.

In the absence of vitamin C, vitamin E could do more harm than good. We know that vitamin E works in synergy with the endogenous antioxidant glutathione in blocking the lipid peroxidation. In carrying out this action, glutathione needs the mineral selenium, which "stops" the lipid radicals in order to allow the action of glutathione. Selenium is also required for the correct action of vitamin E. **Vitamin A** is an essential nutrient for life, however, doses of vitamin A exceeding 10,000 IU can accumulate in the body until reaching toxic levels. Our body can easily form vitamin A starting from beta-carotene, which, by virtue of its non-toxic properties, is therefore more preferred than vitamin A. However, the antioxidant functions of beta-carotene are independent of its role as a precursor of vitamin A, so taking beta-carotene has a double advantage. **Beta-carotene** neutralizes some types of radicals better than vitamin C and vitamin E, and this action alone justifies its inclusion in sports antioxidants. Furthermore, carotenoids work with vitamin E and selenium to inhibit the peroxyl radicals, thus helping to prevent the lipid peroxidation on the membranes. We have already mentioned selenium as a mineral which is capable of reducing the levels of free radicals in the cell membrane, but other mineral antioxidants act inside the cell. Among these we can mention **copper** and **zinc**, which favor the action of superoxide dismutase (SOD), the enzyme that neutralizes superoxide radicals, producing hydrogen peroxide. **Flavonoids** are a subclass of plant substances called *polyphenols*. They are a great source of potent antioxidants, some of which are likely essential to health. By way of example, let us recall how solar radiation represents the main cause of premature skin aging as it is responsible for the formation of free radicals at the level of keratinocytes. In particular, the photo-oxidation processes induced radically by UVA and UVB radiation lead to the degradation of the membrane polyunsaturated fatty acids, with the formation of radical species and peroxidated intermediates which contribute to the induction and propagation of the erythematogenic response and subsequently to premature skin aging. Most nutritionists recommend eating plenty of fruits and vegetables, precisely because these foods provide large doses of antioxidants. Citrus fruits and tomatoes contain vitamin C; yellow and orange vegetables contain considerable quantities of beta-carotene; fruits provide flavonoids, and many natural foods, especially wheat, contain vitamin E. However, over the years, the usefulness of taking extra doses of antioxidants in the form of supplements has been confirmed. Which ones to choose then? We have seen that the ones we know best are vitamin C and vitamin E, beta-carotene and a family of substances called flavonoids, which are undoubtedly among the best antioxidants, but there is another substance that has all the characteristics to become the ideal antioxidant: **alpha-lipoic acid**. We have already seen how oxidized vitamin E is reconstituted from vitamin C and in turn vitamin C is recycled by glutathione, an endogenous antioxidant produced in the body. The cycle continues with another antioxidant, **NADH**, which is a coenzyme necessary for the action of other enzymes that recycle glutathione. In spite of this precise understanding of the antioxidant cycle, it is difficult to find a way to increase the glutathione levels. Glutathione cannot be taken orally like vitamins C and E, because it is destroyed in the stomach before it can reach the blood. Lipoic acid is the missing link. Not only is it a powerful antioxidant itself, but it also stimulates the production of glutathione, thus having a double effect. It is also easily absorbed when taken orally and, once it gets inside the cells, it is rapidly transformed into its most powerful derivative, which is **dihydrolipoic acid**. Since both alpha-lipoic acid and dihydrolipoic acid are antioxidants, their combined action determines the greatest antioxidant power known in nature. In addition, there is another property of alpha-lipoic acid that makes it a powerful antioxidant. Since it is soluble in both water and fat, which means that it is both water-soluble and fat-soluble, it can move in all parts of the cell to neutralize the free radicals. Vitamin C, in other words, is limited to the water-soluble parts of the cells because it is soluble only in water, while vitamin E is soluble only in fat and therefore can only protect the lipid parts of the cells. The effect of alpha-lipoic acid is not limited only on the antioxidant one, as it plays an important role in the cellular metabolism and in the production of energy within the cells. Without lipoic acid, the cells cannot use glucose for energy and lipoic acid also tends to favor the accumulation of glucose in the muscle cell to the detriment of the accumulation of fat in the adipose cell. In addition, alpha-lipoic acid also has a significant lipolytic effect, especially in situations of intense physical activity. In short, a new dimension is being configured for antioxidants, intended not only as a defense against free radicals, but also as a control system for cellular energy production systems: a new perspective that is increasingly interesting for the possibilities and for its possible applications in the sports field.

Evidence

If it is clear that **the use of antioxidants is certainly necessary when it comes to aerobic training of extreme endurance**, given the high production of ROS (Reactive Oxygen Species), i.e. of oxygen free radicals, there is instead **less evidence when we look at the anaerobic training, where they could have a negative effect on the muscle growth**. As we have already said, physical exercise increases the production of ROS by promoting the expression of specific proteins which, within the cell, are able to counteract the oxidative stress.

As a result of the excessive consumption of antioxidants, the activation of these important protein molecules that promote organic adaptation is inhibited. For example, the consumption of antioxidants has been shown to inhibit the upregulation of superoxide dismutase, a very important endogenous antioxidant enzyme that neutralizes free radicals and decreases their damage. The production of free radicals through the production of these proteins stimulates the production of more mitochondria. The increased production of mitochondria allows to meet the higher energy demands during the physical exercise, decreasing the further production of ROS; a higher number of mitochondria increases the cell's ability to produce more energy, promotes the athletic performance, recovery and muscle growth.

In a study by Gomez-Cabrera et al. it was found that the administration of vitamin C inhibited the normal exercise-induced expression of the PGC-1 protein in muscle cells, preventing the production of mitochondria. Vitamin C also inhibited the exercise-induced expression of some antioxidant enzymes in the muscles.

In another study by Ristow et al., 40 people performed a specific exercise regimen that included 40 minutes of circuit training, followed by 20 minutes of stationary bikes, five times a week. Twenty people took 1000 mg of vitamin C and 400 IU of vitamin E, while the other twenty took a placebo. In the end, the study showed that that dose of vitamin C and E is able to decrease the ability of ROS to generate the production of PGC-1 and new mitochondria. Intense weight training, especially with an eccentric prevalence, causes damage to the muscles that require some time to restore the full muscle functions. In order to establish the role of ROS in the muscle recovery, Close et al. conducted a study in which some subjects were given 1000 mg of vitamin C for 14 days after a downhill run, and the other subjects took a placebo. The presence of DOMS (Delayed Onset Muscle Soreness) was found in both groups, as well as an impaired muscle function following the downhill run, but the group that received vitamin C as a supplement showed a more delayed recovery.

Since vitamin C decreased the ROS production following the exercise, it is believed that ROS are involved in the recovery process and that high-dose vitamin C can slow it down. Other studies indicate that of vitamin C supplementation of 1000 mg, taken before training, can reduce the muscle soreness and it also accelerates the recovery after training. At this point, one might think that vitamin C is useful before exercise to reduce the damage caused from free radicals and to lower the cortisol levels, but instead, after the training, it limits the stimulating effect on the regeneration induced by ROS. Given that vitamin C has a fairly short half-life, the timing of its intake could be decisive.

Anthocyanins are a group of flavonoids with very strong antioxidant characteristics. In one study, anthocyanins of black currant were administered to 30 men and women in the form of black currant extract, at a dosage of 0.8 to 3 mg per kg of body weight, and it was seen that they began to circulate in the blood after 30 minutes, peaking after 2 hours. Subsequently, one hour after taking a placebo or the same dosage of black currant, the subjects performed a rowing exercise for 30 minutes at 70% of their VO_{2max}. The subjects who had taken black currants had significantly lower levels of oxidative stress 2 hours after the exercise, compared to the placebo group. They also had a higher amount of white blood cells, indicative of a better immune situation, and a lower heart rate.

Dosages
The dosages of vitamin C and E, which should not negatively affect the modulation of ROS production during the exercise, should be 200 mg and 100 mg, respectively.

Effectiveness

Strength	Resistant strength	Mass	Endurance	Slimming	Concentration	Recovery
++	+	+	++	++	++	+++

ARGININE

Description
Arginine is one of the amino acids that builds up proteins. From a chemical point of view, arginine is an aliphatic alpha-amino acid, of a basic nature due to the presence of the guanidine group. It is also a chiral molecule whose L-enantiomer falls within the 20 ordinary amino acids; for this reason, it is better known as L-arginine.

Due to the importance and the number of biological and therapeutic functions that it performs in the body, arginine is considered a "conditionally" essential or dispensable amino acid, that is, essential in certain circumstances and dispensable due to the inability of the organism, in certain situations, to synthesize it from other amino acids. In fact, in a healthy adult man, arginine is synthesized endogenously in sufficient quantities to respond to the physiological demands of the body. The endogenous synthesis of arginine mainly involves the intestinal-renal axis; citrulline is synthesized from glutamine, glutamate and proline in the mitochondria of the enterocytes, released from the small intestine into the circulation and from there they are extracted by the kidney and converted into arginine.

Enzymes that catalyze the synthesis of arginine starting from citrulline, as well as in the kidney, are present in different types of cells, including adipocytes, endothelial cells, enterocytes, macrophages, neurons and myocytes, indicating the ubiquity of this amino acid in metabolism. Nutrition also plays a key role in maintaining the optimal levels of arginine which are necessary to perform the multiple biological functions of this amino acid.

Several foods, in fact, contain significant quantities. It has been shown that, as a rule, a person should consume 3 to 6 g of arginine per day with their diet, mainly through meat, nuts and plant foods rich in proteins, such as legumes, soy protein isolate (6.07 g), egg white powder (4.4 g) and salted cod (3.75 g).

Therefore, the regulation of arginine homeostasis, which depends on the dietary intake of arginine, the turnover of proteins, the speed of the synthesis and the catabolism of arginine, as well as on the state of health of the individual, is of considerable nutritional and physiological significance. Over the years, various studies aimed at investigating the metabolism of arginine have shown its complexity due to the compartmentalization of various enzymes in the different organs (liver, small intestine, kidney) and in the different subcellular fractions (cytoplasm, mitochondria), as well as for the changes in the expression of these enzymes, during the development and in response to the diet, hormones and other factors.

Properties

After ingestion, arginine can have different metabolic fates; a relatively small amount of arginine is metabolized by enterocytes and the liver, while the remainder reaches the systemic circulation by entering the cells of various organs, which also possess the enzymes that are necessary for the metabolism of this amino acid.

Once inside the cells, arginine can be involved in various metabolic pathways. A recent review highlighted the important contributions of arginine to the metabolism, not only in terms of protein synthesis in cells and tissues, but also in the synthesis of urea, NO, creatine, agmatine, ornithine, glutamate, and its influence in the hormonal release and polyamine synthesis. All these factors place arginine and its precursors and metabolites at the center of different metabolic pathways, through interorganic communication. It follows that arginine, with different but often simultaneous modalities, plays different roles in the disposal of protein metabolic wastes, in muscle metabolism, in vascular regulation, in the immune system, in neurotransmission, up to being involved in the synthesis of RNA and in the regulation of hormones.

From a physiological point of view, arginine is part of the protein synthesis, allowing a correct turnover of both structural proteins and enzymatic proteins, as well as in the nitrogenous substances detoxification process, being an active part in the urea cycle. It is able to produce energy in the absence of carbohydrates, thanks to its glucogenic property, and participates in the synthesis of metabolically active molecules such as NO, a powerful vasodilator.

The probable properties of this amino acid emerge from the results of the studies of this complex metabolism; not all the properties that have been studied have scientific evidence, but it is certain that arginine is an amino acid with a fundamentally important role for the performance of many metabolic functions.

The increase in the daily requirement of this amino acid in order to improve the athletic performance, very common among athletes of various disciplines, as well as in the medical field for some pathologies such as protein-caloric malnutrition, trauma, surgery, hormonal dysfunctions and alterations of the immune system, seems to be satisfied by the use of specific supplements.

It is important to remember that 40% of the amount of the exogenous arginine, introduced with specific foods or supplements, does not enter the systemic circulation but is degraded by the small intestine in the early stages of metabolism; the bioavailability of this amino acid taken orally is therefore 60%. Of this 60%, up to 50% of the orally ingested arginine can be converted into ornithine through the action of the arginase enzyme.

Evidence

In sports, the supplementation of arginine can be used for its possible ergogenic properties, especially the anabolic and anti-catabolic ones.

First of all, arginine, being an intermediate in the urea cycle, has a detoxifying action leading to the elimination of ammonia, a compound that is toxic for the cells of our body, through the synthesis of urea, which is then excreted in the urine. Ammonia can be introduced into our body through proteins, but it is also a product of the deamination of AMP (adenosine monophosphate) by the muscle, and it is formed following intense muscular work and is responsible for the onset of the sense of fatigue. Several authors recommend the intake of arginine to those who perform physical activity of a certain intensity (endurance running, cycling, cross-country skiing, triathlon, etc.), in which there is a high production of ammonia. The process of eliminating ammonia from the body can be favored if sufficient quantities of arginine contained in food or in a specific food supplement are introduced into our body.

Arginine also plays an important role in the synthesis of amino acids and **glucose**. Arginine is a **precursor of creatine and increases the speed of its synthesis**; this property could **positively influence the athletic performance** due to the effects of creatine. Creatine is synthesized starting from arginine and glycine, with the formation of guanidine acetate; the reaction between guanidine acetate and ornithine leads to the production of creatine, the direct supplier of ATP, the energy currency with which the muscles work.

Research has shown that the percentage of creatine in the muscles was significantly increased by the supplementation of arginine, which in this case was associated with glycine. **It is involved in the synthesis of glucose**, acting in this sense as a gluconeogenetic amino acid; arginine can be metabolized to produce energy when glucose stocks are at a minimum after physical activity.

It also seems to be able to increase the immune response in humans; some studies have shown an *in vitro* increase in the activity of T cells when increasing arginine concentrations. This effect has been confirmed in various conditions, such as trauma, surgery, protein-calorie malnutrition, situations in which the immune system is altered, particularly when the T cell system is damaged. Due to these effects on the immune system, it could prove useful for increasing the anabolic processes of the physical exercise, improving the training, recovery, immunological responses and modulation of immunosuppressive conditions after intense physical exercises.

The ability of arginine to induce **an increase in nitric oxide (NO) synthesis** is contributing to the ergogenic effect, with a consequent vasodilator effect, useful for optimizing the muscle vascularization. Due to its vasodilatory properties, arginine could also be useful in the **treatment of cardiovascular diseases** (hypertension, atherosclerosis, angina and hypercholesterolemia) and in erectile dysfunction, by dilating the blood vessels that fill the corpora cavernosa and thus favoring the erection of the penis.

This property of arginine has been confirmed by studies in which high doses of arginine were taken intravenously in fasting healthy humans. As for the oral intake of arginine, at doses that are tolerable for the body, most of the studies do not confirm the same vasodilatory effect. This result is probably due to gastric stress induced by oral arginine intake, which can reduce the assimilated amount, and to the fact that oral arginine has a bioavailability of only 60%, and up to 50% of this can be converted in ornithine.

Furthermore, the potential ergogenic effects of arginine would result in acute effects, which result in a higher exercise capacity after ingestion, and in a chronic effect resulting from the stimulation of the muscle protein synthesis and therefore with an anabolic function. But, while it is clear that exogenous amino acids stimulate the muscle protein synthesis at rest, following resistance exercises and also in a variety of clinical conditions, including burns, sarcopenia and cachexia, the evidence regarding the ergogenic effects of supplementation with single amino acids such as arginine are equivocal. The potential role of arginine as a precursor for the muscle protein synthesis, as well as for the nitric oxide synthesis, can interact in terms of the net effect of arginine on the muscle protein synthesis.

Therefore, considering that the administration of arginine alone does not appear to be effective in stimulating the muscle protein synthesis, it may be useful to take it in combination with other amino acids or, possibly, with meals. This may be related to a greater influx of amino acids to the muscle as a result of the NO synthesis induced by arginine, or to a more direct effect on the muscle protein synthesis, which requires the concomitant increase of other amino acids as well. There is also scientific evidence according to which the integration of arginine in sports promotes the muscle development induced by physical power activities, increasing the lean mass at the expense of fat mass; this effect also seems to be related to the discussed ability to **increase the secretion of GH induced by physical exercise**.

In addition to its role as a precursor in the production of NO and in protein synthesis, arginine can act as a secretagogue, promoting the release of growth hormone (GH) which has an anabolic effect, by inhibiting the secretion of somatostatin. In fact, taking arginine by parenteral and enteral routes has been shown to be effective in enhancing the secretion of GH and insulin.

In one study, oral absorption of arginine resulted in an insulin-mediated anabolic state, with changes that included a decrease in serum leucine and isoleucine, a decrease in blood glucose and free fatty acid percentages, as well as an increase in serum insulin levels.

Especially when combined with other amino acids, for example lysine, it appears to be effective in increasing GH levels, even when taken orally. In a study of 16 men who were given arginine and lysine (1500 mg) before performing a short, intense weight training session, GH levels increased, albeit not significantly compared to the increase in GH induced by exercise alone. However, it seems that GH levels have risen significantly in resting conditions and 60 minutes after the training, when compared with a placebo. In another study, oral administration of arginine (250 mg/kg/day) for seven days increased the nocturnal secretion of growth hormone by 60% in healthy male volunteers, aged between 20 and 30 years. GH stimulates the production of IGF-1 (Insulin-like Growth Factor-1), which acts as an anabolic hormone, stimulating the protein synthesis. Most of the research has found that the effect of arginine on the stimulation of growth hormone seems to be enhanced by taking it in combinations with other amino acids, in particular **ornithine**, another important GH stimulator. Arginine and ornithine are particularly connected, as the former is used by the body to synthesize the latter, through the action of the arginase enzyme. In 1989 Elam et al. concluded that the concomitant intake of 1 g of ornithine and 1 g of arginine, in combination with a weight training program, can increase the muscle strength and lean mass over a period of five weeks. The two amino acids favored the recovery from chronic stress by suppressing the catabolic processes and by lowering the urinary hydroxyproline levels.

In another recent study, trained athletes took a mix of 3000 mg of arginine and 2200 mg of ornithine twice a day, three times a week, while training with weights. The results showed that the intake of the two amino acids produced a higher increase in post-exercise GH levels compared to the placebo group, as well as higher levels of IGF-1. The synergistic intake of ornithine and arginine could also have a favorable effect on the **reduction of the body fat**, as was shown in a study in which a group of men, after taking a mix of ornithine and arginine, in combination with the exercise with weights, had a greater reduction in their fat mass than the group that did not take them.

The results of these researches deserve a careful analysis, but could partly confirm that even low dosages of these two amino acids, when taken in synergy, can bring various benefits, in terms of a higher secretion of GH and IGF-1, a greater suppression of the stress symptoms and a greater improvement in the body composition.

The synthesis of glycogen in the muscle can be optimized by the increased absorption of glucose by the muscle, which is favored by the translocation that occurs because of the glucose transporters GLUT4, from the intracellular vesicles to the cell membrane in response to insulin. A study has shown that a systemic intravenous infusion of arginine in healthy subjects can increase the blood flow in the legs, an effect associated with an increase in endogenous insulin. However, oral arginine supplementation did not significantly affect the insulin levels compared to the placebo group. The dosage of the supplement and the route of administration may have influenced the lack of significant changes in insulin levels after arginine supplementation, probably also due to the reduced bioavailability of the oral administration. Other studies that recognize this effect have been carried out with an oral intake of high doses of arginine, intolerable ones.

In addition to all these potentially improving effects on the muscle performance, some studies have suggested an additional effect that can **promote muscle development**. This new function is linked to the conversion of arginine into compounds known as *polyamines*. Polyamines, such as putrescine and spermine, are natural compounds synthesized in the body from arginine and play an important role in the muscle growth, as recent studies have shown.

Arginine, even at minimal doses but prolonged for at least four weeks, is able to significantly improve both the anaerobic threshold and the time to exhaustion.

However, studies on the effects of arginine supplementation on sports performance show controversial results. While it has been shown that the administration of arginine as part of a multinutrient supplement is able to increase the tolerance to high intensity exercise, in other studies the supplementation with pure arginine has not shown clear effects and to date, its ergogenic effect has never been demonstrated in professional athletes.

The intake of arginine and antioxidants seems to increase the anaerobic threshold by 16%, delaying the feeling of fatigue.

Another possible association is the one with branched-chain amino acids; in fact, a study shows how the supplementation of 2 g of BCAA with 0.5 g of arginine can reduce the proteolysis that follows intense muscle exercises.

Arginine supplementation immediately or for a few days, regardless of the used dose, seems too short to cause changes in the physiological variables and in the physical performance; however, if taken for a longer period of time, it seems to be capable of improving the sports performance.

In 2018 Mor et al. studied the effect of prolonged L-arginine supplementation on the physical performance by recruiting 28 male amateur football players, between 18 and 30 years old, who trained regularly. The subjects were randomly assigned to an experimental group or a placebo group. For 14 days, the experimental group consumed 6 g of arginine and the placebo group consumed 6 g of wheat bran. Then they measured anthropometric, biochemical and recovery capacity parameters after the anaerobic tests, both before and after supplementation, by measuring the lactic acid levels and heart rate up to the 10th minute of the recovery.

The results of this study suggest that the supplementation of L-arginine led to a reduction in the body mass index (BMI) and a faster recovery capacity from the 5th to the 10th minute.

In the experimental group, compared to the placebo group, the subjects' heart rate was reduced more, both at rest and during the 1st minute of recovery. Compared to the placebo group, lactic acid levels in the subjects who supplemented with L-arginine decreased more rapidly by the 5th to 10th minute of recovery. At the end of the study, the subjects of the experimental group also showed a reduction in the levels of aspartate aminotransferase (AST), alanine aminotransferase (ALT), lactate dehydrogenase (LDH) and body mass index (BMI).

This suggests that arginine supplementation accelerates the elimination of lactic acid from the body and also the recovery, with a positive impact on the anaerobic sports performance. In a 2017 study (Pahlavani et. al.), the effect of L-arginine supplementation on sports performance and body composition was analyzed in 56 male soccer players, between the ages of 16 and 35. The subjects were given 2 g per day of an L-arginine supplement or the same amount of maltodextrin (placebo) for 45 days.

At the beginning and at the end of the study, BMI, fat mass (BFM) and lean mass (LBM) were measured, in addition to evaluating the sports performance.

Additionally, 3-day dietary records were collected at three different time points (before, during, and at the end of the study). The results showed that sports performance (VO_{2max}) was more increased in the experimental group that took L-arginine, compared to the placebo group. However, in this study, no significant effect of L-arginine supplementation on anthropometric measurements was found (weight, BMI, BFM and LBM).

Dosages

In studies where positive results were obtained in improving athletic performance, arginine administration generally ranged between 2 and 8 g per day, although the most commonly used dosage appears to be 3 g per day. The intake should be divided into several times and it should be continued for a period of at least 3-4 weeks, given the absence of the positive effects following an acute administration of this amino acid; the best results, in fact, are observed after a period of supplementation of at least three weeks. Intestinal absorption is optimized when the intake is made on an empty stomach, while the biological activity of the amino acid, especially if oriented towards the sustenance of the protein synthesis, reaches its maximum following the intake of simple sugars and other amino acids. Studies that demonstrate an inducing effect on GH secretion describe the assumption of arginine in a single administration before the night sleep and with much higher dosages than those recommended, which can be dangerous and with potential side effects.

A study by Forbes et al. at the University of Alberta, Canada, has shown that when given before weight training, arginine decreases the GH levels, so if your goal is gaining mass via the GH stimulation, it is best not to take it close to the training.

The most common side effects, recorded at large doses, are vomiting, diarrhea and abdominal cramps at doses above 10 g per day.

Effectiveness

Strength	Resistant strength	Mass	Endurance	Slimming	Concentration	Recovery
+	++	++	+++	+++	–	++

ARGININE ALPHA-KETOGLUTARATE (AAKG) AS A PRECURSOR OF NITRIC OXIDE (NO)

Description

Nitric oxide is such an important molecule that in 1998 the Nobel Prize in Medicine was awarded to three Americans for their studies on it. More than 10,000 articles in leading scientific journals have been published in the last decade on the broad-spectrum effects on health and other functions of nitric oxide in the body. Nitric oxide has many effects in the body: it acts as a regulator of the blood pressure, as a substance released by white blood cells to destroy bacteria and cancer cells, as a messenger molecule in the brain, as well as being involved in the processes of regulating the inflammation and the immune system. It seems that the increased supplementation of this amino acid is able to reverse the changes in the vascular reactivity, to reduce the thickening of the intima in atherosclerosis, as a precursor of the endothelial relaxation factor. At an ergogenic level, it facilitates the arrival of oxygen and other nutrients in the muscle cell, with a possible increase in muscle hypertrophy and strength, and at the same time it protects the muscle fibers from the damage induced by intense physical activity. It also causes the release of the growth hormone which in turn stimulates muscle growth and fat elimination. NO is also necessary for the erection and for the vaginal response, regulates the blood flow, improves the lung airflow, reduces total and LDL cholesterol, improves long-term memory and has a powerful antioxidant action.

Properties

Nitric oxide is a stable free radical, present in the form of gas, produced in most of the body's cells. It has the ability to freely cross cell membranes and therefore to act easily within them. NO is synthesized in the body from the amino acid L-arginine through the action of the enzyme nitric oxide synthase (NOS). NOS exists in three forms, or isoforms: neuronal NOS (NOS-1), inducible NOS (NOS-2), endothelial NOS (NOS-3). Depending on where they are located, they produce different effects. For example, NOS-1 acts as a neurotransmitter in the gastrointestinal tract, and animal studies show that it is involved in regulating the sense of appetite. This isoform is also involved in the penile erection. NOS-2 is particularly active in immune reactions and is part of the response to the inflammatory reaction. However, it tends to be the "bad guy" of the three enzymes: being capable of producing too much NO at the wrong time can cause damage. NOS-3, on the other hand, regulates the blood flow and pressure, as well as the platelet inhibition, which is responsible for blood clotting. Muscles also constantly produce NO and some studies indicate that it has a fundamental role in muscle growth. **NO is responsible for maintaining optimal levels of protein synthesis in the muscles.**

Its inhibition (in training subjects) decreases the rate of muscle growth by about 50%. This is the first reason why the athlete who requires a quick protein change or a better protein synthesis in order to increase their muscle mass, should strongly consider NO supplements. All three NOS isoforms can be found in the skeletal muscle; however, the one we find more often is the neuronal NOS. NO, therefore, not only increases the blood flow to the muscles, but also increases their strength and their ability to contract. This implies that a lack of NO can lead to a poor muscle performance. Constant training allows the muscles to become more efficient in producing NO thanks to the increase in NOS, which forms NO from arginine. This last amino acid is very important for the formation of NO.

- Without NO, IGF-1 loses a part of its anabolic function.
- NO is an activator of satellite cells that play an important role in muscle growth.
- NO allows an adequate release of the growth factor IGF-1 (locally released in muscles), which is essential for the fusion between satellite cells and those that are already developed.
- It is able to increase the muscle strength (useful before training).
- Optimizes tendon repair.
- NO also allows (thanks to its vasodilating properties) a higher blood flow to the muscle, improving the transport of oxygen and other nutrients. This substance is an important modulator of the vascular response, promoting an increase in the cyclic GMP molecule (cyclic guanosine monophosphate). An increase in blood flow creates a pumping effect on the muscles, similar to what you get after a workout. The pumping effect is always combined with an increase in muscle volume. The increase in nutrient transport and

volume at the cellular level creates favorable conditions for the formation of new muscle tissue, because it represents a stimulus signal for protein synthesis.
- NO is particularly effective for the treatment of erectile dysfunction and can restore the sex drive.
- NO also affects the secretion of some endocrine glands. For example, it stimulates:
  - the secretion of GnRH (Gonadotropin-Releasing Hormone) from the hypothalamus;
  - the secretion of pancreatic amylase from the exocrine secretion portion of the pancreas;
  - the release of adrenaline, which leads to a greater stimulus in training.

NO, by increasing the blood flow and the transport of nutrients, also promotes a complete recovery after intense workouts; Furthermore, since it also possesses anti-inflammatory properties, it also reduces the post-workout muscle pain and promotes the cellular repair.

Another important molecule to associate with arginine for the production of NO and for vasodilation is vitamin B3 or niacin. Niacin is effective for the circulation and lowering the cholesterol level in the blood. It is vital for a proper nervous system activity, for maintaining skin and tongue health, and for the formation of digestive system tissues. It is necessary for the synthesis of sex hormones and enters the composition of the fundamental enzymes, of oxidative metabolism. Niacin is essential for the synthesis of two enzymes: NAD (Nicotinamide Adenine Dinucleotide) and NADP (Nicotinamide Adenine Dinucleotide Phosphate). NAD is an essential enzyme for the production of NO starting from arginine; therefore, it is necessary to ensure an adequate quantity of this vitamin, which is easily destroyed or used for other purposes.

To optimize the endogenous production, it is useful to:
- decrease the production of cortisol which inhibits the formation of NO (phosphatidylserine: 400-800 mg);
- train constantly with weights (contracting and stretching the muscles produces more NO);
- take arginine AKG (3 g), which is the best form of arginine to stimulate NO production;
- take 100 mg of niacin, a vitamin necessary for the formation of NAD;
- take vitamins C, E and beta-carotene at the same time (500 mg; 400 IU; 5000 IU);
- take ginsenosides (3-9 g of ginseng with 4% ginsenosides) which have properties that stimulate the production of NO in the immune system cells, in the endothelial cells of the vascular system, in the arteries and in the tissues with erectile capacity;
- take the polyphenols, contained in red wine and green tea, which can not only safeguard the functions of NO, but can also prevent an excessive inflammation resulting from an excess of NOS activity.

Evidence

In an attempt to optimize the biological effectiveness of arginine, supplements of this amino acid have been developed in more structurally stable forms. Arginine alpha-ketoglutarate (AAKG) comes in the form of arginine salt, obtained by combining two molecules of arginine and one of alpha-ketoglutarate. In addition to improving its stability in an aqueous environment, alpha-ketoglutarate, an intermediate of the Krebs cycle, improves the ergogenic capacity of arginine and appears to increase its absorption and promote its transport into muscle cells. Alpha-ketoglutarate is, in fact, a very important keto acid from a metabolic point of view, since it represents a crossroads between catabolic and anabolic reactions. As mentioned above, this molecule is part of the Krebs cycle, thus favoring the production of energy, but it is also part of the gluconeogenic process, allowing the synthesis of glucose starting from non-carbohydrate sources such as amino acids; finally, it is also part of the synthesis of some amino acids such as glutamate (hence glutamine), proline and arginine itself. However, there are numerous studies that are testing the potential of this keto acid, with important results relating to the possibility of preserving the protein component in patients with kidney disease, reducing the urinary nitrogen secretion, as well as improving collagen synthesis in elderly patients, with a consequent prevention against some pathologies such as osteoporosis, atherosclerosis and arthritis. Studies show how this form can also guarantee a better protection of the muscular structures, preventing the negativization of the nitrogen balance. Furthermore, these arginine alpha-ketoglutarate (AAKG) supplements have an enhanced ability to produce NO and vasodilation, compared to arginine alone, facilitating, as already mentioned, the distribution of oxygen and nutrients to the muscle and improving the physiological response during the exercise and post-exercise recovery.

An initial study examined blood levels of arginine and its assimilation time to determine if it improved the maintenance of blood levels of arginine over a period of time. This study was aimed at verifying the claim that AAKG favored a special mechanism for releasing arginine into the blood stream, resulting in constant pumping or hemodilation, but the study yielded unsatisfactory results. The second study evaluated the effects of AAKG on the body composition, muscle strength and endurance. Interestingly, the group that took AAKG had an improvement in their performance, with an increased maximal capacity in resistance activities (weight lifting), but without showing a change in muscle mass. These objectives are underlying the observed biological effect and, in particular, the involvement of this amino acid in the synthesis of NO.

This powerful biological mediator, in fact, by promoting vasodilation, should facilitate the supply of oxygen and nutrients to the muscles, allowing us to support the athletic performance longer and more intensely. The metabolic effects of arginine and alpha-ketoglutarate could also be useful in energetically supporting the cell and improving the muscle recovery phase, preserving from proteolysis and increasing the protein synthesis. In the literature, there are different opinions on the actual potential of AAKG supplementation.

Numerous studies seem to agree that oral supplementation with arginine alpha-ketoglutarate can have a metabolic-energetic effect by supporting the athletic performance, delaying the onset of anaerobic metabolism, with an **increase in the peak of maximum strength and a higher resistance to physical exercise**.

One study showed that AAKG increased the strength in the bench press; no significant differences in body mass, lean mass, or body fat percentage were demonstrated between athletes who took AAKG and those who took a placebo. Most studies agree that the simultaneous administration of other amino acids, such as creatine, can lead to a better ergogenic boost, with a relative improvement in muscle endurance and maximum peak strength.

Dosages

The normally recommended dosage is 3 g per dose, preferably 30 minutes before training. An additional dose can be taken in the morning on an empty stomach or in the evening before bedtime. In the case of erectile dysfunction, the administration of 9 g per day divided into three administrations, or in a single dose 30-60 minutes before intercourse, may be useful.

Effectiveness

Strength	Resistant strength	Mass	Endurance	Slimming	Concentration	Recovery
+++	+++	+	+	++	−	++

ASHWAGANDHA (WITHANIA SOMNIFERA)

Description

Withania somnifera, more commonly known as Ashwagandha or Indian ginseng, is a plant that belongs to the *Solanaceae* family which grows mainly in the dry subtropical areas of India and has been used for many years in Ayurvedic medicine. In fact, it belongs to the group of rejuvenating preparations called Rasayanas. According to Hindu healers, this plant "infuses new youth, strengthens the memory and the intellect, prevents the flesh from becoming flabby, revives the complexion and gives a horse's strength". More recently, its use in the form of a food supplement is spreading in the Western world, mainly for its beneficial properties in countering the aging process, oxidative stress and neurodegenerative diseases.

Bioactive molecules called withanolides are obtained from the roots of the plant. Their chemical structure belongs to steroid lactones, to which most of its beneficial effects are due. It is known that this plant is able to support and help the body in case of stress, anxiety disorders, neurodegenerative diseases, depression, obesity, fertility problems, hormonal imbalances, immune system dysfunctions, thyroid dysfunction, insulin sensitivity and impaired glycemic control, memory and concentration problems.

Properties

Various active ingredients with beneficial properties can be found in the leaves and roots of Ashwagandha. Scientists attributed most of the effects to withanoside VI and withaferin A; even if the mechanism of action is not yet fully understood, and it is assumed that the plant is able to modulate the neuronal stimulation induced by stress.

The plant is classified as an adaptogenic herb, as it rebalances the body when it is faced with stressful situations, exerting a calming action in case of strong tension or a stimulating effect during depressive episodes. For these functions, Ayurvedic medicine uses the roots of this plant to regulate the immune functions and improve sexual activity, thus acting on two aspects that, during periods of high stress, are put to the test. Initially the plant was studied for its support functions for the nervous system and the immune system: it is in fact able to reduce stress levels by modulating the production of cortisol in chronically stressed subjects; furthermore, the decrease in cortisol levels is directly related to an improvement in the functions of the immune system, which, in conditions of prolonged stress, is seriously compromised. In fact, the plant, in addition to exerting this important anti-stress effect, is also able to modulate the functionality of the immune system, strengthening the defenses of our organism and regulating its mechanisms. Its effect, in particular, has been demonstrated at the level of T lymphocytes and IgM and IgG immunoglobulins, which play a very important role in the development of food intolerances; the latter represent an increasingly emerging problem in our current society and typically arise in periods of strong mental and physical stress. Its use could prove invaluable in athletes during sports training: periods during which long, frequent and intense workouts are practiced, and especially when the recovery is not adequate, the immune system is compromised and Ashwagandha has shown its effectiveness precisely in these contexts.

Another consequence of the increase in stress hormone levels is a decrease the production of sex hormones, which leads to a decrease in libido and sexual desire. Cortisol and testosterone, in fact, are produced starting from a common precursor and, when situations of strong stress occur, the biochemical reactions are unbalanced towards the production of cortisol, causing a lowering of testosterone levels; Ashwagandha has the ability to lower the cortisol levels when it is in excess. Consequently, the restoration of the corticosteroid production leads to greater production of testosterone, which is the male sex hormone par excellence. Some studies have also reported a beneficial effect on the female libido and on the rebalancing of sex hormones in women.

Another feature of this plant is the ability to support the recovery of the musculoskeletal system and to improve the physical performance. In fact, many studies have shown that supplementation with Ashwagandha root and leaf extracts is able to increase the muscle mass, even in the absence of a training stimulus; if a weight training program is performed together with the supplement, in addition to the increase in the muscle mass, there is also an increase in the contractile and explosive force. Still in the sporting context, the plant also has the ability to optimize the performance in endurance athletes, increasing the parameters related to endurance and delaying the onset of fatigue. In addition, Ashwagandha is able to support the bone health by stimulating the proliferation of osteoblasts; whitaferin A, in particular, is able to increase the bone mineralization rates and for this reason it can be used by athletes, in case of trauma or injury, to accelerate the healing process.

Many studies have analyzed the effect of Ashwagandha and its active ingredients on the nervous system; currently, its extracts are used to support the treatments of neurodegenerative diseases, as they are able to induce the regeneration of nerve cells, by regenerating damaged endings and stimulating the formation of new synapses and neuronal connections; the increase in the performance of strength sports could also be attributable to an improvement in the mind-muscle connection.

Furthermore, Ashwagandha is known to induce an improvement in the metabolic state in general: it increases the insulin sensitivity and decreases the levels of glucose, cholesterol and triglycerides in the blood, both in healthy subjects and in patients suffering from the metabolic syndrome or type diabetes 2. The cholesterol-lowering action has been explained by a mechanism similar to that of sterol plants: it seems that the root extract is able to increase the fecal excretion of cholesterol. Ashwagandha is able to support weight loss, inducing an improvement in the body composition: following the intake of supplements based on its extracts, it is possible to obtain not only an increase in muscle mass, but also a decrease in fat mass. It seems, in fact, that it is able to induce apoptosis of the adipose tissue cells, in particular pre-adipocytes (which are immature adipocytes).

Finally, the plant has a powerful antioxidant effect that helps increase the body's defenses from oxidative stress; intense physical exercises produce an enormous amount of free radicals, which are counteracted thanks to the presence of numerous endogenous antioxidant systems; the antioxidant defenses of the body of a sports subject, in order to function properly, require a higher intake of antioxidant micronutrients, such as vitamins and minerals; in this sense, the intake of Ashwagandha could support the antioxidant defenses and decrease the oxidative stress.

Evidence

Studies have shown a positive effect of the plant on cortisol, the stress hormone: there is a lowering of cortisol levels following the intake of the active ingredients. A study published in the *Indian Journal of Psychological Medicine* analyzed the effect of a highly concentrated extract of the plant on stress and anxiety. The scientists divided 64 women and men into two groups: one group took a placebo, the other took 300 mg of full-spectrum extract twice a day. After a 60-day intake period, both groups were compared with each other. Participants who took Ashwagandha showed significantly lower cortisol levels (up to 27.9% less than the control group). Furthermore, the results of the study reported that the plant extract is able to reduce the physical exhaustion during sports and no side effects were reported in the study participants.

The use of Ashwagandha as an antidepressant is widespread in Ayurvedic medicine and is also supported by numerous scientific studies, which have shown that the plant extract is able to induce a positive effect on brain neurotransmitters.

The antidepressant effect seems to be due to an improvement in the sensitivity of the receptors: in fact, in one study it was found that the administration of Ashwagandha extract improved the sensitivity of the 5-hydroxytryptophan (5-HTP) receptors. These receptors are the ones to which serotonin, also known as the "happiness hormone", binds. Most antidepressant treatments aim to normalize the serotonin levels, and that's exactly what this plant is going to do. In chronically stressed individuals who frequently suffer from depressive symptoms and anxiety, the administration of 300 mg of Ashwagandha extract reduced the symptoms of depression by almost 80%, without inducing side effects.

Ashwagandha is also known for its properties in the perspective of weight loss. It is definitely not a popular supplement for this function, but it can be supportive in many cases. Several processes can explain its function in this sense: the stress reduction effect promotes the weight loss. In fact, when cortisol is produced in excess it can prevent weight loss, exerting a catabolic effect on the muscle mass and a lipogenic effect on the adipose tissue, especially on the abdominal one.

Stress, leading to a condition of chronic fatigue, demotivates people, for which there is less motivation to practice sports and to maintain healthy eating habits (remember that low concentrations of tryptophan in the brain can be the cause of the "craving of carbohydrates and sugars ", or the desire for sweet and high-calorie foods that cause immediate gratification at the central level). A 2018 study highlights how prolonged stress, in fact, favors abdominal obesity. Therefore, since Ashwagandha lowers cortisol levels when it is in excess, it can promote weight loss by rebalancing the organism and by restoring correct eating habits. This was confirmed by a study published in 2017 in the *Journal of Evidence-based Complementary and Alternative Medicine*, in which 52 overweight men with chronic stress participated. These men were divided into two groups. The first group received a placebo, while the second received Ashwagandha dry extract at a dose of 300 mg, twice a day. After 8 weeks of treatment, the scientists compared the two groups. Body weight, body mass index and cortisol levels were significantly lower in the group that took Ashwagandha. In addition, the extract had a positive influence on the desire for food and on the general state of well-being perceived by the subjects. No side effects were reported.

Also in the context of weight loss, a study has shown how the withaferin A lactone, present in the leaves of the plant, can lower the vitality of the adipose tissue cells and induce their apoptosis.

A research conducted in 2015 showed that the plant is capable of improving the body composition. The 8-week study involved 57 young men who received a placebo or Ashwagandha extract at a dose of 300 mg twice daily. During this trial period, the participants performed weight training sessions.

Comparing the two groups, the scientists found that the group that took the Ashwagandha supplement had an increase in their muscle mass and muscle strength; training-induced damage was also reduced, improving the muscle recovery. Furthermore, participants belonging to the experimental group lost 2% more fat mass than the placebo group.

Recently, Ashwagandha has also become very popular in the sports world; many athletes, in fact, use it to improve their sports performance. Studies confirm this effect. The plant, in fact, is able to increase the muscle strength, muscle mass and endurance. A study conducted on untrained and sedentary subjects found a positive effect on muscle strength. The study, published in the *Journal of Ayurveda and Integrative Medicine*, involved 18 men with a sedentary lifestyle; the subjects were not involved in training programs, however the use of Ashwagandha had positive effects on health, as stated by the researchers: "In this study, Ashwagandha supplements showed a positive effect on muscle strength, on the lipid profile in the blood and in the sleep quality".

Muscle strength of back and quadriceps muscles increased by 15.4 and 21.5%, respectively; fat mass was also decreased.

Another study analyzed the synergistic effects of weight training and the administration of Ashwagandha: 57 participants took a standardized Ashwagandha extract (300 mg with 5% withanolide) or a placebo. After 8 weeks the two groups were compared: in the subjects belonging to the experimental group, there was a greater increase in muscle mass and strength than in the placebo group. The difference was 20 kg for the flat bench press and 4.5 kg for the leg extension. Also in this study, no side effects were reported.

Performance in endurance sports can also improve with the intake of Ashwagandha. In an 8-week study of professional cyclists, 1 g of root extract improved their performance. The cyclists were divided as always into two groups, an experimental one (taking 500 mg of root extract twice a day) and a placebo group. At the end of the study, the scientists reported that the use of the extract had caused an increase in VO_{2max} (maximum respiratory volume) of 12.5% and also an increase in fatigue time of 7.2% compared to the control group.

The plant is also used for the treatment of male sexual dysfunctions and in cases where there are low levels of testosterone in men. In Indian medicine, Ashwagandha is used in synergy with other plants to improve male (but also female) sexual health. One of the first studies was conducted in 2009 in mice, in which an increase in testosterone levels was reported. Human studies are somewhat conflicting: in some subjects it has shown a positive effect on raising the levels of testosterone, in others, however, it was not possible to demonstrate any effect. However, a study conducted on infertile men reported beneficial effects following the intake of Ashwagandha: the subjects that were recruited in this study had infertility problems, and there was an increased sperm count following the intake of the plant extract.

However, there are many studies in the literature to support the fact that the use of Ashwagandha may be beneficial for improving sexual performance and to increase the levels of sex hormones. This appears to be mainly due to the antioxidant properties of the active ingredients found in the leaves and roots of the plant. In fact, it has been observed in several studies that the intake of antioxidants in sterile men leads to an increase in sex hormones in the blood. Another interesting aspect in relation to the action on testosterone is reported by a study in which Ashwagandha extract was shown to increase testosterone levels in healthy men undergoing weight training. Over an 8-week period, men taking the supplement had an increase in their testosterone levels by 15% compared to the placebo group.

This improvement is certainly due to the anti-stress effect induced by the plant: it is known, in fact, that stress lowers the immune system and reduces the activity of the immune system; it seems that withanolide A is able to compensate for the weakening of the immune defenses induced by stress. To prove this hypothesis, some scientists analyzed the effect of the plant on dexamethasone, a drug that attenuates the immune response and counteracts the inflammatory processes by suppressing the activity of Th1 cells (which belong to the category of T helper lymphocytes, which regulate the inflammatory processes).

In mice, withanolide A has been shown to compensate for the immunosuppressive effect induced by the drug. The drug has a structure similar to endogenous cortisol, so its mechanism of action is comparable to the modulation of cortisol levels, although the exact mechanism is yet to be clarified. In addition, other studies have shown a regulation of the production of immunoglobulins, in particular those belonging to IgM and IgG class, which perform important functions in the immune system and are also responsible for the phenomenon of food intolerance.

If it's true that physical exercise strengthens the immune system, it is also true that an excess of physical activity can weaken it. Athletes who devote a lot of time to training could therefore profit by the use of Ashwgandha, especially in the most intense preparation periods.

Some studies have shown positive effects of the plant also on the glycemic/lipid profile; in other words, it seems that Ashwagandha is able to lower blood sugar levels, improve insulin sensitivity and lower triglyceride levels; a study conducted on men suffering from metabolic syndrome and type 2 diabetes reported the metabolic benefits, which are attributable to the antioxidant effect and to the modulation of the production of cortisol carried out by this plant.

Dosages

The optimal dosage of Ashwagandha depends on your personal goals. A dose of 300-500 mg per day may be sufficient. For acute disorders such as chronic stress, the intake can be increased up to 1000 mg per day. According to current studies, up to this dosage, no side effects or addiction are found, so the supplement can be taken daily. The best time to take it is in the morning, at breakfast, when cortisol levels are physiologically higher.

Effectiveness

Strength	Resistant strength	Mass	Endurance	Slimming	Concentration	Recovery
++	++	+	++	+++	+	++

ATP

Description

ATP (adenosine triphosphate) is the compound that provides the cell with the energy it needs to carry out any type of biological work. From a chemical point of view, it is a triphosphate nucleotide consisting of a nucleotide, adenine, a sugar, ribose, and three phosphate groups indicated with alpha, beta and gamma. In the cell, the energy obtained from the demolition processes (catabolic or exergonic) is temporarily stored in the ATP and subsequently used for synthesis processes (anabolic or endoergonic) which require energy. The phosphate groups, in fact, are very reactive, in the sense that their hydrolysis or their transfer to another molecule occur with the release of energy. When cells need energy, the phosphate groups are detached from the ATP molecule, first forming adenosine diphosphate (ADP), then adenosine monophosphate (AMP) and finally simply adenosine, which is further hydrolyzed by the cell. About 80-100 g of total ATP are stored in the human body; being an acid, its concentration must be limited in order not to lower the cellular pH too much. The total amount of ATP in the body is sufficient to support maximum work lasting a few seconds. Once the stocks of ATP are exhausted, this molecule must be re-synthesized through anaerobic metabolism (creatine phosphate and anaerobic lactacid) and aerobic metabolism (burning of glucose, fatty acids and proteins with oxygen).

Properties

ATP is the main human metabolite for the intracellular energy and is absolutely essential as a regulator of multiple physiological functions at the extracellular level.

One of the molecular mechanisms in which ATP is used as an energy source is the muscle contraction, which is the result of a series of events that occur inside the cell and that involve a metameric structure called sarcomere, the morphofunctional and contractile unit of the skeletal and cardiac striated muscle. The main peptide components of the sarcomere are: thick filaments of myosin, thin filaments of actin and other structural proteins that stabilize the structure (dystrophin, troponin and tropomyosin). The thick filament of myosin is characterized by the presence of a head that has the ability to hydrolyze ATP in the presence of calcium, and to use the released energy for the contraction process. ATP is linked to myosin when the muscle fiber is relaxed. When the fiber is stimulated, calcium ions activate the hydrolysis of ATP which becomes ADP by releasing a phosphate group. The myosin head, supplied with potential energy, can bind to actin in a configuration known as a "cross bridge".

In the meantime, the ADP and the phosphate group are released and the myosin head "pulls" the actin, causing it to flow towards the center of the sarcomere. As long as another ATP molecule does not bind to the myosin head, the latter remains bound in the cross-bridge configuration. When another ATP molecule becomes available, the mechanism repeats itself, resulting in the progressive shortening of the sarcomere and, ultimately, of the entire myofibril and muscle fiber.

Although oral ingestion of ATP results in its rapid degradation, by removing the high-energy phosphoric bonds and thus compromising its energy value, various studies indicate that oral administration is still able to produce improvements in strength and in the athletic performance. This depends on the extracellular functions of ATP that have nothing to do with the production of energy. In fact, these extracellular functions of ATP require quantities as much as hundreds of times lower than those necessary to perform the intracellular energy functions. Therefore, they are not negatively affected by oral administration. **The extracellular functions that affect the muscle performance are the increase in vasodilation, the facilitation of muscle contraction and the decreased perception of pain.**

These effects occur thanks to the interaction of ATP with the adenosine receptors at the cell membrane level, which triggers a series of cascade reactions that produce the ergogenic effects mentioned above.

Adequate levels of ATP are essential for our health, for the physical effort and also for the functioning of the organs. In fact, the reduction of the quantity of ATP in the blood negatively affects blood pressure and the vascular health.

Evidence

Our metabolism naturally and constantly produces ATP, but there are some factors, such as age, exercise and other stress factors, which can quickly deplete its levels or slow down its synthesis. A variety of clinical and pre-clinical studies carried out on humans show how extracellular ATP and its main degradation product, adenosine, activate specific ATP and adenosine receptors on the cells that line the walls of blood vessels. This interaction determines an improvement in the tone of the vessels, favoring vasodilation through the stimulation of NO production, and also favoring the flow of blood to the heart and to the peripheral organs (in particular the liver and skeletal muscles), promoting the transport of glucose, nutrients and oxygen to the working muscles and the removal of catabolic residues, such as lactic acid and ammonia. ATP would also improve the blood flow in the brain, postponing mental fatigue, maintaining clarity and decreasing the perception of fatigue during exercise.

These effects are expected to impact the muscle endurance. In a study conducted by Rathmacher et al., in which 400 mg of ATP were administered each day for two weeks, there was a significant improvement especially in the last sets of high intensity exercises.

In one study, rodents received 5 mg per kg of body weight of an oral ATP supplement and they showed an increase in the absorption and production of this molecule. It was therefore assumed that these benefits also apply to humans and a series of subsequent studies were carried out. In particular, a study conducted by Jordan et al., carried out on humans, compared the effects of ATP supplementation between a group that took a higher dose of ATP (225 mg) and a group that took a lower dose of ATP (150 mg). The result showed no differences, neither in the levels of ATP in the blood, nor in strength or duration during the bench press. There were no differences immediately after taking the supplement and not even after 14 days of treatment. The supplement did not change the maximum power, nor the average power during the anaerobic training session. However, unlike the placebo group, those who took ATP experienced a significant increase in the number of reps performed in the bench press during the first set and a 22% increase in training volume after 14 days. Another study by Wilson et al. showed that 12 weeks of supplementing with 400 mg per day of ATP during weight training resulted in increased strength and full body muscle measurements. In the same study, it was observed that subjects who overtrained voluntarily had a lower muscle catabolism.

Overall, the results of Jordan et al. suggested that dosages of 225 mg or less of oral ATP supplementation, as a dietary supplement, may have been too low to demonstrate any substantial improvement in the physical performance in humans.

Taking ATP and HMB (β-hydroxy-β-methyl-butyric acid) supplements during a weight training program for 12 weeks increased strength and power, while also preventing the effects of overtraining, as suggested in a study by Led Lowery of the Department of Health Sciences and Human Performance at the University of Tampa, Florida. The test subjects underwent an 8-week weight training program, followed by an intense 2-week program designed to cause overtraining, and then by 2 weeks in which the workload was reduced. Subjects took 3 g of free HMB and 400 mg of ATP or a placebo daily, for the whole duration of the study. Subjects who had taken HMB/ATP showed a gain in strength and power throughout the entire study. The placebo group had far fewer gains and regressed during the 2-week overtraining phase. The supplementation of ATP and HMB during an intense training increases strength and power more than just training and, in addition, it also prevents the worsening of the performance during periods of intense training.

The mechanism by which extracellular ATP can improve the muscle contraction seems to be linked to its ability to stimulate the entry of calcium into the muscle cell, and we know that calcium facilitates the interaction between muscle proteins actin and myosin, by triggering muscle contraction.

In addition, by stimulating the entry of calcium into the muscle cell, the entry of glucose is also stimulated, which can make up for the energy demands of the muscle. This facilitation also occurs in the liver, where the increased level of calcium promotes glycogenolysis, thus making more glucose available to be used by the muscle. To conclude, some studies have shown the ability to decrease the pain perception in patients with acute post-surgical pain or in those that suffer from chronic neuropathic pain, and this ability to increase the pain threshold can obviously be useful when performing particularly hard workouts.

Dosages
Studies indicate that the effective dosage should be between 300 and 400 mg per day. A sublingual oral intake would probably be preferred.

Effectiveness

Strength	Resistant strength	Mass	Endurance	Slimming	Concentration	Recovery
++	++++	++	+	+	+++	−

BACOPA

Description
Bacopa monnieri is the scientific name of water hyssop, a plant used for thousands of years in India in the traditional Ayurvedic medicine and also in TCM (Traditional Chinese Medicine), which is called Brahmi in India. It is considered one of the main plants with rejuvenating and revitalizing effects on the central nervous system. Its name derives from that of the god

Brahma, the creator of the Hindu deities, who heals and ensures good health. It is a perennial plant native to the areas of southern and eastern India, Australia, Europe, Africa, Asia, North and South America, and it belongs to the *Scrophulariaceae* family.

It is a plant with small white flowers that grows up to 20 cm in height; its stem remains below the water level, while the leaves and flowers remain above. In fact, it grows in humid and marshy environments, near lakes, streams and waterholes.

Properties

Bacopa monnieri acts as a neuroprotective agent on various aspects at the brain level, through a combined action on metabolism, circulation and directly at the cellular level; it is effective against some cognitive or mood disorders (anxiety, attention problems, depression, etc.); it improves the memory and the cognitive skills. It is endowed with antioxidant and anti-inflammatory effects, due to some active ingredients that are contained in its leaves.

These bioactive compounds are made up of flavonoids (luteolin, apigenin, jujubogenin, cucurbitacins), alkaloids, vitamin C and, above all, of the triterpenoid saponins and bacosides (A and B) contained in them. *Bacopa* prolongs the life of neurons, particularly in the hippocampus, which is the region of the brain associated with long-term memory. Several actions of this Ayurvedic plant are also beneficial in the cholinergic, dopaminergic and serotonergic neuronal pathways, modulating the functionality of these neurotransmitters. A positive action was observed on acetylcholine levels (a neurotransmitter responsible for the transmission of nerve signals to the memory center) in the hippocampus. In particular, *Bacopa* would positively affect the cholinergic system through the modulation of serotonin receptors. *Bacopa* increases the mental, cognitive and memory functions and improves the brain plasticity, i.e. the ability of the brain to adapt its structure and functions according to the activity of its neurons (neuronal plasticity), following stimuli received from the external environment, in reaction to stressful events, traumatic injuries or pathological changes, but also in relation to the individual development process. For all these reasons, *Bacopa* is particularly useful for enhancing the memory and for counteracting cognitive decline, and it is also an excellent natural anxiolytic that counteracts stress, depression and anxiety. One of the active ingredients, herpestine, is an alkaloid that has been shown to have a relaxing effect, known as a sedative-like substance.

Recently *Bacopa* has also shown interesting effects in improving the sports performance, including the ability to relieve the muscle fatigue and to improve motor functions. To obtain an optimal sports performance, it is also important to intervene on some "cognitive" aspects, including the reaction speed, attention, spatial memory, executive functions and focus on the goal, and *Bacopa* has been shown to be capable of doing all of them.

Evidence

Bacopa and in particular bacosides have antioxidant (lipid peroxidation reduction), anti-inflammatory and antimicrobial effects (Mathur et al., 2010; Simpson et al., 2015). The biological effects of *Bacopa* are also well documented by the scientific literature, which is focused mainly on bacosides as the main responsible substance for the actions on the nervous system. A 2017 American study by the University of Montana demonstrated the anti-inflammatory properties of various preparations (tea, infusions, alkaloids, bacoside A) based on *Bacopa* extracts. Specifically, these extracts are able to inhibit (in vitro) the production of pro-inflammatory cytokines (TNF-α and IL-6), starting from a line of activated microglial cells which, notably, participate in the cerebral inflammatory process. In a study published in 2017 in *Psychiatry Investigation*, other researchers evaluated the effects of a daily oral administration of *Bacopa* extract in depressed rats for 28 days, at a dose of 80 mg/kg. The results show that the treatment is sufficient to restore the levels of BDNF, a protein that acts as a brain neurotrophic factor in the hippocampus, and is responsible for the growth and the survival of developing neurons, and for the maintenance of mature neurons. Recently, some researchers have evaluated the effect of a *Bacopa* ethanolic extract in a model of Parkinson's disease that causes alterations of the so-called nigrostriatal circuit, a dopaminergic neuronal pathway. Not only does the extract reverse the motor deficits, but it also increases the dopamine levels significantly. A standardized natural *Bacopa* extract has also been shown to have positive effects on the memory. In fact, a 2016 study published in the *Pharmacognosy* journal showed that this extract inhibits enzymes such as catechol-O-methyl-transferase (COMT) and prolyl-endopeptidase (PEP). Moreover, the COMT enzyme is involved in the modulation of memory by influencing the metabolism of dopamine: by inhibiting its activity, *Bacopa* extract would improve the memory. The PEP enzyme is known for its neuropeptidase activity, involved in the cognitive decline. In fact, the PEP enzyme eliminates neuropeptides such as arginine-vasopressin, oxytocin, neurotensin or substance P, molecules that play a key role in positive reinforcement, in social interactions, in emotions or even in the response to stress. In these conditions, the inhibitory action of *Bacopa* compounds could therefore have a beneficial effect against cognitive decline, strengthening the cognitive abilities. The neuroprotective effect was demonstrated in a study published in 2006 in *Neuroscience*, in which researchers identified bacoside A as a neuroprotective agent against the death (apoptosis) of neuronal cells in a cigarette smoke-induced toxicity model; a 2014 study also reported the neuroprotective effect of a *Bacopa* extract on aluminum-induced toxicity in the hippocampus of rats.

From a physiological point of view, it is able to increase glycogen reserves and improve the energy metabolism, thus helping to increase the performance (Chen Zhidan, et al., 2017). *Bacopa* speeds up the processing of information (reduces the latency of evoked potentials), increasing alertness, reaction speed, attention, spatial and working memory, thus optimizing the executive functions and the focus towards the goal (Kennedy, 2018; Peth-Nui et al., 2012).

Dosages

The daily doses of *Bacopa* that are generally recommended in traditional practice are 5-10 g of non-standardized powder, 8-16 mL of infusion and 30 mL of syrup per day. For extracts standardized to 20% bacoside A and B, the dosage is 200-400 mg per day for adults, in divided doses. As for possible side effects, these include thyroid disorders and intestinal tract problems. Furthermore, the possible interactions with some drugs are still being studied, such as sedatives, chlorpromazine and thyroid hormones, whose effects could increase.

Effectiveness

Strength	Resistant strength	Mass	Endurance	Slimming	Concentration	Recovery
–	+	+	++	+	+++	–

BETA-ALANINE

Description

Beta-alanine is a non-proteinogenic amino acid produced endogenously by the human body. It is also present in nature, especially in protein foods such as red and white meats or in fish, but not in its free form. In fact, it is bound as a constituent of certain peptides which, through degradation, release beta-alanine into the circulation. The endogenous synthesis of beta-alanine occurs in the liver, starting from the irreversible degradation of pyrimidines (thymine, cytosine and uracil). Once synthesized, it is transported to muscle cells where it crosses the sarcolemic pathway by means of Na^+ and Cl^- dependent transporters (Artoli et al., 2009). Beta-alanine is captured by the various muscle fibers by means of co-transporters for molecules with a structure similar to beta-alanine, such as glycine, taurine and GABA. This process suggested that the supplementation of this amino acid limited or dysregulated the normal uptake of these substances; in reality, there are no studies that prove this hypothesis, therefore the administration of beta-alanine in sports is considered safe and effective.

Properties

Beta-alanine has various functions at the nervous level, acting as a neurotransmitter and neuromodulator for the binding sites of NMDA, GABA-A, GABA-C and glycine receptors (present in the hippocampus), helping in the learning process. Its function in the muscle is closely linked with carnosine, the main buffer system possessed by our muscle cells to counteract the effects of lactic acid. Carnosine, or more chemically speaking β-alanyl-L-histidine, is a dipeptide that is naturally present in muscle fibers. Carnosine is mainly produced in muscle cells from beta-alanine and histidine, a reaction carried out by carnosine synthetase. Between these two amino acids, the one that decreases their synthesis or the limiting molecule is precisely beta-alanine; a reduced amount of this amino acid reduces the production of muscle carnosine. In the intracellular environment, beta-alanine levels have a great impact on the activity of carnosine synthase enzyme, and its deficiency limits this activity. For this reason, beta-alanine appears to be the limiting factor of carnosine synthesis (Harris et al., 2012).

This reaction is catalyzed by carnosine synthetase enzyme and its formation occurs primarily in the muscle cells, just as the levels of this dipeptide in the bloodstream are negligible due to the catalytic action of carnosinases.

The synthesis of carnosine is regulated by three factors:

- the degree of beta-alanine uptake in muscle fibers;
- the serum activity of carnosine synthetase, in the absence of a sufficient concentration of beta-alanine in the diet;
- the hepatic synthesis of amino acids and their transport into the skeletal muscles.

Carnosine is a stable molecule; its intramuscular concentration usually shows a constant level or slight declines over time. Intracellular carnosine levels are higher in men than in women, and higher in type II (white) fibers compared to type I (red) fibers; these levels decrease with age due to the depletion of glycolytic action or due to the loss of type II fibers. One hypothesis for this decrease is attributable to the decline in testosterone levels, which normally occurs with advancing age (Stout et al., 2008; Derave et al., 2007).

Evidence

Carnosine acts mainly as an intracellular buffer of lactate when there is a short-term demand for ATP, which is produced from glucose in the absence of oxygen, through anaerobic glycolysis.

The condition in which these chemical reactions take place, in the presence of sub- or supramaximal efforts, is known as metabolic acidosis and it is concomitant with a decrease in the aerobic capacity of the muscles. Since the mitochondrion needs to extrude the protons for energy production, in conditions of acidosis the intracellular stocks of ATP decrease by about 40%, with a consequent total depletion of phosphocreatine at the expense of an increase in lactic acid and H^+ ions. The excess of these ions causes physiological changes within the muscle, such as the inhibition of phosphofructokinase, the reduction of phosphocreatine resynthesis, a lower muscle glycolytic capacity and a competitive inhibition of Ca^{2+} ions in troponin C subunits, with the consequent delay in the reuptake of Ca^{2+} by the endoplasmic reticulum and the resulting muscle relaxation (Hobson et al., 2012; Hoffmann et al., 2008).

Furthermore, high levels of H⁺ can alter the epigenetic balance by acting on the acetylation of chromatin. Beta-alanine, by maintaining the physiological pH, limits the excessive deacetylation of DNA and the consequent competition of acetate and lactate for the MCT transporter (McBrian et al., 2013).

All these changes compromise the recovery capacity of the muscle, particularly after intense and/or maximal activity; for this reason, the body has buffer and transporter systems that remove lactic acid and H⁺ ions from the muscle. Monocarboxylated transporters, such as MCT1 and MCT4, facilitate the efflux of lactate and H⁺, while carnosine is the most effective buffer system (it has a buffer capacity of 10%). During a particularly intense exercise that induces metabolic acidosis, carnosine acts as an acceptor of H⁺ ions, thanks to its imidazole ring, with a consequent change of its acid dissociation constant (pKa) to 6.83, which allows the maintenance of the intracellular pH and the reduction of the sense of fatigue.

To implement this buffer system, beta-alanine is the best molecule, as it raises the intracellular concentration of carnosine. A 2006 study conducted in humans showed that a repeated intake of 10 mg/kg of beta-alanine (about 2.5 g per day), divided into three daily intakes, induced slight increases in the carnosine concentration, which were decreasing towards basal levels before the next administration. The same study also showed that a prolonged intake (4 weeks) of 3.2 g and 6.4 g of beta-alanine per day, before carrying out the training session, increased the intramuscular carnosine concentration by 42 and 64%. Moreover, the buffering capacity of the muscle increased, reaching values of 12.6 and 18% against the basal value, which normally stands at around 10%.

However, other studies have found that, with a daily administration of high doses of beta-alanine (4-6 g/day) for at least 4 weeks, the intramuscular carnosine concentration increases by about 60%, while at low doses (<4 g/day) this concentration increases by approximately 50%. **This process is enhanced by insulin, which is stimulated by the ingestion of carbohydrates.**

The main ergogenic effect of beta-alanine, by increasing the carnosine concentration, is obtained with a dosage of more than 3 g per day (3.2 g), taken continuously for a period of at least 4 weeks. In competitive sportsmen, such as cyclists, it has been seen that the combination of beta-alanine (65 mg/kg) and sodium bicarbonate ($NaHCO_3$) (300 mg/kg) for 28 days increases the intra- and extracellular buffering capacity, compared to a simple intake of only $NaHCO_3$.

A 2012 study conducted on trained subjects quantified the food timing of beta-alanine and recorded how the intake in a single administration, 20 minutes before the sporting activity, increased the carnosine stores and the buffering power of the muscle long enough to cover the entire training session. The examined subjects recorded a **decrease in the sense of fatigue and, therefore, an increase in the resistant force** (Spradley et al., 2012).

At least four high-quality studies have shown an **increase in lean body mass** in the beta-alanine group compared to the placebo group.

Some other effects of beta-alanine belong purely to the sports field, such as the increase in the athletic performance in sprinters who used a protocol of 6 g/day for 28 days, recording an increase in the training volume and quality. In addition, it was noted that lactate levels after training were perfectly within the normal range, while the values of VO_{2max} and heart rate were increased, a clear sign of an improvement in the aerobic capacity of the subjects under examination (Jordan et al., 2010; Del Favero et al., 2012).

In 2017, a Brazilian study evaluated the supplementation of beta-alanine in 12 judo athletes who engaged in both national and international competitions. In this study, it emerged that in judo, a sport that mainly requires an anaerobic metabolism (glycolysis), 4 g of beta- alanine had the ability to increase the endurance of effort by increasing the total number of throws of the opponent in the game, during the default time.

To support the results obtained from the performance studies requiring the contribution of glycolysis, we refer to the meta-analysis by Hobson et al. (2012), in which it is shown that beta-alanine works optimally on performances lasting between 1 and 4 minutes. In a study on female athletes who belonged to the master category, beta-alanine supplementation for 28 days resulted in an increased strength in the lower body muscles and a higher exercise capacity compared the placebo group (Jordan Glenn et al., *Journal Strength Conditioning Research*, 2016).

As for the possible adverse effects, it is reported that beta-alanine, even at moderate dosages of 3-4 g, can lead to tingling and paraesthesia, especially in the limbs. This particular effect is given by the binding of beta-alanine with MrgD receptors, mainly expressed in the sensory ganglions of the dorsal roots.

Although the perception of tingling is translated as feedback of the supplement's effectiveness, in other cases it could be annoying. A study by Church published in *Journal of the American College of Nutrition*, demonstrates how a gradual release dosage of 12 g of beta-alanine divided into 3 daily intakes of 4 g each, in addition to not causing paresthesia, allows a significant increase in intramuscular carnosine reserves in 2 weeks of supplementation, which is equal to what would have been obtained in 4 weeks with 6 g/day.

This demonstrates how the correct formulation can fill carnosine stocks in less time, with the classic benefits provided by this molecule. Varanoske et al. (2019) demonstrated how the slow release formulation, in addition to speeding up the carnosine concentration, limits the decline of histidine, which could be problematic under certain conditions. Although there were no significant changes in either serum or intramuscular histidine levels during the 2-week study, Blancquaert et al. (2017), in their study, showed how after a supplementation with beta-alanine equal to 6 g/day, histidine levels could undergo a non-negligible drop which, in the case of certain pathologies, such as for example anemia, bone marrow hypoplasia or other disorders affecting the erythrocytes, could make its supplementation not optimal unless there is included a supplementation of histidine equal to 3.5 g/day.

In conclusion, beta-alanine is an excellent supplement, especially for athletes who perform intense activities lasting between 1 and 4 minutes. The improvement of the buffering capacity of the muscle allows to extend the training time and consequently to improve all the parameters related to the endurance: aerobic capacity, resistant strength and resistance, especially in physical activities ranging from 30 seconds to 10 minutes (Saunders et al., 2017). Furthermore, by acting directly on the energy systems, beta-alanine saves more muscle creatine, therefore produces more metabolic energy (ATP) and also increases the intensity of the training. It can also prevent mental fatigue by improving the cognitive functions in situations of physical stress.

Dosages

Effective dosages vary from 3 to 6 g, depending on the weight and on the sporting activity. Usually, taking 6 g a day of beta-alanine is fine for a short period of at least 4 weeks, in such a way as to suddenly raise the concentration of carnosine as a function of a race (of any kind); if you opt for a lower dosage (3-4 g per day), then it is advisable to prolong the supplementation for at least 8-12 weeks, after which a dosage of 1.5 g per day is sufficient to keep carnosine levels around 50% higher than the baseline value.

Effectiveness

Strength	Resistant strength	Mass	Endurance	Slimming	Concentration	Recovery
−	++++	++	+++	−	++	−

BETA-ECDYSTERONE

Description
Ecdysteroids are arthropod steroid hormones that regulate the process of moulting, metamorphosis and reproduction. They are present in 5-6% of botanical species, in which they play the role of deterrent substances, keeping away predatory insects and parasites. The parent molecule, present in both animal and plant kingdoms, is 20-hydroxyecdysone, from which other similar compounds derive through esterification, hydroxylation and glycosylation. In plants, it is present as a phytoecdysteroid, produced by different species such as *Cyanotis vaga*, *Rhaponticum carthamoides*, suma and maca. Numerous preparations containing ecdisteroids can be found on the market, some containing pure 20-ecdysterone, others containing miscellaneous mixtures of ecdisteroids.

Properties
Ecdisteroids are endowed with numerous therapeutic activities described by various authors, which however require further research to be confirmed. In mammals, they intervene in the main metabolic pathways of proteins, fats and carbohydrates, acting as anabolic, hepatoprotector, antioxidant, immunoprotector and hypoglycemic agents. Furthermore, by acting as adaptogens, in addition to improving the athletic performance, they improve stress tolerance and they also have an anti-aging effect. A considerable amount of data has demonstrated the anabolic effect of ecdysteroids and the absence of side effects. The mechanism of action does not involve the androgen receptor and this effect seems to be due to the increase in the concentration of calcium and potassium ions in the muscle cells, thus catalyzing the process of protein synthesis with the relative advantage that this way, they **do not inhibit the synthesis of testosterone or other hormones**. On the contrary, they stabilize the cortisol levels.

Another way through which it is believed that the ecdysteroids can exert an anabolic effect at the muscle level, is through the activation of the signal mediated by the PI3K/Akt pathway. With aging, the degree of protein synthesis in the muscle decreases due to the reduction in the activation of this signal, leading to the condition known as the "anabolic resistance". More recent studies seem to have identified an estrogen receptor, ER-beta, as a possible ecdysterone receptor, the activation of which exerts an anabolic effect. Among other things, ecdysterone is able to stimulate the gene expression of the estrogen receptor in a dose-dependent manner. It also increases the serum concentration of 17-beta-estradiol, which in turn activates ER-beta.

Another potential effect of ecdisteroids is the ability to influence positively the cellular repair process following muscle injuries. The anti-inflammatory and antifibrinolytic properties of these compounds can provide additional benefits, in addition to those stimulating hypertrophy, as excessive inflammation and related fibrosis of the muscle tissue compromise the functional healing. However, studies have yet to be carried out.

Evidence
The first studies on the possible use of beta-ecdysterone as a supplement were carried out in the 1970s by Russian scholars, who noted an increase in protein synthesis and a possible anabolic activity following the consumption of the molecule, subsequently confirmed by another study in which they compared the effects of beta-ecdysterone itself and of the steroid meta-androsterone on protein synthesis, revealing a higher greater efficacy of the former. Other studies, this time in animals (rats), have suggested the same anabolic effects.

The problem is that most of the studies conducted in Eastern European countries were published in Russian and therefore, the articles are not easy to access, also in order to verify the correct procedure. Demin et al. (1976) reported a significant increase in the athletic performance, including strength, duration and coordination, after taking *Rhaponticum carthamoides* (RCE). According to Petkov et al. (1984), RCE considerably increases the working capacity of the already fatigued muscle fibers, and it increases the concentration of glycogen, ATP and creatine phosphate. Portugalov et al. (1996) reported the effects of three preparations containing ecdisteroids on the protein balance and on the training capacity, concluding that these preparations possessed an anabolic, anti-catabolic and a recovering capacity. In 1998, a study by Simakin et al. evaluated the coupled effect of taking ecdysterone together with a high protein diet. The results showed mean increases of 6-7% in lean mass and 10% reductions in fat mass in the test subjects; moreover, ecdysterone seemed to be able to reduce the circulating glucose levels without altering the insulin levels.

However, there are more recent studies which have not shown such effects. For example, in 2006, a double-blind placebo study by Wilborn et al. conducted on 45 athletes for 8 weeks, evaluating the possible effects on the increase of protein synthesis and on the increase of sports performance, did not show any correlation between the intake of doses of 200 mg/day of ecdysterone and the effects on chemical indicators related to protein synthesis or to hormonal changes, nor to the increase in the athletic performance or changes in the body composition.

Another study conducted on rats evaluated the increase in muscle mass in the whole body and in specific muscle groups after the administration of 20-hydroxyecdysterone (5 mg/kg/day). It showed a significant increase in triceps brachialis after only 5 days of treatment compared to the control cases, and genome analyzes of the treated rats revealed gene expression changes related to the triceps muscle. They identified 16 genes involved particularly in the muscle development. Some researchers, always analyzing the effects of 20-hydroxyecdysterone supplements in rats, have reported further increases in both size and diameter of the soleus muscle, suggesting with higher hypertrophic/anabolic effects compared to compounds that are considered doping, always administered to rats as control cases (metandienone, estradienedione, SARM S-1), all in doses of 5 mg/day for 21 days.

Dosages
In any case, beta-ecdysterone does not seem to have side effects even at fairly consistent dosages. The suggested doses are at least 200-300 mg/day, taken close to meals. To maximize its effects, it will also be important to follow a diet that meets the individual's protein needs.

Effectiveness

Strength	Resistant strength	Mass	Endurance	Slimming	Concentration	Recovery
+	++	++	+	+	+	++

BETAINE

Description
Betaine is a natural substance that has been found in sugar beets. Chemically, it is a small N-trimethylated amino acid and a neutral compound, with a positively charged functional cation group and a negatively charged functional group, also known as trimethylglycine. It is a natural organic osmolyte that serves to protect cells from dehydration by increasing the water retention through its osmotic effect, without disturbing the enzymatic functionality, the structure of proteins and the integrity of the cell membrane.

In addition to being produced by the liver and kidneys thanks to the choline oxidase enzyme, it is widely present in spinach and quinoa, and abundant quantities have also been found in bran and fish. The average intake is around 100-400 mg/day and a dosage of 2.5 g/day is sufficient to evaluate its effects on the performance and on the body composition.

Furthermore, it is a methyl donor and is therefore important in the transmethylation processes that occur in the liver during the detoxification phases. It also favors the conversion of homocysteine into methionine, with the consequent formation of SAM-e.

Properties

Betaine's ability to maintain the hydration at the cellular level reduces the negative impact that dehydration can have on the athletic performance, such as tachycardia, increased rate of glycogen breakdown, increased body temperature in the muscles and the increased concentration of lactic acid. Furthermore, this ability to hydrate the muscle cell seems to favor the protein synthesis and lower the catabolism, as if the cell were stimulated to increase its size at a structural level.

This mechanism also appears to be at the basis of the effectiveness of other supplements, such as creatine, glutamine and also of drugs such as anabolic steroids. Furthermore, since betaine is a methyl donor, it contributes to the synthesis of s-adenosylmethionine, which is, together with arginine and glycine, a constituent necessary for the synthesis of the tripeptide creatine. Further *in vitro* and *in vivo* studies have shown that betaine is able to stimulate the production of IGF-1, which is a potent anabolic peptide hormone, increasing the lean mass and reducing the abdominal fat.

In addition to being used for the improvement of the athletic performance, betaine's ability to lower homocysteine levels, limit oxidative stress, allow creatine synthesis and DNA repair, and decrease the side effects of TMAO, mean that this supplement can also be a candidate in cardiovascular, neurodegenerative, neoplastic and musculoskeletal diseases.

Evidence

Betaine, given its ability to prevent dehydration, has been considered as a supplement for runners and cyclists, for whom dehydration is a very serious problem. However, at the moment, most of the studies have not demonstrated any efficacy of betaine in improving aerobic performance. Conversely, an increase in maximum leg strength was found in cyclists after aerobic training. Specifically, in one study two groups of cyclists trained for two hours at 60-70% of their maximum aerobic capacity and then a 15-minute "trial" was carried out on bikes followed by an isometric leg strength test.

The first group consumed a carbohydrate drink, while the second group consumed a carbohydrate drink plus betaine. Well, the group that took betaine showed an improvement in the cycling trial, indicating that betaine, by limiting dehydration, has a positive effect on performance. Additionally, the group taking betaine had a **significant increase in strength** compared to the carbohydrate-only group. In a study by Marsh et al., it was found that 14 days of supplementing with 2.5 g of betaine per day produced significant improvements in bench press and vertical jump tests. In fact, these results could be mediated by the action of creatine and there are no studies demonstrating an additive effect of betaine added to creatine. **Betaine supplementation also increased IGF-1 values by 7.8% and decreased cortisol values by 6.1%**, thus creating a better anabolic situation from an endocrine point of view. In a study by Apicella et al., 12 trained men took betaine or a placebo for two weeks, after which a blood sample was taken immediately after a workout and different markers related to muscle development were measured. The results demonstrated an increase in IGF-1 activity and a decrease in the catabolic effect of AMPK, thus configuring a better anabolic situation which favors the muscle growth.

Armstrong et al. found that betaine reduces thirst and the sensation of heat during the final sprint after 75 minutes of running, and Hoffman et al. found a significant increase in the anaerobic power and strength, as well as a **reduced perception of fatigue**, during a high volume workout with a supplementation of 2.5 g of betaine.

More recently, in 2018, Cholewa et al. published a study in which they demonstrated the effects of betaine supplements in non-sedentary normal weight women, aged between 18 and 35 years. Subjects were asked to practice weight training three times a week for 8 weeks. The study, although carried out meticulously by respecting several criteria (standardized nutrition, monitored hydration, non-bulky clothing), showed only an improvement in fat mass ($-3.3 \pm 1.9\%$) compared to the placebo ($-1.7 \pm 1.6\%$) and in the total weekly work volume, while no significant results were found on the 1RM squat and bench press strength or in power (vertical jump) and lean mass tests.

Even though several studies have found more consistent improvements in strength and in the endurance performance, probably due to betaine's ability to maintain a constant hydration, to prevent the oxidation of the myosin chain and the affinity between Ca^{2+} and troponin, and to ensure a thermodynamic protection of mitochondrial citrate synthase, it should however be considered that women, in addition to having a smaller amount of intramuscular betaine (40% less), also have a greater amount of estradiol and cortisol, which must necessarily be eliminated through the BHMT enzyme. The latter, using betaine, strongly limits the intracellular osmotic effect. In addition, the study did not comply with the standard low-calorie regime protein quantities recommended by the International Society of Sport Nutrition, equal to approximately 1.8-2.2 g/kg of body weight.

Returning to the function of betaine as a methyl donor, it can intervene in the synthesis of neurotransmitters such as dopamine and hormones such as adrenaline, which are very important for coping with strenuous and intense exercises. Dopamine promotes a **higher mental charge and concentration**, while adrenaline, also called epinephrine, favors the use of substrates such as glucose and fatty acids for energy purposes. This increased adrenaline production can improve the athletic performance.

Also due to its property as a methyl donor, we have already said that betaine favors the conversion of homocysteine, which is a known cardiovascular risk factor, into methionine, favoring the availability of the latter for the production of creatine, lowering homocysteine levels and sparing the use of choline, which is used as a precursor for plasmatic and mitochondrial membranes. Furthermore, betaine supplementation is able to limit the excess of homocysteine derived from a previous load of methionine, which normally occurs in some individuals with mutation of the MTHFR gene who consume excessive quantities of foods containing this amino acid (red meat or sulfur foods). Furthermore, betaine can be used as a protector against the reductive stress, a form of cell damage derived from the reaction of iron with hydrogen peroxide (Fenton reaction); this characteristic is given by the fact that it contains positively charged N groups, also present in SAM-e, carnitine, phosphatidylcholine and sphingomyelin, which make the adjacent methyl group devoid of an electron and, therefore, able to be accepted by $NADH^+$, widely present in cases of mitochondrial dysfunction.

Since homocysteine worsens the insulin sensitivity, a lower homocysteine level will favor a better uptake of glucose and creatine by muscle cells, and a greater synthesis of glycogen and creatine phosphate, with a positive impact on the athletic performance, especially the anaerobic one.

Dosages

The best time to take betaine is probably before and after training, in two doses, 1.25-2 g at a time. It is best to take betaine with simple carbohydrates to increase the muscle uptake. A study showed that taking 6 g of betaine per day increases cholesterol levels, so it is advisable not to exceed the recommended dose.

Effectiveness

Strength	Resistant strength	Mass	Endurance	Slimming	Concentration	Recovery
+++	+	++	+	+	++	++

BRANCHED AMINO ACIDS

Description
Among the amino acids that make up the protein chain, the ones we know best are undoubtedly the so-called branched or BCAAs (Branched Chain Aminoacids), regarding the branching of their molecular structure. Leucine, valine and isoleucine are essential amino acids and must be introduced with the diet; they are distinguished from other amino acids as they are the only ones that do not undergo modifications when passing through the liver, thus reaching the organs responsible for their metabolization "unharmed" (muscle tissue is the primary place of BCAA degradation). The muscles are able to use BCAAs directly for any need, both during the catabolic phase during stress or physical activity, and during the anabolic phase. Numerous experiments conducted on isolated muscles (both *in vitro* and *in vivo*) have highlighted the proteo-anabolic and anti-catabolic properties of BCAAs. A lack of these amino acids causes the beginning of the catabolic process, promoting a decrease in the protein content of the muscle. Particular attention should be paid to leucine, as it is responsible for the majority of the stimulus needed for the protein synthesis.

Properties
BCAAs represent a maximum of 20% of the dietary proteins, while their very high turnover means that they represent the dominant share of circulating amino acids used after a protein meal. Following a protein meal, BCAAs are easily absorbed in the intestine and reach the liver, where, unlike other amino acids, they do not undergo chemical changes. Following appropriate stimuli, the liver releases the BCAAs, which reach the various organs through the circulation, where their utilization and metabolization takes place, in particular in the muscle tissue.

In muscles, BCAAs make up 20% of contractile proteins and can be:
- oxidized for energy purposes (especially leucine can be used in this way, resulting in a precious glucose saving);
- used for the synthesis of proteins in muscle;
- used in the synthesis of alanine, an amino acid of fundamental importance for neoglucogenesis;
- re-released into the circulation without being metabolized to be used electively in the brain.

These events suggest that the serum concentrations of BCAAs are effectively regulated and that those who exercise need greater amounts of these amino acids.

The catabolism of BCAAs occurs in the mitochondria of the cell. BCAAs undergo reversible conversion into their α-ketoderivatives (known as branched-chain α-keto acids) via the branched-chain aminotransferase (BCAT) enzyme and are then irreversibly metabolized (oxidative decarboxylation) via the branched-chain enzyme α-keto acid dehydrogenase (BCKDH), which is thought to be the limiting factor in the breakdown of BCAAs.

Given the high concentration of BCAT and BCKDH in the skeletal muscles and their low concentration in the liver, the catabolism of BCAAs tends to occur in the skeletal muscle, hence their susceptibility to physical exercise. Both valine and isoleucine are neoglucogenic amino acids and can be converted into glucose in the human body, while leucine is a ketogenic amino acid and can produce ketone bodies by its metabolization. The branched chain amino acids found in protein foods, and in particular leucine, stimulate muscle protein synthesis through signals involving mTOR (target of rapamycin in mammals) in a dose-response manner; mTOR is commonly referred to as the main metabolic target of leucine, but it can also be activated by physical exercise alone. The mTOR pathway is regulated by stimuli from a variety of cellular signals, including mitogens, growth factors (such as IGF-1 and IGF-2), hormones such as insulin, nutrients (amino acids, glucose), the levels of the cellular energy and stressful conditions.

Leucine can also stimulate the insulin secretion, which in turn can induce the phosphorylation of mTOR through the activation of its receptor. So, the same way branched-chain amino acids and leucine regulate protein synthesis via the mTOR/Akt axis, insulin does too. The use of norleucine, which shares the properties of leucine with reference to mTOR but not in the ability to secrete insulin, has shown that insulin *itself* is not so necessary to achieve adequate levels of the protein synthesis.

There is also a competition at the level of transport and absorption systems of the blood-brain barrier with the aromatic amino acids (phenylalanine, tyrosine, tryptophan).

The branched chain amino acids and the aromatic ones (tryptophan, tyrosine) compete for the active transport system (L-carrier) across the blood brain barrier. The passage from the bloodstream to the brain of varying amounts of one or the other amino acid, based on their concentration is extremely important because aromatic amino acids are precursors of hormones/neurotransmitters such as catecholamines (dopamine) or serotonin.

An increase in catecholamines, which derive from tyrosine, is functional to a state of alarm; serotonin, which derives from tryptophan, is the mediator that characterizes the mood and promotes relaxation. In physical exercise, especially if intense, it is believed that the change in brain serotonin concentration is dependent on the large increase in the proportion of free plasma tryptophan due to the selective uptake of BCAAs by the muscle, and it is responsible for the central fatigue state that occurs. It is characterized by drowsiness, moodiness, a sense of tiredness with difficulty in continuing the commitment.

Regarding the fatigue related to ammonia formation during exercise, one must be careful not to take too many branched chain amino acids in the pre-activity period, as an excess of BCAAs could lead to an increase in plasma ammonia rather than a decrease, which happens if the quantities of BCAAs are not high. Along with the decrease in plasma ammonia there is also a lower accumulation of lactate, which benefits the performance.

Over the years, more and more scientific studies have demonstrated the validity of BCAAs in improving the performance, as they have found the following properties:

- BCAAs are able to counteract the passage of tryptophan in the brain, which can be followed by the transformation into serotonin, the neurotransmitter responsible for the sensation of fatigue;
- the administration of BCAAs before exertion allows a better respiratory performance for the athlete, thanks to the "buffer" action exerted on metabolic acidosis resulting from the muscular work;
- the regular administration of BCAAs during training, prevents the decline
- of glutamine linked to repeated and prolonged efforts, a primary index of a decrease in the immune system's defenses;
- they positivize the nitrogen balance and have a stimulating action on the protein-muscle synthesis in sports activities;
- they have an anti-catabolic action and a saving effect on protein substrates;
- they favor a higher use of fats for energy purposes.

During sporting activity, BCAAs are able to inhibit the oxidation of glucose in the muscle, favoring the use of fats, resulting in a saving of glycogen and thus improving the endurance performance; Furthermore, it should be considered that, in addition to the combustion of carbohydrates and lipids, there also occurs a combustion of amino acids deriving from the catabolism of muscle proteins, which is intended to supply the glucose formation (albeit in a reduced form), through hepatic neoglucogenesis (a series of studies attributes a consumption charged to amino acids for a value ranging from 5 to 15% of the energy needs, and leucine is one of the most used). One of the fundamental factors for maintaining an efficient neoglucogenesis is the availability of alanine, an amino acid whose synthesis is improved significantly by BCAAs. Recent studies have shown that these amino acids provide the pyruvic acid, a substance used by the Krebs cycle to produce energy. Another important role played by BCAAs is represented by the intervention in the neutralization mechanisms of amino radicals, whose accumulation in the body is highly toxic, both for the brain and for the cellular functioning in general. Unlike the liver, skeletal muscle lacks the enzymes that eliminate ammonium such as urea; to overcome this drawback, BCAAs in muscle and adipose tissue stimulate the synthesis of alanine and glutamine, scavenger amino acids capable of neutralizing the amino radicals. Both alanine and glutamine are not essential amino acids, but BCAAs represent the fundamental precursors of their synthesis. Some studies show an action of branched chain amino acids as a stimulus for raising the testosterone levels. The most recent study on this issue involved 10 men between the ages of 20 and 25. The subjects received BCAA supplementation or a placebo for 3 weeks, then performed a week of weight training (four workouts), while continuing the intake of the supplement. Blood tests were performed at time zero, at the end of the third week, on the second and fourth days of the training, and finally 36 hours after the last training session. The subjects who had taken BCAAs showed significantly higher testosterone levels, as well as a decrease in cortisol and the CPK enzyme levels (which highlights the damage to the muscle cell). A BCAA deficiency is determined not only by the physical exercise, but also by various pathological or paraphysiological conditions. For example, the resumption of an adequate muscular trophism in the re-education phase following trauma to the locomotor system, burns, weight loss following surgery or particularly debilitating diseases, cirrhosis (which frequently causes hepatic encephalopathy), and senile age (in which there is a generally reduced propensity to consume meat) are all conditions that recommend an adequate supplementation of BCAA reserves.

Evidence

The numerous studies conducted on the subject have finally confirmed the effectiveness of oral administration of BCAAs in terms of tolerance, absorption and an adequate distribution of amino acids in the body.

In a study published in the scientific journal *Medicina dello Sport* that evaluated the effects of branched chain amino acids on the performance capacity in endurance sports, 24 male cross-country skiers were divided into two groups: one group took 14.4 g/day of branched chain amino acids for 60 days, while the other was given a placebo substance containing only sugar.

The classic double-blind experimental design was used to try to separate the modifications induced by branched chain amino acids from those caused by the normal training.

During the 60 days of the investigation, blood tests and urine samples were taken on three occasions: at the beginning (T0), after 30 days (T30) and after 60 days (T60).

The tests that were carried out were the following:

1. The aerobic power test (maximum oxygen consumption, submaximal test around the anaerobic threshold of 40 mm, time to exhaustion) using a conveyor belt.
2. The test of strength and the anaerobic power of the lower limbs using the ergojump.
3. The test for determining the lean muscle mass.

4. An evaluation of blood ammonia and urea excretion in urine in the 24 hours following the aerobic power test.

The results of this research indicate an **improvement in the aerobic performance** (oxygen consumption, heart rate, oxygen pulse), as well as in the absolute performance, given the longer time to exhaustion found in the group treated with branched chain amino acids.

As for the effect of the treatment on the strength and power of the lower limbs, there is **an increase of 7-8% in the lactacid power performance**. From the examination of the lean mass, a tendency to muscle mass loss was noted in both groups, but it was significantly higher in the untreated group.

It is therefore appropriate to draw attention to the protection that athletes treated with branched chain amino acids seem to have towards the slow but progressive loss of muscle tissue that occurs after 60 days of training. This protection also appears to be more evident in athletes who endure greater workloads (2-3 hours per day). Finally, blood and urine samples showed a tendency to produce less ammonia and urea under treatment with branched chain amino acids. The same group of researchers evaluated the recovery in athletes treated with branched amino acids after a demanding 40 km uphill race in the days following the competition, comparing it with the control group athletes. It has been shown that the administration of 15 g/day of branched chain amino acids leads to a lower production of ammonia and urea, and a faster disposal of these toxic substances in the nervous system during the following days, thus detoxifying the body. This would be in full agreement with the feelings of the athletes who report that they endure greater workloads. At the end of this study, it can be stated that the administration of branched amino acids in endurance sports determines a better adaptation to the training, which is evident in all performed tests: in this perspective, the increase in the lower limb strength, the increase in the time to exhaustion in the aerobic test, the lower level of ammonium ions and the lower excretion of nitrogen, indices of a lower protein catabolism after the test.

Finally, let's talk about the timing of the daily intake of branched chain amino acids. The best time to take them is definitely during the first 40 minutes after the training, since in this period of time, the concentrations of the growth hormone and testosterone remain high, which favor the transformation of amino acids into proteins and therefore into muscular tissue.

By treating some subjects in a 21-day trek, at an altitude above 3000 meters with BCAA supplementation, some researchers found a significantly lower loss of the lean mass compared to the placebo group.

Other interesting studies have observed the acute response to exercise following oral administration of BCAAs in athletes that practice power sports. The rather modest dose was 5 g per day for 5 weeks, combined with a high-protein diet. The obtained responses confirmed the net decrease in the muscle catabolism and allowed us to hypothesize an influence of BCAAs on plasma growth hormone levels. Finally, two very recent studies have shown the usefulness of BCAA supplementation in programs aimed at reducing body fat, as well as their ability to prolong the physical activity of men and women in very hot environmental conditions. According to what emerged from the most recent acquisitions, the use of BCAAs is justified in the most diverse sports, from power to endurance sports, but also in team sports with alternating aerobic-anaerobic commitment.

We have already mentioned how a lack of these amino acids determines the start of the catabolic processes in the muscles, promoting a decrease of the protein content in the muscle.

Among these three amino acids, particular attention should be paid to leucine, as it improves the effect of insulin, and it inhibits the formation of hepatic urea and ammonia. But what is even more important for athletes, is the fact that leucine is the most involved amino acid in inhibiting the degradation of muscle proteins and in promoting their synthesis (as can be seen from Table 44.1).

Table 44.1 From this table, it emerges that leucine alone has an anticatabolic action almost equal to the one expressed by the three branched altogether, and it also shows a good ability to stimulate the protein synthesis (10% higher than the isoleucine-valine combinaton). It has a greater influence in the improvement of the protein-muscle patrimony, compared to the other two branched amino acids. Furthermore, leucine is easily oxidizable and therefore represents an excellent energy source for the muscle, the value of which varies according to the diet protein content and the state of rest or exercise

Amino acids	Protein synthesis	Protein degradation	Net change
Leucine Isoleucine Valine	(% of the increase) 47%	(% of the decrease) 28%	(% of the increase) 75%
Leucine	25%	25%	50%
Isoleucine, valine	16%	22%	38%

Care must be taken in choosing BCAA-based supplements: all scientific studies that have demonstrated the validity of their use have been performed by administering preparations that contain leucine, isoleucine and valine in the optimal 2:1:1 ratio. It must also be said that the initial formulation of the BCAAs was made respecting the balance defined through studies carried out mainly on cirrhotic patients. Studies concerning sports medicine and the use of amino acids in various sports have instead indicated that the consumption of leucine is higher, especially in intense physical activity; hence the need to increase the quantity of this amino acid in the formulation of branched supplements, immediately recognized by the companies in the sector, which competed to place on the market formulations of BCAA with a higher proportion of leucine than valine and isoleucine , starting from 4-1-1 all the way to 12-1-1, and I think the upside race will continue for a while. But, apart from the obvious marketing reasons behind this trend, which exploit the now consolidated credibility of the BCAA "brand" in the sports sector, given that at this point it would be worth taking leucine alone, it actually becomes appropriate to consider the reason why the BCAAs are taken, and consequently consider the timing of the consumption. We have seen how **all BCAAs stimulate the protein synthesis, and leucine is by far the best**. Consequently, a competition with the other BCAAs can only decrease their anabolic effect, which occurs especially in the post-workout phase. It is at this moment that these new formulations of BCAAs or leucine alone can be useful, even if, in reality, the best protein synthesis requires the presence of the other branched amino acids too or, to be honest, of all essential amino acids, because an unbalanced ratio in favor of leucine would have a negative effect on the protein synthesis. Conversely, taking leucine before the training can only be useful for endurance activities due to its glycogen-saving effect. On the contrary, isoleucine increases the flow of glucose within the muscle cell, favoring its use for energy purposes and can therefore reasonably improve the performance where there is an involvement of the anaerobic lactacid or high intensity aerobic metabolism.

In BCAA formulations, isoleucine appears to play a role in improving the fat metabolism.

Japanese researchers found that mice that were given isoleucine while eating a high-fat diet, accumulated much less fat than mice that did not consume isoleucine. This is due to the ability of isoleucine to activate some special receptors known as **PPAR**, which increase the fat burning and inhibit their storage.

PPARs help increase the activity of genes that stimulate greater fat burning in the body, reducing the activity of genes that normally increase their accumulation. This leads to a greater ability to burn fat, with less chance of storing it.

As for valine, its ergogenic effect is partly due to its mechanism of competition with tryptophan, whereby, by decreasing the concentration of tryptophan in the brain it decreases the production of serotonin, which is a neurotransmitter that increases the sensation of fatigue. But the feeling of fatigue is also reduced by another neurotransmitter, dopamine, which is instead decreased, with a competitive mechanism, by leucine. So, if on the one hand, by taking BCAAs we lower serotonin thanks to valine, on the other hand, we run the risk of nullifying its effects due to leucine, which lowers dopamine, because, in reality, what matters is the serotonin/dopamine ratio.

The BCAAs work together, they need each other to be able to enter the anabolic and catabolic processes. They share the same conversion pathways and enzymes. In addition to the dosage, if one of the BCAAs is out of the physiological ratio, it can unbalance the conversion pathways of all three essential amino acids, by competing with the others.

An excess of leucine over valine and isoleucine will result in a decrease in their quantities in the tissues, as leucine will occupy more enzymes and transporters, displacing the other two.

In the body, the transport of leucine, isoleucine and valine is carried out by a system of common transporters, so in certain conditions a competition can arise between these three amino acids. Activation of BCAA dehydrogenase by leucine, with the consequent stimulation of BCAA degradation and the increase of tissue protein synthesis, together with the decrease of tissue proteins in the presence of high concentrations of leucine, is believed to contribute to a decrease in the blood and muscle reserves of valine and isoleucine, especially after fluid infusions or consumption of diets that contain high levels of leucine.

These interactions between BCAAs can provide an explanation for the nutritional antagonism between leucine, isoleucine and valine. **The administration of large quantities of one of the BCAAs can create imbalances in the concentrations of the other BCAAs, favoring their degradation**; this implies the need to consider a balanced ratio between the three BCAAs if they are used in the treatment of clinical problems, but also in high-level sports and beyond.

It is interesting to note that, in association with intense exercise, the use of proteins extracted from rice has been shown to be more anabolic than the use of whey proteins. The leucine content was studied, and the serum was found to have higher levels of BCAAs and leucine, but the bioavailability of leucine was found to be higher and faster with rice proteins, and the timing of entry into the bloodstream may actually be more important than the dose. This is a starting point, but more research is still needed.

Another reasoning that can be done (although it is supported by little scientific evidence) is that **leucine is a ketogenic amino acid**, so it can be converted into ketones which, in turn, can be used as fuel and muscle mass savers. Unfortunately, these ketones also save fat, as an excess in leucine, converted into ketones instead of fat, will slow down the lipolysis. This also happens because ketones are not always good for the body, so when they rise quickly this goes into alarm state. Valine, on the other hand, can be converted and used as a sugar. Isoleucine can do both. We need **these amino acids to be balanced when used as an energy source, so as not to compromise the ability to burn fat**.

Another interesting finding is that the bioavailability of BCAAs and leucine alone is much better when we take low amounts and when they are supplemented with other amino acids. BCAAs taken through food are absorbed in rates of 40-60%, compared to 14-18% when taken as supplements.

In this regard, **vitamin B12** is essential for the metabolism and the conversion of BCAAs. The deficiency of vitamin B12, in fact, can cause defects in the metabolism of BCAAs. In summary, before an endurance activity, the 2-1-1 formulations can work well, because they have the right balance between energetic, anti-catabolic and psychotropic effects; instead, for power sports, it is better to take 1-1-1 formulations and after training the 4-1-1 formulations or just leucine, together with EAAs or hydrolyzed proteins.

Another important role of BCAAs is **to enhance the immune defenses**, especially in athletes of long-term disciplines (triathlon, marathon, ultramarathon, ultratrial, etc.), where it has been seen that their administration is able to decrease the inflammatory cytokines and interleukins.

Dosages

The dosages for sports supplementation range from 1 to 2 g (depending on the type of activity, weight and commitment) per 10 kg of body weight, divided equally before and after the training, bearing in mind that the dose of leucine that is necessary for the stimulation of protein synthesis is about 3 g. During prolonged and energy-intensive sports activities, you can take a dose even during mid-performance, to improve the muscle endurance. Some authors recommend its use even before the night rest, in relation to the nocturnal secretion of GH, responsible for a stimulating action on the protein synthesis.

A little attention must be paid to hyperadrenergic subjects: taken before going to sleep, branched chain amino acids could have effects on nerve stimulation, causing insomnia, precisely because BCAAs have an inhibiting effect on serotonin. In the evening, it would be better not to make these subjects take too many protein sources that are rich in tyrosine and BCAAs in order to avoid problems during the night rest.

Effectiveness

Strength	Resistant strength	Mass	Endurance	Slimming	Concentration	Recovery
++	+++	++++	+++	++	++	++

CAFFEINE

Description

Caffeine (1,3,7-trimethylxanthine) is a natural alkaloid derived from xanthine and is present in various plant species, including coffee, cocoa, tea, cola, guarana and mate plants, and therefore in the drinks obtained from them. It is considered a psychoactive drug, entering the category of psychostimulants. Today, in addition to its psychoactive and stimulating properties, coffee is also consumed to mark the rhythms of the day: it inaugurates the morning, closes meals, marks the meetings between people, fills the breaks of conferences and lectures, excluding those parts of the world in which its place is taken by tea, which also contains caffeine.

Table 44.2 The quantities of caffeine contained in some of the most common beverages and foods

Product	Quantity	Caffeine
1 espresso (coffee)	5 cl	100 mg
1 energy drink can	25 cl	80-100 mg
1 instant coffee	1 dose	57 mg
1 cup of black tea	25 cl	20-70 mg
1 cup of green tea	25 cl	8-50 mg
1 can of cola	33 cl	35 mg
1 decaffeinated coffee	5 cl	10 mg
1 square of chocolate	10 g	5 mg

Properties

Caffeine is well absorbed orally: significant levels are found in the plasma after 30 minutes following its intake, with a maximum plasma peak within 90 minutes, and it is rapidly distributed in all tissues, it crosses the blood brain barrier and the placenta. The half-life in the body is about 4 hours (but varies from 2 to 10 hours). It can be present in breast milk, so special precautions must be taken in case of pregnancy and breastfeeding. By acting on the central nervous system, caffeine stimulates the mental abilities, reduces drowsiness, fatigue, enhances the memory, learning and concentration abilities, facilitates the perception of sensory stimuli, improves the reaction time, space-visual processing and verbal memory, and also alleviates headaches and migraines in general. Other effects of caffeine are: an increased coronary flow, cardiac output, systolic pressure, an increased muscular, renal and skin blood flow, metabolism, secretion of gastric juices; an improvement in the functioning of the respiratory tract; an increased synthesis of gonadotropins; an increased lipolysis through stimulation of catecholamines and cortisol; a stimulating action on nerve cells; an improved recruitment of the muscle fibers; an analgesic and diuretic action.

Evidence

The ability of caffeine to **increase the alert threshold and to sustain attention** for longer has been well documented and its main mechanism of action as an ergogenic substance and stimulant of the central nervous system is given by its antagonistic action against adenosine, a chemical substance produced naturally by the body, to which various roles are attributed. We can mention, at the cardiac level, the slowing of atrioventricular conduction (with a decrease in the contractile force, heart rate and therefore blood pressure) and, at the CNS level, a sedative and anticonvulsant effect. For these and other reasons, adenosine is known as the "fatigue molecule". The beneficial action of caffeine is therefore linked to the blocking of adenosine receptors present in the nervous, heart and muscle tissue. Through this molecular mechanism, caffeine can enhance the ability to make a physical and mental effort before fatigue occurs, by maintaining the state of wakefulness. The blocking of adenosine receptors in the CNS may also be responsible for constricting the blood vessels, which reduces the symptoms of migraines and headaches, and explains why caffeine is contained in many analgesics.

The relationship **between caffeine and sports performance** has been investigated several times. Several studies are conducted since the middle of the last century and they have shown how this substance has positive effects both in **endurance** sports and, according to more recent analyzes, in short duration and high intensity exercises.

The ergogenic effect of caffeine in endurance activities is expressed through two actions: one direct and one indirect. The direct action, as already mentioned above, is linked to the ability of this molecule to act as a competitive antagonist against adenosine receptors, reducing the sensation of perceived effort, while the indirect action is due to its ability to stimulate the release of catecholamines (adrenaline and noradrenaline) by the adrenal medulla, with effects on muscle, adipose and vascular tissue, and also on the metabolic system. In particular, following a series of complex cellular mechanisms, caffeine causes a greater contraction force even at low stimulation frequencies, an **increase in lipolysis and a saving of muscle glycogen** (due to the increase in the oxidation of free fatty acids), an increased coronary flow (increased blood supply to the heart), an increased cardiac output (increased blood flow to the tissues) and an increased systolic blood pressure. In addition, caffeine and its metabolites, rapidly crossing the blood brain barrier, improve the neuronal excitability and facilitate the recruitment of motor neurons, facilitating signal transmission between the central and peripheral nervous systems.

These properties of caffeine are particularly valuable in endurance exercises, where any glycogen depletion could limit the effectiveness or the speed of the performance. Caffeine is also able to increase the accumulation of glycogen in the muscles, functioning as a carbohydrate-partitioning agent, when taken both before and after the training. A study conducted on this subject shows the benefits of caffeine in the swimming performance: 11 athletes, 7 males and 4 females, consumed caffeine (6 mg/kg body weight) 2.5 hours before a 1500m swimming race. On average, the swimming speed was higher than the controls. After the caffeine intake, the subjects reached the same distance covered by the control cases but in a shorter time.

Another reason why caffeine is able to increase the endurance performance may be due to the fact that it is able to increase the performance of slow red fibers faster than fast white fibers (6% versus 3% respectively).

Regarding the effects of caffeine on maximal high-intensity efforts, there have been quite controversial opinions for years, but recent studies have shown that **caffeine can exert a beneficial effect during short-duration, high-intensity exercises**. For example, a 2009 review of the effects of caffeine on the performance during anaerobic exercise, compared trained participants and untrained participants, habitual versus non-habitual caffeine users, participants with slow or fast caffeine metabolism, with different dosages (fixed doses of caffeine vs. mg per kg of body weight), as well as different types of tests. The overall results showed that caffeine can exert beneficial effects in some types of short duration and high intensity exercises, in trained athletes who have refrained from consuming caffeine before the event and in cases where it is ingested in discrete doses (beyond above a certain threshold, but not excessively high). These aspects have also been evaluated and confirmed by Dr. Michael Colgan, world-renowned sports nutritionist, who recognizes the positive effects of caffeine in weight training, but with some exceptions. "The first mistake," says the scholar, "is to assume that the sedentary person pushed to exercise, reacts to caffeine the same way as an athlete". Dr. Luke Bucci, quoted by him, conducted a study on the effects of caffeine in sedentary subjects and athletes, concluding that the only beneficiaries of caffeine effects would be athletes.

In reality, as can be seen in the chapter on concentration (to be kept as a reference for the number of studies mentioned), elite athletes receive the greatest benefits, but Bucci's claims are too cutting! Many researches carried out after what Colgan wrote have shown that even "normal" subjects obtain good results, albeit inferior, as demonstrated by the very recent study by Jodra et al. (2020).

"The second mistake," continues Colgan, "which is commonly made in research, is to confuse subjects who habitually use coffee, tea, cocoa, soft drinks or chocolate, with subjects who have a low daily intake of caffeine". In short, caffeine addicts would not derive any help from caffeine in the improvement if their sports activities. "It would be like pretending to get drunk with a glass of wine while you are able to drink a liter without any side effects". **The only way to obtain benefits from caffeine would therefore consist in eliminating it from everyday life.** The celebrated nutritionist states that there are at least three reliable studies showing that at least 4 days of caffeine abstinence are required to be able to appreciate any improvement in your performance. Otherwise, for those who usually consume three to five cups of coffee a day, there is no improvement obtained from caffeine intake. In this case, to obtain a significant effect, an abnormal quantity (12 mg/mL) should be taken: 1200 mg of caffeine, equal to about 10 cups of coffee; an amount that, among other things, would cause major intestinal problems.

Even in this situation, however, this is not quite the case... Overlooking the comparison related to alcohol, apart from the fact that an **alcoholic with a liver damaged** by years of drinking develops a reverse tolerance that makes them sensitive to even a small dose of alcohol, a whole series of recent studies have given opposite results (van Soeren et al., Irwin et al., to name two): therefore, Colgan is partly right, but staying up to date is essential in order to have the widest possible range of knowledge!

A recent University of Birmingham study on 20 hockey players which was published in the *Current Biology* journal showed that athletic performance can vary by 26% throughout the day and that the best time to perform an athletic performance is in the late afternoon. However, there is a system, used unconsciously by most of us, which alters the biological clock and which can drastically increase our athletic performance: caffeine! To test the promising ability of caffeine to enhance the athletic performance in the morning, Rodriguez et al. tested 12 trained men during the execution of the squat and horizontal bench press, at 75% of the maximum weight, at different times of the day, with or without caffeine, in a double-blind placebo experiment. The result was that the group that trained in the afternoon without caffeine was significantly stronger than the morning group, which was given the placebo, confirming the negative impact of training in the morning. When both groups received caffeine, there were no significant differences in either squat or bench press, indicating that caffeine was able to close the "gap" in performance between morning and afternoon. The same pool of scholars, with Rodriguez as first author, achieved similar results in another trial in 2015. Caffeine is able to trigger the AMPK enzyme, an energy regulator at the cellular level, which in turn activates SIRT 1, an enzyme normally activated by low energy levels (for example a low-calorie diet) that accelerates the energy production starting from fats and glucose. SIRT 1 is able to regulate the biological clock by inhibiting the CLOCK protein, which represents the central biological clock, rhythmically activated according to a circadian rhythm. The CLOCK protein is deactivated when energy consumption is low, thus promoting the accumulation of energy at the cellular level and not its production; this is why in the morning, upon waking up, since energy consumption is still low after a morning rest, the effect of the CLOCK protein, which decreases the energy production, is responsible for the lower muscle performance, due to a decrease in energy availability for the muscle contraction. In conclusion, the ability of caffeine to stimulate SIRT 1, which inhibits the CLOCK protein, promotes a better biological clock for the morning training. Among other things, a study carried out by researchers at the University of Toledo (Spain) found that caffeine improves the performance of bench press and squats when administered in the morning rather than in the afternoon. Therefore, **caffeine in the morning is more effective and has fewer side effects**, perhaps because in the morning the cortisol is already naturally high, while taking caffeine in the afternoon or evening raises the cortisol at a time when it should be physiologically lower.

In recent years, in the world, there has been a considerable increase in the consumption of energy drinks, canned drinks containing caffeine (generally in quantities greater than or equivalent to 80-85 mg) and, at times, they also contain other substances, such as guarana or ginseng. Numerous researches have shown how caffeinated energy drinks can actually increase the performance of the athletes by providing them with energy.

Furthermore, several studies show the effectiveness of chewing gums containing caffeine, guarana and other stimulating herbs. They are widespread, especially in the United States, especially in all those categories of workers who require attention and clarity for many hours, and are even supplied to the US army. A fairly recent report shows that the use of caffeine chewing gum would improve the performance of both male and female cyclists during the last 10 km, especially through an increase in the activation of the central nervous system. Again, some studies have been cited in the previous chapters.

Australian researchers from a collaborative consortium between the Garvan Institute of Medical Research in Sydney, St. Vincent's Institute of Medical Research in Fitzroye and the Royal Melbourne Institute of Technology University (RMIT) in Bundoora, found that the supply of glycogen occurs more rapidly if athletes ingest both carbohydrates and caffeine after exertion.

The research was conducted on seven well-trained cyclists who exerted themselves to exhaustion with a cycle ergometer and then ate a low-carb dinner, in order to minimize the glycogen stores in sight of the experimental tests the next day. After a second session aimed at depleting the glycogen stores, the athletes consumed a drink containing only carbohydrates or carbohydrates plus caffeine (8 mg/kg body weight). In the following hours, the researchers carried out some muscle biopsies and blood samples to measure the amount of glycogen that had been reconstituted, together with the concentrations of metabolites and hormones that regulate glucose levels, including insulin.

According to the results of the study, with this combination, 4 hours after the end of training, the amount of glycogen in the muscles was 66% higher than in athletes who had only taken carbohydrates. Some of the subjects subsequently had problems falling asleep, and this obviously can negatively affect the recovery; moreover, it is known that caffeine, in this aspect, causes different responses according to the subjects. Further studies would be desirable to see if lower dosages are equally effective.

In some studies, caffeine has shown the ability to increase testosterone levels, but in a study published in 2018 in *Cancer Causes and Control* ("Consumption of caffeinated beverages and serum concentrations of sex steroid hormones in US men"), they found a positive correlation between coffee consumption and SHBG (Sex Hormone-Binding Globulin), which is the protein that binds sex hormones and which, therefore, makes them not bioavailable. 1410 men over the age of 20 were recruited into the study. Daily caffeine intake was estimated by multiplying the concentration of caffeine per cup by the frequency of coffee, tea or soft drinks consumed daily. The study showed a positive correlation between consumption of coffee and SHBG, while no correlation was observed between SHBG and consumption of tea or soft drinks that contain caffeine. Probably, there is something in coffee and not in caffeine, that increases the blood concentration of SHBG.

Dosages

A very important note: the effects of caffeine are variable because people eliminate it at different rates.

Nutrigenetic research has shown that the population is divided in half between slow and fast metabolisers. Slow ones are more sensitive to caffeine and its side effects. In any case, given the results of the studies cited above, the prolonged use of caffeine can lead to tolerance by the body and can cause addiction: the consumption of large quantities of caffeine – generally more than 600 mg per day (equivalent of about seven to eight cups of espresso) – could lead some people to the condition known as caffeinism, in which caffeine addiction is combined with a broad spectrum of unpleasant physical and mental effects, such as nervousness, irritability, agitation, insomnia, headache and heart palpitations. If you consume a quantity of caffeine close to 600 mg per day, it should be divided into two or three intakes spaced throughout the day. The LD_{50} of caffeine (lethal quantity for 50% of the population) corresponds to 150 mg/kg of body weight, well 30 times above the recommended dosages: in fact, **moderate amounts of caffeine** are enough (3-6 mg/kg of body weight) in order to have **positive effects** both in endurance sports and, from the latest evidence, in mixed sports, as we have also amply seen in the chapter on concentration.

Advice on how to take caffeine to take advantage of its maximum effects is provided by Graham, a marathon scientist and, to date, one of the world's leading caffeine experts: according to him, the best results are obtained with the ingestion of caffeine pills. In reality, the alternative forms to the drink have different assimilation times, but the results are not too different, and in any case the studies are less numerous than those relating to the classic cup. Therefore, it will also depend on the situations... in cases where the liquid form proves to be impractical, other methods can be used.

Effectiveness

Strength	Resistant strength	Mass	Endurance	Slimming	Concentration	Recovery
++	+++	+	+++	+++	++++	++

CAPSAICIN

Description

Capsaicin (trans-8-methyl-N-vanillyl-6-nonenamide-$C_{18}H_{27}NO_3$) is a natural substance derived from plants of the *Capsicum* genus, *Solanaceae* family.

The *Capsicum* genus consists of about 25 wild and five domestic species. The five domestic species are *Capsicum annuum, C. baccatum, C. chinense, C. frutescens* and *C. pubescens*. Among the domestic species, *C. chinense* gives the spiciest type of fruit. The "spicy" principles of chilli are capsaicinoids, which are alkaloids that accumulate in the placenta of the ripening *Capsicum* (chilli pods) and have wide applications in the nutritional, medical and pharmaceutical field. About 80-90% of the capsaicinoids present in *Capsicum* consist of capsaicin and dihydrocapsaicin, in a ratio of approximately 1:1 and 2:1, respectively. The remainder is composed of nordihydrocapsaicin, homodihydrocapsaicin, homocapsaicin, norcapsaicin and nornorcapsaicin.

Capsaicin and capsaicinoids are incredibly stable alkaloids, in fact they remain unchanged for a long time, even after cooking and freezing. Capsaicin was discovered in 1816 by P.A. Bucholtz, who isolated the spicy substance from macerated peppers using organic solvents. In 1846 L.T. Thresh synthesized it in a crystalline form and baptized it with the name of capsaicin. In 1878, the Hungarian Endre Hogyes also obtained capsaicin in crystals, which he called capsicule, and demonstrated that the substance is able to stimulate the mucous membranes of mouth and stomach, increasing the production of gastric juices.

A small parenthesis: capsaicin is a lipophilic substance, which means it has an affinity for fats and not for water; this explains why it is useless to drink water when consuming a spicy food: in fact, the water does nothing but better distribute the molecule in the mouth. One way to counteract the severe burning that you feel is, for example, to eat yogurt.

Properties

Like all capsaicinoids, capsaicin is an irritant in mammals, including humans, and produces a burning sensation in the mucous membranes, including the mouth, where it dissolves and stimulates the VR1 (Vanilloid Receptor type 1) receptors, which activate the VRL-1 (Vanilloid Receptor-Like 1) protein. These receptors are activated respectively, in "normal" conditions, at temperatures of about 43 and 52° C and are present in the mouth, stomach and anus. What they do is send a signal to the brain as if our mouth or stomach is "burning", so the effect of pain and burning is completely virtual.

Infinitesimal dosages of capsaicin are sufficient to cause a strong burning sensation. The sensation of the "mouth on fire" feeling, therefore, is not real, in the sense that there is no real increase in the temperature of the mouth. Capsaicin, in fact, simply interacts with the aforementioned thermoreceptors present in the mouth (VR1 and VRL-1, responsible for signaling the brain when the temperature exceeds respectively 43 and 52° C) and triggers them as if the temperature rise in the mouth is real. This stress causes a **rapid release of adrenaline, giving the body a burst of energy**. This first hormonal discharge is followed by the release of endorphins, endogenous opioids with a powerful analgesic and exciting activity. Capsaicin is a gastric stimulant, antirheumatic and intestinal antifermentative.

The capsaicin receptor, called the transient vanilloid potential receptor 1 (TVPR1), was cloned in 1997 from rat dorsal root ganglia (DRG) using a functional screening strategy to isolate complementary DNA (cDNA) clones. This newly cloned cDNA was initially named VR1, for the vanilloid receptor subtype 1. Subsequently, VR1 was identified as a member of the (TRP) cation potential channel transient receptor family and the TRPV1 nomenclature was adopted to indicate this association.

To date, TRPV1 has been cloned from human, guinea pig, rabbit, mouse and pig tissues. Its distribution has been studied mainly in the tissues and organs of humans, rats and mice, but also in many other mammals. By reverse transcription polymerase chain reaction (RT-PCR), TRPV1 has been localized in human DRGs, brain, kidney, pancreas, testis, uterus, spleen, stomach, small intestine, lung and liver.

Initial studies on isolated cells showed that capsaicin and other natural substances, as well as some physical activators, activate TRPV1. Broadly speaking, and in the more complex context *in vivo*, TRPV1 has been linked to thermosensation (heat), autonomous thermoregulation, nociception, regulation of food intake and multiple functions in the gastrointestinal tract. Specifically, in the central nervous system, the receptor was also involved in driving the growth cone, in long-term depression, in endocannabinoid signaling and in osmosensing, the latter with a particular variant of TRPV1. Notably, TRPV1 is also implicated in several human pathological conditions, including vulvodynia, gastrointestinal inflammation, Crohn's disease and ulcerative colitis. In light of the above observations, it is not surprising that capsaicin has been clinically used and has been shown to be of some benefit in obesity, cardiovascular and gastrointestinal conditions, various types of cancers, neurogenic bladder and some dermatological conditions, although in many of these conditions, the effects appeared to be independent of TRPV1.

The spiciness of chilli was created in nature as a repellent substance and has been transformed for cultural reasons into a pleasant chemesthetic experience, relating to the people who use it. A completely similar path was followed by other deterrent molecules that were developed by plants to interact with the somatosensory system of animals, such as those of Sichuan pepper. In some cases, these phenomena have in fact well-defined the responsible chemical and it is through a specific mechanism, as in the case of capsaicin and menthol, that they interfere respectively with the TRPV1 and TRPM8 receptors, causing a sensation of burning heat or coolness in the mouth and on the skin, even in the absence of fire or ice.

More precisely, according to recent evidence, capsaicin could:

- be effective as an anti-inflammatory agent, especially if used topically;
- exercise a noteworthy immunomodulatory action;
- be valuable in the management of inflammatory diseases such as rheumatoid arthritis;
- act as an analgesic substance;
- improve physical endurance skills;
- assist in weight loss;
- act as a modest anti-cancer substance.

Specifically, **capsaicin** has a thermogenic effect capable of increasing the caloric expenditure for a few hours, by increasing adrenaline levels. Most studies have shown that capsaicin increases the daily calorie consumption by 4 to 5% and increases the use of fat by 10 to 16%. Furthermore, capsaicin has a pro-apoptotic effect against fat cells, which means, it promotes their self-destruction. In one study, the administration of 10 mg of capsainoid increased the adrenergic activity and energy expenditure, with a greater utilization of fat in resting conditions but not during the physical exercise and during the recovery phase, and therefore, it is a supplement that can be useful for slimming. Furthermore, capsaicin, being a vasodilator and a blood thinner, and by lowering the blood pressure, can be safely used even by those people who normally should avoid thermogenics that stimulate the central nervous and cardiovascular system.

Both capsaicin and its analogues have been used in medicine for centuries, but have recently been extensively studied for their analgesic, antioxidant, anti-inflammatory and antiobesity properties and, more recently, for their antitumoral activity against a variety of cancers.

Evidence

It has recently been shown that capsaicin induces apoptosis in many types of cancer cell lines, including colon adenocarcinoma, pancreatic cancer, hepatocellular carcinoma, prostate cancer, breast cancer and many others, leaving normal cells unharmed. The molecular mechanism by which capsaicin induces apoptosis in cancer cells is not fully understood, however it involves an increase in intracellular calcium and ROS, a disruption of the mitochondrial membrane transition potential and an activation of transcription factors such as NF-κB and STATS.

Let's now go into the correlation between capsaicin and weight loss and capsaicin and sport.

The growing epidemic of obesity and metabolic diseases requires the development of new prevention and treatment strategies. A 2016 study by **Baskaran et al.** suggests that the browning of the white adipose tissue (browning effect: white adipose tissue, by increasing the number of mitochondria and consequently cytochromes, takes on a darker color and can be defined as "beige", thus becoming a tissue with a thermogenic activity similar to Brown Adipose Tissue [BAT]) increases the energy expenditure to counteract obesity and, specifically, the activation of TRPV1 channels counteracts obesity.

The effect of capsaicin in the diet was therefore evaluated in inducing the browning process of the white adipose tissue, activating the TRPV1 channels to prevent diet-induced obesity with the use of wild-type and TRPV1 mouse models. The significant results showed that capsaicin stimulated the expression of the uncoupling protein 1, endowed with a thermogenic effect, specific to brown fat. It also stimulated the bone morphogenetic protein-8B in white adipose tissue, triggered the browning of the white adipose tissue by promoting the expression and activity of sirtuin 1 which, is related to well-being and longevity. It increased the expression of the coactivator PPARγ 1, improved the metabolic activity, stimulated the sirtuin-1-dependent deacetylation of PPARγ and the transcription PRDM-16 and, finally, facilitated the PPARγ -PRDM-16 interaction to induce the browning of white adipose tissue. On the contrary, dietary capsaicin did not protect TRPV1 mice from obesity.

In conclusion, the results show for the first time that the activation of TRPV1 channels by dietary capsaicin triggers the browning of the white adipose tissue to counteract obesity, so the data suggest that the activation of TRPV1 channels is a promising strategy for countering obesity.

Capsaicin has been shown to enhance the production of mitochondrial biogenesis and adenosine triphosphate (ATP). In fact, the study by **Hsu et al.** (2016) provided evidence on capsaicin effects on physical fatigue and physical performance.

The aim of this study was to evaluate the potential beneficial effects of capsaicin on the anti-fatigue and ergogenic functions, following a physiological challenge. Some mice were divided in four groups (n= 8 per group) and were administered oral capsaicin for 4 weeks at doses of 0, 205, 410 and 1025 mg/kg/day and were identified as control groups. These groups were named CAP-1X, CAP-2X and CAP-5X, respectively. The anti-fatigue activity and the exercise performance were assessed using forelimb grip strength, swim time to exhaustion, the levels of serum lactate, ammonia, glucose, BUN (Blood Urea Nitrogen) and creatine kinase (CK) after a 15-minute swimming exercise.

Grip strength and swim-to-exhaustion time in the CAP-5X group were significantly higher than in other groups. The supplemental dose of capsaicin dependently reduced serum lactate, ammonia, BUN and CK levels and increased glucose concentration after the 15-minute swim test. Additionally, capsaicin also increased the hepatic glycogen content. In conclusion, these results suggest that the supplementation of capsaicin may have a broad spectrum of bioactivity in improving the general health, the performance and fatigue.

Recently, it has been seen that the acute supplementation of capsaicin improves the performance of the 1500 running time trial and the rate of the perceived exertion in physically active adults. The purpose of this study was to examine the acute effect of capsaicin supplementation on the performance, the Rate of Perceived Exertion (RPE) and blood lactate concentrations during short-term running in physically active adults. Ten physically active men (age = 23.5 ± 1.9 years; mass = 78.3 ± 12.4 kg; height = 177.9 ± 5.9 cm) completed two randomized double-blind studies: capsaicin condition (12 mg) or placebo. Forty-five minutes after consuming the supplements, participants performed a 1500 m time trial run. The blood lactate concentration was analyzed at rest, immediately after exercise, and 5, 10 and 30 minutes during the recovery phase after the exercise (RPE).

Time was significantly shorter in the capsaicin group (371.6 ± 40.8 seconds) than in the placebo group (376.7 ± 39 seconds). The perceived exertion rate was significantly lower in the capsaicin group than in the placebo group, while lactate increased over time for both conditions with no significant differences. In summary, it was concluded that acute capsaicin supplementation is able to improve the running performance at medium distance (1500 m) and it also reduces RPE in physically active adults.

Dosages

With capsaicin supplementation, energy expenditure, lipid oxidation increase and satiety increase, while the energy intake is reduced. Clinical studies are multiple and they have shown a safe dose of up to 33 mg/day for 4 weeks, or 4 mg/day for 12 weeks. Potential adverse effects are: gastrointestinal upset, increased insulin levels and decreased high density lipoprotein (HDL) levels.

Effectiveness

Strength	Resistant strength	Mass	Endurance	Slimming	Concentration	Recovery
+	++	−	+	++++	−	+

CARNITINE

Description

Carnitine (L-carnitine) is a dipeptide whose synthesis within the human body occurs in the liver and partly in the kidney and brain.

It performs its primary function in the metabolism of fats (as a transporter of fatty acids) and its endogenous synthesis requires two essential amino acids (lysine and methionine) and the presence of optimal quantities of vitamins C, B6 and iron. For these reasons, vegetarians may have lower carnitine levels than omnivores.

Carnitine has a centuries-old history. It was identified as early as 1905 by Gulewitsch and Krimberg in beef extracts (present also in the cardiac level), but its chemical structure was unknown until 1927. In 1935, Strack highlighted the structural and biological analogies between carnitine and acetylcholine (an important neurotransmitter).

Properties

Carnitine supplementation could be effective for various reasons, including improving the stimulus of the hematopoiesis and preventing programmed cell death of immune cells; it has been shown to have a direct influence at the level of genes (e.g. carnitine-acyltransferase), thus modulating the concentration of long-chain fatty acids at the cellular level. The same study also evaluates its effectiveness in decreasing the production of lactic acid after intense workouts.

The ergogenic effect of carnitine is mainly linked to the transport of long-chain fatty acids within the mitochondria, where they will be used for energy purposes. Furthermore, carnitine supplementation positively affects the muscle recovery and also has the ability to increase the availability of androgen receptors. An important property of carnitine is that of improving the oxygenation capacity in the muscles and therefore, it is effective in improving the performance, specifically in long-lasting workouts.

In endurance sports (aerobic type) it allows a better use of fats, a better function of the heart muscle (carnitine is in fact more present in the heart and skeletal muscle) and therefore a constant supply of energy. In power sports (purely anaerobic) it favors glycogen savings and a reduced formation of ammonia and lactic acid, which translates into a prolonged athletic performance and a reduction in fatigue symptoms.

Recent studies have begun to shed light on the beneficial effects of carnitine when used in various clinical therapies. Because carnitine and its esters help reduce the oxidative stress, they have been proposed as a treatment for many conditions, such as heart failure, angina, and weight loss. Further research is needed in order to evaluate the biochemical, pharmacological and physiological determinants of the response to carnitine supplementation, as well as to determine the potential benefits of carnitine supplements in specific categories of subjects who do not have fatty acid oxidation defects.

Evidence

In 2002, a study on healthy adults was carried out for the first time, confirming the **lipolytic properties** of carnitine, previously only theorized. In 2004, the lipolytic property of carnitine was confirmed (it allows an oxidation of fats of about 4% more than the placebo) and the way this amino acid can help preserve the loss of lean mass was highlighted. Subsequent studies confirmed this aspect of carnitine; in particular, a research conducted in 2006 which also shows an **"anti-fattening"** property of carnitine, obtained from its role in suppressing the adipogenesis gene (increase in adipose tissue cells).

The increase in lipolysis induced by this supplement allows for a higher energy availability (from fat burning) and improves the retention of nitrogen (greater protein synthesis and/or less catabolism) by the body. In fact, carnitine supplementation has shown its ability to increase nitric oxide levels in the plasma with doses of 1-3 g per day, regardless of physical exercise, which could be linked to **the increase in the oxygenation of the muscle tissues**.

A review collected and evaluated studies on the efficacy of carnitine in obesity, diabetes and physical performance. It has been seen that in obese subjects, carnitine **helps with weight loss and helps normalize the lipid profile** (especially triglycerides). In one animal study, carnitine lowered leptin levels and abdominal fat in subjects on a high-fat diet. In those who play sports, carnitine can be useful for its effect on the muscle recovery and for lowering the blood fats (the heart suffers less and the blood flow is smoother with a better oxygen transport).

Insulin sensitivity in obese people, in those with an impaired glucose tolerance (as in pre-diabetes) or with a metabolic syndrome, can be increased with carnitine supplementation. The improvements in insulin sensitivity were also noted only after 10 days of a carnitine supplementation, in the amount of 2 g, although this particular study involved a low-calorie diet combined with the supplementation. At the same time, increases in the availability of glucose in certain brain regions were detected 25 days after the oral ingestion of 500 mg/kg in juvenile mice. Finally, it has been shown that carnitine can reduce the risk of gestational diabetes by preventing an increase in the free fatty acids in the plasma, which has been seen to be the main cause of the gestational diabetes and the consequent insulin resistance.

Another interesting aspect is that diabetic patients often suffer from muscle cramps. The study by Imbe et al. in 2018 aimed to compare the quality of life (QOL) of diabetic patients with and without muscle cramps, and to study the effect of carnitine supplementation. 91

patients with diabetes were enrolled in this study: 69 patients with muscle cramps and 22 patients without muscle cramps. In the prospective part of the study, 25 diabetic patients with muscle cramps received carnitine supplementation (600 mg/day orally) for 4 months.

The questionnaires were administered before and after the supplementation. Scores in diabetic patients with muscle cramps were lower than those in patients without muscle cramps, including the physical function, physical role, body pain, vitality, general health, and social function subscales. Meanwhile, 25 patients with muscle cramps who underwent a supplementation with carnitine had a reduced monthly frequency of muscle cramps and pain rating scale scores. The scores of the following parameters improved after supplementation with carnitine: body pain, vitality, social function and emotional role.

Recent research has been focused on the role of carnitine in the athletic performance, without focusing on its effect on fat metabolism. One study evaluated the effect of carnitine on the recovery of athletes who trained with weights. After three weeks of supplementing with 2 g per day, muscle damage was significantly lower than in those who took the placebo. An Italian study showed the effects of carnitine on post-workout muscle pain, noting its **protective effect on the pain caused by eccentric contractions.**

Given its key role in the oxidation of fatty acids and in the energy metabolism, carnitine has been studied as an ergogenic aid in improving the exercise capacity in the healthy athletic population. Early research indicates its beneficial effects on the acute physical performance, such as an increase in maximum oxygen consumption and an increased energy production. Subsequent studies indicate the positive impact of dietary carnitine supplementation on the recovery process after the exercise.

Carnitine has been shown to relieve the muscle damage and reduce the markers of cell damage and free radical formation, accompanied by the alleviation of muscle pain. It is therefore suggested to take it in order to improve the blood flow and the supply of oxygen to muscle tissue, which is achieved through a better endothelial function, thus reducing the cellular and biochemical disruptions induced by hypoxia.

Studies conducted in older adults have also shown that taking carnitine can lead to an increase in muscle mass, accompanied by a reduction in body weight and a reduction in the physical and mental fatigue. Based on current animal studies, as written in *Nutrients* in 2018, they have identified the role of carnitine in preventing the degradation of muscle proteins associated with age and in regulating the mitochondrial homeostasis.

In a study by Koozehchian et al. of 2018, they observed that carnitine was capable of improving the performance of various exercises and it speed up the recovery process by reducing the oxidative stress. This study aimed to examine the effects of a 9-week carnitine supplementation on the exercise performance, anaerobic capacity and exercise-induced oxidative stress markers, in trained males, using weights.

In a double-blind, randomized, placebo-controlled treatment, 23 men (age 25 ± 2 years; weight, 81.2 ± 8.31 kg; body fat 17.1 ± 5.9%) took a placebo (2 g/day, $n = 11$) or carnitine (2 g/day, $n = 12$) for 9 weeks, in combination with weight training. The primary outcome measurements were analyzed at the baseline and after 3, 6, and 9 weeks. The participants underwent similar weight training (4 days/week, upper/lower body split) over a 9-week period.

The conclusions showed significant increases in the bench press lift volume at week 6 and week 9 in the carnitine group. A similar trend was observed for the leg press. In addition, significant increases in mean power and peak power, post-exercise reductions in blood lactate levels, and beneficial changes in total antioxidant capacity occurred in the carnitine group.

In conclusion, it has been found that carnitine supplementation is able to improve the exercise performance by attenuating blood lactate levels and oxidative stress responses to weight training.

A not inconsiderable aspect is that elderly people can suffer from a relative lack of carnitine. Serum carnitine levels tend to increase up to about 70 years, and then undergo a decrease for reasons that are still unclear, although the loss of muscle mass that occurs with aging seems to be involved. In these subjects, a supplementation of 2 g of carnitine is associated with a **decrease in fatigue** and a better body composition, as well as an increase in the muscle function.

In dialysis patients, carnitine intake led to an increase in the production of red blood cells and hemoglobin, a decrease in the amount of the administered erythropoietin and a decrease of the inflammatory parameters such as C-reactive protein (CRP).

GPLC (glycine-propionyl-L-carnitine) is formed from a glycine amino acid, linked to a molecule of carnitine which is esterified to a short-chain fatty acid.

When propionyl-L-carnitine reaches the mitochondria, it is metabolized into L-carnitine and propionyl-coenzyme A. Propionyl-coenzyme A is relevant as it is converted into succinyl coenzyme A and then into succinate, which is an intermediate of the Krebs cycle.

The initial phases of metabolism are subjected to the *carnitine acetyltransferase* enzyme, the same that mediates the breakdown of ALCAR (acetyl-L-carnitine) into L-carnitine. In practice, propionyl-L-carnitine appears to be more effective than L-carnitine in situations involving blood flow problems and/or regulations. GPLC has also been shown to be effective in increasing the production of nitric oxide in sedentary men and athletes at doses of about 3-4 g/day.

Carnitine, in the form of propionyl-L-carnitine (PLC), has been shown to improve the symptoms of *claudicatio intermittentis*. Supplementation with PLC at a dose of 1-3 g/day appears to reliably increase the maximum walking time in people suffering from *claudicatio intermittentis* and improve their quality of life. PLC helps people with peripheral arterial disease in general, as it increases the peripheral microcirculation. In people with peripheral arterial disease, PLC supplementation can increase their strength and improve their physical performance.

In another study production in males during a workout according to the Wingate test, used to measure a subject's power and anaerobic capacity, acute GPLC supplementation was shown to produce a greater anaerobic work capacity, with reduced lactate levels. However, it is not known what the effects of chronic GPLC supplementation are, so the purpose of this study was to examine the long-term effects of different dosages of GPLC on repeated sprint performance from Wingate high intensity tests.

Forty-five trained men participated in a double-blind controlled study. All subjects completed two test sessions, 7 days apart, 90 minutes after oral ingestion of 4.5 g of GPLC or 4.5 g of cellulose (PL), in random order. The stress test protocol consisted of five 10 second Wingate test sprints, separated by 1-minute active recovery periods. After the completion of the second testing session, all 45 subjects were randomly assigned to receive GPLC at a dose of 1.5g, 3.0g, or 4.5g per day, for a period of 28 days.

Subjects completed a third testing session after 4 weeks of GPLC supplementation, using the same testing protocol. The values of peak power (PP), mean power (MP) and percentage decrease in power (DEC) were determined and standardized regarding their body mass. Heart rate (HR) and blood lactate (LAC) were measured before, during and after the five sprint bouts.

The results did not reveal any significant condition effects or significant interaction effects for PP and MP. However, the data obtained indicated that sprints three, four and five produced 2-5% lower values of PP and lower values of MP (3-7%), with GPLC at 3.0 or 4.5 g per day. On the other hand, 1.5 g of GPLC produced higher PP values (3 to 6%) and higher MP values (2 to 5%), compared to baseline PL values.

DEC values were significantly higher (15-20%) over the five sprint periods with 3.0 g or 4.5 g GPLC, but supplementation of 1.5 g GPLC produced DEC values of −5%, −3%, +4%,

+5% and +2% compared to baseline PL values. The 1.5 g group showed a statistically significant reduction of 24% in the accumulation of net lactate per unit of delivered power ($p < 0.05$).

In conclusion, it can be stated that the **effects of GPLC supplementation** on the anaerobic work capacity and lactate accumulation **appear to be dose-dependent**. Specifically, 4 weeks of GPLC supplementation at 3.0 and 4.5 g/day resulted in reduced mean values of delivered power, with higher DEC rates than baseline, **while 1.5 g/day** produced mean values were higher than MP and PP, with modest increases in DEC. The supplementation of 1.5 g/day also produced a significantly lower rate of lactate accumulation per unit of delivered power, compared to 3.0 and 4.5 g/day.

In conclusion, GPLC appears to be a useful dietary supplement for improving the anaerobic working capacity and potentially the sports performance, but apparently the dosage must be determined specifically for the intensity and the duration of the exercise.

It is now known that the endothelial dysfunction compromises the cutaneous microvascular blood flow by inducing an imbalance between vasodilation and vasoconstriction, as a result of the reduced production of nitric oxide (NO) and the increase in oxidative stress and inflammation. Propionyl-L-carnitine (PLC), as a natural derivative of carnitine, has been reported to improve the post-ischemic blood flow recovery. The results show that PLC treatment is able to improve post-ischemic injury recovery and its beneficial effects probably derive from the improvement of the mitochondrial oxidation, the reduction of oxidative stress and Nox4-mediated endothelial dysfunction.

Obesity contributes significantly to insulin resistance, which leads to the development of type 2 diabetes and cardiovascular alterations. The PLC plays a key role in the energy control. The aim of this study was to evaluate the metabolic and cardiovascular effects of PLC in obese mice with a diet-induced obesity.

C57BL/6 mice were fed a high-fat diet for 9 weeks and then they were divided into two groups, receiving either pure water (vehicle HF) or PLC (200 mg/kg/day) for an additional 4 weeks. "Standard" animals were used as lean controls (ST vehicle). Body weight and food intake were monitored and glucose and insulin tolerance tests were evaluated, as well as HOMA index, serum lipid profile, hepatic and muscle mitochondrial activity, **oxide release nitric in the tissues (NO)** and, finally, the systolic blood pressure and the cardiac and endothelial functions.

The HF vehicle showed a greater increase in weight, while in the group that had taken PLC it was noticed that the supplement improved the state of insulin resistance and inhibited the increase in total cholesterol levels. The HF vehicle then showed a reduced ratio between cardiac output/body weight, a reduced endothelial dysfunction and a tissue decrease in NO production. All these parameters improved in the PLC group. Finally, the reduction in hepatic mitochondrial activity by the high-fat diet was increased in the group that took PLC.

In conclusion, the oral administration of PLC may be able to improve the insulin resistance developed in obese animals and decrease the cardiovascular risk, probably through the correction of the mitochondrial function.

Returning to carnitine, its action at the cellular and muscle level appears to be optimized by high levels of insulin; this is why it may be recommended to consume it with carbohydrates (however, the goal of supplementation must be evaluated as it is known that high levels of insulin block the release and the oxidation of fats). In a study carried out at the University of Nottingham (UK), published in the *American Journal of Clinical Nutrition* in 2016, it was found that the simultaneous intake of whey protein decreases the carnitine uptake in the muscles.

Today, much attention is paid to the study of the immune regulation disorders and to the methods for effective immune correction in athletes. In this regard, the use of sports foods, containing nutrients with immunomodulating properties, is of particular relevance in youth sports. Indeed, the purpose of the work published in 2019 by Trushina et al. was to study the immunomodulatory activity of carnitine and also of coenzyme Q10 in junior athletes, during the training period. The subjects of this study were 30 junior athletes (sports masters and candidates for sports masters in swimming), aged between 14 and 18, including 9 girls and 21 boys.

The athletes were divided into three groups of 10 people each. The athletes in the 1st and 2nd groups received carnitine (600 mg/day) and coenzyme Q10 (60 mg/day), respectively, in addition to the basic diet, for 4 weeks. Athletes in the 3rd (control) group received only a basic diet without any sports supplementations.

As a result of a comprehensive survey of the junior athletes, it was observed a positive effect of carnitine intake on the erythrocyte hemoglobin content (30.2 ± 0.4 pg *vs.* 28.3 ± 0.3 pg at the beginning). The relative content of basophilic leukocytes in athletes of groups 1 and 2 decreased significantly by the end of the observation period: in the carnitine group, from 0.64 ± 0.05 to 0.45 ± 0.04%, in the coenzyme Q10 group, from 0.66 ± 0.07 to 0.50 ± 0.04%, **which indicated an increase in the body's resistance to allergic reactions**. To sum up, the biomarkers of the immunotropic effect of carnitine and coenzyme Q10 are: a decrease in the expression of the apoptotic marker CD95/Fas on peripheral blood lymphocytes and the suppression of the production of proinflammatory cytokines synthesized by Th1 lymphocytes, with switching of the response to humoral immunity. This, therefore, is proof of the effectiveness of the use of carnitine and coenzyme Q10 in sports nutrition, in order to restore the immune function and the adaptive potential of junior athletes.

Dosages
At least in carnitine deficiency states, the recommended dose (which may not be fully applicable to healthy humans) is 100-200 mg/kg body weight. As a supplement, dosages of 1-2 g per day are normally recommended.

Effectiveness

Strength	Resistant strength	Mass	Endurance	Slimming	Concentration	Recovery
−	+	−	+++	+++	+	++

CARNOSINE

Description
Carnosine, from a chemical point of view, is made up of two amino acids (it is a dipeptide): beta-alanine and histidine. We began to study this molecule when its presence was highlighted exclusively in the muscles and in the brain. In particular, muscles with a higher quantity of fast-twitch white fibers (where anaerobic metabolism plays a very important role) contain more carnosine than the red-fiber muscles, which are more suitable for aerobic and oxidative works.

One of the most important functions of carnosine is linked to its antioxidant and buffering properties, as it is able to counteract the reduction of intracellular pH due to the production of lactic acid. Both in the terrestrial and in the aquatic world, there are animals that enlighten us on the importance of the buffering effect of carnosine. For example, aquatic mammals, such as the whale, which due to their habitat are forced (and therefore genetically predisposed) to long hypoxia, would be subject to a high production of lactic acid with a consequent metabolic acidosis. On the contrary, this situation is obviated by the presence carnosine. This molecule is also present in humans, but in limited quantities, capable of justifying the limitation of the performance and the early fatigue when intense activities with lactacid anaerobic characteristics are carried out (i.e. in the presence of low oxygen and lactic acid production).

Properties

Carnosine is absorbed intact through a specific transport mechanism in the small intestine. Subsequently, it is transported in the bloodstream at the level of peripheral tissues or hydrolyzed to beta-alanine and histidine by the carnosinase enzyme present in the blood, liver and kidney (the latter seems to be the main responsible factor for the catabolism and excretion of this dipeptide). Admitting a dietary intake of 0.05-0.25 g of carnosine for a diet including 100 g of beef, pork or chicken, the quantitative data on its absorption, transport, distribution and catabolism are still uncertain. Of course, some changes in the eating habits, lifestyle or an intake of food supplements can affect the concentration of muscle carnosine.

As for its content in animal species, it varies in relation to the type of the muscle that is being considered and analyzed. As reiterated previously, it is the muscle with a high percentage of white fibers that contains higher quantities of this dipeptide, and this is confirmed by the presence of a quantity of carnosine that happens to be six times higher in the chicken breast (2.7 g/kg) than in the thigh. (0.5 g/kg). Pork (2.8 g/kg), turkey and beef (1.5 g/kg) also contain a good amount of carnosine, unlike salmon, which is almost devoid of it. Cooking does not have a significant influence on the concentration of this molecule in the food.

Recent studies have shown that the buffering effect of carnosine is achieved thanks to its particular chemical structure and more specifically, because of the presence of the imidazole ring. Furthermore, carnosine helps prevent glycation, which is the non-enzymatic reaction between blood sugars and proteins that leads to the production of AGEs (Advanced Glycation End products), which favor the tissue degeneration and the aging processes.

When performing an anaerobic activity, inadequate oxygenation of the skeletal muscles causes the accumulation of hydrogen ions (H^+), with the formation of lactic acid. This increase in acidity which is not readily buffered, can lead to muscle fatigue in a short time, since it does not allow for a sufficient production of ATP; this causes a decrease in the contractile capacity of the skeletal muscle and therefore, it worsens the quality of the performance.

Carnosine works by capturing lactic acid's hydrogen atom, allowing it to be converted into pyruvic acid in order to produce new energy, and allowing the buffering of the muscle pH. The consequent synthesis of ATP will be available to allow a greater amount of muscle contractions, by delaying the sense of local fatigue as much as possible.

As for the antioxidant properties, carnosine is able to reduce the lipid peroxidation of the sarcoplasmic reticulum. This function is linked to its ability to chelate the transition metals and to perform a scavenger function against some free radicals. Carnosine binds both copper and iron in particular, and it is able to inactivate the hydroxyl radicals (very dangerous) produced by the reaction between hydrogen peroxide (H_2O_2) and iron with ionizing radiations. It can inactivate a single oxygen, but it is not able to react with the superoxide radical.

Evidence

The intake of carnosine requires the presence of vitamins A, C, E, also known as excellent antioxidants. For athletes, the antioxidant action of carnosine is very important as it **prevents the tissue damage induced by training**, helps and speeds up the muscle recovery and allows the disposal and inactivation of the free radicals produced during exercise and involved in the processes of degenerative diseases, related to aging, and the development of chronic diseases.

The confirmation of the antioxidant capacity of carnosine, even indirectly, has been endorsed by data that indicate that, in the absence of vitamin E, this dipeptide is "consumed" in greater quantities by the muscles. Carnosine is also able to inhibit the oxidation of bad

LDL cholesterol (it has been seen that in the onset of cardiovascular diseases, the quantity of oxidized LDL is almost more important than the absolute quantity) and the experimental induction of breast cancer by the metabolites of anthracene in animals with vitamin E deficiency, therefore it can be adopted as a valid dietary antioxidant.

Although carnosine is not involved in the classic metabolic pathways of the synthesis of adenosine triphosphate (ATP), these results suggest an important role of the dipeptide in the cell energy homeostasis. In fact, another important function of carnosine is to participate in the activation of myosin ATP-asis, an enzyme that allows a **faster release of energy** and a better contractility of myofibrils.

High levels of carnosine are found in elite sprinters; this is an important factor for the metabolism involved in their discipline, and it is not known precisely whether it is more linked to a genetic issue or if it is a consequence of all the years of specific high-level training. In women, the amount of carnosine contained in the muscles is lower than in men, and it also decreases with age in both sexes. **Carnosine levels are more likely to be lower in vegetarians.**

The exogenous intake of carnosine was found to be effective in improving the performance in those **sports that involve lactacid metabolisms** (particular phases of cycling races, training with loads that allow for 15-20 repetitions, sprints from 200-400 m, etc.).

Some studies have shown, through the Wingate test (cycle ergometer test that measures the maximum anaerobic power), an improvement in the recovery capacity. As shown by recent publications, oral ingestion of beta-alanine can significantly increase (up to 80%) the carnosine content in the human skeletal muscle, with improvements in the performance in high intensity exercises, in both untrained and trained individuals. A deficiency of the amino acid histidine in an experimental diet leads to a reduction in the concentration of carnosine in the muscles, while a dietary supplementation of 1% of histidine does not increase the levels of carnosine in the muscles. However it can increase its presence in the liver; a dietary supplementation of 5% of histidine is instead capable of increasing muscle carnosine by 2.8 times.

In 2016, the *International Journal of Sports Physiology and Performance* published the results of a study that aimed to evaluate the effects of a combined carnosine and beta-alanine (Carn-BA) supplementation on dynamic and isometric exercises.

This study involved 12 healthy participants, who performed maximum voluntary knee extensor contractions (MVC) and counter-movement jumps (CMJ), before and after a strenuous protocol (continuous 45-second CMJ). The isometric and dynamic tests were performed 4 hours after the ingestion of 2 g of carnosine and 2 g of beta-alanine or a placebo, in a randomized manner. After the fatigue protocol, the concentration of lactate in the blood, the effort received and the muscle pain were evaluated.

The mean contact time and jump height were respectively lower and higher in the subjects who took had taken the supplements than in the subjects who had taken the placebo. Overall perceived effort was lower and muscle pain was higher in the Carn-BA group than in the placebo group. Muscle RPE and lactate did not differentiate between the conditions.

In a randomized double-blind study, 15 overweight or obese subjects were given 2 g of carnosine for 12 weeks, and another 15 subjects were given a placebo. In both groups, insulin sensitivity and insulin secretion, glucose tolerance, blood pressure, plasma lipid profile and carnosine levels in the urine were measured. The data obtained suggested that the concentration of carnosine in the urine increases after the supplementation. **Subjects treated with carnosine showed an improvement in the insulin resistance and lower levels of insulin and glucose compared to placebo**, regardless of age, sex and weight variables.

Another study published in 2018 showed for the first time that supplementation with carnosine is able to reduce the concentration of resistin and leptin in the serum of overweight and obese non-diabetic subjects. The study was carried out in a double-blind manner, involving 30 sedentary, non-smoking, non-diabetic, overweight or obese adults (BMI ≥25). They were given 1 g of carnosine twice a day or a placebo, for 12 weeks. After this period, the serum resistin and leptin levels changed significantly between the placebo and carnosine groups, indicating a reduction in resistin and leptin in the carnosine group. This research therefore indicates the **potential role of carnosine in the prevention and treatment of heart and metabolic disorders related to obesity in healthy adults**.

Dosages
The limiting factor for the spread of this molecule as a supplement in sports is the high production cost, which affects the sales cost, also in relation to the useful amount of intake. The latter, in fact, varies from a minimum of 400 mg, up to 5 g per day, according to individual needs, lifestyle, body weight, etc. It can be taken 30-60 minutes before the athletic performance or even in the days before the competition (a kind of "carnosine load"), in order to increase the concentration of carnosine in the skeletal muscles.

Effectiveness

Strength	Resistant strength	Mass	Endurance	Slimming	Concentration	Recovery
++	++++	+	+++	–	–	++

CELLFOOD®
by Giorgio Terziani

Description
Cellfood® is a multifunctional food supplement of a colloidal nature that contains a complex mixture of amino acids, enzymes and trace elements (in particular selenium), dissolved in an aqueous dispersing phase, obtained from algae of the *Lithothamnium calcareum* species. An original patented process, lasting nine months, which provides for the enrichment of the initial marine extract with further mineral components, such as deuterium sulphate, obtained from the emanations of geysers, ultimately leads to the so-called "Everett-Storey formula", also referred to as "Deutrosulfazyme®" (literally "deuterium sulfate and enzymes"), which is the basis of the product currently marketed as Cellfood®.

Cellfood® is currently proposed as a physiological modulator, potentially able to provide bioavailable oxygen "on demand" – in the right quantity and at the right time – to tissues at risk of hypoxia and, at the same time, to prevent any excess gases that can be transformed into ROS, which generate the characteristic oxidative stress lesions, in the most varied clinical conditions. Rapid and complete absorption and a maximum bioavailability at low dosage allow the distribution of the active ingredients in the various tissues, according to the real metabolic needs.

Properties
Oxygen is considered the vital element par excellence: in fact, by accepting the reducing equivalents from flavin and pyridine dehydrogenases during the catabolism, it allows mitochondria to generate ATP, which is essential for all cellular functions.

Not surprisingly, the famous American physiologist Guyton, stated that "any state of suffering, pain or disease, depends on a lack of oxygen at the cellular level". Today, confirming his intuitions and his studies that have their roots in the sensational discoveries of Otto Warburg, Nobel Prize for Medicine in 1931 – it is practically established that an altered bioavailability of oxygen and, in particular, hypoxia (i.e. lowering the pO_2 below the critical threshold of 60 mmHg) can trigger a series of undesirable events at the microcirculation level, with negative repercussions at a local and/or systemic level.

A reduction in the bioavailability of oxygen, if not promptly and effectively controlled, leads, through acidosis and the release of iron from plasma proteins, to the splitting of hydroperoxides and, therefore, to the generation of reactive oxygen species (ROS). The latter play important biological roles, but, if produced in excess, they can cause damage. For this reason, the level of hydroperoxides, from which they largely derive, is strictly controlled by glutathione (GSH) through glutathione peroxidase (GPx). Unfortunately, the disruption of this physiological and delicate balance between the production and elimination by the antioxidant defense systems, from ROS and other oxidizing species, can lead to an oxidative stress condition.

Oxidative stress is now considered an emerging risk factor for our health, as it is associated not only with a premature aging, but also with numerous diseases, often linked to lifestyle, such as obesity, dyslipidemia, diabetes mellitus, cardiovascular diseases, neurodegenerative disorders and many forms of cancer. Particularly insidious, because it does not give rise to specific clinical manifestations, it can be diagnosed only by putting the subject (who is probably affected) under specific biochemical tests, unfortunately not yet available in all laboratories.

Evidence

Improving the bioavailability of oxygen in the cellular sites where it is used the most, that is the mitochondria, while preventing, at the same time, the undesirable effects of a possible exuberant production of ROS, is one of the priority objectives of any preventive medicine intervention, especially in subjects who carry out a particularly demanding sporting activity.

In fact, regular physical activity can prevent or attenuate the oxidative stress both through the release, by endothelial cells, of nitric oxide (NO), a free radical with a vasodilating and anti-inflammatory action, and through neosynthesis in the muscle cells by antioxidant enzymes (mainly superoxide dismutase and catalase). However, particularly demanding physical activities – for workload and/or duration, such as the aerobic one – especially in inadequately trained subjects, can trigger or aggravate the oxidative balance imbalances through the enhancement of the mitochondrial metabolism on the one hand, and through the activation of cytosolic xanthine oxidase on the other.

In particular, the damage to the level of mitochondrial bilayers reduces the efficiency of the respiratory chain, while the lowering of ATP levels and the corresponding increase in the concentration of adenyl nucleosides, substrates of xanthine oxidase, lays the biochemical basis for ischemic-reperfusion lesions.

This is a trigger of a vicious cycle, in which **ROS, produced by the following incongruous physical activity at the level of the respiratory chain, ends up damaging the mitochondria themselves**, favoring the further "escape" of the reducing equivalents and, therefore, the propagation of oxidative stress.

These statements are now supported by a series of clinical and experimental evidence, provided for the first time by the famous "Studio Pretoria". In this double-blind, placebo-controlled, cross-arm trial, performed at the Institute of Sports Science of the University of Pretoria (South Africa), on a group of 45 marathon runners, the intake of Cellfood® at doses object of evaluation (25, 35 or 40 drops per day), appeared to be associated with a statistically significant reduction in the mean heart rate, compared to the placebo, measured at the speed of 17 km/h (162 vs. 180 beats/min): in practice, this effect translates into a prolongation of the filling times of the heart chambers and, therefore, in a better performance of the myocardium, as required by a prolonged physical effort.

From a statistical point of view, respiratory performance was also significantly improved, with a lowering of the frequency of the respiratory acts, **an increase in the absolute maximum oxygen volume (VO_{2max}) and a reduction in the respiratory quotient (RQ)**, all measured at VO_{2max}. The lowering of the respiratory rate, particularly evident at the lowest of the dosages tested (−14% vs. −1%), indicates an improvement in the pulmonary ventilation, while the increase in VO_{2max} is equivalent to putting the athlete in optimal conditions in order to increase the ability to produce energy and, therefore, the efficiency of the muscular effort. The concomitant, significant lowering of the RQ, i.e. the ratio between the volume of exhaled carbon dioxide and the volume of inspired oxygen, which reflects the metabolic exchange of gases in the organism and which is dictated by the use of substrates, confirms the potential of the formulation in improving the physical performance. **These effects resulted in a significant increase, compared to the placebo, in hematocrit (E 46.41 vs. 41.38), in the number of erythrocytes (5.04×10^6 vs. 4.55×10^6) and in the level hemoglobin** (16.65 vs. 14.09 g/dL), with a statistically significant reduction in serum lactate levels, especially at the average dose (35 drops per day), at 12 km/h (-26, 2% vs. + 3.7%, range −10 −26.2 vs. +0.1 + 30.4%). Overall, the results of the "Pretoria Study" indicate that Cellfood® induces a series of functional variations that all combine to predispose the body to an optimal use of oxygen, with an aerobic change in the metabolism and a very significant decrease in the production of lactate, resulting in an improvement in the athletic performance.

It is noteworthy that, about 10 years after this study, another clinical trial, controlled with a placebo, performed at the Slovenian universities of Ljubljana and Primorska, on professional cyclists, trained to a regimen of eight sessions/week, substantially confirmed the previous observations showing that, even in this category of athletes, the intake of Cellfood® at a dosage of 12 drops/3 times/day is accompanied by a statistically significant increase in VO_{2max} and maximal power at 5 weeks, with no significant changes in either maximal heart rate or serum lactate levels. These favorable effects on the oxygen consumption somehow reflect what was observed, with the same formulation, in a group of asthmatics (increased peak expiratory flow and oxygen saturation).

Obviously, as mentioned in the beginning, excessive oxygen consumption, as required by strenuous physical exercise, increases the risk of oxidative stress and it is interesting to note that in a preliminary study carried out on a group of 20 athletes, the intake of Cellfood® at the normally suggested dose of 8 drops/3 times/day for 6 weeks, was accompanied, compared to baseline, by a significant decrease in the plasma oxidizing capacity measured by the d-ROMs test, with more marked effects in the group aged 18 and 30 years (303 ± 23 vs. 418 ± 35 U CARR). Similar effects were observed on other subjects at risk of oxidative stress, such as smokers, obese and fibromyalgia sufferers.

Summarizing the published works, the antioxidant activity of the Cellfood® supplement has been documented in recent years by various experimental evidence, both *in vitro* and *in vivo*.

The first *in vitro* studies have shown that Cellfood® has a high antioxidant capacity and is able to protect both biomolecules (glutathione and DNA) and cells (erythrocytes and lymphocytes) from oxidative damage induced by ROS. At the same time, studies on endothelial cells in culture have shown that Cellfood® increases the consumption of oxygen and the production of ATP, thus promoting the mitochondrial oxidative activity. Overall, Cellfood® is able to modulate oxygen at the cellular level, allowing all possible benefits to be derived from cellular oxygenation, without intervening in the oxidative processes associated with it.

These *in vitro* findings have also been confirmed by some in vivo studies. In fact, supplementation with Cellfood® has been shown to be effective in reducing the serum levels of ROS in subjects at risk of oxidative stress, such as athletes, smokers and overweight subjects. In patients with osteopenia, the administration of Cellfood® has made it possible to significantly reduce the serum levels of the oxidized lipoproteins, involved in the onset of the atheromatous plaque. Similarly, in patients with neurodegenerative diseases, treatment with Cellfood® significantly reduced serum ROS levels, with a concomitant increase in plasma antioxidant capacity and in glutathione levels.

The high antioxidant action of Cellfood® and its ability to promote mitochondrial oxidative activity could also be the basis of the clinical benefits observed both in patients with fibromyalgia and in professional athletes. In fibromyalgia patients, treatment with Cellfood® significantly alleviates the painful symptoms, muscle weakness, tiredness upon awakening and in general mood disorders. In marathon runners and professional cyclists, Cellfood® increases the availability of oxygen, with an improved cardiorespiratory performance and physical performance, with benefits also in the adaptation process during the training period.

In conclusion, the scientific studies carried out so far suggest that Cellfood® can be a valid adjuvant in the prevention and treatment of various physiological and pathological conditions related to oxidative stress: competitive sports, cellular aging, neurodegeneration, up to cancer. In fact, thanks to its antioxidant, oxygenating and proapoptotic properties, Cellfood® could be a good candidate in cancer prevention and it can bring important clinical benefits in association with standard antineoplastic therapies.

Dosages

The latest research conducted at the universities of Urbino and Milan is shedding new light on the biochemical basis of the clinical effects of Cellfood®. In particular, the ability to inhibit the oxidation of GSH, its depletion in erythrocytes (of extreme importance in the prevention of athlete's anemia) and the ability to stimulate not only the aerobic metabolism, but also the expression of mitochondrial SOD in endothelial cells humans, allows us to conclude that Cellfood®, taken regularly up to maximum daily doses varying from 24 to 36 drops per day, is potentially capable of putting the body and, in particular its muscle machinery, in the optimal metabolic conditions to develop the best performance, without the risks associated with acidosis and, therefore, oxidative stress.

Effectiveness

Strength	Resistant strength	Mass	Endurance	Slimming	Concentration	Recovery
–	++	–	++++	++	++	++

CITRATES

Description

Citrates are elements that inhibit the crystallization, growth and aggregation of dissolved salts in urine and their administration increases urinary excretion and concentration.

The acid-base balance can undergo changes that lead to a sudden drop in blood pH as a result. This can manifest itself clearly, as for example in the case of respiratory and metabolic acidosis; at other times, however, milder or even latent forms may occur, where the blood pH is still within the normal range but its buffer function is compromised. Every single system, apparatus or organic tissue works optimally with certain pH values that are kept constant by the tissue pH. Feeling of tiredness and fatigue, migraines, muscle stiffness and joint pain are just some of the symptoms that highlight a state of bodily acidosis. Tissue pH is an evaluation index of the state of well-being of our tissues and varies according to the type of diet, caloric intake, drug intake, type and intensity of training, alcohol intake, smoking status, therefore in general to the lifestyle you follow. An accumulation of acidic metabolic waste, which our organs are unable to dispose of quickly, leads to an alteration of the tissue pH.

Minerals such as magnesium, potassium, sodium and calcium, which are alkaline, play an important role in maintaining the balance of a latent acidosis. Among the mineral salts, citrates are those that have a greater bioavailability as they do not act on the alkalinization of the stomach but in the intestine, where citric acid serves as an activator of the Krebs cycle, also facilitating the purification of the intestine.

Properties
Potassium citrate
Potassium citrate is the potassium salt of citric acid which can be found in tripotassium, dipotassium and monopotassium forms. Both of its constituents, potassium and citric acid, are widely found in nature and within our body; at room temperature it is presented in the form of a white crystalline powder, devoid of color and with a saline taste. Potassium is very important for maintaining the acid-base balance and the blood pressure, and for the muscle contraction (heart and smooth muscles). Citric acid is a key molecule of metabolic processes that take place inside the cells of our body, such as the Krebs cycle (called the tricarboxylic acid cycle or citric acid cycle), a metabolic cycle of fundamental importance in all cells that use oxygen in the process of cellular respiration. In these aerobic organisms, the Krebs cycle is the link of the metabolic pathways responsible for the degradation (catabolism) of carbohydrates, fats and proteins into carbon dioxide and water, with the formation of chemical energy. It is an amphibolic metabolic pathway, since it participates in both catabolic and anabolic processes and also provides many precursors for the production of some amino acids (for example alpha-ketoglutarate and oxaloacetate) and other molecules which are essential for the cell. As a food additive, potassium citrate is used as a buffering agent, as a metal ion chelator, and as a yeast nutrient in some fermented foods. In the pharmaceutical field and in the field of supplements, it is used as an antacid to combat heartburn, digestive difficulties and gastric hyperacidity, since, being a weak acid, potassium citrate acts as a base in contact with the hydrochloric acid of the stomach. As an alkalizing agent, it is used to make urine alkaline and to counteract metabolic acidosis.

Sodium citrate
Sodium citrate is the salt of citric acid found in the form of trisodium citrate, disodium citrate and monosodium citrate. At room temperature it appears as a white solid with a salty, slightly sour and odorless taste. Sodium is very important for the regulation of blood pressure, for the control of blood volume and extracellular fluids, for exchanges at the cellular level, for the maintenance of the acid-base balance and finally for the transmission of nerve impulses and for the muscle contraction. Like potassium citrate, sodium citrate is also used in foods as a corrector of acidity and flavor, as an antioxidant to prevent oxidation and the consequent browning of some preserved foods, such as fruits, as a metallic ion chelator and as a yeast nutrient in fermented foods; in the pharmaceutical field, it is used as an alkalizer for the treatment of metabolic, gastric and urinary acidosis and for the prevention of urinary stones due to an excess of uric acid. The use of sodium citrate is also very useful in sports for improving the athletic performance, especially in sports conducted at the anaerobic lactacid threshold, thanks to the buffering action of sodium citrate on the muscles.

Evidence
Sodium citrate is an agent capable of increasing the extracellular buffering capacity. After its intake, it is rapidly dissociated into its constituent ions; the nitrate anion is expelled from the plasma, thus inducing a change in the electrical balance. To recover this equilibrium,

a decrease of H^+ (hydrogen) in the plasma results in a consequent increase of $HCO3^-$ (hydrogen carbonate or sodium bicarbonate), **thus improving the extracellular buffer capacity**. The increase in blood pH through the supplementation of sodium citrate facilitates a greater efflux of hydrogen and lactate from the muscles, by means of a monocarboxylate protein transporter that transports the monocarboxylate across the cell membrane. A study by Potteiger et al. showed that following an intake of 0.5/g/kg of sodium citrate, after 100-120 minutes there was a peak in blood pH and hydrogen carbonate values; this gives indications on what might be the correct timing of intake to make the extracellular buffer capacity more effective, although the most effective dose remains to be defined. A study carried out by McNaughton and Cedaro has shown that the intake of 0.5 g/kg of sodium citrate is the most favorable dosage to optimize the anaerobic performance, and indeed, they have shown that this dose of sodium citrate **significantly improves a high intensity cycling performance with a duration of 120-240 seconds**. During the execution of a shorter performance (10 and 30 seconds cycling training protocol), the same dosage did not lead to an improvement in the performance, probably because the buffer capacity is not critical in such short duration protocols. Subsequent studies carried out by both McNaughton and Linossier, Dormois, Brégère et al., and later also by Van Someren, Fulcher, McCarthy et al., showed that the ergogenic effect of sodium citrate in high intensity cycling performance with a duration of 1-4 minutes was further proven by using a supramaximal test. Van Montfoort, Van Dieren, Hopking et al., in a study conducted to evaluate the effects of bicarbonate, citrate, and lactate intake in those who practice sprinting, showed that the effects of sodium citrate administration in runners appear to be more uncertain; a dosage of 0.5 g/kg of body mass showed an improvement in the resistance to fatigue in only 50% of the athletes.

Additional protocols gave more equivocal results. Tiryaki and Atterbom showed that a lower dosage (0.3 g/kg) did not improve the performance of athletes and non-athletes during a 600-meter run. Shave, Whyte, Siemann et al. instead showed that a higher dose (0.5 g/kg) improved the performance of male and female athletes during a 3,000 meter run and also the performance of highly trained college runners during a 5,000 meter run, as reported from a study by Oöpik, Saaremenets, Medijainen et al. However, further research by the same team did not show the same effects when taking the same dose of sodium citrate (0.4 g/kg) in a group of male runners during a 5 km time trial run, and in middle-distance athletes in 1500 m performances. A study carried out by Cox and Jenkins showed that sodium citrate was unable to improve the performance in moderately active males who performed series of repeated 60-second sprints. The evaluation of the data reported in the literature shows that there is a variable response during the execution of sports performances, both in the protocols used in cycling and in those used for running, following the administration of sodium citrate, and therefore, when we interpret the results, caution should be used and the different dosages must be taken into account. Further studies should be done to better evaluate the real effectiveness of an ergogenic administration of sodium citrate.

In 2018, ten young tennis players participated in a double-blind case-control study with the aim of evaluating the effects of sodium citrate supplementation on their performance. The subjects took sodium citrate (0.5 g/kg) or a placebo. Through the blood analysis it was noted that all the metabolic parameters observed, namely the pH and bicarbonate and lactate levels, were increased in the subjects who had taken sodium citrate compared to those who had taken the placebo. It is interesting to note that the increase in lactate occurred despite the increase in pH. However, there are other induced alkalosis studies that show the concomitant increase in pH and lactate. In conclusion, the intake of sodium citrate, as opposed to placebo, has been linked to **better performance for tennis players: greater consistency in the shot and greater number of games won**.

During the same year, a study on 20 cyclists was published with the aim of evaluating whether the ingestion of an alkalizing substance, such as sodium citrate, after a dehydrating exercise, was able to reduce the blood levels of stress hormones during 40 successive km of cycling carried out in warm temperatures. Male athletes first lost 4% of their body mass by exercising in the heat; then, during a recovery period of 16 hours, they took 0.6 g/kg of sodium citrate or placebo and then did 40 km of cycling at 32° C. Compared to the group that took the placebo, **after the cycling performance there were recorded lower levels of cortisol and aldosterone in subjects that had taken sodium citrate**. Therefore, this study seems to indicate that **taking sodium citrate during the recovery after a dehydrating exercise can relieve stress, allowing you to better prepare for the next effort**.

Dosages

Both potassium citrate and sodium citrate should be taken with a 250 mL glass of water, immediately after meals, in order to reduce their slightly corrosive effect on teeth and upper digestive tract mucosa, which may also be associated with a feeling of nausea, vomiting, stomach cramps and diarrhea. Both potassium citrate and sodium citrate promote diuresis, which is therefore useful in the presence of cystitis or in cases with a tendency to urinary stones. The dosage that is generally considered useful for improving the performance is around 0.5 g/kg. As for sodium citrate, it should be remembered that the daily sodium intake, considering that provided by water, drugs, supplements and foods, should not exceed the 3 g, especially in people with hypertension or heart failure. In the presence of hypokalaemia or predisposing situations, such as nausea, vomiting, use of thiazide diuretics, sweating etc., it is preferable to use potassium citrate. In general, in the presence of a good state of health, it is preferable to use sodium citrate, both for the best tolerance in the stomach and for the taste.

Effectiveness

Strength	Resistant strength	Mass	Endurance	Slimming	Concentration	Recovery
−	+++	++	++	−	−	++

CITRULINE

Description

Citrulline is a non-essential neutral amino acid. Its name derives from the food in which it was first isolated in the 1930s, namely watermelon (*Citrullus vulgaris* in Latin). Originally it was thought that citrulline was just a simple intermediate compound of various metabolic processes, and in particular of the urea cycle, without giving any importance to its multiple effects on the body. This amino acid has never been given much importance, as it does not participate in the synthesis of proteins. At the endogenous level, citrulline is synthesized mainly from arginine by means of the arginine deaminase enzyme.

Subsequent studies have shown that citrulline not only presides over the control of ammonia, as a shuttle between mitochondrion and cytosol, but also has important qualities as an antioxidant (Akashi et al., 2001), as a regulator of the cardiovascular functions (Romero et al., 2006), as a regulator of the immunity (Norris et al., 1995), it facilitates muscle recovery, but above all, it plays a key role in regulating nitrogen homeostasis (Osowska et al., 2004, 2006).

Properties

The urea cycle has the main purpose of detoxifying the human body from ammonia, which is metabolized into urea. Within the mitochondria of hepatocytes, citrulline is synthesized starting from ornithine and carbamyl phosphate by the enzyme ornithine-carbamyl-phosphate transferase. In turn, carbamyl phosphate is synthesized by carbamyl phosphatase I, from ammonia and bicarbonate. Once synthesized, citrulline is transported from the mitochondrion to the cytosol, through transporters that carry ornithine inside and citrulline outside the mitochondrion.

In the cytosol, citrulline, under the action of argininosuccinate synthase, binds aspartic acid to form argininosuccinate. Subsequently, the argininosuccinate is transformed into arginine under the action of argininosuccinate lyase to form the fumarate. Arginine is metabolized into ornithine by arginase, which releases a urea molecule. Ornithine returns to the mitochondrion to be metabolized by ornithine-carbamylphosphate transferase, while the urea molecule leaves the liver and is captured by the kidneys to be expelled through the urine (Cynober, 2013).

Evidence

Physiologically, all the citrulline produced by the liver is reused by the hepatic metabolism.

In 1981 Windemueller and Spaeth discovered that citrulline is released into our body from the intestine. The endogenous synthesis of citrulline comes from arginine and glutamine. In enterocytes, about 40% of arginine is converted into ornithine (Castillo et al., 1993). The same goes for glutamine (ornithine amino transferase enzyme). The ornithine produced is metabolized into citrulline by ornithine-carbamyl phosphate transferase. When arginine levels are very low, ornithine becomes the direct precursor of citrulline (Marini et al., 2011). Proline is also a precursor of citrulline, in fact, in the small intestine, this amino acid is converted into P5C (delta 1-L-pyrroline-5-carboxylate), which will subsequently be converted into ornithine. About 80% of the citrulline produced by the liver is captured in the portal vein and reaches the kidneys, where it is converted into arginine, increasing its blood levels.

This arginine/glutamine-ornithine-citrulline cycle is an important endogenous source of arginine (about 60%) and also presides over nitrogen homeastasis. However, the citrulline produced by arginine and glutamine serves to stem the flow of these two amino acids towards the portal blood, to be captured later by the liver, to form urea. This action serves to prevent the over-activation of ureogenesis, which would lead to an inappropriate increase in the amino acid catabolism; this process would lead to a reduced level of amino acids in the blood, which would cause a reduction in the protein synthesis.

Citrulline works well in **preventing amino acid catabolism in the presence of restrictive diets with a low protein** or arginine **content**. Numerous studies (Shang and Taylor, 2011; Moinard et al., 2006; Osowska et al., 2006; Faure et al., 2013) have shown how the administration of citrulline in older mice with a restrictive diet, prevented muscle the loss and the mechanisms of protein oxidation that are the basis of proteolysis, and therefore of muscle catabolism. From these studies, it emerged that this amino acid blocks the expression of the proteolysis activator protein (subunit 1 of the proteasome activator complex).

Another effect to mention is the **antioxidant activity of citrulline**. Oxidative stress, inflammation processes and nitrogen homeostasis are closely related and governed by the activation of NF-κB (Nuclear Factor bappa-light-chain-enhancer of activated B cells), which governs the gene expression of proinflammatory molecules. The antioxidant power of citrulline has been proven to be a powerful scavenger, which protects the DNA and the enzymes from the attack of ROS (Reactive Oxygen Species), especially by the hydroxyl radical OH^- (Akashi et al., 2001; Matsugo et al., 1995).

In sports, citrulline has been shown to be an effective supplement, working on the increase of plasma arginine, accelerating the clearance of lactate and plasma ammonia through the urea cycle, and finally increasing muscle function (Briand et al., 1992; Verleye et al., 1995; Giannesini et al., 2011). Citrulline increases the production of nitric oxide and it can be more effective than arginine, as it has a higher absorption rate and is therefore able to restore the nitric oxide production more quickly. A study by van Wick et al. showed that the supplementation of 10 g of citrulline, taken one hour before a bike ride, at 70% of maximum effort, limited injuries to the intestine more than the placebo group.

In a study by Bailey et al. at the University of Exeter (UK), it was shown that 6 g of citrulline per day increased the use of oxygen during the exercise, **improved the endurance performance and increased the tolerance to high intensity exercise.**

Further studies have shown that short-term supplementation with L-citrulline in addition to watermelon juice reduced the perception of post-exercise muscle pain.

A study by Martínez-Díaz et al., evaluated the effect of watermelon juice enriched with L-citrulline (3.45 g of L-citrulline/500 mL of juice) on the physical performance and biochemical markers after a half marathon race; The results of the study showed that watermelon juice with L-citrulline reduced the perception of muscle pain 24 to 72 hours after the competition and had kept the plasma lactate concentration lower after the strenuous exercise. The conversion of L-citrulline into argininosuccinate and L-arginine through a *de novo* synthesis seems to be a possible mechanism of action to explain these results, and this increase in the bioavailability of L-arginine would increase the blood flow, decreasing the perception of muscle pain.

In two other recent studies, the effect of taking L-citrulline with watermelon juice over a prolonged time of 14 or 16 days, was tested with doses from 980 mL (juice only) to 6.0 g (juice added) respectively in cyclists and physically active men.

This supplementation demonstrated an increase in plasma nitrate concentrations, a mechanism that could be associated with an increase in NO production by NO synthase.

In addition, during exercises of moderate intensity, while the pulmonary O_2 did not show significant changes, muscle oxygenation improved after taking the watermelon juice; this result could imply that watermelon juice improves the balance between the supply of O_2 and the muscle demand for O_2 during exercises of moderate intensity.

In the study by Shanely et al., the intake of watermelon juice was associated with a higher score on the RPE scale, an increase in plasma levels of L-citrulline and L-arginine, as well as an increase in antioxidant capacity and total nitrates, albeit without evident acute effects on post-exercise inflammation and on the immune function.

Other studies have also evaluated the effects on the physical performance of a prolonged supplementation, between 6 and 14 days, of L-citrulline, with dosages ranging from 2.4 to 6.0 g.

In general, it was observed a significant increase in the bioavailability of NO, an increase in blood flow, a reduction in the time of speed tests, reduced muscle pain after physical exertion and an increase in the rate of VO_{2max}.

Gonzales et al. found that supplementation with L-citrulline increased the blood flow in the femoral artery by 11% and the femoral vascular conductance by 14%, when performing lower limb exercises in elderly men, while they were not observed changes in women of the same age.

This modest improvement in the muscle blood flow during submaximal exercise could imply a greater tolerance to physical exercise in elderly men, following a prolonged supplementation of L-citrulline.

In another study by Ahsley et al., 7 days of L-citrulline supplementation did not improve the oxygen consumption in moderate-intensity walking in young or elder subject, although an improvement in oxygen uptake kinetics was noted in men, but not in women.

In another study conducted by Benjamin Wax at the State University of Mississippi (USA), it was found that citrulline improved the resistant strength in the execution of exercises such as: pull-ups, pull-ups with reverse grip and pushups, in college students.

The association between citrulline and malic acid amplifies all these functions and increases their absorption in the intestine. In fact, malic acid is an intermediate of the Krebs cycle and its presence increases the energy production, especially in situations of prolonged effort (Bendahan et al., 2002; Wagenmarkers et al., 1998). Furthermore, their association increases ATP levels in the muscle during the training and increases phosphocreatine levels during the post-workout.

A 2010 study verified the use of citrulline malate, with a single dose of 8 g before training, during an upper body training session. The researchers measured muscle soreness and fatigue after 24 and 48 hours of high-intensity training. The authors found that the administration of citrulline malate **significantly increased (21%) the repetitions for each exercise and also reduced the muscle soreness, compared to the placebo group**.

Another 2015 study, by Wax et al., verified the ergogenic effect of citrulline malate on experienced weightlifters who engaged in lower body exercises (leg press, leg extension, hack squat). This double-blind study involved 12 subjects and consisted of three daily training sessions, repeated 48-72 hours apart, for one week. The first session was aimed at determining the maximum, while sessions 2 and 3 were used to quantify the number of series that can be performed for each exercise until failure.

Sixty minutes prior to these two sessions, subjects were randomly given 8 g of citrulline or a placebo. The protocol consisted of two series with submaximal loads and after a three-minute recovery, the series were performed with 60% of the maximum up to failure, with one-minute recoveries. The results showed that the experimental group was able to perform a significantly higher number of series compared to the control group, while the concentration of lactic acid and the measurement of blood pressure levels (systolic and diastolic) and heart rate, show no significant differences. The results showed that supplementation with citrulline malate had reduced the sense of fatigue in athletes who used it; the researchers hypothesize that the ergogenic effect is due to the synergy between these two compounds.

Malic acid is an intermediate of the Krebs cycle and increases the production of the metabolic energy (ATP); moreover, malate acts as a shuttle between the mitochondrion and the sarcoplasm, thus reducing the formation of lactic acid and increasing the formation of pyruvate (an important activator of the tricarboxylic acid cycle). Citrulline, on the other hand, acts mainly on the synthesis of nitric oxide, which increases the contractile function of the muscle and, by increasing blood flow, favors the arrival of nutrients in the muscle areas. Furthermore, citrulline improves the cell repair processes through the activation of satellite cells and myotrophic factors.

Several studies from 2016 to now show a positive effect of the short-term supplementation of citrulline malate on the sports performance. The main benefit of this supplement is the reduction of the RPE score and muscle pain, following a physical exertion.

In this sense, the study by Pérez-Guisado et al. showed that there was a reduced perception of muscle pain at 24 and 48 hours after the exertion in the subjects who had taken citrulline malate, compared to the placebo.

Similarly, Glenn et al. also showed a reduction in the score on the RPE scale after the supplementation of 8 g of citrulline malate.

The lower perception of post-exercise muscle pain seems to be due to the ability of citrulline malate to buffer the acidosis, reducing the concentration of lactic acid and ammonia.

Short-term supplementation with citrulline malate led to increased repetitions, increased upper and lower body weight exercises, grip strength, vertical power and performance test in master tennis players at Wingate, one hour after taking citrulline malate.

According to these studies, the effect of short-term supplementation with citrulline malate on physical performance results in the reduction of the muscle fatigue and the perception of post-exercise pain, and an increase in the number of repetitions during strength training.

In the study by Kiyici et al., the effect of a prolonged citrulline malate supplementation (3 g per day, divided according to the meals) was examined in handball players subjected to intense strength and technical training for 4 weeks, four times a week.

At the end of the study, a reduction in the concentration of lactic acid in the blood of the players who had taken the supplement was observed and this result suggested that the prolonged supplementation with citrulline malate can improve the physical performance by delaying the onset of muscle fatigue.

Dosages

Dosages recommended to obtain an ergogenic effect vary from 3 to 8 g/day. If, on the other hand, you want to use it in synergy with arginine, then only 2 g is enough. If you want to use citrulline as an anticatabolic molecule in periods of low nutrient intake (definition), you must take at least 3 g per day.

Effectiveness

Strength	Resistant strength	Mass	Endurance	Slimming	Concentration	Recovery
++	+++	++	++	+++	–	++

CITRUS AURANTIUM

Description

Citrus aurantium, also called bitter orange, is a small citrus tree with white and fragrant flowers, native to subtropical Asia and the Indian regions, also cultivated in Spain for over 800 years, where it is used in various food products including jams, syrups and juices. *Citrus aurantium* has a long tradition of use in the traditional Chinese medicine, where it was better known as "Zhi Shi" and was used to stimulate the circulation and the congestive phenomena of the respiratory system. All parts of the plant are used for different purposes: for example, the flowers are used in teas, for the preparation of an essential oil useful for the production of orange blossom perfumes and liqueurs (such as Triple Sec, Grand Marnier, Cointreau and Curaçao) or as a flavoring for sweets; in aromatherapy, the essential oil is also applied to the skin or inhaled for its stimulating effects.

Properties

Thermogenesis is a physiological process that takes place mainly in muscles and in the brown adipose tissue. It takes place through a series of chemical and biochemical reactions intended to metabolize the molecules of fats or their derivatives, releasing energy. The thermogenic process is triggered by the activation of the beta-adrenergic receptors closely connected to the enzymatic system of adenylate cyclase. The activation of adenylate cyclase, modulated by G-proteins with a stimulatory action, increases the intracellular levels of the second cyclic AMP messenger. Thanks to this increase in cyclic AMP, there is an increase in lipolysis and an increase in mitochondrial oxygen consumption, an indication of an increased thermogenic activity (heat is produced instead of work).

The mechanism of thermogenesis is linked to metabolism and varies from individual to individual as it depends on genetic factors. These factors affect the amount of "brown fat" (brown adipose tissue) which is a tissue capable of producing heat and energy by "burning" fat in greater quantities than any other area of the body.

Some molecules have the ability to interact with beta-3 receptors located at the level of brown fat deposits and they can activate the thermogenic process. The unripe and dried fruits of *Citrus aurantium* contain a mixture of sympathomimetic amines such as synephrine, N-methyltyramine, hordenine, octopamine and tyramine, which stimulate the processes of thermogenesis by activating the beta oxidation of fats and by improving the ratio of lean mass to fat mass. The concentrations of these molecules are sufficient to activate the beta-3 receptors and to stimulate the lipolysis without causing side effects on the nervous system and on the heart, as is the case for other substances with a thermogenic effect, including ephedrine.

In fact, many studies have investigated the safety of synephrine due to its structural similarity with ephedrine. A recent review that focused on human, animal, *in vitro* and even mechanistic studies (mechanism of action) concluded that both *Citrus aurantium* and synephrine are safe for use in supplements and foods.

Some studies in the past, reported potential adverse cardiovascular effects for the use of *Citrus aurantium* extract and synephrine, but the same review, analyzing them, reported that many of these studies did not consider the composition of the supplements used in the subjects' diet, in which synephrine was present in association with other components, so it was not possible to conclude that the causative agent was the extract of *Citrus aurantium* and synephrine. It should also be remembered that possible cardiovascular effects occurred in rats from the use of synephrine in combination with caffeine, since the binding of synephrine with the adrenergic receptor is ten times greater, which would explain these effects observed in rodents, compared to humans.

In addition to the ability to increase fat burning, synephrine is able (again thanks to its beta-agonist action) to keep the muscles toned and to preserve them from the loss of muscle mass, sometimes associated with low-calorie diets.

Octopamine is chemically similar to synephrine and noradrenaline and is able to stimulate beta-3 receptors, present on brown fat, thus activating lipolysis, increasing the metabolism and promoting the transport of glucose (insulin-like effect).

Synephrine is certainly best known for its thermogenic activity, but the *Citrus aurantium* extract proved to be much more than a simple thermogenic, as it increases the metabolic activity by improving the body's physical performance through a marked increase in beta oxidation of fatty acids in the muscles.

To confirm this, there is a further study (Gutiérrez-Hellín et al., 2016), in which it was found that the intake of synephrine as a pre-workout contributed to an increase in the beta oxidation of fatty acids, allowing for greater use of the latter for energy purposes at the mitochondrial level, while reducing the use of carbohydrates as a substrate, and therefore their oxidation rate during low and moderate intensity exercises.

Citrus aurantium is usually associated with other thermogenic substances such as caffeine and willow extract, although recent research has shown encouraging results using only its extract. The case of *Citrus aurantium* once again confirms the rule that the administration of a phytocomplex (i.e. the extract of the plant) is more effective than the individual components.

Evidence

In one study, it was seen that the use of *Citrus aurantium* is much more useful for increasing thermogenesis in women than in men, if taken in conjunction with a meal, while the best effectiveness in men was found if it was taken alone. Its use, however, did not cause increases in the blood pressure or heart rate.

According to research by McGill University (but also in other researches), a reason for the effects of *Citrus aurantium* is that **it stimulates certain receptors (called beta-3 adrenergic) that are specific for the adipose tissue, which promote lipolysis**. At the same time, this stimulation helps to increase the levels of the resting metabolism without causing an increase in blood pressure and/or tachycardia, to the extent that other classes of adrenergic receptors are not stimulated.

In addition to its slimming effects, *Citrus aurantium* also finds a valid use in increasing sports performance due to its adrenergic action, without the effect of increasing the blood pressure and heart rate.

Research conducted in 2008 (Haller, Duan, Jacob, Benowitz; Br J Clin Pharmacol) highlights how **the supplementation of *Citrus aurantium* and caffeine decreases the perception of fatigue during the exercise, compared to a placebo group**.

A study is available in which "citrus + caffeine + St. John's Wort" were used in combination for 6 weeks, in subjects with an 1800 Kcal diet, to evaluate the effect of this combination on body composition, metabolic changes, lipidemia and mood, in healthy and overweight adults.

In this research, 23 subjects with BMI > 25 kg/m^2 were divided into three groups: *group A* received 975 mg of CA extract (*Citrus aurantium*), 528 mg of caffeine and 900 mg of St. John's wort per day; *group B* received maltodextrin as a placebo; *group C* served as the control group. For 6 weeks, the subjects were subjected to a caloric regimen of 1800 Kcal per day, and 3 days a week they had to perform scheduled physical exercises under supervision and psychological tests.

During the exercise sessions, the subjects reached 70% of the maximum heartbeats produced for the corresponding age. Compared with the subjects treated with a placebo and with the control group, the treated subjects lost more body weight (-1.4 kg) and, in addition, a significant amount of body fat (on average 2, 9%). In other words, the fat loss of the subjects in group A was significantly important; furthermore, the control group showed a greater tendency to recover the lost fat.

On the other hand, the variations in the results on mood profiles and on the tests for fatigue and vigor were not significant. For group A, there were no significant changes in cholesterol and triglyceridemia. Changes in blood pressure, heart rate, electrocardiographic report, serum and urine chemical analyzes were not known in each group.

Based on the obtained results, it can be concluded that the combination of *Citrus aurantium* extract, caffeine and St. John's wort is safe for that period of time and that the effects combined with a calorie restriction and exercise promote weight and fat loss in healthy and obese adults.

Subsequent studies (Jung et al., 2017) have further investigated the possible effects induced by the acute ingestion of a pre-workout supplement (among other components, there was also caffeine), with and without the addition of synephrine, on body composition, muscle endurance and strength, resting metabolism, blood chemistry, heart rate and cognitive function. The participants in the study had been chosen and selected, among the various characteristics, also for their experience on weight training (resistance training) for at least 6 months.

From these studies, it emerged what had already been found in previous studies, namely the intake of a pre-workout supplement with the addition of synephrine (20 mg) led to an increase in metabolism at rest and an improvement in the perception of the execution of the exercise, with no significant changes in blood chemistry, blood pressure and heart rate. At the same time, the effects on muscle endurance were limited and there was no effect on the anaerobic sprint capacity. Among the positive effects, one of the most important was that of improving the cognitive function, which theoretically is fundamental during the last stages of a competition, as it improves the performance, especially in events that require a quick decision-making process.

The 50 mg dose of synephrine can increase the metabolic rate by approximately 65 Kcal, compared to the placebo (which instead caused a decrease of 30 Kcal; measurements taken when fasting for more than 75 minutes), and the addition of 600 mg of naringenin enhances this increase in the metabolic rate to 129 Kcal, as it slows down the metabolization rate in the liver. If 100 mg of hesperidin were also added to the first two ingredients, the increase in caloric expenditure would reach 183 Kcal.

Higher levels of hesperidin have not been shown to be effective in further increasing the rate of energy expenditure.

As with ephedrine, synephrine shows a marked synergy with caffeine, more evident in those who rarely consume coffee.

A recent study has instead revealed the underlying mechanism of the anti-adipogenic effect of *Citrus aurantium*, where AMPK is the crucial factor. The study involved the treatment of mice with *Citrus aurantium* for 8 weeks, subjects in which obesity had been induced with a high-fat diet. This treatment resulted in a reduction in body weight, a decrease in the adipose tissue and a decrease in serum cholesterol levels. In addition, peroxisomal proliferator-activated receptors (PPARs) and CCAAT enhancer-binding proteins, both key regulators of the adipogenesis process, were inhibited by *Citrus aurantium*. Therefore, their inhibition can be a strategy for the control of obesity and the excessive growth of white adipose tissue which, in obese individuals, has been suggested to be the cause of the proliferation and the hypertrpohy of adipocytes. Furthermore, the treatment with *Citrus aurantium* also activated the thermogenesis and the differentiation of the brown adipose tissue, but not of the white adipose tissue. The activation of brown adipose tissue, as well as the adipogenesis process, also depended on AMPK. This suggests that *Citrus aurantium* is a potential anti-obesity agent, capable of inducing thermogenesis in brown adipose tissue and inhibiting adipogenesis in the white adipose tissue, by activating AMPK.

Dosages

Usually a maximum dosage of synephrine of 30 mg/day, as a substance is present in supplements. Ready preparations or materials for galenic preparations are available based on dry extract titrated at 4 or 6% synephrine. Even though *Citrus aurantium* extract does not modify the cardiovascular activity and, due to its physico-chemical characteristics, does not pass the blood brain barrier, it is still not recommended for those suffering from cardiovascular disease, hypertension or anxiety disorders.

Effectiveness

Strength	Resistant strength	Mass	Endurance	Slimming	Concentration	Recovery
+	+	+	++	+++	++	–

COENZYME Q10

Description

Coenzyme Q10, or ubiquinone, is a compound with ubiquitous distribution as it is present in the mitochondria of all cells of the body. It is lipophilic, insoluble in water and essential for the life of every cell, being involved in the production of energy. Foods with a higher ubiquinone content are sardines, tuna, spinach, peanuts and beef. Identified by Moore and colleagues in 1940, coenzyme Q10 was isolated more than ten years later by Dr. Frederick Crane of the

University of Wisconsin (USA), who worked on the bull's heart. Since the 1960s, many studies have been carried out to support its properties for the body; in 1978, Professor Peter Mitchell was awarded the Nobel Prize in Chemistry for highlighting its important functions, but especially in recent years, coenzyme Q10 has assumed a considerable role in the nutritional supplementation world, both for the antiaging effect and for the prevention of cardiomyopathies, hypertension, degenerative diseases, ulcers, migraines and a wide range of other diseases. Numerous studies have in fact shown that our body cannot survive without it: a 25% reduction of the normal levels causes a series of serious problems, including high blood pressure, angina, heart attacks, periodontal problems, an immune system depression, lack of energy, abnormal weight gain and even premature death. A 75% reduction leads to certain death.

Properties

The main benefits that can be obtained by CoQ10 supplementation concern in particular: the increase in energy production, the stimulation of the immune system and the prevention of aging. Ubiquinone is an integral part of the mitochondria membrane, intracellular particles that produce 95% of the body's total energy; in them, ubiquinone is responsible for the synthesis of ATP, the fundamental molecule for the production of energy. In particular, CoQ10 is recognized as an indispensable element for the health of all those tissues where energy consumption is higher, such as the heart, the vascular system and the nervous system, and is therefore extremely useful for the physical exercise as, acting as a cofactor in cellular energy production, it **improves the endurance and the aerobic capacity, and it also reduces the body fat**. Today's life is increasingly characterized by environmental pollution and high forms of stress which, in addition to causing an overload in demand for energy, can undoubtedly favor the formation of very unstable and reactive molecules called free radicals, responsible for important damage to the structural elements of the cells. The attack of free radicals on the cell membrane, for example, causes a loss of elasticity, rigidity, a decrease in the permeability of water and nutrients, causing cell aging and subsequently death. Ubiquinone acts at this point by promoting the stabilization of the cell membrane and, acting as an **antioxidant agent**, it protects the cells from the damage caused by free radicals. In addition, exogenous ubiquinone appears to have inhibitory activity on phospholipase, the enzyme responsible for the degeneration of the cell membrane. In fact, exogenous administration of ubiquinone causes a powerful brake on lipoperoxidation, a process that occurs when free radicals attack membrane phospholipids, compromising the cellular stability. The concentration of **CoQ10 tends to decrease with aging**; low levels are also recorded in the presence of particular chronic diseases, such as those resulting from heart problems, Parkinson's disease, muscular dystrophy, diabetes, cancer and AIDS. Even some drugs, such as statins and metformin, which are used in the control of hypercholesterolemia and blood sugar, can lower CoQ10 levels.

Evidence

As suggested by numerous studies, supplementation with some antioxidants, such as vitamin C, vitamin E, carotenoids, alpha-lipoic acid, etc., allows to prevent or limit the "damage" caused by physical exercise and guarantees a faster recovery. In a group of 18 elite athletes who performed martial arts for 5.5 hours a day, 10 of them were given a dose of 300 mg/day and the other eight took a placebo. Those who had taken the CoQ10 supplementation had a decrease in the levels of CPK and lipid peroxidation, indices of less damage to the membrane of the muscle cell. The ergogenic effects caused by supplementation with CoQ10 have been studied in both rats and humans, and they have been demonstrated only in the recent years. The human body is able to produce CoQ10 autonomously, but its synthesis is reduced in the event of diseases and, above all, progressively decreases from the age of 21. Therefore, it could be said that starting from this age, a physical decline begins: it is no coincidence that many of the records held in sports that require intense physical performance and a very efficient metabolism are obtained by very young athletes. The reason for this decline is not difficult to understand: a lower amount of available CoQ10 leads to a lower efficiency in the production of ATP by the mitochondria, the energy plants of the cells, and therefore less efficiency in withstanding extreme efforts at the muscular level. The function performed by the coenzyme therefore allows to obtain really interesting results, in particular for people who practice sports. Athletes and people wishing to increase their level of physical endurance can take CoQ10 supplements and thus obtain a higher energy level and greater tolerance to physical effort, counteracting the typical symptoms of fatigue. The activity of CoQ10 at the skeletal muscle level, expressed as the ability to improve the energy production at the cellular level, has led to the use of CoQ10 also in sports medicine, where some studies carried out on professional cycling and cross-country skiing athletes have demonstrated the positive effect on the physical performance and on muscle tone indices.

Intense physical exercises and hyperthermia can induce an oxidative stress and adverse effects on the myocardial function. The aim of the study by Emami et al. carried out in 2018, was to study the effect of coenzyme Q10 supplementation on creatine kinase-MB (CK-MB), cardiac troponin I (cTnI), myoglobin (Mb), lactate dehydrogenase (LD), total antioxidant capacity (TAC), lipid peroxidation (LPO) and CoQ10 concentration in elite swimmers. During an 18-session protocol in the morning and in the evening, subjects participated in speed and endurance swimming training sessions, 5km in each session. Blood was collected before (two phases) and after (two phases) the administration of CoQ10. There was a significant increase in the levels of CK-MB, cTnI, Mb, LD and LPO in the control group compared to the group that had taken the supplement. Consequently, it was concluded that through supplementation with CoQ10, it is possible to prevent the myocardial damage and the oxidative stress during the swimming competition phase.

In a Finnish study, 25 cross-country skiers were treated with CoQ10 or a placebo; **the results showed an improvement in all physical performance indices**. 94% of the athletes treated with CoQ10 had an improvement in their time and in their performance, while in the group treated with the placebo, only 33% of the subjects experienced this result. Furthermore, CoQ10 can also **be effective for weight loss**, as, thanks to its ability to generate cellular energy, it increases the metabolism, improves the body's ability to convert food into energy and affects the regulation of fats and sugars which are already present in the blood. Obviously, CoQ10 supplementation has proven to be even more effective when it is taken in combination with a healthy diet and an exercise program.

Insulin-like growth factor 1 (IGF-1) has a multitude of effects beyond those on cell growth and metabolism. The reports also indicate anti-inflammatory and antioxidant effects and it is important to emphasize that IGF-1 concentrations decrease with age, especially if our organism is inflamed. Since selenium and coenzyme Q10 are involved in both antioxidant defense and inflammatory response, Alehagen et al. on 2017 conducted a study whose aim was to examine the effects of supplementation with selenium and coenzyme Q10 on the concentrations of IGF-1 and on its IGFBP-1 binding protein, in a population that had shown a reduction in the cardiovascular mortality following such supplementation. 215 people were included and, after supplementation with selenium and coenzyme Q10, applying group mean assessments, significantly higher IGF-1 levels were found in the active treatment group, while a decrease in concentration of the same biomarkers was found in the placebo group. Supplementation with selenium and coenzyme Q10, therefore, resulted in an increase in postprandial IGF-1 and IGFBP-1 levels and an increase in age-corrected IGF-1 levels, compared to the placebo. These effects could be included in the mechanistic explanation behind the surprisingly positive clinical effects on cardiovascular morbidity and mortality previously reported by this form of supplementation.

Many neurodegenerative diseases are linked to the presence of damage in the functionality of the energy metabolism and in particular to mitochondrial functions. Some bioenergetic agents, such as CoQ10, nicotinamide, riboflavin, creatine, carnitine and lipoic acid, are able to give benefits and exert neuroprotective effects in the examined subjects. Even though the use of CoQ10 in Parkinson's is still being studied, a first important indication of its activity comes from a randomized, double-blind, placebo-controlled study conducted in 80 patients with Parkinson's disease, whose goal was to evaluate the ability of CoQ10 on slowing the progression of the disease. All 80 patients recruited for this study had early-stage Parkinson's disease; some received CoQ10 treatment at various daily dosages (300, 600, 1200 mg), while others took a placebo.

All subjects were assessed using the Unified Parkinson Disease Rating Scale (UPDRS) at 1, 4, 8, 12 and 16 months after the initial visit. The primary end point was the change from the baseline of the UPDRS score at the last visit. The analysis of the data collected at the end of the study allowed the authors to conclude that CoQ10 appears to be able to slow the progression of the disease in patients with Parkinson's disease, without significant side effects. Another study in 28 Parkinson's disease patients treated with 360 mg of CoQ10 per day led to the same conclusions, demonstrating an improvement in symptoms in patients treated with this supplement.

The ability to maintain the cell membrane and the mitochondrial membrane in good efficiency, the ability to neutralize free radicals (where it has been demonstrated an efficacy 50 times higher than that of vitamin E) and the ability to act as a carrier for oxygen, make CoQ10 a useful supplement for cancer prevention as well.

As we have seen, the heart is the organ in which the highest concentration of CoQ10 is found. In 1994, a study published by the University of Texas showed a significant improvement in cardiopaths treated with doses of CoQ10 from 80 to 600 mg per day. Other research has shown that heart attacks tend to occur when CoQ10 supplies are particularly low, and that in people who have suffered a heart attack, administering high doses of CoQ10 helps restore the heart function. Among other things, CoQ10 demonstrates the ability to protect the heart from oxygen deprivation in ischemic patients, allowing them to live much longer. In patients undergoing open heart surgery who are pretreated with CoQ10 administrations, there is a higher rate of success for the intervention and a much shorter recovery time than in untreated ones, demonstrating the ability of ubiquinone in improving the oxygenation of the heart muscle and, consequently, also of the organism in general.

People with diabetes have a higher risk of having cardiovascular diseases; in this case, CoQ10 has been shown to have properties that ensure an improvement in the cardiovascular functions and in the management of diabetes. Also, type 2 diabetes is often associated with high cholesterol levels that lead many diabetics to take statins. Researchers coordinated by B.J. Lee, of the Taichung Veterans General Hospital in Taichung (Taiwan), assuming that high oxidative stress and chronic inflammation can contribute to the pathogenesis of diseases affecting the coronary arteries, have shown that the addition of CoQ10 significantly improves the activity of antioxidant enzymes and reduces the inflammatory state in patients with CAD (Coronary Artery Disease) during statin therapy. Knowing, in fact, that CoQ10 is an endogenous fat-soluble antioxidant and that statin therapy can reduce its biosynthesis, the researchers wanted to study the effects of supplementation with CoQ10 (300 mg/day; 150 mg/2 times a day) as an antioxidant and as an anti-inflammatory, in patients with CAD who were already being treated with statins. Fifty-one patients identified by coronary angiography (coronary artery stenosis of at least 50%) and treated with statins for at least one month, were randomly divided into two subgroups: one taking a placebo, the other taking CoQ10, for a period of 12 weeks. After this period, they evaluated the concentrations of CoQ10 and vitamin E, the activity of antioxidant enzymes (superoxide dismutase, catalase and glutathione peroxidase) and the inflammatory markers [C-reactive protein (CRP), Tumor Necrosis Factor-alpha (TNF-α) and interleukin-6 (IL-6)]. The plasma levels of CoQ10 and enzymes with antioxidant activity were significantly higher after CoQ10 supplementation, while the levels of inflammatory markers (TNF-α, $P = 0.039$) were significantly lower. In the same group, vitamin E levels and antioxidant enzyme activities were significantly higher than in the placebo group.

Dosages
CoQ10 can be taken as a supplement, either in capsule form or in drinking vials. In healthy adult subjects, the recommended daily dose is 50 mg/day (30 to 60 mg/day), up to a maximum of 100 mg/day, but, in the presence of pathologies, the dose may be higher. For example, for patients on statin therapy or in those who are recovering from heart failure, the dosage can reach up to 150 mg/day, taken under medical supervision. The only precaution to be taken concerns patients suffering from gastric hypoacidity: for this reason, they are subjected to *Candida* infections in the upper bowel area, so they must avoid taking ubiquinone by mouth, because the latter favors the development of *Candida* in a low acid environment.

Effectiveness

Strength	Resistant strength	Mass	Endurance	Slimming	Concentration	Recovery
−	+	−	+++	++	+	+

COLOSTRUM

Description
"Colostrum" is the term that indicates the milk secreted by mammals in the first phase of lactation, i.e. during the first 5-7 days. It is also the name of the first milk and has a very dense consistency and a yellowish color; this is due to the fact that some carotenoids are present in high quantities in its composition. Colostrum, compared to other types of milk (including mature milk), has a higher quantity of proteins (about 25%), and it is precisely the quality of these proteins that gives it its importance. In fact, in addition to containing several essential amino acids, colostrum is rich in peptide components of whey and caseins. It also contains a fair amount of lactose, which is useful for buffering the state of hypoglycemia of the newborn in the period immediately after birth. This milk is very rich in immune factors, such as lactoferrin, lactoperoxidase, lysozyme and type G- and type A-immunoglobulins; the latter have a protective action on the intestinal cells, as well as counteracting possible infectious processes affecting the intestine. Furthermore, it is very rich in albumin, the main carrier protein, in mineral salts and in numerous growth factors, including IGF-1 and IGF-2 (Francis et al., 1988).

Properties
Bovine colostrum acts and mediates numerous metabolic pathways in the human body; some have been identified and confirmed, others are still under study.

In bovine colostrum, the concentration of growth factors is particularly high, in fact the concentration of IGF-1 varies from 7 to 67 nmol/L, compared to 0.3 nmol/L of the normal milk. IGF-1 is one of the most important mediators of anabolism, for both muscles and bones.

This growth factor is mainly regulated by the calorie intake and the physical training. In fact, a diet that is too low in calories and above all in carbohydrates and/or proteins significantly reduces the production of IGF-1, with a consequent reduction in the protein synthesis and an increase in proteolysis.

Other positive effects of colostrum are recorded at the gastrointestinal level, at the immune level and at the endocrine level. In fact, it has been shown that the administration of colostrum improves the intestinal absorption by reducing its permeability. From an endocrine point of view, it has been observed that colostrum promotes the maturation of the hypothalamus-pituitary-somatotropic hormone axis. Colostrum proteins are transported directly into the cerebrospinal fluid, arriving in the brain and stimulating the production of anabolic hormones such as GH and sex hormones at the hypothalamic and pituitary level. In addition, maternal colostrum, unlike the supplement, contains purely sex hormones (GnRH, LH, testosterone), somatotropic and glucocorticoids, useful for forming and maturing the endocrine system of the newborn.

At the immune level, bovine colostrum plays a positive role by stimulating the synthesis of immunoglobulins. Several studies have confirmed that colostrum increased serum and salivary IgA concentrations. These studies were focused on measuring the incidence of diseases related to the upper airways in athletes. The administration of 60 g of colostrum daily for eight weeks, led to a reduction of this type of infections in about 12% of endurance athletes, compared to the placebo group. Other studies on dairy animals have shown how the administration of colostrum in doses of 1-5 g per day, for at least three weeks, increased the gene expression on the production of Peyer's plaques; in addition, in vitro studies have shown how colostrum has a reduction action on the pro-inflammatory cytokines, with a consequent reduction of TNF-α, IL-6 and IL-4.

Another effect (albeit of lesser importance) of colostrum is recorded on the thyroid metabolism: the presence of a significant concentration of iodine and selenium improves its metabolism, increases the production of thyroid hormones and improves the immune function of the thyroid.

Evidence

A 2002 study conducted on 30 adult athletes, compared the effects of using colostrum for two weeks to a placebo consisting of maltodextrin, on IGF-1 values and immunoglobulin levels. The supplementation was divided into four dosages throughout the day and the subjects also had a training session every day; after two weeks, it was noted that the serum values of IGF-1 had increased by 17% and the salivary concentration of IgA had increased by 33%, compared to the placebo group.

As for the quantities of immunoglobulin G, there were no significant changes between the experimental and control groups.

This very important increase in these growth factors is attributable to the fact that bovine colostrum contains a very high quantity of IGF-1, which is perfectly identical (same amino acid sequence) to the human one, and it is assumed that this increase in its concentration is due to a higher intestinal absorption, as well as an increase in the stimulation of its synthesis.

On the other hand, for immunoglobulins, the study showed that IgA was increased more than IgG; this may be due to the fact that IgA plays a fundamental role in the protection of the intestinal mucosa against viruses and bacteria, and since the first immune defenses that are formed in newborns are those in the stomach and intestines, colostrum first increases these defenses at the expense of the others, since in the new individuals, the formation and protection of the intestinal tract is of primary importance, both regarding the absorption of nutrients and for the engraftment and growth of the intestinal bacterial flora.

As for the ergogenic effect of colostrum, numerous studies since 1997 have shown how a massive supplementation of colostrum (60 g/day) increased the maximal strength and also the endurance. Regarding the anaerobic capacity, there are very few studies showing that colostrum supplementation improves the buffer capacity towards excess H^+ ions. Brinkworth et al. (2002) have shown how the rate of intramuscular acidosis, following intense exercise, was significantly decreased after the administration of colostrum. The dose they used was 60 g/day, for nine weeks. The buffering capacity was assessed by the difference between blood lactate concentration and blood pH, at the start and at the end of the training. At the end of the study, there was a significant increase in the buffering capacity in the group using the experimental protocol. However, this increase in the buffering capacity was not matched by an increase in the athletic performance. This is probably due to the fact that in the athletes under study, there was already an increase in the hemoglobin's ability to buffer H^+ ions, or an increase in the concentration of intracellular phosphates, which represent one of the most effective endogenous buffer systems.

In a 2014 study by Philip Chilibeck and Whitney Duff et al. at the University of Saskatchewan (CA), it was found that the administration of colostrum in adult subjects with an average age of 59 years (in the original study it was written "elderly adults", but I felt this was too strong and I removed "elderly", A/N), both men and women, involved in weight training, produced a greater increase in leg strength and less bone resorption, compared to the administration of 30 g of whey protein.

The increase in the intestinal permeability is a condition that occurs frequently in athletes and can be caused by various factors. From various studies, it has emerged that colostrum is able to improve the intestinal permeability; in a study conducted in 2017, 16 athletes took a colostrum supplement during 2 weeks of pre-competition training. The study was conducted in a double-blind fashion: one group took a placebo (whey protein) and the other took 500 mg of bovine colostrum. The integrity of the intestine was assessed through the differential absorption of lactulose and mannitol and through the dosage of zonulin in the faeces. At the beginning of the study, 75% of the subjects showed an increased intestinal permeability; after the supplementation period, the values of the lactulose/mannitol test returned to the normal range and were significantly lower than in the placebo group. Zonulin levels also decreased significantly compared to the control group. This study therefore demonstrated the efficiency of colostrum supplementation in reducing the intestinal permeability in athletes.

Another research analyzed the effects of colostrum supplementation in a group of athletes. The 10-week study involved 29 male cyclists who performed a high intensity training program (5 High Intensity Trainings, HIT, per week). At the end of this period, the researchers compared the placebo group to the experimental group and identified an improvement in the performance in the group that had taken colostrum: the parameters relating to VO_{2max} were improved.

Dosages

Colostrum turns out to be a supplement that can be used for increasing the muscle mass, for improving the sports performance and also for those who want to implement their immune system. The effective dosage at which all the capabilities of colostrum are met is 20 g/day, divided into two or three intakes. Lower dosages (5 g/day) help stimulate the production of immunoglobulins, lactoferrin and several immune system mediators. On the contrary, higher dosages, such as 60 g/day, stimulate protein synthesis and IGF-1 production. To be effective, supplementation must be continued for at least 4-6 weeks.

Effectiveness

Strength	Resistant strength	Mass	Endurance	Slimming	Concentration	Recovery
++	++	++	+	+	–	+

CONJUGATED LINOLEIC ACID (CLA)

Description
The "conjugated linoleic acid" term does not refer to a single fatty acid, but to a mix of fatty acids characterized by the same structure as linoleic acid (a carbon skeleton of 18 atoms and two double bonds). While maintaining the same carbonaceous constitution, CLA differs from linoleic acid in the position of the two double bonds; the most studied and most often referred to isoforms in scientific studies are *c9t11* (cis-9, trans-11, which is the one that is found mostly in natural food sources and which represents at least 75% of total CLA, also known as rumenic acid) and *t10c12* (trans-10, cis-12, which is biologically more active).

The conjugated linoleic acid is a fatty acid naturally present in various foods, particularly in animal meat, almost exclusively from ruminants, and in milk, especially in dairy products. The synthesis of CLA in animals, which takes place through the rumen biohydrogenation process (a process consisting of a series of chemical reactions by the digestive microbiota, which effects the fermentation of rumen and leads to the formation of intermediate products, including rumenic acid), is higher if these animals have been raised on pasture by eating grass and not fed with cereal derivatives; if they are raised in the wild, CLA production is even higher.

There are two ways of synthesis of the *c9t11* isomer (rumenic acid), which include: isomerization of linoleic acid by the enzyme α-desaturase, or the endogenous synthesis pathway at the level of the mammary gland. Since the biohydrogenation process is not 100% efficient, many cis-trans fatty acids (as intermediates) are transferred from the bloodstream to the mammary gland, therefore the percentage of endogenous origin makes at least 60% of the total amount found in milk.

Generally, we already take 1 g of CLA per day by eating normally, but to reach an effective amount we would need to consume higher quantities, thus also introducing an excess of proteins, fats and other substances that could be harmful to the body. For example, cheeses contain an average of 2.9-7.1 mg of CLA for each gram of fat: to get at least close to the dose (4 g) that appears to be effective, we should eat a few pounds a day. It is therefore more logical to consume CLA supplements, which contain a high concentration of this particular fatty acid.

Properties
Conjugated linoleic acid belongs to the family of fatty acids called omega-6 (polyunsaturated fatty acids); it is an important factor involved in multiple functions of the body, for example it intervenes in the inflammation process, in the interaction between glucose and lipid metabolism, and in the disposal of fats. In addition, laboratory tests have shown its powerful antioxidant properties and have confirmed its effects, the stimulation of the immune system, anticarcinogen properties, the stimulation of lean mass and the reduction of fat. In particular, regarding the reduction of fat mass, scholars have hypothesized three different mechanisms of action of CLA: 1) direct action on fat metabolism with an improvement in the use of fat for energy purposes and a saving of muscle glycogen; 2) counteracting the adverse effects of catabolic hormones such as cortisol, which, as we know, destroys muscle proteins and increases fat deposits; 3) increasing the production of E1 prostaglandins which increase the somatotropic hormone brain levels, with obvious advantages for athletes in increasing muscle growth and increasing the blood flow to the muscles, brain and other organs.

Among the countless properties of CLA, a recent study has shown that it also acts as an anti-atherosclerotic agent, thus assuming a preventive role in cardiovascular diseases. Although the consumption of trans fatty acids found in foods has been linked to a higher incidence of cardiovascular diseases, previous studies have probably ignored the role of individual isomers. In fact, a relationship has been identified between vaccenic acid (C18:*1t11*), an intermediate of biohydrogenation and a precursor of the *c9t11* isomer (rumenic ac.), and cardiovascular diseases. In fact, in oral toxicity tests in rats fed with milk fat enriched with vaccenic acid, the plasma triglyceride content was significantly reduced. Hence the importance of vaccenic acid as a precursor of rumenic acid (*c9t11*), one of the most relevant bioactive compounds in milk fat.

Evidence

Dr. Yann Rougier, M.D. (a leading European sports doctor) believes that CLA "is the key to muscle growth". He believes that, in some way, the antioxidant properties of CLA can "clean the lock" of the nutrient transport system through the membrane of the muscle cell, favoring the flow of nutrients to the cells and causing a significant muscle growth. Most of the research was conducted on animals (cattle, pigs, chickens) and found **positive effects on the body composition (more muscle and less fat)**. Other studies indicate that a purified isomer of CLA, t10c12, is effective in increasing the resistance to exercise in mice thanks to its ability to stimulate the use of fatty acids instead to glucose, with a consequent saving of muscle and liver glycogen.

A further study in middle-aged male mice, fed with a diet rich in fatty acids, examined the effects induced by the simultaneous administration of CLA and omega-3 (ω3) fatty acids, with or without a weight training program. The study involved the subdivision into four experimental groups, respectively: a control group with only a diet rich in fatty acids, a group with diet and weight training, a group with a diet rich in fat and supplementation with CLA/ω3 and, finally, a group with a high-fat diet, weight training and supplementation with CLA/ω3. The aim was to investigate the induced effects on the body composition, musculoskeletal properties and functional capacities of mice. Comparing the various groups, the results showed that the administration of CLA/ω3 attenuates the increase in fat mass and improves the myogenic capacity by increasing the satellite cells; however, there were no significant effects on strength and muscle mass; however, at the same time, despite the catabolic environment created by a diet rich in fatty acids, weight training attenuated the loss of muscle mass because it increased the myogenic capacity and the anti-inflammatory effect of CLA. There was an improvement in the sensorimotor capacity thanks to the combination of CLA/ω3 and weight training, although the greatest effect was due to training. Furthermore, treatment with CLA/ω3 has also been shown to improve the anabolic signaling during the catabolism, induced by a diet rich in fatty acids. This resulted in an increase in the expression of IL-15 mRNA, a cytokine with anti-inflammatory, anabolic and anti-catabolic properties, in the groups treated with CLA/ω3 and especially in that combined with weight training.

In a human study, CLA was administered for 6 weeks during an endurance training program and there was no effect on the stationary bike endurance capacity, in the number of sit-ups performed or in long jump from standing.

Another study, on the other hand, investigated the effect of supplementing with CLA on endurance training, but above all on the possible anti-fatigue effect, directly on male athletes, for a period of 14 days. The results, even if the study was performed on a small number of subjects (10 male students), showed a significant increase in the exercise duration, while the rate of the perceived exertion tended to decrease, indicating the possibility of reducing the exercise-induced fatigue.

Ultimately, there are various studies on the ability of CLA to increase the metabolic rate; some of these correlate the increase in the calorie expenditure to the increased amount of muscle mass that occurs when the consumed calories are increased (re-nutrition after diet) and at the same time a CLA supplement is taken.

Oral supplementation with t10c12 has been shown to acutely induce an insulin resistance in obese men, probably due to an increase in lipid peroxidation with a relative increase in circulating free fatty acids that are capable of worsening insulin sensitivity (a form of oxidative stress) in conjunction with a mean weight reduction of 1.5 kg compared to the placebo. In particular, the ability of t10c12 to induce the lipid peroxidation, assessed by urinary measurement of 8-iso-PGF2α, is much greater than that of c9t11: increases of up to 578% compared to baseline levels were observed with t10c12 alone, while a 25% increase occurred with the same amount of c9t11.

Both isomers, however, seem to have positive effects on antioxidant enzymes, by acting as modulators of the expression of a transcription factor, NF-κB (although for now only *in vitro*): this modulation also gives the combination of isomers an anti-inflammatory effect. In conclusion: while the studies on animals are positive, the results in humans are still controversial.

Probably the concentration of CLA used in animal studies could also be a limitation. In animal tests, in fact, particularly in those involving the intake of foods enriched with the c9t11 isomer (rumenic acid), the concentrations were high, which is a determining factor. To date, intervention studies on the human diet are still scarce.

Dosages

The effective dose is about 3 to 5 g of CLA per day. The studies were carried out on both adults and children. The supplementation was well tolerated, and the effects varied: some subjects lost fat and not weight (so they showed a simultaneous increase in muscle mass), others lost both weight and body fat. Studies generally range from 4 to 16 weeks of supplementation up to a few months, and often without an adequate dietary control for weight loss. Positive results were also obtained in obese and diabetic women, in postmenopausal women, in overweight subjects and in those that suffer from the metabolic syndrome, where the supplement was about 4 g of CLA. Other studies would prove the poor efficacy of this supplement in determining a slimming effect; in this regard, it is important to consider the existence of genetic or individual variables that can cause different effects for different subjects at the same dose. For example, for highly overweight subjects, the best results are obtained with quantities of 6.4 g per day.

Effectiveness

Strength	Resistant strength	Mass	Endurance	Slimming	Concentration	Recovery
−	+	++	−	+++	−	−

CORDYCEPS SINENSIS

Description

Cordyceps sinensis is a native mushroom of China, widespread on the Tibetan highlands, used regularly in traditional Chinese medicine. Numerous properties are attributed to this mushroom that amplifies the functionality of the body and the athletic performance. Its media peak came during the Beijing National Games in 1993, when numerous swimming records were broken.

The athletes subjected to doping control were all negative and the federal leaders gave the credit for these results to nutrition and supplementation based on medical herbs, including *Cordyceps*.

From a chemical point of view, this mushroom is composed of about 60% of unsaturated (oleic and linoleic acid) and saturated (palmitic acid) fatty acids, 30% of proteins and 10% of minerals, vitamins and polysaccharides.

Properties

The most important compounds of *Cordyceps* are cordycepin, cordycepic acid and numerous bioactive molecules, such as nucleosides (adenosine, guanosine and uracil) and phytosterols, including ergosterol, a precursor of vitamin D2. As micronutrients, zinc, magnesium and manganese are very abundant, very important for the development and the homeostasis of steroid hormones and gonads. The effects of *Cordyceps* on the body are manifold; for example, it was found that they have immunomodulatory, antihypertensive, hepatoprotective, hypocholesterolemic and aphrodisiac effects. The most important, which affects sports, is the increase in the oxygenation of various tissues through the relaxation of the bronchial muscles and the increase in the heart flow, with an improved aerobic capacity, VO_{2max} and endurance.

Evidence

Unfortunately, there are very few reliable studies on humans and these results have emerged in studies conducted *in vitro* or on laboratory animals.

A 2011 Indian study investigated the role of *Cordyceps sinensis* in improving the sports performance, endurance and antioxidant effect. In this study, 24 mice were divided into four groups: a control group given a placebo (C), an experimental group given a 200 mg/kg/day *Cordyceps* solution over a period of 15 days (CSS), a group that performed the routine exercise without *Cordyceps* supplementation (E) and a group that exercised regularly given *Cordyceps* (CSS + E). The training protocol consisted of 30 minutes of progressive swimming, up to one hour of training.

The results showed how the supplementation of this mushroom significantly improved performance, increasing the endurance capacity, both in trained and untrained subjects, compared to control group. To fully understand how *Cordyceps* improves the metabolic abilities, the researchers tested the protein expression levels of the main metabolic regulators AMPK, PGC-1 and PPARδ. In the supplemented groups, both trained and untrained, the expression levels of these regulators were significantly higher than in the control.

This shows how *Cordyceps* implements the expression of these metabolic regulators regardless of training. All these parameters show how the improvement of the aerobic capacity (AMPK), fat oxidation (PPARδ) and muscle oxidative capacity (PCG1) are stimulated at the level of gene expression. In fact, the groups supplemented with *Cordyceps* showed a higher gene expression of these proteins, and the striking fact was that this change did not derive from the physical activity, but from the mere ingestion of the fungus.

The synergy of these proteins allows a significant improvement in the oxidative capacity of the fatty acids and therefore a greater increase in metabolic energy (remember how cordycepin has a chemical structure similar to that of the nucleoside adenosine, the structural component of ATP, which increases the production of adenosine triphosphate), with a consequent increase in the resistance to effort and an improvement in endurance.

The activity on lactic acid, the antioxidant activity and the muscle uptake of glucose were also evaluated and the researchers saw that the lactate transporters MCT1 and MCT4, the expression of superoxide dismutase 1 (SOD1) and the expression of GLUT4 glucose transporters were significantly increased in the *Cordyceps*-fed groups. This shows how the components of this fungus, especially some polysaccharides, are able to increase the antioxidant activity of cells in general (SOD1 is expressed in almost all the cells of the body) and improve the ability of the muscles to capture and use glucose as an energy source (increase GLUT4 expression), thus increasing the insulin sensitivity.

A 2014 Italian study investigated the use of *Cordyceps sinensis* as a hormone modulator, and more specifically on the **regulation of testosterone and cortisol levels during a sporting performance** (before and after the competition). It has been known for many decades that the ratio between testosterone and cortisol (T/C) is one of the fundamental markers of the stress induced by physical activity. If this ratio decreases by more than 30% from the baseline value, or the value measured before the sporting activity, then we can say with certainty that we are in an overtraining situation. In this study, the levels (via salivary swabs) of these hormones were measured in seven amateur cyclists, who traveled about 300 km weekly, both in the resting phase and before and after the cycling sessions.

The supplementation protocol involved the combined use of 1335 mg of *Cordyceps sinensis* (standardized extract) and 1170 mg of **Ganoderma lucidum** or **reishi** (a parasitic mushroom with hypocortisolic properties) per day. The results were truly striking.

After three months of supplementation with the mycetal mix, testosterone levels were significantly increased from the baseline, in both the placebo group (0.08 ± 0.02 ng/mL *vs.* 0.052 ± 0.01 ng/mL) and in the experimental group (0.12 ± 0.04 ng/mL *versus* 0.035 ± 0.01 ng/mL), registering a 3.4-fold increase, and these results were evidently related to the training effect.

A similar argument applies to cortisol, except that the increase in the experimental group was significantly lower, thus resulting in a striking increase in the testosterone to cortisol ratio, which is the true indicator of the athlete's hormonal recovery. In this study, the T/C ratio in the placebo group decreased by 69.3%, that is, clearly exceeding the overtraining threshold (−30%), while in the experimental group it decreased by only 8.7 percentage points. This shows how the intake of these two mushrooms significantly helps the athletic performance by delaying the sense of fatigue and therefore improving the endurance and the sports performance.

A 2019 study by Liao et al., published in *Nutrients*, evaluated the effect of *Cordyceps* on the aerobic capacity (VO_{2max}), body composition (fat mass, weight, BMI), blood parameters (including insulin, glucose, cholesterol, triglycerides), oxidative and antioxidant capacity (TBARS and TAC). The subjects of this study (control and experimental) underwent 8 weeks of training on the cycle ergometer with a variation in intensity from 60% (first week) to 75% (eighth week).

The experimental group was administered a mix of *Rhodiola crenulata* and *Cordyceps sinensis* with a dosage of 20 mg/kg of body weight, therefore a range between 1000 and 1800 mg/day, with a ratio of 6: 4 between *Rhodiola* and *Cordyceps*. The mix was taken at breakfast for 5 days in a row, each week for 8 weeks. The results showed that the experimental group achieved significant improvements in all parameters, compared to the control group. The implemented values were the aerobic capacity (VO_{2max} + 4.1 mL/kg/min) and the glycemic control capacity (glucose −6.8 mg/dL and insulin −5.1 µIU/mL), as well as a marked improvement in the fat mass and lean mass (especially in the lower part of the body, since the training was practically performed by the lower body).

As for the antioxidant capacity, normally both Rhodiola and especially Cordyceps improve this capacity, by increasing the capacity and functionality of the main antioxidant systems (SOD, GSH, catalase); no such improvement as noted in this study, as the dosage of the two extracts was probably too low (usually about 1000 mg for both of them).

Dosages

Summarizing, from an ergogenic point of view, *Cordyceps sinensis* increases both the aerobic and antioxidant capacity in trained subjects (both in a state of rest and in conjunction with a sporting performance), bringing out its role as a tonic substance. Dosages vary from 500 mg to 1.5 g/day, although numerous studies have shown that in sports, the best results are obtained with 1500 mg per day.

Effectiveness

Strength	Resistant strength	Mass	Endurance	Slimming	Concentration	Recovery
−	+++	+	++++	+	−	++

CREATINE

Description
Creatine is perhaps the most famous dietary supplement in the field of power sports and bodybuilding and, after protein, it is the supplement that contributes most to the turnover of the food supplement industry. It was discovered by the French chemist Michel Eugène Chevreul, who isolated it from meat broth in 1832 (hence the name, from the Greek *kreas* = meat). Later, it was the German Justus von Liebig who confirmed that creatine was a normal constituent of meat. In particular, the muscle of wild foxes contained a quantity of this molecule ten times higher than that of foxes kept in captivity; he thus came to the conclusion that motor activity tends to increase its muscle concentration. Creatine is both synthesized by the human body and normally ingested with food or, in our case, taken through specific supplements. Of this part, about 94% is localized in the skeletal muscles, where it is stored in both free and phosphorylated form (40% and 60% respectively).

Properties
Endogenous creatine is synthesized by the liver, kidney and pancreas (1 g/day) from arginine, S-Adenosyl-Methionine and glycine (amino acids) and is a fundamental compound of the anaerobic alactacid metabolism. This metabolism has certain characteristics that limit the field of use of this substance. Alactacid anaerobic metabolism is an immediate metabolism (activates very quickly), very powerful (develops a lot of energy), easily exhausted (lasts 6-10 seconds), does not require oxygen (anaerobic) and does not produce lactic acid (alactacid). The average total creatine *pool* (PC + free creatine) of the skeletal muscles is about 120 g for a 70 kg individual. However, muscle tissue has the ability to deposit up to about 160 g of creatine (values related to the surface and body composition of the subject of course).

At a biochemical level, the phosphorylation reaction of ADP into ATP of this metabolism almost completely depends on the amount of PC (phosphocreatine) stored in the mitochondrial membrane and on the concomitance of magnesium (Mg^{++}) as a cofactor. During intense exercise, the PC concentration drops, making the system less available for the resynthesis of ATP, which is needed to continue a high-intensity exercise. Creatine supplementation would intervene at this level by increasing the quantities of high-energy substrates that are ready for use in the muscle cell. As we said in the opening words, creatine is mostly present in meat and, in particular, 900 g of red meat contain about 3 g of creatine (vegetarians, for example, have lower phosphocreatine levels and, if given creatine supplements, their muscles will capture it very well). So, once in the blood, creatine is absorbed by the striated muscle and phosphorylated by the creatine phosphokinase enzyme, so that it remains in the cell as a source of energy. Creatine phosphokinase (intracellular enzyme) can be measured in the blood in its different isoforms and can be considered an index of the tissue damage, and therefore a rise in the serum levels same is common, for example, following intense training. Subsequently, this energy is transferred to create ATP, which is used for muscle contraction, at the end of which almost all the free molecules of creatine and phosphate residing in the muscle come together again to regenerate creatine phosphate, and this process requires oxygen to pay the debt incurred during the exercise in anaerobiosis. During the recovery part, the free creatine is rephosphorylated in 60 seconds; another part is regenerated during a five-minute rest period, and the remaining small amount is metabolized by the muscles as creatinine. The body breaks down approximately 1-2% of the total creatine *pool* into creatinine daily, which will then be eliminated from the blood in the urine.

Evidence

During maximal exertion, our muscles have enough ATP for only a few seconds of high-intensity workouts and consequently the creatine phosphate (PC) system is activated, which allows the cell to immediately resynthesize more ATP. This metabolism will therefore intervene in high intensity and short duration sports, and it will be these that will benefit most from a creatine-based supplementation. The effects of supplementing with creatine are direct and indirect. It directly favors a **greater availability of phosphates for the resynthesis of ATP** through PC and therefore it helps produce more energy (increases in power), prolong its use a few more seconds (increases in resistance) and speed up the recovery times (less lactate accumulation). This molecule also acts as a buffer for the intracellular acidity that is formed during the exercise; in a 2014 study by Jonathan Oliver et al. of the Christian University of Texas (USA), 20 g of creatine per day, divided into four doses, delayed the lactate threshold during an incremental test on a cycle ergometer, demonstrating that creatine can also improve the performance in endurance sports. The indirect effect of creatine occurs through **a greater accumulation of glycogen** in the muscle, which attracts water; this effect is sought above all in bodybuilding and fitness due to the phenomenon of volumization of the muscle mass. Many studies in the literature have evaluated the effects of creatine supplementation on muscle physiology and exercise capacity in healthy, trained but also pathological subjects. Short periods of taking this supplement increase the organic pool of creatine by 10-30% and phosphocreatine by 10-40%. Many studies have evaluated the potential ergogenic effect of creatine. Approximately 70% reported an **increase in maximal power and strength (5-15%)**, in the work performed in sets of maximal muscle contractions (5-15%), in single sprint performance (1-5%) and in repeated sprints (from 5-15%). In addition, creatine supplementation during training has been seen to promote **significant gains in lean mass**. This property is partly linked to its ability to support workouts with higher loads and shorter breaks. In addition, every athlete knows that one of their main enemies is muscle catabolism, even induced by a restrictive diet and overtraining. There are also studies that evaluate the supplementation of creatine monohydrate and carbohydrates versus only carbohydrates, regarding the secretion of cortisol. Combining carbohydrate with creatine appears to significantly reduce post-workout cortisol in power swimmers. Cortisol is a hormone that cannibalizes the lean mass, so its management is essential in the body's economy, especially for the athletes. Another hormone modulating effect of creatine is its ability to increase the levels of DHT (dehydrotestosterone), which is the most biologically active form of testosterone. In a South African study of veteran rugby players, creatine supplementation (20g per day for seven days) increased DHT by 57% and remained elevated 40% above baseline during the maintenance phase (5 g per day). These results would go in the same direction as other studies on muscle atrophy and sarcopenia in the elderly, in which a creatine supplementation, even at low doses, would slow down the loss of lean mass.

Furthermore, creatine stimulates the increase of muscle mass by activating various cellular mechanisms, including myogenesis, that is, the formation of new muscle cells, and the increase in the synthesis of myosin, a muscle protein.

Creatine and the female universe

The creatine/phosphocreatine/creatine kinase circuit is essential for maintaining an ATP turnover in those tissues which, given their function, require high energy to meet organic needs (heart, muscles, brain).

Table 44.3 The energy expenditure of different tissues/organs

Organ or tissue	Metabolic rate (Kcal/kg/day)	% Total metabolism at rest	Weight (kg)	% of total body weight
Adipose tissue	4.5	4	15	21.4
Others (bone tissue, skin, intestines, glands)	12	16	23.2	33.1
Muscles	13	22	28	40.0
Liver	200	21	1.8	2.6
Brain	240	22	1.4	2.0
Heart	400	9	0.3	0.5
Kidneys	400	8	0.3	0.5

From: Aragon et al. *Journal of the International Society of Sports Nutrition* (2017) 14:16.

The main role in the human being is to bridge the muscle catabolism through its strong osmotic capabilities which allow, through hydration, an anti-catabolic effect that promotes the protein synthesis. In 2015, Ellery et al. described the effects of creatine according to the different phases of the menstrual cycle. The collapse of progesterone levels during the menstrual phase of the cycle, leads to a degeneration of the extracellular matrix with a consequent loss of enzymes. Under these conditions, the extracellular levels of creatine kinase (CK) are decidedly higher than those analyzed during the other phases of the menstrual cycle, assuming a decrease in performance due to the lower synthesis of phosphocreatine, which occurs exclusively in the mitochondrial compartment.

Women, in addition to having 30% less muscle mass than men, they consume a much smaller amount of meat, the food that has a high content of creatine. If we reasoned with homeostatic logic, creatine in women should have a decidedly positive ergogenic effect, given the low intracellular reserves.

However, a lower amount of IGF-1 and T3 (triiodiothyronine) present in women does not allow for optimal upregulation of the sodium channels, which are responsible for creatine uptake (SLC6A8), thus flattening the effects of the tripeptide.

An important role of creatine in favor of women is observed during the delicate period of pregnancy, in which, although the muscle tissue of the woman contains less creatine than men, the placenta, throughout pregnancy, through the production of estrogen and progesterone, increases intracellular levels of CK in order to improve the energy production for the fetal well-being.

Furthermore, during the pregnancy, the fetus is unable to synthesize the creatine necessary for its own development by itself, and it is precisely here that a supplement of 3 g per day can help the fetal development by saving choline and maintaining an important mediation of DNA, which has always been indispensable for a safe intrauterine development.

Since, as seen above, it is precisely estrogen that stimulates the synthesis of creatine, its supplementation could be very useful for women with low levels of estrogen and DHEA and, in general, during the last phase of the menstrual cycle, especially if special sports performances are required.

In a study conducted by Sremi et al. and published in 2009 in *Molecular and Cellular Endocrinology*, creatine was shown to cause a **decrease in myostatin levels** in muscle cells, leading to a significant increase in muscle growth. The double-blind study involved 27 young males divided into two groups. One group trained with weights and took creatine (0.3 g/kg of body weight per day, for a week, then 0.05 g for the rest of the study, which lasted eight weeks), while the other group just trained with weights. At the end of the study, both groups showed a significant drop in myostatin levels, but the creatine group had a markedly greater decrease, associated with greater gains in strength and muscle mass. It should be noted that the most consistent drop in myostatin occurred in the fourth week, in agreement with a previous study by Volek et al., which had shown that creatine supplementation caused the greatest hypertrophic stimulus at the fourth week of intake. In a 2014 study by Mobley, Fox et al. it has been shown that the combination of creatine and leucine is able to inhibit the negative effect of myostatin on the muscle growth. Myostatin is able to block the muscle growth by blocking the formation of new muscle fibers and by inhibiting the mTOR pathway that activates the protein synthesis. In another 2014 study conducted by researchers from the University of Sao Paulo (Brazil), it was found that by administering 20 g of creatine per day, for 11 days, there was no decrease in strength following an endurance exercise (5 km running on the treadmill), thus demonstrating that creatine helps maintain strength in training programs that include both weights and aerobics. In a recent 2015 study by Brazilian researchers, they found that creatine monohydrate supplementation (20 g for five days) decreased oxygen consumption in the initial stages of a one-kilometer cycling race, evidently favoring the use of creatine phosphate and promoting a **saving of the muscle glycogen**. To broaden the range of effects of creatine, a recent study conducted by Stefano di Biase (2019) outlined the importance of creatine on the immune surveillance by CD8 + type T lymphocytes.

CD8 T lymphocytes are killer cells against pathogens that generate a response only after binding to the cell that possesses a receptor containing a class I histocompatibility factor, called MHC-I.

The study showed how, in the event of inflammation, immune cells up-regulate creatine transporters to support a much more efficient defense.

The ability of this supplement to allow a rapid regeneration of ATP allows the lymphocyte receptor not only to better recognize the threat, but also to activate a signaling strong enough to counter it. This protective effect of creatine can be used to speed up the recovery during a bout of flu, during a particularly intense training period or during the change of seasons, when the immune defenses are particularly low.

A creatine supplement can also be considered in the event of exposure to endocrine disruptors or environmental pollutants capable of altering the structure of the mRNA. In outdoor training conditions, especially if you are in a particularly polluted city, the intake of creatine can be very useful in order to maintain an adequate protein synthesis, thanks to the protection exercised by the mRNA, without which we could not synthesize proteins. In correlation with its effect on mRNA, we find the association with beta-alanine, advantageous for its ability to act as a foundation for the synthesis of purine nucleic acids.

Since creatine reserves are rapidly depleted in all conditions in which high oxidative stress is present, its use should be evaluated in all cases where cellular redox functionality could compromise the muscular (cardiac and skeletal) health, nervous (neurons, oligodendrocytes) and immune (macrophages, lymphocytes) systems, both in physiological conditions and especially in diseases such as Parkinson's, Alzheimer's, fibromyalgia, heart failure and spinocerebellar ataxia.

Its ability to improve the production of ATP allows a bioenergetic advantage that can speed up the mitochondrial function and indirectly limit the cytoplasmic accumulation of H^+.

In fact, the refosphorylation of ADP into ATP requires the flow of H^+ ions into the mitochondrion, with a consequent rebalancing of the cell's pH.

Brazilian researchers, in a study on mice, found that creatine supplementation reduced the catabolic effects of corticosteroids. They injected the corticosteroid dexamethasone to mimic a catabolic overload, which causes muscle wasting and decreases the motor skills. Creatine reduced the destructive effects of dexamethasone by limiting the decrease in muscle mass and in the physical capacity. Creatine supplements may reduce the catabolism that is normally triggered by corticosteroids. Therefore, it would be a good idea to take creatine during a steroid therapy.

Since creatine is particularly prone to conversion to creatinine, we tried to create forms that would minimize its conversion. The following are all forms of creatine that are intended to increase its bioavailability. However, the studies by Mc Call (2008) and Cannon (1927) show that, at a pH equal to 1-2, the conversion of creatine into creatinine is about 2%, a value that is not significant to leave out the supplementation of creatine monohydrate.

New forms of creatine, other than creatine monohydrate, which appeared from the beginning, have been continuously introduced to the market, which are credited with the best physical and chemical properties, bioavailability, efficacy and/or safety:

- effervescent creatine: creatine monohydrate is combined with potassium bicarbonate and citric acid. This solution neutralizes the gastric acidity, promoting a better absorption;
- microionized creatine: being made up of particles with a diameter of less than about 20 times of that of creatine, it is more soluble and more easily absorbed;
- creatine taurinate: represents a basic creatine salt which, by increasing the pH in the stomach, promotes its solubility and absorption;
- creatine malate: malic acid associated with creatine should activate the production of energy on the muscle level;
- alkaline creatine: also known as Kre-Alkalin, is alkalized and therefore has a higher pH. With a higher pH, the creatine molecule is more stable, less converted into creatinine and more easily absorbed;
- creatine ethyl-ester: it is a more advanced form of creatine monohydrate, which, with the addition of ester salts, becomes more absorbable by the cells;
- creatine decanoate: it is a rapidly absorbed form of creatine, but, as it contains only 50% of creatine, double dosages are required;
- creatine gluconate: is a creatine molecule linked to a glucose molecule. Glucose acts as a transport molecule by elevating the absorption capacity in the muscles;
- chelated magnesium creatine: it is transported using a different channel and combines the benefits of creatine supplementation with those of magnesium supplementation, promoting a higher hydration in the muscles;
- creatine HCL: creatine hydrochloride is more soluble and this should improve the absorption and any possible swelling;
- PEG-creatine: glycosylated polyethylene creatine is a form in which creatine is combined with a glucosidic chain; this makes it more stable and more absorbable, allowing for lower dosages.

Despite this, currently, there is no significant evidence that any of these new forms of creatine are more effective or healthier than creatine monohydrate, therefore, given the higher cost, the choice must be conditioned by evaluations on the subjective tolerability. As for the safety of its use, currently, the vast majority of studies do not show any deleterious effects on healthy subjects, but given the overwhelming number of unrecognized kidney diseases, it would be advisable to evaluate the renal function before starting the intake.

A further way to maximize its assimilation is through the concomitant ingestion of glucose. Although the mechanisms are still under investigation, the ability of glucose to decrease creatine clearance has been documented by Pittas et al. (2010). The stimulation of insulin secretion and the slowing of gastric emptying resulting from the intake of glucose allow a higher muscle retention of creatine, resulting in a higher bioavailability. Furthermore, as for muscle sodium transporters, the effect of insulin on the externalization of neuronal creatine transporters should not be overlooked, in which it is observed an increase in cerebral creatine from 5% to 15% of the baseline, with supplementation (cell swelling).

Dosages

The recruitment protocols are different in the literature and mostly related to the use of creatine monohydrate. There are many other formulations on the market that boast various qualities, such as a better intestinal absorption (diarrhea is a known problem in those who exceed recommended doses) or a better uptake in striated muscle cells. However, the literature regarding these new products is very scarce for now. The most famous scheme of taking the monohydrate form is that of loading and maintenance: loading of 0.3 g/kg/day or of 20 g/day for five to seven days, followed by the maintenance of 3-5 g/day. The same results over a longer period of time are obtained with the no-load protocol: a constant intake of 3-5 g/day. Another mode of intake in the literature is the cyclic loading protocol: load of 0.3 g/kg/day or of 20 g/day for 5-7 days, followed by maintenance of 3-5 g/day, and a new loading phase every 3-4 weeks.

As for the timing of the intake, creatine can be used both before and after the training, even if the window obtained in the post-workout seems to be the best for the muscle uptake. To verify this, in a 2014 study by Antonio and Ciccone, 19 healthy, male bodybuilders, with an average age of 23, who had been training regularly for at least a year, were randomly divided into two groups: a group was taking 5 g of creatine right before the training and the other group was taking it right after. The subjects exercised five days a week for four weeks, following a split bodybuilding routine and also taking creatine on rest days. The results, although not "robust" from a statistical point of view, demonstrated **a greater effect in strength and muscle growth by taking creatine after the training**. In a more recent 2015 study by Candow et al., carried out on healthy elderly adults, 8 g of creatine or a placebo were administered before or after a weight training. The results showed a greater increase in muscle mass in the group that had taken creatine after the training and, on the other hand, the strength gains did not show significant differences in the groups that had taken creatine before or after the training.

This effect could be due to the higher concentration of intramuscular creatine that occurs with the intake of creatine after training, which by increasing hydration at the cellular level, stimulates the protein synthesis and reduces the catabolism of muscle proteins, which is induced by weight training and lasts for a few hours after the training. Furthermore, the depletion of energy substrates linked to an anaerobic alactacid metabolism during resistance training would create an excellent substrate for the supercompensation of inorganic phosphates. In particular, the usual post-workout carbohydrate intake in conjunction with creatine, increases its absorption in the muscles (true limiting stage of the cycle).

Therefore, the concomitant secretion of insulin is fundamental, which must push this supplement into the muscles, but whose work must be short-lived to have a maximum anabolic effect. Too generous or multiple repeated doses of simple carbohydrates, in combination with creatine, tend to limit its ergogenic effect. Creatine, carbohydrate and protein formulas with lower carbohydrates, have been shown to be just as effective as creatine and carbohydrate-only ones. This approach would maintain a high cellular uptake of creatine, without increasing the blood glucose excessively.

Effectiveness

Strength	Resistant strength	Mass	Endurance	Slimming	Concentration	Recovery
+++	++++	++++	+++	++	++	+++

CYCLODEXTRINS

Description
Cyclodextrins, as can be understood from the name, are carbohydrates in which the glucose monomers are arranged to form non-linear, closed cyclical structures. They are obtained from corn starch amylopectin, through a reaction catalyzed by the enzyme called cyclodextrin glycosyltransferase.

Thanks to their particular structure, cyclodextrins are used as a chemical tool to convey active ingredients, improving their solubility, absorption and bioavailability.

Some characteristics of cyclodextrins:

- high molecular weight (150,000 Da);
- excellent water solubility;
- low osmolarity, which translates into a reduction in gastrointestinal side effects;
- good resistance to oxidative phenomena;
- they are thermally stable;
- do not absorb humidity (non-hygroscopic): storage stability;
- they are completely and rapidly broken down into glucose in the intestine;
- very low DE (dextrose equivalence): <10;
- they are not very sweet compared to a high DE maltodextrin.

Properties
Cyclodextrins, being rapidly absorbed and rapidly assimilated carbohydrates, have several advantages, including: rapid stimulation of plasma insulin production, rapid blocking of catabolic mechanisms (gluconeogenesis), an anticortisolemic effect, they are promoters of glycogenosynthesis, they are a vehicle for amino acids and others molecules taken together with them and, finally, they have a minimal impact on water retention, which is higher for glucose. Furthermore, being high molecular weight molecules, they do not cause intestinal discomfort, as happens with other carbohydrates.

Evidence
In the mid-1990s, the process for obtaining highly branched cyclodextrins (HBCD) was patented and the product was given the name of Cluster Dextrin®.

Structurally, Cluster Dextrin® carbohydrate is characterized by a high molecular weight, but also a tighter molecular weight distribution curve. This means that the finished product contains almost all cyclic dextrin molecules characterized by the same weight, and is therefore homogeneous. This is the consequence of the high specificity of the branching enzyme from which it is produced.

High solubility
The Cluster Dextrin® solution, compared to solutions containing maltodextrins of various DEs, is remarkably clear and this reflects the high solubility that characterizes highly branched cyclodextrins, thanks to their molecular structure and also to the homogeneity discussed above.

Rapid gastric emptying
What makes the preference for one carbohydrate over another, a fundamental factor in sports, is the gastric emptying time that characterizes it. Cluster Dextrin® has a rapid gastric emptying time (GET), so it can be an ideal solution to use during the workout.

This product can be used to maintain muscle hydration even during intense and prolonged weight training, which lasts over 60 minutes, as also suggested by the ISSN guidelines.

Comparison: gastric emptying of various solutions
If we add Cluster Dextrin® to an isotonic solution containing amino acids, electrolytes and vitamins, we will have a faster gastric emptying compared to the isotonic solution in which we added the exact, which corresponds to the carbohydrate source in maltodextrin (DE 16).

Rapid degradation into glucose in the intestine means no discomfort
Cluster Dextrin® has a very low degree of discomfort during the training/competition, almost comparable to water. This makes it an excellent candidate for reserving a part of the daily total carbohydrate in the peri-workout, as it is also quickly absorbed.

We note that maltodextrins also have a rapid gastric emptying, and if used alone, they are excellent in the context of peri-workout and post-workout. Due to the lower bioavailability, they are not recommended for intra-workouts.

Resistance
Highly branched cyclodextrins appear to have positive effects on the endurance: in one study (Takii et al., 1999) an interval swimming test was conducted to monitor the endurance and the swimming time up to maximum fatigue. VO_{2max} was the criterion used to measure the resistance. With the intake of Cluster Dextrin®, the swimming time was 1.5 times higher compared to that of the group that had only taken glucose.

Minor fatigue
A dosage of 15 g of cyclodextrin seems to give clear advantages on the sense of fatigue, when compared with an equal dosage of maltodextrin. This is probably due to the fact that the absorption rate and blood bioavailability of cyclodextrins are more effective. In fact, a study (Takashi et al., 2014) related to the subjective perception of the physical effort over time, with the score obtained by a group of subjects who had taken Cluster Dextrin® after 60 minutes of cycle ergometer, reported a perception of less fatigue compared the group that took maltodextrin.

Cyclodextrins and inflammation
Exercise induces a certain degree of inflammation, which depends on various factors, including the type of exercise, intensity, duration and training state of the subject.

This inflammatory response can be quantified based on the degree of production of certain molecules, such as cytokines and stress-related hormones, which is a completely physiological process. However, if the quantity of these substances is excessive, it can become negative, as it worsens the perception of fatigue and even leads, if not adequately balanced by rest, recovery and nourishment, to injuries and, in the long term, to the exhaustion of the antioxidant capacity of the organism. Here, carbohydrates, from this point of view, can make the difference in the health of a body subjected to a considerable sports stress. Cluster Dextrin® appears to attenuate stress-induced hormone production and inflammatory cytokine production following exhaustion exercises. In a study by Suzuki et al., (2014) it was shown how the post-workout intake of a Cluster Dextrin® drink, compared to the intake of another glucose-based drink, after a duathlon (5 km of running + 40 km of biking + 5 km of running) caused a lower production of norepinephrine, as well as inflammatory cytokines.

Increased bioavailability of branched chain amino acids
Another group of molecules that play a key role in the recovery phase after an exercise, are branched chain amino acids (BCAAs). Its use and significance are widely known, but a study has shown that a concomitant intake of highly branched cyclodextrins and BCAAs seems to

improve, in the first 2 hours after the workout, the absorption and bioavailability of the amino acids themselves, compared to glucose association + BCAA. Plasma measurement of leucine was used as the evaluation criterion. It is assumed that this advantage is extended to the whole group of essential amino acids.

As we said at the beginning, cyclodextrins act as molecules that carry other molecules, and the case in question is an excellent example of this. Direct consequences of a greater availability of amino acids are: an anabolic boost, understood as protein synthesis, a turnover and therefore a protein renewal and hypertrophy; the inhibition of the catabolism and muscle nutrition, also favored by the hyperemia that is created during and in the moments that follow the training.

Dosages
The recommended amount for each intake is 30-40g in 500 mL of water. Given the characteristics listed above, cyclodextrins are well suited to be used before, during or after the training, whether it is for resistance or endurance sports.

Effectiveness

Strength	Resistant strength	Mass	Endurance	Slimming	Concentration	Recovery
–	+++	++	+++	–	–	+++

D-ASPARTIC ACID

Description
Aspartic acid is a non-essential amino acid and it is found in two isomers, L-aspartic and D-aspartic (D-Asp).

Properties
It is supposed to improve athletic performance, testosterone levels and even the muscle mass.

Evidence
In a substantial review by Roshanzamir et al. (2017), there were analyzed almost 400 studies up to 2015, and then the number was narrowed down to thirty, including studies on humans and studies on animals: the conclusion is that, on animals, the results are decidedly good, while on our species they are rather inconsistent and we hope for a greater number of trials (conducted, possibly, with all the trappings of the case).

Some studies have investigated its potential in subjects who practiced training with weights: Melville et al., in 2015, even found a decrease in testosterone in subjects who took 6 g of D-Asp, compared to the placebo group or to the 3 g dosage of D-Asp, precisely after 2 weeks of weight training. More recently, the same group wanted to re-test 6g vs. placebo, but for 3 months, without noting any difference. Willoughby et al. (2018) did not get any feedback after 28 days of weight training and using 3g of D-Asp *vs.* placebo.

However, a group of Italian scholars led by D'Aniello was able to verify excellent results on mouse models, in 1996, while in 2009, this time with Topo as first author, significant improvements were found on the release of LH and testosterone both in men and mice.

Based on these findings, even the prestigious ISSN (Institute of Scientific Sports Nutrition) does not recommend its use.

Dosages
The dosages used in the studies, as seen, range from 3 to 6 g.

Effectiveness

Strength	Resistant strength	Mass	Endurance	Slimming	Concentration	Recovery
–	–	–	–	–	–	–

DHEA (DEHYDROEPIANDROSTERONE)

Description
DHEA and its sulfur derivative, DHEA-S, are the most abundant steroid hormones in our body, but their functions have been less studied than those of cortisol and many consider them primarily as precursors of estrogen and testosterone.

DHEA is produced in the reticular area of the adrenal cortex, but also to a small extent in the gonads and in the brain.

The amount of DHEA present in the body is correlated to the age of the individual: the production of the hormone increases until the age of 25, and then decreases, in parallel with the production of GH, until it reaches a reduction of the synthesis by 80-90%, at the age of 65. The decline of DHEA coincides with the onset of various degenerative pathologies associated with aging.

At the moment DHEA is mostly used in the field of anti-aging medicine and rarely, it is associated with corticosteroid therapies to counteract its catabolic effect.

The WADA (World Anti-Doping Agency) has banned the use of DHEA.

Properties
DHEA is involved in numerous biological functions, which are summarized below:

- decreases cholesterol;
- decreases the formation of fat deposits;
- prevents the formation of blood clots;
- increases bone growth;
- promotes the weight loss;
- increases the brain function, improves the memory and reduces the learning deficit;
- increases the lean body mass;
- increases the sense of well-being;
- helps manage stress;
- supports the immune system;
- helps the body to repair and preserve its tissues;
- decreases allergic reactions;
- decreases triglycerides;
- reduces the risk of cardiovascular disease, osteoporosis and diabetes;
- it is useful in the treatment of Alzheimer's disease, lupus, HIV infection and Epstein-Barr infection, and chronic fatigue syndrome (CFS), whose pathophysiologies are linked to the chronic inflammation;
- improves the GH → IGF-1 axis;
- improves the insulin sensitivity (in diabetic patients it decreases the necessary insulin dosages).

These physiological functions of DHEA are fundamentally highlighted in subjects who, due to pathological problems or related to aging, have low levels of DHEA; currently there is no particular scientific evidence that DHEA administration as a supplement can improve healthy normal subjects.

Evidence

In a double-blind study involving 71 women and 13 men, aged 40 to 70 years, the experimental group was given 50 mg/day of DHEA for 3 months and the control group took a placebo. Within two weeks, the authors of the study found that in subjects who had taken the hormone, the levels of DHEA and DHEA-S were typical of a young subject and that these levels were maintained during all 3 months of treatment. 84% of women and 67% of men reported experiencing a feeling of both physical and mental well-being, of having a better quality of sleep, increased energy levels, better ability to manage stress and an increased sense of relaxation. The researchers also found a significant increase in IGF-1 unrelated to changes in GH levels, probably due to a greater hepatic synthesis, or an increase in the number of GH receptors.

The effects of DHEA on the immune system have emerged in some studies performed on adult rats, in which the administration of DHEA produced a reduction in the activity of monoamine oxidase (MAO), which are the enzymes responsible for the metabolization of catecholamines released in the synaptic space and which, in the treatment of depression, are inhibited with specific drugs, in order to increase the levels of neurotransmitters that promote a good mood. They also cause a decrease in the peroxidation and lipofuxin levels in the brain, all characteristics that are accentuated during aging and in depression.

Some studies show that a supplementation with DHEA may, in fact, help prevent prostate cancer and prostatic hypertrophy, and separate studies at Johns Hopkins University in Baltimore and Humbuldt University Medical School in Berlin, have found significantly lower DHEA levels in prostate cancer patients.

In a study by Gravisse et al. (2018) published in *Int J Sports Med* ("Short-term dehydroepiandrosterone intake and supramaximal exercise in young recreationally-trained women"), 11 young volunteers completed four run-based anaerobic sprint tests, shortly before and after taking an oral placebo treatment or DHEA (100 mg/day for 28 days), following a double-blind, randomized protocol. Their body composition was assessed with the bioelectrical impedance. At rest and after the passive recovery, blood samples were collected for the measurement of lactate, and saliva samples for the analysis of DHEA, testosterone and cortisol.

There were no significant differences in the body composition or in the performance parameters after DHEA administration, despite the trend towards an increased peak power and a decreased fat mass. Further studies are needed to determine whether a higher daily dose would produce an ergogenic effect during anaerobic exercises.

The most amazing results were obtained by investigating the combination of obesity and low levels of DHEA.

In a 1988 study, in which high doses of DHEA (1600 mg/day) were given for 4 weeks, body fat decreased by 31% in four out of five subjects, resulting in a noticeable increase in muscle mass. Some researchers believe that the anti-obesity effect of DHEA is due to its ability to block a specific enzyme called glucose-6-phosphate dehydrogenase (G6PD), which inhibits the storage and formation of fat in the body. Furthermore, DHEA acts at the level of mitochondrial respiration by increasing the thyroid function and by favoring the energy expenditure, rather than the accumulation.

Another mechanism by which DHEA can act against the increase of fat is through its antiglucocorticoid effect (Wright, 1992). By contrasting cortisol (for this reason DHEA also has a remarkable anti-stress effect), it blocks the activity of tyrosine aminotransferase and ornithine decarboxylase enzymes, promoting fat loss. A recent study, on the other hand, would indicate that one of the mechanisms by which DHEA promotes fat loss could be the increase of serotonin in the hypothalamus region, increasing the release of cholecystokinin (CCK), the satiety hormone. Consequently, the lower food intake promotes the loss of body fat.

To conclude, we can therefore think that the beneficial effects of DHEA derive from its antioxidant, antilipogenic and antilipoperoxidative activities, with a consequent antiaging action.

There can be several causes of DHEA deficiency in an individual, such as:

- menopause;
- a decrease in its production;
- stress;
- aging;
- smoking (nicotine inhibits the production of 11-beta-hydroxylase, which is necessary for the production of DHEA).

The daily variations of DHEA are affected in part by the pulsatile rhythm of ACTH and they are more responsive to acute stress situations, compared to the chronic type. The production of DHEA in the adrenal gland appears to be controlled above all by the enzymatic activity of the stimulating CYP-17 and by the inhibitory 3B-HSD2. Some studies have shown an inhibiting action caused by hyperglycemia and hyperinsulinemia. Inflammation, through the production of cytokines (IL-4 and others), also seems to have an inhibiting effect on the production of DHEA, while it increases the production of cortisol.

DHEA's action at the tissue level is mainly in contrast to that of cortisol, improving the insulin sensitivity, positively modulating the immune response by attenuating rather than inhibiting the inflammation, improving the endothelial function and the bone metabolism, protecting the brain structure and exerting a positive effect on the adrenal function. With this in mind, it is advisable to measure DHEA, in addition to cortisol, to evaluate the functionality of the HPA axis and the anabolic/catabolic state of the subject, since, in addition to the specific values of these two hormones, the cortisol/DHEA ratio is very important. If it is unbalanced in favor of cortisol, it favors its negative effect on the tissue level, with a consequent poor adaptation to stress.

This marker can be useful for the evaluation of HPA axis dysfunctions and laboratories often calculate it differently, by reporting it in a single sample at a fixed time (for example in the morning), between the sums of all four cortisol withdrawals and the DHEA value in one sample or their averages, or again by calculating the DHEA/cortisol ratio. Furthermore, although it is known that the cortisol/DHEA ratio increases with age, the reference ranges of the laboratories are normally not parameterized to age. The concentration of DHEA in the central nervous system is six to eight times higher than in the serum, and most of it is believed to be synthesized directly in the brain, rather than the adrenal glands, and this is also because DHEA-S (which is a larger polar molecule), unlike DHEA, is unable to pass the blood brain barrier. For this reason, DHEA has also been defined as a neurosteroid which can have a wide variability of neurobiological and neuropsychiatric effects.

The **fields of use** of DHEA supplementation are:

- increasing the muscle strength and lean mass;
- activating the immune function;
- improving the quality of life;
- improving sleep;
- increasing the feeling of well-being;
- increasing the insulin sensitivity;

- decreasing triglycerides;
- blocking the harmful effects of stress;
- raising growth hormone levels.

Just like its deficiency, the excess also causes some **side effects**, such as:
- fatigue;
- anger;
- depression;
- lowering of the timbre of the voice (in women);
- insomnia;
- weight gain;
- growth of facial hair (especially in women);
- acne (especially in women);
- craving for carbohydrates ("carb-craving");
- restless sleep;
- irritability.

A great deal of caution must be applied when administering DHEA to subjects affected by hormone-sensitive tumors such as:
- breast cancer;
- uterine cancer;
- ovarian cancer;
- prostate cancer.

Dosages

Women are more sensitive to the effects of DHEA and require lower dosages than those given to men. Antiaging dosages range from 25 to 100 mg in men and from 5 to 25 mg in women. It is always better to start with a lower dosage and then increase it progressively.

In light of the above, supplementation of DHEA – since it is a hormone involved in numerous metabolisms which, during the aging process, fail, thus favoring the development of degenerative diseases – must be promoted to a greater extent. In conclusion, as Dr. Samuel Yen, an endocrinologist responsible for a major study on DHEA that was performed at the University of California at San Diego, says, "DHEA would help people age more kindly."

Effectiveness

Strength	Resistant strength	Mass	Endurance	Slimming	Concentration	Recovery
++	+	++	+	++	++	++

DMAA

Description

Dimethylamylamine (DMAA, also known by other names) is a chemical substance with amphetamine-like effects, synthesized in the 1940s by a pharmaceutical company and used as a vasoconstrictor. Some products for sale show a plant extract that would be obtained from the oil of a type of geranium (*Pelargonium graveolens*): many researchers dispute this natural derivation (unlike a pool of Chinese scholars...) and in any case, its chemical synthesis is more common.

Properties
DMAA was recommended as a pre-workout in the 2000s instead of ephedrine, due to its stimulating effects, and is also used to lose weight and to increase sports performance. In rare cases, it has also been also used for the treatment of attention deficit hyperactivity disorder (ADHD).

Evidence
It should be noted immediately that in recent years, the substance has been banned in various countries around the world. In the US, in 2012, the FDA ordered its withdrawal, although some companies continue to include it in their products and the army has imposed its removal from military bases outlets, following the death of some soldiers who had used it.

It is also prohibited in the European Community and is considered doping by sports federations.

In fact, it was the numerous cases of cerebral haemorrhages, deaths or in any case serious illnesses that led to its withdrawal, as we can read especially in Gee's studies, but also in many others: we are talking about atrial fibrillation, myocardial infarction, severe liver injuries and other very serious pathologies.

In reality, the cases described by Gee concern the use of tablets purchased in night clubs, the composition of which is doubtful, to say the least! In these tablets, there would have been who knows what ingredients, as well as a probably excessive amount of DMAA, with the effects that we have partially seen; in fact, from the blood tests carried out in the hospitals, the values of the substance were still quite high after a few hours, signifying its massive ingestion.

However, a very interesting review in Portuguese by Zovico et al., from the Brazilian University of Espirito Santo, comes to our aid, in which the issue is widely examined and it is explained how numerous other studies have instead shown the non-toxicity of DMAA in "normal" dosages: all the studies related to single "severe" acute cases are analyzed, and also the clinical ones, which are more structured, and the authors conclude that there is not enough evidence to determine their danger or safety.

Indeed, even Brown et al. (2013) and Whitehead et al. have published some reviews or direct trials in which it is clearly seen that at a normal dosage (25 mg), the substance does not give particular problems with blood pressure or increased heart rate; others, such as Forrester, have analyzed numerous cases of emergency hospitalizations (which occurred in Texas, specifically), finding minor problems and not directly attributable to DMAA, since they derive from the ingestion of pre-workout preparations consisting of different ingredients.

Dunn, in 2016, while mentioning some cases of intoxication (resolved, however, with the cessation of use), complained that having banned its marketing, it slowed down the possibility of carrying out research with the correct scientific criteria.

Van Hout et al. (2015) in " 'Plant or poison': a netnographic study of the recreational use of 1,3-dimethylamylamine (DMAA)" (we recall what is written above regarding its extraction from some plants) echo what has just been explained, underlining that precisely the 'use as a recreational drug and the subsequent ban from the market have discouraged further technical insights into its use as a supplement, and remarking that many of the published studies are only "case studies".

Bloomer et al. carried out various in-depth analyzes which (2011a/b and 2018), together with the Brazilian study mentioned above, represent the sum of what is known today about

DMAA: American researchers explain in detail what has been written to date and also report their results, specifying that with 25 mg dosages, the negative effects are nil, while at 50 and 75 mg dosages, there is an exponential increase in the blood pressure and heart rate.

Dosages

The Memphis University scholars, despite having been on the payroll of a company that sold a DMAA-based product at the time, were quite objective: at a dose of 0.5 g/kg, the substance does not give major side effects, but not even great results (which is why it is often used in a mix of other substances). Therefore, its use is probably not justified.

A certainty, on the other hand, is that it must not be abused **at all**.

Effectiveness

Strength	Resistant strength	Mass	Endurance	Slimming	Concentration	Recovery
+	+	−	++	+	+	−

DMAE

Description

DMAE, or dimethylaminoethanol, is known in Europe as deanol, an element that is naturally occurring in the brain in low concentrations and it is also found in salmon, sardines and other similar fish.

DMAE is a precursor to the acetylcholine neurotransmitter, at least according to most studies (Pfeiffer et al., Haubric et al., Millington et al., London et al., Jope et al.), while others go in the opposite direction (Zahniser et al.): However, this substance appears to be involved in the metabolism of choline.

Properties

The link with choline and with the synthesis of acetylcholine, important both in brain functions (memory, focus/concentration, neuroprotection) and in muscle contractions, makes it possible for us to be interested in its optimization. It is also useful at an antioxidant level (cerebral, but also cutaneous).

Evidence

It should be noted immediately that many studies date back to a few decades ago and that, in general, the evidence is not exactly clear.

A review compiled by Dean et al. lists the potential of DMAE, underlining how it produces a mild stimulating effect that occurs over a period of several weeks, an aspect also emphasized by other authors, who highlight the difference compared to other nootropics with a faster effect. A further benefit for people who are no longer young (in which, however, the values of acetylcholine decrease with the passing of the years) is represented by its rejuvenating effect at the dermal level (since it slows down the deterioration of the cell membrane and decreases the excess of arachidonic acid, which can cause wrinkles and skin aging) and by its powerful antioxidant action, as recently highlighted by Malanga et al. (2012).

Actually, the DMAE had some success in the 1960s and 1970s, when it was marketed under the name of Deanol: at a certain point, however, the US FDA changed its pharmacological status and required more studies to continue its sale, and the manufacturer withdrew it from the market because the cost/benefit ratio had become unsustainable.

Acetylcholine and its precursor choline have difficulty in passing the blood brain barrier, while DMAE, thanks to a similar but not the same chemical structure, succeeds better and therefore can express a greater nootropic action, as evidenced by Ceder et al.

Some studies have checked the effectiveness of DMAE through the use of the electroencephalogram, verifying tangible results for the substance in question, but not for choline (Goldstein et al.). Dimpfel et al. also used the electroencephalogram to verify the effect of DMAE, this time in combination with some mood tests: the subjects who had taken the substance detected brain wave values such as to prove a better state of alertness and the volunteers "were clearly more active and felt better"; moreover, the results of the questionnaires were clearly superior, "in full agreement with the laboratory tests".

A very interesting work is that of Coleman et al., who managed to highlight the potential of DMAE in a sample of hyperkinetic young people on whom, at the dose of 500 mg/day, it exerted a balancing effect, to show how the substance really optimizes the brain levels of neurotransmitters at 360 degrees, whether starting from a "normal" state or from a hyperactivity one.

A French study (Caille) also showed (with a rather high dosage, 1200 mg) that patients who had taken DMAE showed "a significant and progressive synchronization of the two hemispheres [...] which was correlated with a better neuromotor control and better results in behavioral tasks" on the electroencephalogram. An investigation by Kapoor et al. in 2009, proved the effectiveness of DMAE with regard to memory, learning and brain function, as well as a study by Oettinger, this time in pediatric subjects: it was found an increase in attention and concentration, without any kind of overexcitation or nervousness; Kugel et al. have also found (again on children) significant increases in the energy values.

Lewis and Young carried out an analysis on minors, who used 500 mg of DMAE or 40 mg of the "usual" Ritalin: both, albeit with different nuances, showed improved reaction times and improved results to a series of psychometric tests in 79 patients. Danysz et al. reaffirm the cholinergic properties of the substance in question and recommend it for "mental and physical efficiency in humans"; in 1974, Re carried out a review in which he listed the positive effects of DMAE on concentration, finding better results than Ritalin on 124 students. Geller also reported positive results on the intellectual functioning and the alertness in 75 young people, with a dosage of only 100 mg/day, as did Pfeiffer (1957), who achieved cognitive improvements in two-thirds of the boys and in three-quarters of the girls he examined (a sample of over 100 subjects).

Pfeiffer himself, in 1959, observed 100 patients and found that DMAE was able to relieve chronic fatigue through its effects "on physical energy and motivation", without creating addiction, unlike some chemical preparations. Pieralisi et al. added ginseng to DMAE and administered the compound to some physical education teachers: both the final result on the treadmill (carried out with progressive increases in resistance) and various biological parameters were better in the treated group, especially in the less trained subjects.

Finally, Ray Shaelian, a nutritionist and an author of books covering the full spectrum of supplements that have sold over a million copies, strongly recommends DMAE; in fact, he has included it in his mix of nootropic substances, also reporting a personal experience, shared by other experts: over 350 mg of the substance can cause muscle tension in the neck and shoulders.

Dosages

DMAE dosages range from 100 to 600 mg, although some studies have used higher amounts; however, also bearing in mind what is written a few lines above, it is still advisable to start from the minimum quantities and, probably, stop at 200 mg: the same Pfeiffer, a true pioneer of DMAE, in an old study (1963, not quoted), noted that the individual response, even in this case, was quite varied.

It should also be remembered that the substance can interact with different categories of drugs, so it is recommended not to take it on your own initiative.

Effectiveness

Strength	Resistant strength	Mass	Endurance	Slimming	Concentration	Recovery
+	+	−	+	+	+++	−

DMG

Description
An intermediate of the metabolism of choline, dimethylglycine (DMG) is a methylating agent, that is a donor of methyl groups (CH_3) and it is precisely to this characteristic, that we owe the most important beneficial effects.

The body produces this molecule in the liver from trimethylglycine (TMG), commonly known as betaine, as it was first isolated in beetroot.

Structurally, DMG consists of a glycine molecule (the simplest of the 20 amino acids) with two methyl groups attached.

DMG is involved in the methylation or transmethylation process, which is the process by which CH_3 are transferred from one molecule to another; a biochemical process essential to the life, health and regeneration of the body's cells.

Vitamins, hormones, neurotransmitters, enzymes, nucleic acids (RNA, DNA) and antibodies require the transfer of methyl groups to complete their resynthesis and perform their function in the body.

A note must be made on the use of DMG and TMG as supplements: since TMG (once absorbed) transforms into DMG in the liver, it performs the same functions as DMG, however some studies suggest the use of TMG over DMG, since TMG has the ability to positively influence the cell osmosis.

Properties
DMG is a nutritional supplement with many positive effects, including stress reduction, improving athletic performance, and increasing the cardiovascular, brain and immune function. It represents an adaptogen, which works with other cofactors in the body to counteract the negative effects of physical, emotional and metabolic stress and to help prevent and overcome degenerative diseases. It is capable of normalizing physiological functions and helping to maintain homeostasis (balance) within the body. These physiological functions include the regulation of blood glucose levels, immune response, blood pressure, hypoxic conditions, hormone and cholesterol levels, as well as the regulation of important biologically active molecules such as SAM-e, glutathione and creatine.

- It supports all aspects of the immune response, acting as an anti-virus, anti-bacterial and anti-fungal agent.
- It improves the cardiovascular functions by supporting normal cholesterol and triglyceride levels, reducing the angina, improving the circulation and decreasing homocysteine levels, if they are high.

- It improves the oxygenation, reducing the fatigue and increases the energy to improve the physical and mental performance.
- It supports the neurological function and the mental clarity, acting as a precursor of the amino acids that are used for the synthesis of neurotransmitters.
- Acts as an antioxidant against free radicals.

Most of these benefits are due to its involvement in the methylation processes, where it supplies methyl groups to other molecules, by regulating the processes of modification, construction, detoxification and recycling of many components of the body.

- DMG also functions as a mineral transporter, chelating agent and cellular communicator.
- It helps the detoxification from toxic substances, as it is involved in phase II of the detoxification process that occurs in the liver.

DMG represents a very important component in the human metabolism and in biochemical terms, it can be considered an intermediary metabolite.

As mentioned above, it owes its most important effects to the ability to transfer one or two methyl groups to other molecules. Through this process of transmethylation, for example, it transforms homocysteine into methionine, thus reducing its plasma levels, the value of which is now considered a valid biomarker on the health of the cardiovascular system. Dr Kilmer Mc Cully, a pathologist, has suggested that a high level of homocysteine in humans is a cause of atherosclerosis and cardiovascular disease.

DMG can therefore play an important role in maintaining homocysteine at normal levels.

DMG acts as a continuous source of methionine, reducing the harmful excess of homocysteine, which causes free radical damage to the arterial walls, while at the same time it increases the level of methionine, which can act as a free radical scavenger. For these reasons, DMG is very advantageous for the recovery of patients who are subject to heart disease and for those who want to reduce the risk of cardiovascular diseases related to aging.

Evidence

DMG is assimilated quickly and very effectively by the digestive tract, but above all by the sublingual route. The sublingual intake of DMG ensures that its absorption is extremely rapid; the effects are frequently evident within 20 minutes of taking the product. All the experiments on DMG have shown that it is rapidly metabolized by the liver, and for this reason the body does not store appreciable quantities of the product.

Dimethylglycine can be considered an important anti-stress food supplement according to J.W. Meduski, Ph. D., of the University of Southern California School of Medicine, who called DMG a "metabolic enhancer".

Although the human body produces DMG from choline and betaine, increasing the dietary intake of this dietary supplement can significantly improve the biological adaptation to physical and mental stress, and it also helps the recovery from degenerative diseases.

According to some studies, DMG reduces the concentration of lactic acid in the blood, in response to surgical stress in animals. In particular, a study in DMG-treated horses reported lower plasma lactate concentrations after a treadmill exercise. However, this study raised doubts about the effectiveness of DMG since the model used was not very objective. Pipes demonstrated that DMG significantly improved the performance in a group of athletes.

The group that was treated with dimethylglycine, compared with a group that was given a placebo, showed a 27.5% increase in VO_{2max} and a 23.6% increase in the time to muscle exhaustion. The ergogenic capacity (increased energy) of DMG may be due to several factors, including the better use of oxygen and an improved cellular respiration, a reduced lactic acid peak and an increase in carbolipid metabolism. In another double-blind study on a small group of top-level athletes, Kleinkopf showed that DMG has positive effects on VO_{2max}.

A study carried out by Lytle in 1978, which partly reproduced a work done in Russia, used the DMG in a group of gymnasts and sprinters and demonstrated its effectiveness in normalizing blood sugar levels during a competition. In a cross-over, double-blind study, athletes that took DMG showed a 30% reduction in blood lactate levels when compared to athletes in the control group.

The results of these tests demonstrate the positive effect of DMG in the biological processes during muscle activity and it seems that this molecule can reduce the tissue hypoxia by increasing the use of oxygen.

DMG can also accelerate the recovery during rest periods following the training.

However, there are other studies that show exactly the opposite; for example, a study by Gray and Larry found no significant changes in maximal short-term treadmill performances between a group treated with pangamic acid (calcium gluconate and DMG) and a placebo. There was no improvement in the aerobic and anaerobic performance when 400 mg of DMG per kg of body weight was administered to elite basketball players.

DMG supplementation failed to improve the exhaustion effort made by well-trained young women on treadmills. The authors of this study concluded that there is no evidence to recommend DMG as an ergogenic supplement for endurance athletes.

DMG is often advertised as an immune stimulant; Although it has no role in the body that could explain a direct effect on the immune system, the results of a Graber study suggest that the supplementation with DMG improves the humoral status, as well as the cell-mediated immune responses in humans.

Further work carried out at Clemson University has shown that DMG improves the production of B and T cells, and that it also stimulates the production of cytokines such as interferon, tumor necrosis factor, and a number of interleukins.

Experimental studies have suggested the possible protective effects of DMG on the glucose metabolism.

DMG is degraded to glycine through a reaction catalyzed by the DMG-dehydrogenase (DMGDH) enzyme.

Low plasma levels of DMG were significantly associated with higher levels of glucose and insulin in the blood, defining a state of increased insulin resistance and therefore an increased incidence of diabetes.

Dr. Roger Kendall, considered one of the leading researchers on the effects of DMG, says it may act as an antioxidant due to its ability to protect the body from radiation. The US Army and Clemson University completed some studies that were published in 2000, in which the authors report that DMG, in a dose-dependent manner, reduces the production of lipid peroxides in a rat model.

Kendall also confirms the work done by other colleagues, in which the ameliorative effects of DMG on the immune system are highlighted; he states that, based on his experience, most people - athletes, students, seniors, men under constant stress or struggling with degenerative conditions - would benefit from taking 250-500 mg of DMG per day, in order to strengthen their own immune defenses.

Dosages

DMG, often sold commercially as a hydrochloride salt (dimethylglycine HCL), is also the active part of pangamic acid (the ester of gluconic acid and dimethyl-glycine, also called vitamin B15), another formulation that can be found on the market. While not showing toxic effects even at high doses, AIFA defines the maximum levels of the daily intake as 200 mg. However, research recommends, depending on the specific problem, a dose of DMG of 125 to 500 mg per day. In case you want to strengthen your immune system, you need to take 250 mg/day.

To rapidly reduce lactic acid levels, it is recommended to take 125 mg of DMG sublingually following manifestations of muscle pain or cramps due to the accumulation of lactic acid.

Repeated high dosages over several days could cause irritability, insomnia, restlessness and cardiac arrhythmias.

Effectiveness

Strength	Resistant strength	Mass	Endurance	Slimming	Concentration	Recovery
+	++	–	++	–	++	++

ECHINACEA

Description
Echinacea is a plant native to North America that belongs to the Composite family. These plants show a remarkable ability to adapt to different environmental conditions, growing both in the plains and at altitudes above 1500 meters. The active ingredients present in the root are ketoalkenes, ketoalkynes and polyacetylene derivatives which derive from caffeic acid, such as the echinacoside.

Properties
The medicinal use of this plant dates back to the native populations of North America, who used it to treat wounds, sores, snake bites, etc. In the modern pharmacopoeia, echinacea is used above all for its ability to boost the immune system, although there are few scientific certainties in this regard. The European Medicine Agency (EMA) has approved the use of *Echinacea purpurea* extracts for the short-term prevention and treatment of colds.

Evidence
The effectiveness of echinacea derives in part from its ability to activate the phagocytic action of lymphocytes, by increasing the number of leukocytes, in particular neutrophils and macrophages of the reticulo-endothelial system, which are responsible for destroying the bacteria. In a review of chemical experiments, it was found that **echinacea is able to decrease the chance of catching a cold by 58% and it also reduces its duration from a minimum of one day to a maximum of four**. In endurance sports, such as the marathon, the appearance of URTIs (upper respiratory tract infections) related to a decrease in immune defenses following long-lasting physical activity is very common. In a double-blind, placebo-controlled study, the effect of a daily oral pre-treatment with a juice obtained from *Echinacea purpurea* was examined in 42 triathlon athletes, before and after a competition.

Another group was treated with magnesium. The interesting aspect is that during the 28-day pre-treatment period, no member of the "echinacea" group became ill, compared to three subjects in the magnesium group and four in the placebo group. Recently, echinacea has been taken into consideration not only to mitigate the immunosuppressive effects of endurance sports, but also to increase performance.

As it has been seen in some animal studies, increasing EPO (erythropoietin) levels is in itself capable of improving exercise capacity without increasing the number of red blood cells – – possibly by increasing the ratio of dopamine to serotonin at the brain level, thus decreasing the central fatigue and increasing motivation during exercise – we wanted to verify whether echinacea could also increase EPO and improve the exercise capacity, without affecting the number of red blood cells. In this study, conducted by Whitcherad et al., 24 young men were divided into two groups: one group received 8000 mg of echinacea per day for 28 days, while the control group received a placebo.

At the end of the experiment, the blood samples showed a **significant increase in EPO** only in the group that had taken echinacea, without showing any increase in the number of red blood cells. In a subsequent study, the same University of Arkansas researchers found that the intake of echinacea associated with the increase in EPO, also induced **an improvement in the endurance performance**. In the latter study, the same amount of echinacea was administered to 24 men, for the same period of time.

At the end of the study, there was a natural increase in EPO, which had produced a considerable improvement in the endurance performance, demonstrated by **an increase in maximum oxygen uptake (VO_{2max})** of approximately 1.5% compared to the control group, who had shown no improvement in the endurance. Taken together, these two studies show that echinacea, as a supplement, is able to significantly increase the production of EPO, which improves the aerobic performance, even without increasing the amount of red blood cells.

Dosages

A spoonful of echinacea roots and a cup of water are needed for the preparation of the echinacea decoction. Pour the chopped root into cold water and bring it to a boil. Boil for a few minutes and turn off the heat. Cover it and leave it to infuse for 10 minutes. Filter the infusion and drink it.

As for the dry extract: 500-750 mg in capsules or tablets administered twice a day between meals, or 400 mg once a day, to prevent flu. For the tincture: 30-40 drops twice a day between meals, or 30 drops once a day for the preventive immunostimulating action. To improve the performance, 8000 mg per day, divided into two doses.

Effectiveness

Strength	Resistant strength	Mass	Endurance	Slimming	Concentration	Recovery
−	+	−	+++	+	+++	+

ELEUTEROCOCCUS

Description

Eleutherococcus (*Eleutherococcus senticosus*), also known as the Siberian ginseng, is a shrub suitable for cold climates, belonging to the *Araliaceae* family. It is native to Siberia and Mongolia, where it generally grows in coniferous forests and rarely extends beyond 2 meters in height. In summer, it produces yellow to purple flowers, to which are added dark and fleshy berries. For therapeutic purposes, it is customary to use its roots (in the form of both drops and tablets), where many substances of various chemical nature are concentrated (including triterpenes, sterols, coumarins, flavonoids, polysaccharides, glycosides, etc.). They are important, as they give the plant the typical adaptogenic and anti-fatigue action, which is able to increase the resistance and defenses of the organism against stress factors, in a non-specific way.

Properties

The main components of the eleutherococcus root are eleutherosides, a heterogeneous group of compounds, among which the most important are the eleutherosides A, B1, B2, D, E, K, L, M. In particular, the eleutherosides of group B are absorbed and metabolized quickly, reaching, according to animal models, the maximum concentration after 75 minutes, with a rapid decline within four hours of administration. 90% of eleuteroside B or its metabolites are excreted in the urine after 48 hours and it is found at a concentration of 3% in the faeces. Eleuteroside B has been found in the pancreas, pituitary gland, liver, kidneys, spleen and endocrine glands (pituitary, thymus and adrenal glands).

The greatest concentration, however, is reached in the adrenal glands, at a level three times higher than in the other organs.

Eleutherococcus is known and traditionally used for its stimulating properties, useful for fighting fatigue, for recovering strength and for optimizing energy, by intervening both at the level of the central nervous system and at the immune system.

Acting as an invigorator on the central nervous system, the extract of eleutherococcus root can be useful for dealing with periods of stress, as it helps to concentrate the energy and make thinking more lucid, and it combats the physical fatigue and the drowsiness.

For these reasons, the eleutherococcus is also used to reinvigorate the sexual sphere, especially when difficulties arise not due to physical problems, but due to a decrease in desire or an increase in worries. In fact, in humans, it can have positive effects in dealing with erectile deficit situations, obviously in the absence of pathologies or other clinical evidence. By intervening on the immune system, it seems that the eleutherococcus stimulates the action of T lymphocytes and Natural Killer (NK) cells; for this reason, it is often associated with convalescence due to winter ailments, such as colds and flu. Currently, in fact, the indications related to the use of this plant mainly concern asthenia and convalescence from infectious diseases, but the Siberian ginseng extract can also be useful as an adjunct to other therapies.

However, the ergogenic action of eleutherococcus should not be overlooked: for a long time, it was considered the plant of the sportsman, both for its general toning and immunostimulating properties. Moreover, thanks to its invigorating peculiarities, it can be useful as a remedy for those athletes suffering from low blood pressure, as long as they are not already undergoing another specific drug treatment.

Evidence

Most of the studies carried out so far on the properties of eleutherococcus confirm its biological activities and today, the best known clinical uses described for this supplement are those related to its adaptogenic activity and to an increase in the physical performance. Eleutherococcus is in fact a phytocomplex capable of intervening on the homeostatic mechanisms that allow the body to adapt to situations of psychological or physical stress, in unfavorable environmental conditions that are usually accompanied by anxious states, which result in a weakening of the immune defenses.

The pharmacological properties of the *Eleutherococcus senticosus* leaf have not been well understood. This plant is considered almost as a drug due to the properties found in its leaves. A study by Yamauchi et al. (2019), analyzed the effects of the extract obtained from *E. senticosus* leaves on the memory function of normal mice. Oral administration of the extract for 17 days significantly improved the object recognition memory and the compounds that were found mainly in the plasma and in the cerebral cortex were ciwujianoside C3, eleuteroside M, ciwujianoside B and ciwujianoside A1.

Thereafter, the pure compounds (except ciwujianoside A1) were re-administered orally for 17 days to normal mice and it was observed that ciwujianoside C3, eleuteroside M and ciwujianoside B had significantly improved the recognition memory of the objects. These results showed that an oral administration of *E. senticosus* leaf extract improves the memory function and that the active ingredients contained in the extract, such as ciwujianoside C3, eleuteroside M and ciwujianoside B, are able to penetrate in the brain and to work within it, by promoting an improvement in memory.

The mechanism of action of the eleutherococcus is still to be clarified, but it seems that it exerts its action on the hypothalamus-pituitary-adrenal glands axis. Winterhoff et al., in 1993, had shown how an aqueous extract of eleutherococcus (containing 0.6% of eleutheroside B and 1% of eleutheroside D), acting on the receptors of many steroid hormones, such as corticosteroids, increased their concentration already 30 minutes after its administration. According to some researchers, by interfering with a feedback mechanism, eleutherococcus can cause a **stimulation of the adrenocortical function** in conditions of moderate hypoadrenocorticalism. It is probable that the invigorating and "anti-fatigue" action of this phytocomplex, which leads to **an increase in the physical performance**, is also due to the effects it has on glucose metabolism: in rats, eleutherosides enhance the effect of insulin by increasing the transport and the availability of glucose within the muscle fiber. Experimentally, an increase in the physical activity and a reduction in the sensation of fatigue have been recorded in animals treated with an aqueous extract of eleutherococcus, thus promoting **a greater resistance to the effort**. In a research carried out in China, male Kunming rats were divided into two groups: the test group, which received distilled water with the supplement at various concentrations (100, 200 and 400 mg/kg), and the control group, which received only distilled water.

After four weeks of treatment, both groups were subjected to a forced swimming test, in which rats were forced to swim in a limited space, with no possibility of escape. The parameters evaluated at the end of the test were: azotemia, glycogen and lactate levels. The results confirmed what was expected, namely that the rats in the test group treated with eleutherococcus had a greater tolerance to exercise, with higher levels of muscle glycogen and lower concentrations of lactate and nitrogen in the blood. In the stress context, in a recent 2014 study conducted on young rats, Wistar shows how the extract of the root of *E. senticosus* works by normalizing the altered expression of c-fos (a proto-oncogene responsible for defects in the specific-tissue development, including osteoporosis, delayed gametogenesis, lymphopenia and behavioral abnormalities) and by modulating the activity of the hypothalamic-pituitary-adrenal axis (HPA), which controls our body's ability to adapt to stress.

Numerous experiments have also had positive results in humans. In a recent double-blind clinical trial, 42 subjects who had practiced amateur cycling for at least three years were treated with the dry extract of eleutherococcus titrated at 0.5% eleutherosides, at a dosage of three capsules per day. Before the start of the treatment and on a monthly basis, an ECG, blood pressure measurement, a complete series of blood chemistry tests and a thorough medical examination were performed. Supplementation with eleutherococcus was significantly effective 120 days after the first intake; if the treatment continued beyond this period, the benefits were even greater. A major randomized, placebo-controlled, double-blind cross-over study involving a dozen departments, centers and institutes across China aimed to examine the effects *of E. senticosus* (ES) supplementation on resistance, on the cardiovascular functions and on the metabolism of untrained males. For eight weeks, some of them received 800 mg/day of ES extract, while others received a placebo (P).

During the test, all subjects cycled at 75% until exhaustion. The physiological variables that were examined included: stamina, maximum heart rate during exercise, VO_{2max} and the assessment of the perceived exertion. Biochemical variables, which included plasma (+ free) fatty acids (FFA) and glucose, were measured at rest, after 15 minutes and after 30 minutes. The main result of this study was: VO_{2max} peak was 12% higher, the endurance time was improved by 23% and there was a 4% increase in the maximum heart rate. This is the first well-conducted study, which shows that eight weeks of ES supplementation **improves the** stamina, the cardiovascular functions and shifts the metabolism towards fat burning, favoring the glycogen savings.

However, in humans, the effect of eleutherococcus is particularly evident in conditions of asthenia that accompany and follow influenza or infectious diseases. In a single-blind, placebo-controlled crossover study in healthy volunteers, they examined the improvement in the physical performance using a bicycle exercise test. The subjects were treated orally for eight days with an ethanolic fluid extract of eleutherococcus (4 mL/day) or with a placebo: treatment with eleutherococcus was better than controls for all the evaluated parameters (oxygen consumption, heart rate frequency, ergometric performance and total time).

However, the eleutherococcus extract does not show the same beneficial effects for professional athletes: a clinical trial in athletes treated with eleutherococcus or a placebo, and subjected to five phases of running at a speed of 10 km/h and a maximum test on the treadmill, in the span of eight weeks, showed no difference in the heart rate (HR), oxygen consumption (VO_{2max}), expiratory volume (EV) and other respiratory parameters between athletes treated with eleutherococcus and those treated with the placebo.

In conclusion, eleutherococcus finds its clinical application in cases of convalescence, asthenia, hypotension, overtraining and in untrained individuals. During asthenic states, eleutherococcus improves the power of concentration, sleep and appetite.

Dosages

Toxicological studies attest to the high tolerability of this phytocomplex. The side effects of the use of eleutherococcus reported in the literature include agitation and/or insomnia, arrhythmia (including tachycardia), extrasystoles and hypertonia. The use of eleutherococcus is not recommended in subjects with severe hypertension and in patients with heart diseases under cardiotonic therapy. Since it produces central stimulation effects, it is recommended to take the product in the morning and/or early afternoon, and not to take the eleutherococcus continuously, but by carrying out periodic cycles interspersed with a temporary suspension of the treatment.

If eleutherococcus is used in the form of a dry extract titrated in eleutheroside (>1%), the recommended dosage is 100-200 mg, three times a day; if used in the form of dried root, it can be taken 2-3 g per day as an herbal tea or decoction, in 150 mL of water, which can be divided into three doses throughout the day.

Effectiveness

Strength	Resistant strength	Mass	Endurance	Slimming	Concentration	Recovery
+	+	−	+++	+	+++	++

EPHEDRINE/MA HUANG/PSEUDOEPHEDRINE

Properties

Ma Huang is the Chinese name of a plant (*Ephedra sinica*) that contains various alkaloids, including ephedrine and pseudoephedrine, the extract of which has been used in the East for centuries, usually without particular problems, while in the West there have been some serious problems. Incidentally, numerous other "variants" are included in the genus *Ephedra*.

A series of deaths, in fact, prompted the American FDA to ban it from the market, even if some supplements still contain it (probably the other less effective alkaloids of the chemically produced substance). The fact remains that it is considered doping by WADA and that the European Community has restricted its sale, as it is used as a precursor to other drugs.

However, it is sold with less difficulties as an herbal product "in general", but if on the one hand the content of the active substances is much lower (and therefore the results), on the other hand any impurities due to an uncertain origin can even increase its danger.

Indications
Ephedrine and pseudoephedrine, structurally similar to amphetamines, are sympathetic-mimetic agents with agonist activity, both direct and indirect, against α and β-adrenergic receptors, and therefore stimulating the central nervous system. Ephedrine is believed to be able to increase the mental acuity, improve strength and reduce weight through an increase in the activity of the sympathetic nervous system and thermogenesis.

Evidence
In the 1990s, among bodybuilders, the ECA stack (ephedrine, caffeine, aspirin) was the most popular: the synergy of the three substances is very interesting, and the success met was more deserved than that of others, but some serious cases (strokes, heart attacks, sudden deaths) have relegated this union to oblivion: the deceased subjects were overweight and/or in poor health conditions, or had taken ephedrine in particularly unfavorable climatic situations (excessive heat). However, nervousness, anxiety, palpitations, increased blood pressure, tachycardia, gastrointestinal disturbances, nausea, diarrhea, headache and dizziness, although less drastic, are not so rare side effects...

Several cases of very serious liver toxicity have also been reported, also in the East: in these cases, it is difficult to understand whether the problems are to be attributed to ephedrine itself or to other herbs often used together in the products, perhaps even "homemade", as can happen precisely in the various areas where *Ephedra* is widely used (China, India, Pakistan).

An interesting review by Powers (2001) evaluates the various properties of this substance in a concise but effective way: lipolysis, the increase in endurance, the increase in strength, "grit" and energy, all properties that attract athletes from the most disparate disciplines and overweight subjects (also thanks to the decrease in appetite).

Powers also explains the various mechanisms through which alkaloids perform their activity. We will not list them here, but we should mention the warning issued by the US scholar regarding some commercial products; in one, for example, a capsule was sold as containing only a generic Chinese ginseng, but instead, each capsule consisted of 45 mg of ephedrine and 20 of caffeine: since the recommended dosage was 5 tablets/day, you can well imagine the problems which can be incurred by taking 225 mg of ephedrine (plus the rest) per day! Moreover, often most of the products sold online by sites that do not go back to known companies, do not contain what is written on the labels.

The American scholar does not totally ignore the advantages of the substance but, addressing in particular the sports coaches, points the finger more than anything else on the risk/benefit ratio, which is definitely unbalanced, given that it is a substance indicated as a doping agent.

Interesting ideas can also be found in the literature, such as "Reducing the dose of combined caffeine and ephedrine preserves the ergogenic effect", by Bell et al., and many others.

Given the illegal status of the substance, the number of studies has gradually declined.

Dosages
For the same reasons as above, recommending a dosage does not make much sense; however, exceeding 1 mg/kg/day increases the risk of side effects.

Effectiveness

Strength	Resistant strength	Mass	Endurance	Slimming	Concentration	Recovery
++	+	+	++	++	+	−

ESSENTIAL AMINO ACIDS

Description
Talking about amino acids has become very current and important in recent years. In fact, there are many areas in which a correct use of amino acids can bring improvements, especially in reference to problems such as sarcopenia, which is becoming increasingly present in modern society. Considering an increasingly elderly population and an increasingly pronounced muscle decay in industrialized countries, we can imagine how we are taking long steps towards an increasingly fragile contemporary society that will be increasingly forced into assistance.

It is estimated that the onset of the sarcopenic syndrome (which involves not only the loss of muscle mass, but also of strength) begins between the ages of 40 and 50. At 60 it affects 30% of subjects and the percentage rises to 50% among eighty-year-olds. Strength drops to a lesser extent if you train, and weight exercises are the best way. Strong seniors get sick less frequently, have fewer complications, and are more independent. However, amino acid availability is the fundamental premise for these results. In fact, people over 40 years of age respond less to key amino acids and for this reason they should often consume protein during the day to maintain the muscle mass and prevent atrophy. With aging, the anabolic response is reduced due to low doses of amino acids (brilliant response, however, in the young). The "over 40" subject has a lower response to stimuli that produce muscle improvements (free radicals, insulin, amino acids). While in young people the protein synthesis can be stimulated with the ingestion of amino acids up to 3 hours after training, in older subjects this is no longer possible and the amino acids should be taken immediately after the workout, without adding carbohydrates (this is even recommended for young people).

The commercial offer of amino acids is truly vast and information on this subject can make a difference in terms of performance, health or simply prevention. In the past, we knew only 20 amino acids, but recently they have discovered three new ones (selenocysteine, pyrrolysine and N-formylmethionine). Out of the total of 23 amino acids, there are 8 that must be strictly included in the diet, because the body is unable to produce them: phenylalanine, threonine, tryptophan, methionine, lysine, leucine, isoleucine and valine. The last three are the famous branched chain amino acids (BCAAs) and remember that 35-40% of muscle tissue is made up of leucine, isoleucine and valine. Histidine is also considered an essential amino acid, but only in children, although there are studies that are re-evaluating its importance for adults.

If these essential amino acids are not taken in adequate quantities, they become "amino acids that limit the protein synthesis". This means that if there is a lack of one of these amino acids in quantities greater than 50% of the body's needs to synthesize a certain protein, this is less expressed and can affect various organic functions and even growth itself. Here we can add the conditionally essential amino acids, i.e. those that become fundamental in certain conditions (protracted stress, pathologies, hypercatabolic states, etc.), i.e. arginine, cysteine, glutamine, glycine, proline and tyrosine. The quantity of essential amino acids that a protein contains characterizes its biological value.

High biological value is usually attributed to animal proteins (rich in essential amino acids) and low biological value to vegetable proteins (which have one or more limiting amino acids). The biological value also expresses how similar the protein is to those of the human body and how much the latter ends up retaining and reusing them. Depending on the limiting amino acids of vegetable proteins, they can be combined in order to obtain all the essential amino acids (the concept of protein complementarity – cereals and legumes or cereals and soy etc.), but the ingested quantities must be higher.

To clarify with a classic example, cereals are deficient in tryptophan and lysine (present mainly in legumes), while legumes are deficient in methionine and cysteine (present to a large extent in cereals), so it is a good idea to combine them. Therefore, it is not certain that in order to reach the correct amount of essential amino acids it is mandatory to consume mainly animal proteins, but it is possible (sometimes advisable) to combine different proteins with medium or low biological value (including vegetables, mushrooms, fruits). It should be remembered, however, that this protracted approach (as in vegans, for example) inevitably leads to an increase in the intake of carbohydrates (and therefore the level of physical activity of the subject and the insulin-glycemic pattern must be carefully evaluated), to a drop in saturated fat and cholesterol (and here hormonal levels must be particularly evaluated, especially the steroid line), an excess of fiber (and here the intestinal microbiota, the presence of any fermentative dysbiosis or SIBO, etc.) or an increase of polyunsaturates (which, if excessive, puts the subject at risk of lipid peroxidation of the plasma membranes, etc.).

Properties

Briefly, we will associate each essential amino acid with a recognized main function, in order to fix some concepts:

- **lysine**: important for keratin, therefore for the skin and skin appendages, then for the production of antibodies and post-exercise recovery;
- **phenylalanine**: thyroid metabolism and wakefulness;
- **threonine**: immune system (antibodies and humoral immunity);
- **methionine**: sulphate, purifying capacity;
- **tryptophan**: sleep-wake rhythm, important in recovery and in the sensation of fatigue;
- **leucine**: ketogenic, muscle building;
- **isoleucine**: neoglucogenic, maintenance of glycaemia;
- **valine**: competes with tryptophan, maintains concentration;
- **histidine**: precursor of histamine, vasomotor and immune role.

In situations involving a deficiency of these amino acids, various problems arise: a decrease in the muscle tone and an increased catabolism, susceptibility to infections, skin appendages and brittle hair, water retention, fatigue, etc. The supplementation of these amino acid mixtures is particularly important both in the subject who does intense sporting activity and in the prolongation of orthosympathetic states (very common today).

Regarding the requirement of each essential amino acid, this can be calculated in mg per kg of body weight, per day, as shown in the Table 44.4.

Table 44.4 Essential amino acid requirements in adults*: values in mg/kg/day

Isoleucine	10
Leucine	14
Lisyne	12
Methyonine	13
Phenylalanine	14
Treonine	7
Tryptophan	3.5
Valine	10
Histidine**	(8-12)**

* Source: FAO Committee 1973, modified.
** Histidine: an essential amino acid, especially for the newborn.

For example, for tryptophan, a 70 kg man should take (3.5 × 70 = 245) 245 mg per day (minimum amount).

Evidence

It must be said that there are numerous controversies regarding both essential and branched amino acids. Regarding the essentials, the controversy depends on the fact that they would be represented in both animal and vegetable proteins, but the different concentrations would make them more or less useful for the construction of a given organic protein (supplementation, therefore, would not be necessary because only the presence/absence of the amino acid in question is evaluated). According to this view, strict vegan diets would have no amino acid deficiency. For BCAAs (in the limelight because they are used purely by muscles – primarily used as anti-catabolic in liver diseases), the controversies concern the fact that, lacking the other essential amino acids during their intake, they would not be able to assume the anabolic plastic value that the various claims attribute for over 30 years. Notably, a 2017 review published in the *Journal of the International Society of Sports Nutrition* (Wolfe et al.) concluded that the consumption of BCAAs to increase the anabolic response is unwarranted. A subsequent review in 2019 (Santos et al.) also confirmed this hypothesis. Excluding that the most important factor remains the daily amount of protein taken by the subject in 24 hours, there is still a low tendency of the population to reach even just one gram per kg of body weight of protein (which, among other things, should be adapted at least for athletes and the elderly). In this situation, supplementing with amino acids may remain a good idea. Even if, from the latest studies in the literature, it appears that the BCAAs lack an effective plastic response in the post-workout, it is also true that it is difficult for the subject to take only those during the day and that, as we know, during the post-workout the fundamental stimulus is given by leucine. This is why the market took advantage of this to launch BCAA formulations that contain disproportionate concentrations of this amino acid (4:1:1, 8:1:1, 10:1:1, 12:1:1, they are so popular that the normal 2:1:1 are now hard to find).

In the post-workout, in effect, BCAAs can stimulate the protein synthesis by translating this into a real protein gain only by interacting with the other essential amino acids deriving from the protein catabolism induced by training, or with those that are already present in the circulating pool. During the pre-workout, on the other hand, the branched ones have the advantage of being gluconeogenic (isoleucine and valine), therefore they produce sugar for the physical activity in a gradual manner and without an exaggerated insulin stimulation, which could affect the performance or the workout. To tell the truth, it would be enough to take valine and isoleucine pre-workout (but there are no supplements like this) to maintain the clarity during the training, and take a complete protein source such as whey protein or, in fact, the essential amino acids post-workout. (perhaps with the addition of a little leucine if our goal is gaining muscle mass).

As for the essential amino acids in their entirety, the Journal of the *International Society of Sports Nutrition* still comes to our aid which, again in 2017, when they published a review (Kerksick et al.) in which they discussed the nutrient timing in particular. This review concludes that the consumption of essential amino acids (EAA; about 10 g) in free form or as part of a protein bolus of about 20-40 g has been shown to stimulate the muscle protein synthesis (MPS) to the maximum. Starting from the fact that the protein synthesis depends on the level of essential amino acids and leucine in the blood, it seems that the essentials are the best choice for the post-workout. In fact, a 2018 study (Nakayama et al.) compared the amino acidemia (in particular the concentration of essentials) resulting from the administration of whey proteins with that deriving from essential amino acids alone and found that whey increased it faster (with the same essential content). The discussion of the study explained this result with the fact that a protein can differ from another not only in the amount of essential amino acids it carries, but also depending on how many di-tripeptides it produces during its hydrolysis. The hydrolysis of some proteins will bring in proportion more di-tripeptides and less essential amino acids, while other proteins would give more essential amino acids and less peptides. The latter are absorbed by preferential routes, therefore, while the essentials are transported only in one way, both di-tripeptide and essential channels are available for whey proteins. The result is a more rapid increase of the post-absorption total essential amino acids for whey.

Dosages
For essential amino acids, the doses are 10 g (equivalent to 20-40 g of protein) and can be added to meals to complete the daily intake or in relation to the workout.

Effectiveness

Strength	Resistant strength	Mass	Endurance	Slimming	Concentration	Recovery
++	++	+++	++	++	+	+++

EXOGENOUS KETONES

Description
When the level of carbohydrates in the diet is very low (VLCKD), the body switches from a predominantly glycolytic metabolism to a metabolism uses fats for energy, and the liver begins to convert fat into molecules that can be called the fourth energy nutrient for humans, after carbohydrates, fats and proteins, which are ketone bodies. Most supplements rely on b-hydroxybutyrate (BHB) as a source of exogenous ketone bodies. BHB is the most common exogenous ketone body due to its ease and efficiency in the energy conversion, and it can be converted to acetoacetic acid. It is this acetoacetic acid that will enter the energy path by becoming two molecules of acetyl-CoA. Acetyl-CoA is therefore able to enter the Krebs

cycle in order to generate ATP. The remaining BHB molecules that are not synthesized in acetoacetic acid are then converted to acetone the acetoacetate decarboxylase. Some of these supplements are in the form of salts in which BHB is bound with sodium, potassium or calcium, in order to improve its absorption and its overall bioavailability.

Recently, some exogenous ketones that have been developed for supplementary use, can be also used as a sports drink and have some effectiveness on the sports performance; they consist of a ketone ester (R)-3-hydroxybutyl (R)-3 hydroxybutyrate, which is hydrolyzed to D-β-hydroxybutyric acid and 1,3 butanediol.

Dr. Richard Veech, a leading expert on ketosis, head of the laboratory of the US National Institute of Health (NIH), created a ketone ester that is synthesized from an organic chemical called 1,3 butanediol and a monoester that the body converts in β-hydroxybutyrate (BHB).

Exogenous ketone supplements are normally a combination of BHB salts, MCT powder, and ketogenic amino acids such as leucine and lysine. Foreign ketones also have the effect of lowering ghrelin levels and, therefore, decreasing the appetite.

Properties

A ketone-based drink, even in a person who does not follow a ketogenic diet, can favor the transition from the use of glucose or fatty acids for energy purposes, to the use of ketones.

This mechanism occurs mainly during long distance and duration workouts, in which the muscles end up relying mainly on ketones as their preferred energy source.

Ketosis is essential for survival because the brain can only use glucose and ketone bodies for energy. Therefore, in the absence of glucose, the brain mainly uses ketone bodies. So do the muscles during an aerobic work, thus preserving the muscle mass that would otherwise be attacked by neoglucogenesis in order to transform gluconeogenic amino acids into glucose. However, to facilitate the metabolic shift of the organism towards the use of ketone bodies for nutritional purposes, an alternative to nutritional ketosis can be obtained through the consumption of synthetic or exogenous ketones, such as MCT oil, coconut and other supplements such as ester ketones.

Exogenous ketones are thermodynamically beneficial and easily usable as fuel for the skeletal muscle. During the use of exogenous ketones, the energy metabolism of the exercise is altered, with an increase in fat oxidation and a saving of the intramuscular glycogen. It also has a positive effect on the performance at low and moderate intensity; on the other hand, high-intensity performances that require a rapid use of glycogen can be negatively affected. Proper nutrition for post-workout recovery, along with an ester ketone instead, increases glycogen synthesis and reduces the catabolism.

The increase in glycogen is probably due to the fact that glucose, once inside the muscle cell, is preferably deposited in the form of glycogen due to the inhibitory effect on glycolysis, exerted by exogenous ketones. Training causes a certain degree of muscle catabolism in order to optimize the metabolic processes at the cellular level and this manifests itself with an increase in BCAA levels within the muscle after training; the intake of ester ketones before training reduces the increase in BCAAs within the muscle. The ester ketones increase the activation of the protein synthesis; after the exercise, the mTOR pathway is activated, which triggers the protein synthesis. When athletes combine ester ketones with a carbohydrate-based recovery drink, mTOR is activated even more. The use of exogenous ketones creates a new physiological state in which high levels of ketones and high carbohydrate stores are simultaneously present. However, supplementation with BHB reduces the oxidative stress, inflammation, muscle damage, immune dysfunction and fatigue during the training. All this can have a positive impact on the recovery and on the subsequent performance.

Evidence

In a study published in July 2016 in the *Cell Metabolism* journal, giving a ketone drink of esters to 39 professional athletes, including former Olympic cyclists, showed that they used ketones for energy purposes, producing less lactic acid, and that they could pedal an average of 411 meters more during a 30-minute maximal training test, compared to when they did not take a carbohydrate drink. This equates to a 2% increase in speed.

Peter Hespel, head professor of the Athletic Performance Center at the Catholic University of Leuven, conducted a study by dividing 18 subjects into two groups and by making them pedal for 21 days, in order to simulate the duration of a race like that of the Tour de France. His intention was reaching a level of overreaching or, in any case, a point where the performance expires.

One group took ketones and the other one took a drink containing 16.4 g of MCT, which provided the same calories as the ester ketone drink. After 21 days they were all exhausted, with symptoms of fatigue comparable to those of high-level professional runners after stage races. The difference was that ketone users experienced far fewer symptoms, recovering faster and continuing to eat better.

Therefore, according to the data of this study, it is deduced that:

- the group that used this nutrient managed to increase the training volume by 15% during the third week;
- during the trial, the same exogenous ketone users always obtained a 15% improvement on average, compared to the other group.

Furthermore, the group that had taken the ester ketones did not show the physiological symptoms of overtraining, presenting a regular resting heartbeat and lower levels of the stress hormone GDF15. According to Hespel, the intake of ester ketones acts on the autonomic nervous system which regulates the heartbeat and the reaction to stress; in other words, ester ketones help avoiding the physical effects of overtraining rather than causing an actually increase in the performance.

Youm et al. (2015) found that BHB, but not acetoacetic acid or short-chain fatty acids butyrate and acetate, reduced the inflammatory cytokines IL-1β and IL-18 which are produced in human monocytes, thus blocking the activation of inflammasome.

In two studies published in the *Frontiers in Physiology* journal, adults who took a drink with ketone esters or ketones alone, after one hour, had ketone levels comparable to those of a person after a week of fasting. It should not be thought that ketonuria raised due to the use of exogenous ketones is comparable in metabolic effects to that induced physiologically by fasting or by a VLCKD; if real ketosis promotes weight loss, the use of ketone bodies does so indirectly by its anorectic effect, as it is in any case of an additional intake of calories which, indeed, inhibit the endogenous ketosis.

Dosages

The drinks used for the tests contained approximately 15 to 25 g of β-hydroxybutyric acid or ketone esters.

Effectiveness

Strength	Resistant strength	Mass	Endurance	Slimming	Concentration	Recovery
–	+	–	+++	++	+++	+++

FENUGREEK

Description
Fenugreek (*Trigonella foenum graecum*) belongs to the legume family and looks like an herbaceous plant with a straight and hollow stem, three-pointed leaves and light yellow flowers that have a triangular appearance, hence the geometric name "trigonella". Originally from the Middle East, it arrived in Europe only after the 9th century, where it found an environment and climate that was suitable for its growth.

The seeds, yellow to amber in color, are also widely used in the culinary field in dishes such as soups and vegetables; roasted seeds are used as a spice to enhance the flavor, especially in the Indian continent and in the countries of the Middle East.

Fenugreek is one of the oldest medicinal plants, dating back to the times of the ancient Egyptians, Greeks and Romans, who used it as a medicinal and culinary herb. Among its main components, in fact, we find: vitamins (A, B, C), iron, calcium, lecithin, phosphates, proteins, alkaloids (trigonellin, choline), saponins and sapogenins (diosgenin).

Properties
The fields of application of fenugreek are many. In India fenugreek is used in curry, while in America the oil obtained from the seeds is used in baked goods and ice cream. Its extract is used in the treatment of skin irritations, eczema, boils, ulcers and cellulite (for its anti-inflammatory, antiseptic, emollient, soothing, tonic-stimulating, restructuring properties); it is considered useful for arousing or increasing sexual desire, for relieving menopausal disorders (sexual dysfunction, hot flashes, mood swings, insomnia, vaginal dryness, night sweats, etc.) and is often used as an agent that increases the production of breast milk. This supplement is also used as an ally for the digestive system, thanks to its enzymatic ability to stimulate the metabolism and act in case of indigestion, dyspepsia, stomach ulcers, diarrhea and gastrointestinal spasms.

Fenugreek seeds are particularly recommended for excessively thin or asthenic individuals, as they exhibit strong anabolic and GH-stimulating properties. Due to the presence of some osteogenic factors (vitamin D, calcium, vitamin PP), it is interesting to use fenugreek in some osteopathies (for example osteoporosis), in growth disorders or to help consolidate fractures. In the field of sport, fenugreek is known for its anabolic effects deriving from furostanolic saponins, which contribute to the increase of muscle mass and strength, and allow an improvement of the athletic performance.

Evidence
The **anabolic effect** of fenugreek in sports is linked to its ability to facilitate the accumulation of proteins in the muscles, increasing their mass. Several studies highlight the presence of 4-hydroxy-isoleucine, a rare amino acid (whose main source is precisely an extract of fenugreek seeds), which is a specific molecule that would stimulate the production of insulin by the pancreas (resulting in greater use of sugars by cells) and would increase the cellular sensitivity towards insulin, improving the uptake of nutrients. For example, the increase in the glucose uptake by the muscle can improve the restoration of glycogen after exhaustive exercise.

The ability of 4-hydroxy-isoleucine to increase the insulin sensitivity can also be exploited for the loss of body fat. Some researchers, in fact, consider it an excellent adjuvant in weight loss and it is especially useful for those suffering from the metabolic syndrome, which is now not difficult to find, even in people who are simply overweight (without leading to obesity). Furthermore, 4-hydroxy-isoleucine directly stimulates mTOR, resulting in the activation of the mechanisms of protein synthesis.

A 2019 study reiterates the proven effect of the sensitization to the action of insulin (Rita et al.), and it also reports that the intake of the active component diosgenin, associated with a biological matrix of fenugreek seeds, has a potential adjuvant effect in thyroid diseases. In fact, many studies, in addition to supporting this insulin sensitization action, have revealed that fenugreek seeds can affect the synthesis and functions of other metabolic hormones, such as thyroid hormones. In particular, they have shown themselves capable of reducing the levels of thyroid hormone in the periphery, consequently modifying the T4/T3 ratio, which in healthy people could be a side effect; however, in hypothyroidism, which primarily manifests itself with high levels of TSH, this effect may represent a possible natural alternative to the use of drugs.

But what emerged from the study was above all a careful evaluation of the dose-dependent effects of fenugreek. In the study, carried out on rats that had been induced insulin resistance through a diet rich in fatty acids, different concentrations of diosgenin were used, respectively 1 mg/kg, 10 mg/kg and 50 mg/kg, assigned in a randomized manner to the various groups. The results showed that the beneficial effects of insulin sensitization and the adjuvant effect in thyroid diseases were obtained with the lowest dose; this apparently contradictory response could be explained by the hormesis mechanism, according to which some compounds administered at low doses have a beneficial and stimulating effect, and activate adaptation mechanisms in the organism, while, conversely, high doses do not activate our body's balancing mechanisms, producing an opposite inhibitory effect.

Hence the importance of the correct dosage, since in this case low doses of diosgenin have had beneficial effects, while higher doses have altered the insulin sensitivity and homeostasis of the hormones being analyzed.

In a recent study, fenugreek extract taken by athletes undergoing physical exercise with weights, was shown to be useful **in increasing the upper body strength and favorably modifying the body composition, resulting in a decrease in body fat and an increase in lean mass**. The ergogenic effect of this supplement would be enhanced by creatine: taking 900 mg of fenugreek with 3.5 g of creatine monohydrate for 8 weeks, shows an increase in lean mass and strength, results that are comparable to the same amount of creatine taken together with 70 g of dextrose.

In rats, the oral intake of 10-35 mg/kg of fenugreek furostanol for 4 weeks resulted in an increase in the levator ani muscle weight (used as an indicator of the anabolic action in males), with no significant influence on the level of circulating testosterone or alterations of the prostate. In healthy men, however, studies on the relationship between fenugreek and testosterone have produced mixed and sometimes discordant results.

In a first study, by administering 500 mg fenugreek (trade name Testofen) over an 8-week period, **serum testosterone in males who trained with resistance exercises was increased**, compared to testosterone levels of those who took the placebo (who instead had experienced a drop in testosterone from baseline). Another similar research, which involved taking 600 mg of Testofen for a period of 6 weeks, found a decrease in DHT, a metabolite of testosterone, probably with an inhibitory action on 5 alpha-reductase, but it was not able to demonstrate a significant influence on the total testosterone.

A further study examined Testofen with the same dosage in male subjects, always subjected to weight training, reaffirming the anabolic effect of androgens and also in this case detecting an increase in free testosterone, without reducing the total levels; moreover, there was a significant improvement in the body composition in favor of lean mass, without reducing the muscle strength, which resulted in beneficial effects in terms of repetitions until exhaustion in weight training exercises.

In another study, however, it did not only cause an increase in free testosterone levels, but thanks to the intake of a fenugreek seed extract there was also an improvement in both the profile and morphology of the spermatozoa, as well as an improvement in libido, mood and mental alertness. Finally, a very recent study has shown that the hydrolysate proteins of fenugreek seeds have an antioxidant activity, since they are able to reduce the intracellular levels of ROS.

Dosages
If fenugreek is taken in the form of dried and pulverized powder, a daily dose of 6 g is recommended; for example, if taken as an infusion, it is recommended distribute it in two to three doses a day, using 6 g of powder.

If fenugreek is taken in the form of dry extract, it is recommended to take 300 mg of product twice a day; while if this supplement is taken in the form of soft extract, it is possible to take 500 mg twice a day.

Effectiveness

Strength	Resistant strength	Mass	Endurance	Slimming	Concentration	Recovery
+	−	+++	−	+	−	++

FORSKOLIN (COLEUS FORSKHOLII)

Description
Coleus forskohlii is a perennial herbaceous plant belonging to the *Lamiaceae* family that grows in the mountains of Asia, in particular in the subtropical areas of India, Nepal, Burma and Thailand. It is characterized by light green leaves with jagged edges and violet, indigo and turquoise colored flowers. The active ingredient, which takes the name of forskolin, and other substances which are recognized for various beneficial and curative properties are obtained from the fleshy and aromatic roots.

This plant, also known as Indian coleus, has always been known and used in Ayurvedic medicine, both as a spice to accompany foods and as a natural remedy for the treatment of disorders affecting the cardiovascular, respiratory and digestive systems. In the Western World, it is known and mainly used as a food supplement capable of stimulating lipolysis and the metabolism.

Properties
The plant has several active ingredients, among which **forskolin** is the best known, but there are also diterpenes and triterpenes, rosmarinic acid and beta-sitosterols.

Forskolin acts directly on adenylate cyclase, an enzyme that positively influences other enzymes present in our body, which regulate the energy metabolism, muscle growth and fat loss. In fact, adenylate cyclase is able to activate intracellular cyclic AMP (cAMP), which acts as a second messenger in numerous intracellular biochemical reactions, regulating their speed and efficiency. In this way, forskolin is able to perform various functions: it regulates the body's thermogenic response following the ingestion of food, increases the basal metabolism and stimulates the thyroid function.

Its best known and studied function is the stimulation of lipolysis by stimulating hormone-sensitive lipase, thus promoting the breakdown of triglycerides present in adipose tissue, by stimulating the release of free fatty acids; the latter can be used by the muscles for energy purposes or can be partially dispersed as energy in the form of heat by activating the UCP-3 uncoupling proteins. Basically, forskolin, by increasing the production of cAMP, directly stimulates the lipolysis.

Evidence

In cell physiology studies and research, forskolin has been shown to be able to increase cAMP levels. The effects of forskolin on cAMP were already described in detail in the 1980s, and can be observed in isolated cell preparations and intact tissues. More recently, *in vivo* studies have shown that the mechanism is also preserved in humans, showing that, hormone-sensitive lipase activation occurs and consequently lipolysis increases following the ingestion of forskolin. To date, therefore, in the scientific literature, it is possible to find a huge number of researches that have shown that the intake of forskolin is able to effectively stimulate lipolysis through cAMP.

In one study, 30 obese men took forskolin supplements (250 mg of extract titrated to 10%), twice a day for 12 weeks. The results showed that the use of forskolin caused favorable changes in their body composition (determined by DEXA): fat mass was significantly reduced by 11.23% compared to the 1.73% reduction observed in the placebo group.

Other researchers conducted a study, published in the *Journal of the International Society of Sports Nutrition*, with the aim of studying the efficacy and safety of forskolin intake in overweight women. Scientists evaluated the effect on adipose tissue, appetite regulation and energy levels, and verified the appearance of any side or adverse effects. The randomized double-blind study divided the subjects into two groups: one group took 250 mg of forskolin titrated to 10%, twice a day for a period of 12 weeks; the other group took a placebo pill.

Body composition parameters (determined by DEXA) and anthropometric parameters were recorded at the beginning and after 2, 8 and 12 weeks, to evaluate the slimming effect; to highlight any side effects, blood samples were taken at the beginning and at the end of the study. All the participants also kept a food diary in order to study the possible anorectic effect induced by the supplement.

The results showed that women who took forskolin had a decrease of their fat mass and reported less hunger (resulting in less daily calorie intake), more energy and less fatigue during workouts. No statistically significant differences were reported, however, with regard to blood markers related to the lipid profile, liver and kidney function, blood pressure and electrolyte levels, there were no side effects reported during the intake, demonstrating the efficacy and the safety of using the product.

Another study, on the other hand, analyzed the effect of forskolin on the thyroid metabolism. Thyroid hormones are produced by the thyroid gland in the presence of thyroid stimulating hormone (TSH) produced by the adenohypophysis, which therefore represents the main stimulus for the production of the two forms of hormones, T4 (the less active) and T3 (biologically more active). Therefore, some researchers have studied the effect of forskolin on the thyroid metabolism by comparing it precisely with that induced by stimulation with TSH. The study, published as far back as March 1984, was conducted on the thyroid lobes of dogs, in which it was perfused an equal dose of forskolin and TSH.

The results reported that both agents induced increases in cAMP, but the forskolin response was much more effective than the one induced by TSH. Following the increase in cAMP, after 20 minutes, there was an increase in the secretion of T4 and T3, and the initial phase of hormone secretion was significantly faster after stimulation with forskolin rather than with TSH. However, the response to forskolin has a less lasting and stable effect over time (hence the recommendation to supplement with different daily intakes). In particular, the authors stated that with forskolin, there was a higher increase in the production of T3 than that of T4.

Some studies also suggest that forskolin, acting as a vasodilator, is able to produce beneficial effects on the cardiovascular system: it reduces the blood pressure, inhibits platelet aggregation (less clot formation) and exerts an ionotropic action on the heart (increased contractile force); these properties are interesting in terms of cardiovascular disease prevention in overweight subjects with hypertension (hyperlipogenetics), but also in sports subjects, who, in addition to fat loss, seek an improvement in the sports performance and an increase in muscle mass.

In all these studies, the researchers directly analyzed the effect of taking forskolin-based supplements and the results are quite consistent: the active ingredient is able to promote the body recomposition, decreasing the percentage of adipose tissue and preserving the lean mass at the same time. For these properties, forskolin turns out to be an excellent supplement, able to effectively support weight loss, especially in a context of low-calorie diet and physical activity, but it should be emphasized that the active ingredient has also proved effective in studies in which nutrition and physical activity were not included, showing that the molecule is able to promote weight loss even individually. Obviously, its effects can be enhanced in association with an ad hoc diet and an adequate physical activity.

Dosages
A good *Coleus forskholii* supplement should be standardized to a minimum of 10% forskolin in order to achieve the desired effects. Scientific studies show that the effective dosage ranges from 165 to 250 mg, for three or four daily intakes.

Effectiveness

Strength	Resistant strength	Mass	Endurance	Slimming	Concentration	Recovery
–	+	+	+	+++	–	–

FUCOXANTHIN

Description
Fucoxanthin is a carotenoid, a fat-soluble pigment without vitamin activity, with chemical formula $C_{42}H5_8O_6$ and characterized by the presence of a single allene ring.

This pigment is characteristic of diatoms and many edible brown algae, such as Undaria pinnatifida (better known as Wakame seaweed) and Laminaria japonica (or Ma-Kombu).

Taken in the diet, it is hydrolyzed to fucoxantinol in the gastrointestinal tract, thanks to digestive enzymes such as lipases, and then converted to amarouciaxanthin A in the liver. It is this metabolite, amarouciaxanthin A, that is the biologically active form of fucoxanthin.

Fucoxanthin can be stored in abdominal adipose tissue, whereas fucoxantinol is stored in other tissues.

Properties
First of all, like carotenoids in general, it has an antioxidant action, able to reduce the markers of oxidative stress, also stimulated by exercise. In addition, fucoxanthin, by increasing the levels of Nrf2 protein, is able to restore the levels of reduced glutathione, one of the most powerful endogenous antioxidants of our body.

It should be added that the antioxidant action of this carotenoid is particularly significant at the hepatic level, where it protects HepG2 cells (Xiao H. et al., 2020).

In fucoxanthin, the scavenger activity of singlet oxygen and ROS in general is combined with an important anti-inflammatory action.

This is expressed:
- thanks to the beneficial interaction, recently recognized, between the carotenoid and the intestinal flora;
- through the inhibition of the over-regulation of important pro-inflammatory cytokines such as IL-6, IL-1β, TNFα, COX-2 and iNOS;
- through the inhibition of UVB-induced apoptosis (Xiao H. et al., 2020).

Such features making this molecule very effective in optimizing the recovery phase.

Fucoxanthin also has important slimming properties.

First, it acts as an antiobesogen (Koo S. et al., 2019), able to inhibit adipogenesis and food intake, depending on the high content of mucilage (satiating element).

In addition, it has an antidiabetic effect, specifically, fucoxanthin and its metabolites were found to be effective in modulating the expression of PAI-1, linked to increased insulin resistance, and PPAR-γ receptor, also linked to insulin resistance as well as lipogenesis (Koo S.Y. et al., 2019).

Finally, a diet containing fucoxanthin promotes blood glucose uptake into muscle cells by increased translocation of GLUT4 to the plasma membrane and generally activating the insulin signaling pathway (Nishikawa S. et al., 2012).

Evidence

In 2010, Abidov M. et al. conducted a double-blind 16-week experimental study on a group of obese women, randomly divided into a study group and a control group (Abidov M. et al., 2010). The study showed that the administration of fucoxanthin and a preparation consisting of fucoxanthin and pomegranate seed oil is able to increase energy expenditure at rest, measured by resting calorimetry. The study recorded a reduction in body weight, fat and blood pressure in the treated subjects.

In another 2010 study, a significant alteration of PPAR receptors was demonstrated following fucoxanthin supplementation, again by a dose-dependent mechanism (Matsumoto M. et al., 2010).

Dosages

The study, conducted by Abidov et al. in 2010 in women, showed that an overall dosage of fucoxanthin greater than 4 mg has significant effects on resting energy expenditure.

In general, the clinical studies reviewed report a dosage in men of between 2.4 and 8 mg per day.

Effectiveness

Strength	Resistant strength	Mass	Endurance	Slimming	Concentration	Recovery
++	++	+	++	++++	−	+++

GABA

Description

GABA (gamma-aminobutyric acid) is one of the most potent neurotransmitters in the human brain tissue and is the main inhibitory mediator. The sensations given by the action of GABA are relaxation and calmness.

The human body is able to synthesize it directly from the excitatory neurotransmitter glutamate (glutamic acid), using the glutamate decarboxylase enzyme and it can be converted back into glutamate, then entering the Krebs cycle as succinate. It regulates many depressive and sedative actions in the brain tissue and is critical for relaxation: it is involved in a wide range of repressive and depressive functions associated with the parasympathetic nervous system (PNS) physiology.

GABA is an endogenous molecule and the nervous system regulates its absorption with a negative feedback mechanism: when the levels are already high, its further absorption is inhibited, which, on the contrary, increases if the concentration decreases. However, this inhibition is not such as to prevent a possible overload of GABA: the brain is able to expel excess GABA and about 80% of it can be blocked, so 20% would still be able to be transported to the brain by passive diffusion.

Properties

GABA is used as a supplement, as a relaxant and as a muscle relaxant, to combat disorders such as anxiety, insomnia, difficulty falling asleep and even mood disorders. It is also widely used in the world of sports, as it is a promoter of the growth hormone production.

Evidence

As for the action on the secretion of GH hormone, the existence of an immunoreactive growth hormone (irGH) and an immunofunctional growth hormone (ifGH) was discovered. These are two analogues that seem to be influenced by the oral administration of GABA, which stimulates their release. This action would therefore improve the muscle function, especially in relation to sports/strength exercises (resistance training).

Furthermore, it appears to induce these changes also through reactions mediated by the release of dopamine at the suprapituitary level.

It is interesting to note that increases in GH production were recorded 30 minutes after an intense physical exercise, following the intake of GABA. These effects can also be traced to the fact that physical exercise promotes the production of nitric oxide: the latter facilitates the passage of GABA, taken orally, beyond the blood brain barrier.

In this regard, we can also note that in hypertension, where there are decreases in nitric oxide, there can also be a worsening of the well-being and mental balance, with signs such as difficulty falling asleep and anxiety related disorders. This could be a link between the cardiovascular function and the influence of the nervous system on it.

Dosages

GABA, as a supplement, in order to improve the indirect production of growth hormone is recommended in dosages ranging from 3000 to 5000 mg per day, in conjunction with intense exercise or before bedtime; as a relaxant, the dosages are 750-1500 mg are recommended. To be able to take it correctly during the training, it is necessary to test the subjective sensitivity: the effect depends on the amount of adrenaline that the subject produces following a physical activity. If this is not enough, it may be necessary to add stimulants such as caffeine.

Conversely, it is also true that, in the case of a person who produces an excessive amount of adrenaline, GABA could help to avoid the exacerbation of its catabolic effects. This can be particularly useful in the case of a calorie restriction.

It is very interesting to note that sometimes, in some subjects, excitatory effects can be observed following the intake of GABA. It is therefore important not only to test the subjective sensitivity, but also to contextualize its use in training and food plans.

Effectiveness

Strength	Resistant strength	Mass	Endurance	Slimming	Concentration	Recovery
–	–	+	–	++	++	+

GINKGO BILOBA

Description

Ginkgo biloba ("ginkgo" is a term that derives from the Japanese Yin-Kuo, which means "golden apricot", while "biloba" refers to the two-lobed shape of the leaf) is a plant of the *Ginkgoaceae* family native to Central Asia, resistant to very low temperatures (down to –35° C), lack of water and attack by toxic substances and parasites; for this reason, it is considered a living fossil. It is a tree with a wide crown and a pyramidal or oval shape, depending on the age, and can reach up to 40 m in height. It has fan-shaped bilobed leaves that contain flavonoids, non-glycosidic bioflavonoids, catechins, proanthocyanidins and terpene derivatives.

It has both male and female reproductive structures (dioecious plant), separated on different plants, and its fruits, with their yellow and smelly pulp, contain the seeds.

Properties

The leaves contain terpenes, the most important of which is ginkgolide B, which has a strong action as an inhibitor of the platelet aggregation factor, therefore, it is very useful in preventing the formation of thrombi and atherogenic plaques. Among the active molecules contained in the leaves, there are mainly flavonoids, quercetin, coumaric acid, catechins and proanthocyanidins, performing a contrast function against free radicals, which are responsible for the cellular damage and aging. *Ginkgo biloba* extract can help increase the activity of antioxidant enzymes in the liver tissue, reducing the damage from lipid peroxidation caused by free radicals. Although further research is still needed regarding the properties and effects deriving from the use of this plant, it has been seen that the use of the extract has positive effects in the treatment of cerebrovascular insufficiency with deterioration of brain functions (for example atherosclerosis and dementia); it is useful in reducing the negative effects in patients undergoing chemotherapy treatments; associated with CoQ10, it seems to improve the quality of life of people with fibromyalgia; associated with *Rhodiola crenulata*, it improves the durability and the sports performance. Being an antioxidant, it can reduce the toxicity associated with iodine-131 therapy in patients with thyroid disorders. *Ginkgo biloba* is particularly known for its use in cases of symptoms of arterial vascular insufficiency (useful in the prevention and complementary treatment of venous thrombosis and in the prevention of phlebopathies), in vascular tone alterations (for example, in Raynaud's disease, it acts effectively by reducing the frequency of arterial spasm episodes, followed by a vasodilation in the arteries of the hands, which occur following cold or emotional stimuli, improving the circulation) and in the presence of high blood sugar levels or glucose intolerance in people with type 2 diabetes.

Evidence

Treatment with single plant extracts has proven to be effective for various problems. A 2010 study of 48 mice divided into two groups, one exercising and one resting, in turn divided into subgroups, including a control group and a group given *Ginkgo biloba* extract, showed that the supplementation can increase the resistance to exercise and delay tiredness and fatigue; in addition, *Ginkgo biloba* extract can help increase the activity of antioxidant enzymes in the liver tissue, reduce lipid peroxidation caused by free radicals and improve the athletic abilities and the post-exercise recovery.

Studies have shown that it increases the blood flow in the cerebral cortex, increases alpha wave patterns in the brain, related to alertness, as well as increases brain ATP synthesis and the glucose uptake. In a 2009 study, 67 healthy subjects were divided into two groups: the test group, consisting of 34 subjects taking *Rhodiola* and *Ginkgo biloba* capsules, and the control group, consisting of 33 subjects taking a placebo. Both groups underwent the treatment for approximately 7 weeks. At the end of the study, the results showed that in subjects treated with *Rhodiola* and *Ginkgo biloba* capsules, there was a greater increase in the oxygen consumption compared to the placebo group; blood cortisol levels remained unchanged in subjects treated with the supplement, while they increased significantly in the placebo group.

So, in conclusion, supplementation with a combined *Rhodiola* and *Ginkgo biloba* supplement could improve the endurance performance, increase oxygen consumption, and protect against the negative effect of excessive cortisol production. A 2009 study showed that supplementation with *Ginkgo biloba* would promote the capillarization of the calf muscle, thus helping to improve the treadmill walking assistance in patients with *intermittent claudication*.

As for the properties of *Ginkgo biloba* regarding the concentration and cognitive abilities, please refer to the paragraph in the chapter on the diets for concentration, to avoid repetition.

Dosages

Ginkgo biloba is available in the form of drops or in capsules and tablets that contain the standardized extract with a content of flavonoids and terpene derivatives of 22-27% and 5-7% respectively. The recommended daily intake is 120-200 mg per day, perhaps cycling it over the course of the year: many studies, however, have used higher dosages.

Effectiveness

Strength	Resistant strength	Mass	Endurance	Slimming	Concentration	Recovery
–	–	–	++	+	++	+

GLUCOSAMINE AND CHONDROITIN SULFATE

Description

From a chemical point of view, **glucosamine** is a molecule formed by a combination of glucose and the amino acid glutamine, naturally present in the human body, and is the starting point for the synthesis of many important macromolecules, such as glycoproteins, glycolipids, mucopolysaccharides. It is necessary for the production of an important family of macromolecules called glycosaminoglycans (GAGs), which represent the components of numerous tissues in the digestive and respiratory tract, in some structures of the eye, blood, heart valves, and found in large quantities in the synovial fluid, tendons, ligaments and joints.

At the joint level, it inhibits the synthesis of cleavage enzymes called metalloproteases, with a consequent reduction in the degradation of proteoglycans. Glucosamine limits the inflammatory process as well as the apoptosis of chondrocytes (it would produce an increase in both TGF-β1 and in the connective tissue growth factor [CTGF]).

Chondroitin sulfate is the main component of the cartilage, it is a polymer of glucuronic acid and N-acetyl-galactosamine sulfate and can be found in numerous tissues, including tendons, bones, vertebral discs, cornea and heart valves. Over the years, chondroitin sulphate production from chondrocytes decreases, resulting in an increasingly weakened cartilage. Therefore, taking chondroitin sulfate can help increase the concentration of glycosaminoglycans in the cartilage and limit its excessive degradation.

Properties

In a healthy joint, the cartilage performs some functions, for example it acts as a shock absorber to reduce the impact on the bones and at the same time provides a surface that serves as a "friction" for a smooth, soft and painless joint movement. When we exert a weight overload or a mechanical stress on the joints, the cartilage squeezes the synovial fluid, an oily substance produced by the synovial membrane, into the synovial capsule; if the pressure is released, the cartilage absorbs the synovial fluid like a sponge: this nourishing ebb and flow acts as a buffer and lubricates every movement we make. Joint pain affects the world population, heavily modifying their quality of life; joint cartilages are affected, often with pain, swelling and muscle stiffness.

The mechanical overload from repeated impacts is another problem at the joint level, due to the technical gestures of various sports (for example tennis, baseball, rowing, running, etc.). But even working out in the gym consists of repeated exercises, especially on the shoulder joint (shoulder), precisely because it is the one that intervenes in almost all movements. In particular, glucosamine is essential as it stimulates the formation of glycosaminoglycans (GAG, important proteins that bind water to the cartilage matrix) and for the production of proteoglycans by chondrocytes. Chondroitin sulphate acts synergistically with glucosamine, as it draws water into the proteoglycans, allowing greater lubrication and better transport of nutrients, essential for the cartilage health, inhibiting the destructive action of enzymes that prematurely devour the cartilage, hindering other enzymes which can cause the interruption of the transport of nutrients to the matrix, etc.

Evidence

In recent years, there has been an increasing interest in non-pharmacological chondroprotective agents (therefore as food supplements) for osteoarticular treatment and/or prevention. The optimal characteristics that this category of supplements should have are the stimulation of chondrocytes to produce collagen and proteoglycans, and the inhibition of cartilage degradation (for example by inhibiting enzymes).

The compounds that have been shown to have these characteristics are those naturally present in the cartilage, including hyaluronic acid, glucosamine and chondroitin sulfate.

In a relevant study on the effects of glucosamine, half of the patients (106 people) were treated with oral glucosamine sulfate (1500 mg per day in a single dose), while the other half (106 patients) were randomly treated with a placebo. As a diagnostic reference, the evaluation of structural modifications ("structure modifying" effect) was carried out through magnetic resonance and radiographic examinations, with particular attention to the reduction of the joint space and to the evaluation of painful symptoms ("symptom modifying" effect) through the WOMAC (Western Ontario and McMaster Universities) index. This index is used internationally to assess osteoarthritis and provides questions relating to joint pain, joint stiffness and functional limitations.

From the structural modification point of view, glucosamine sulphate has proved **effective in limiting the phenomenon of joint space reduction**: patients treated with this molecule, after three years of administration, did not show any reduction of the joint space, compared to a decrease of 0.31 mm in those people who were given a placebo.

Glucosamine sulfate has also been shown to be effective in reducing painful symptoms and functional limitations. According to the WOMAC algofunctional index, the reduction of painful symptoms and functional limitations, after three years of treatment with glucosamine sulphate, was 24.3%, compared with an increase of 9.8% in the placebo group.

Both glucosamine and chondroitin sulfate are neither analgesics nor classic anti-inflammatories, as they do not directly inhibit the synthesis of prostaglandins. However, some studies have shown that their intake determines a mild anti-inflammatory effect (probably due to a block of free radicals).

In particular, in a major study with over 200 participants, chondroitin was no**t only responsible for a significant reduction in pain**, but its anti-inflammatory action allowed the participants to move the affected joints more freely. The pain-relieving effect in the presence of joint problems obviously translates into the possibility of using greater workloads and carrying out exercises that would otherwise be too annoying, all this leads to the advantage of a better workout. In addition to this, chondroitin sulfate has also shown a significant action against gout, contributing to the reduction of uric acid production (also probably linked to the antioxidant effect).

A 2015 study carried out at the Rheumatology Research Institute in Montreal, Canada, led by Jean-Pierre Pelletier, showed that taking 1200 mg of chondroitin sulfate per day for 2 years was able to delay the progression of joint diseases and degeneration, improving the functional capacity and decreasing pain in patients with osteoarthritis to a greater extent than celecoxib 200 mg (a non-steroidal anti-inflammatory drug [NSAID]).

A recent meta-analysis (Zhu et al., 2018) evaluated the effectiveness of the oral intake of chondroitin sulfate and glucosamine, and their use in combination in the treatment of knee and hip arthrosis. In this meta-analysis, respectively, chondroitin sulfate managed joint pain more effectively, while glucosamine improved the joint stiffness more. What should be noted, however, is that this meta-analysis did not record any improvement when the two molecules were used in combination. This meta-analysis actually records some biases related to the quality of the studies taken into consideration, the quality of the molecules used and the different intervention designs that a meta-analysis study must attempt to summarize. However, another double-blind, randomized multicentre study from 2016 (Roman-Blas et al.) had already reached the same conclusions by evaluating the association of the two molecules in the treatment of knee osteoarthritis.

Returning to the variability of the quality of the formulations and the heterogeneity in the design of clinical studies concerning glucosamine sulfate and chondroitin sulfate, the current guidelines for the treatment of arthrosis of the American College of Rheumatology (ACR) and of the Osteoarthritis Research Society International (OARSI) do not recommend the use of such molecules. In Europe, however, the European Medicines Agency (EMA) has approved the use of glucosamine sulfate and chondroitin sulfate formulations that follow the pharmaceutical quality standards and their use is recommended as a first-line treatment for the osteoarthritis of the knee. In Brazil, the general agreement of the Sociedade Brasileira de Rheumatologia certifies the use of glucosamine sulfate as a possible symptomatic treatment for osteoarthritis.

Dosages

Another consideration is that often, the beneficial effects of glucosamine and chondroitin sulfate are not noticed immediately, and it may be necessary to wait 2 to 6 months before seeing the results. As for the effects of the two supplements taken in combination, further studies are needed to fully validate their use, given that the same scientific societies do not have a common vision. Some studies have considered other supplements, such as vitamin C, bioflavonoids, selenium, zinc and vitamin E for the treatment of cartilage degeneration, but the most recent research does not include such use.

Another association is that fish oil: taken with glucosamine and chondroitin sulfate, it would seem to reduce the inflammation markers by 22% and even more than the placebo, as demonstrated in a study that took C-reactive protein (CRP) as a reference. The doses of glucosamine and chondroitin are calculated according to the body weight: if it is less than 54 kg, 1000 mg for glucosamine and 800 mg for chondroitin sulphate; if it is between 54 and 90 kg, 1500 mg for glucosamine and 1200 mg for chondroitin sulfate; if it is greater than 90 kg, 2000 mg for glucosamine and 1600 mg for chondroitin sulfate.

These dosages are only indicative, as they should be evaluated case by case and adjusted according to the pain and the degree of mobility of the joint.

Effectiveness

Strength	Resistant strength	Mass	Endurance	Slimming	Concentration	Recovery
++	++	+	–	–	–	–

GLUTAMINE

Description
Already more than 35 years ago I was commissioned by the LPA (Laboratory for Amino Acids) to study a new formulation of amino acids that could give something more for energy than the usual branched amino acids. Thus was born Aminature Six, a new formula containing leucine, valine, isoleucine (the usual branched ones), glycine, alanine and glutamine. At that time, I had already evaluated the enormous potential of a multivalent amino acid such as glutamine, which only after many years entered the market as a food supplement. Glutamine is an amino acid defined as non-essential, as it can be synthesized by our body.

The amino acid glutamine makes up about 65% of all amino acids present in the skeletal muscles, especially at the cytoplasmic level, and is the predominant amino acid in the cerebrospinal fluid and blood. Although it can be synthesized from other amino acids, under certain stressful conditions (for example, training), our body requires more of it than it can actually produce, as it performs multiple functions (all very important) in our body. Glutamine, in fact, provides cellular energy reserves in some tissues (including muscles), strengthens the immune system, increases the muscle cell volume, directly regulates the protein synthesis and the activity of the immune system cells.

Properties
Never had a non-essential amino acid such as glutamine found such a high consensus by athletes (and not only) as a "do-it-all" supplement. In fact, supplementation with this supplement:

- has a detoxifying action, managing to neutralize excess acids and dispose of the toxins that are produced during intense exercise sessions, such as weight training or sprinting, and which in many cases are the limiting factor of performance;
- increases the volume of muscle cells, improving hydration and also promoting the passage of nutrients and electrolytes that facilitate and accelerate all the biochemical and anabolic processes that take place within it, improving its functions, energy efficiency and general metabolism;
- intervenes in the energy metabolisms;
- performs a hepatoprotective, anti-inflammatory and pain-relieving action;

- allows you to accelerate the "fat burning" and at the same time preserve lean muscle mass from catabolism. There is clear and documented evidence that maintaining a high intramuscular glutamine level is essential to prevent the tissue degradation;
- acts in the brain with important functions, thanks to the ability to easily cross the blood brain barrier (a sort of barrier designed to defend the brain from substances that could damage it). Once this "obstacle" has been overcome, glutamine can be transformed into glutamic acid, an excellent brain fuel, which helps to maintain clarity and alertness even during physical activities or in situations of psychophysical stress. This allows to raise the threshold of perception of fatigue, while maintaining a high mental concentration. Glutamine detoxifies the body from ammonium, which on the contrary leads to a sleepy state. Furthermore, its neoglucogenic function allows the production of glucose helping the brain itself not to run into that dulling situation that is often felt after intense and protracted physical exercises;
- in the brain, glutamine also acts on the hunger center by stimulating the sense of satiety; this is especially useful for those who undergo low-calorie diets. This important action depends on the fact that this amino acid helps to maintain the glucose homeostasis and attenuates the changes in blood sugar induced by insulin, without establishing the typical sensations of hypoglycemic hunger that occur when blood sugar levels drop below a certain value;
- is able to raise the levels of the growth hormone (GH) in a sufficient, lasting but not excessive way, avoiding the occurrence of adverse situations such as hyperglycemia and the resulting consequences;
- plays an important role in the synthesis process of brain neurotransmitters;
- strengthens the body's immune defenses by directly stimulating the immunocytes; this is very important for those athletes who undergo long and continuous training, followed by reduced or no recovery periods (i.e. in a state of chronic overtraining) and who tend to get sick very easily precisely because they have put their defenses in crisis by impoverishing their immune system;
- constitutes the preferred source of energy for the rapid breakdown of cells, such as enterocytes (intestinal cells) and lymphocytes (white blood cells).

Evidence

All the experiments conducted on athletes and concerning the metabolism of glutamine under exercise, but also in conditions of rest and recovery from physical exercise, have proved very important, as they have led scholars to reconsider the role of glutamine in sports practice to the point that some researchers today define this substance as a "conditional essential amino acid". Recent studies highlight the importance of the roles played by glutamine in sports and muscle growth. For example, the effect that glutamine has on the sugar metabolism is of great importance. A recent study conducted by the University of Rochester in New York demonstrated the importance of glutamine as a **regulator of gluconeogenesis** (the formation of glucose from other substrates). In particular, it was found that in humans, glutamine is directly converted into glucose (probably in the kidneys), but without causing changes in the profile of insulin and glucagon, the two antagonistic hormones that intervene in the regulation of blood sugar. The results of this discovery can be particularly useful for bodybuilders who, in the pre-competition period, want to dispose of up to the last gram of their subcutaneous fat. In this circumstance, managing the insulinemic response that follows the ingestion of carbohydrates becomes very complex: high insulin levels, in fact, inhibit lipolysis and predispose to the accumulation of fat, and it is for this reason that we tend to keep the blood levels of this hormone very low. Since one of the multiple functions of glucose is to save and safeguard muscle proteins, the problem arises when we drastically reduce the consumption of carbohydrates, because there is a risk of favoring the breakdown of these proteins (catabolism). In this rather critical situation, the "wildcard" glutamine can come into play, which can be converted into glucose, which in turn is able to perform the fuel function for the brain and thus save glycogen and the muscle proteins. Since the conversion does not lead to an increase in insulin (on the contrary, it has been seen that **glutamine is able to modulate blood glucose levels causing a lower release of insulin**), the antilipolytic effect typically associated with it is not encountered.

From an ergogenic point of view, glutamine showed no particular effects. A study by Canow et al. who included athletes following strength training found that, even after 6 weeks of treatment, there was no improvement in either strength or muscle mass, compared to athletes who did not train. In addition, other studies have shown the ineffectiveness of glutamine in improving the resistant strength. In one of these studies, glutamine supplementation was unable to increase the number of repetitions performed on the leg press or bench press.

An important effect in the use of glutamine is related to the regulation of body weight. In a study carried out on mice that were fed a high-fat diet, supplementation with glutamine showed the ability of regulating the amount of the accumulated fat. Both glutamine and alanine added to the high-fat diet produced less body weight gain than that associated with the same diet, but without the amino acids.

Prolonged exercise and periods of intense training are associated with a decrease in the plasma concentration of glutamine; this could be a potential cause of the impairment of the immune system induced by intense exercise. Several studies have shown that supplementation with glutamine allows you to maintain its plasma concentration at constant levels following intense and prolonged exercises. Glutamine is essential for the functioning of the immune system, as it is required for the proliferation of lymphocytes; when glutamine concentrations decrease, the functions of the immune system can be compromised, increasing the susceptibility to infections. Acute oral intake of glutamine of about 20-30 g (doses up to 0.65 g/kg body weight) is well tolerated by subjects and does not lead to abnormal plasma ammonia levels, ensuring the safety of the supplement.

Glutamine is not an essential amino acid, but however, some studies have shown that when it is taken in a post-workout amino acid blend, it is able to increase the glycogen synthesis (essential for a proper muscle recovery) and also the protein synthesis. One study compared the post-workout administration of a carbohydrate blend and a carbohydrate blend with the addition of 8 g of glutamine. The results reported that 2 hours after the intake of carbohydrates and glutamine, muscle glycogen reserves increased by 25% compared to the group that had only taken carbohydrates, demonstrating the anti-catabolic and muscle recovery effect of this amino acid.

Another study looked at the effect of consuming a mixture of carbohydrates, proteins and glutamine in the 2-hour period after the training (100g of carbohydrates, 20g of protein, 8g of glutamine): the results reported an increase in the resynthesis of muscle glycogen and an increase in the protein synthesis, underlining the importance of the synergistic effect of the three compounds for muscle recovery. In addition, another study showed that glutamine can raise GH levels in the blood by four times: 2 g of glutamine taken after weight training results in a four-fold increase in GH levels 90 minutes after the administration.

In conclusion, supplementation with glutamine in sports subjects can be beneficial for supporting the immune system, for increasing the glycogen synthesis and for its important anti-catabolic effect.

In 2012, a study conducted by researchers from the Department of Experimental Medicine of the University of Parma, revealed that the combined intake of BCAA and glutamine preserves lean mass more than the intake of BCAAs alone, since the synergistic action of branched chain amino acids and glutamine manages to reduce the oxidation of the BCAAs themselves (in particular of leucine), as well as accelerates the muscle hypertrophy.

As has been amply demonstrated by several studies, leucine is the amino acid that mostly stimulates the activity of mTOR, which accelerates the protein synthesis, but to activate this synthesis, leucine needs a "help" which, according to the researchers of the University of Leicester and Louisiana State University, is glutamine. In fact, the intake of glutamine pre- and post-workout is useful, as the cells, before training, must have substantial reserves of glutamine to allow the absorption of leucine and the hypertrophy of the cells themselves. Reduced mTOR activity has been noted in glutamine-deficient cells, although leucine and other essential amino acids are present in adequate quantities.

In conclusion, the researchers believe that glutamine can stimulate mTOR in a different way from leucine, but if they are combined, these amino acids are able to increase their efficiency. This hypothesis was recently confirmed by researchers at the University of Basel, in Switzerland, who also specified that glutamine is metabolized through a glutaminolysis process that signals mTOR to accelerate the protein synthesis. Ultimately, glutamine deficiency, in addition to causing a reduction in the cell volume, negatively influences the stimulation of protein synthesis by leucine.

Dosages

The recommended intake doses are generally 3-6 g per day, usually to be taken after the training, perhaps together with creatine, BCAAs, lipoic acid and dextrose (if you want to enhance its volumizing properties). An amount of 2 to 5 g taken before falling asleep (possibly on an empty stomach and on low blood sugar levels), possibly associated with arginine and ornithine, may be useful in promoting a greater nocturnal release of growth hormone. For those who want to increase or restore their immune defenses, glutamine may be useful if taken as follows: 3 g in the morning, 3 g in the early afternoon or before training, 3 g immediately after the training (if it is done) and 3 g before falling asleep (the doses are related to the severity of the decrease in immune defenses).

Another intake methodology is the one recommended by Dr. Eric Serrano, an expert in the field of supplementation, who argues that the pre- and post-workout are the two crucial moments for the intake of glutamine and that the daily amount (divided between these two moments on training days) can be 0.17 g/kg of body weight. On rest days, 5-6 g/day seems to be a good dosage, which will need to be slightly increased (over a period of 7-10 days) if you are sick or if you are overtraining.

What is the best and safest form of glutamine to take? Some studies have shown that, unfortunately, between 50 and 85% of glutamine introduced orally does not reach the bloodstream (and therefore is not transported to the muscles and brain to detoxify it) because it is immediately used in the intestine, by the liver and from the immune system, especially in people under psychophysical stress who need to recover and have a better state of health before increasing their muscle mass. The problem is given by the fact that the athlete who has just finished a hard training or a competitive race, and who therefore has to recover the lost energy and repair the damage caused by an intense physical activity, is in a state of psychophysical stress. We can well understand how supplementation with glutamine in its free form can meet (in part) the demands of the intestine, liver and immune system, but certainly not those for muscle repair and growth.

At this point, research show how glutamine peptide can act as an optimizer of glutamine absorption, allowing it to increase its passage into the bloodstream and therefore it will be more likely to be used by the muscles.

Glutamine peptides, in addition to making this amino acid more stable in aqueous solutions (it degrades less easily into glutamic acid and ammonium ion, losing its effectiveness), are more assimilable than glutamine in its free form. It is known that amino acids can be absorbed more quickly if they are derived from small peptides rather than from an equivalent free form amino acid solution.

Furthermore, it seems that the individual amino acids do not interfere with the absorption of peptides, making us understand that there are two separate transport systems. The transport system of di- and tripeptides within the intestinal cell is carrier-mediated and requires energy. The absorption of peptides can have further advantages: their transport increases the absorption efficiency of the products of the digestion of proteins by the intestinal mucosa; moreover, if the absorption of amino acids is compromised during prolonged fasting in humans, that of peptides is still preserved (opposes the catabolism induced by low-calorie diets).

Effectiveness

Strength	Resistant strength	Mass	Endurance	Slimming	Concentration	Recovery
–	–	++	++	+++	+++	++

GLUTATHIONE

Description

Glutathione (GSH) is a tripeptide consisting of cysteine, glutamate and glycine, which is formed mainly in the liver but is contained intracellularly in practically every cell of the organism (this should underline the importance of this molecule from an evolutionary point of view). In fact, GSH, together with selenium, forms the enzyme glutathione peroxidase, a powerful antioxidant, but it can also be used as a chelator of toxic metals, helping to eliminate them from the body (therefore it mainly takes part in controlling the redox balance and intracellular organic detoxification). There is a marked variability between subjects in GSH levels in the blood and tissues, and low levels can be associated with exposure to pro-oxidants, drugs, toxins, poor diets, etc.

Even partial depletion of GSH impairs the immune function and increases the susceptibility to a wide range of xenobiotics and to oxidative damage. Low GSH levels are associated with an increased risk of numerous diseases, including cancer, cardiovascular disease, arthritis and diabetes.

Increasing endogenous GSH would represent a potentially important approach to counteract the disorders associated with its exhaustion, to improve the detoxification capacity and to protect against diseases.

The limiting factor in its production seems to be the lack of cysteine (common in situations of fasting or in diets with a low intake of meat and legumes). Intracellular levels of GSH can be reduced in some tissues, including the liver, even during short periods of fasting, such as that which occurs at night.

To stimulate its production, it is usual to use N-acetyl-cysteine, a molecule used both as an antidote to toxins and as a mucolytic (the reaction limiting precursor is provided), however there are formulations of glutathione which, if used for detoxifying purposes, should be taken just before going to bed, possibly sublingual.

Properties

Intracellular concentrations of glutathione vary between 0.5 and 10 mmol, while extracellular concentrations of glutathione are significantly lower, with values estimated in the micromolar range (this suggests a purely intracellular use and storage). Here, glutathione is found mainly in its reduced state (GSH) or in the form of its most commonly observed oxidation product, GSSG (oxidized glutathione), which is made up of two glutathione molecules linked by a disulfide bond. The GSH/GSSG redox system maintains an overall **reducing** environment in the cell, with GSH/GSSG ratios of 30-100:1 in the cytosol, nucleus and mitochondria.

This ratio is considerably lower in the endoplasmic reticulum, with reported values of 1-3:1, conditions in which disulfide bonds are generated in proteins that cross the secretory pathway (here the GSH would take part in the post-transductional control of the protein). GSSG is then converted back to its reduced state by glutathione reductase, using the NADPH that is generated mainly by the pentose phosphate pathway (it is an alternative glucose oxidation pathway to glycolysis and is essential for the production of essential molecules for the cell, such as NADPH and pentoses, and to direct pentoses towards glycolysis or gluconeogenesis).

Reduced glutathione is easily oxidized by reactive oxygen species produced from the cellular metabolism and subsequently reduced again by glutathione reductase. The redox balance of glutathione has been used as a marker of the antioxidant status in various conditions. Exercise reduces the reduced form and increases the oxidized form of glutathione. Furthermore, prolonged exercise reduces the total content of plasma and tissue glutathione over time, which suggests that glutathione may be associated with the aerobic energy metabolism and with the maintenance of muscle contraction.

Evidence

There are studies that would attest to the effectiveness of the oral administration of glutathione in increasing endogenous GSH levels. In 2014, for example, Richie et al. subjected healthy non-smoking adults aged 30-79 years to oral GSH administration for a period of 6 months (randomized double-blind), divided into three study groups with different doses (placebo, 250 mg and 1000 mg of oral GSH). Results: Blood GSH levels increased after 1, 3, and 6 months from the baseline, with both GSH doses. At 6 months, mean GSH levels increased by 30-35% in erythrocytes, plasma and lymphocytes and by 260% in buccal cells in the high-dose group ($p < 0.05$). GSH levels increased by 17 and 29% in blood and erythrocytes, respectively, in the low-dose group ($p < 0.05$).

A recent study recruited 75 men who were split into three groups and received glutathione and citrulline, citrulline alone, or a placebo per day. The study lasted 8 weeks, during which the subjects followed a weight training program.

Participants regularly completed testing sessions for the body structure and muscle strength, as well as underwent periodic blood tests.

Between the various groups, no significant changes were noted in the total fat mass, while lean mass increased in the glutathione + citrulline group, in comparison with the other two groups, starting from the fourth week of training.

In conclusion, the authors highlight that the administration of glutathione + citrulline improved the lean mass after 4 weeks of weight training; moreover, its intake has been associated with the improvement of muscle strength, all without side effects. In fact, subsequent studies would have demonstrated the usefulness of glutathione in:

- supporting the athlete's antioxidant defenses;
- reducing the concentrations of post-workout muscle damage markers;
- improving the aerobic performance;
- reducing the risk of accidents.

However, it seems that, due to the fragility of this tripeptide (inability to resist the digestive juices), not many studies report results like the one we just mentioned. Other formulations will likely need to be considered to affect the GSH stocks. Obviously, the best form could be an intravenous infusion or intramuscular, but the dosages for these types of administration are reported only as an adjuvant chemotherapy (1.5 g/m^2, corresponding to about 2500 mg).

However, sublingual and liposomal formulations have also been marketed to increase the chances of getting GSH intact into the bloodstream and the results appear to be promising. In 2018 Sinha et al. conducted a 1-month pilot clinical study on the administration of oral liposomal GSH in two doses (500 and 1000 mg of GSH per day) in healthy adults. GSH levels in blood, erythrocytes, plasma and peripheral blood mononuclear cells (PBMCs) of 12 subjects were assessed at baseline and after 1, 2, and 4 weeks of GSH administration. The results: GSH levels increased as early as 1 week, with maximum increases of 40% in the peripheral blood, 25% in erythrocytes, 28% in plasma and 100% in PBMCs, which instead occurred after 2 weeks ($p < 0.05$). The increases in GSH were accompanied by reductions in oxidative stress biomarkers.

Dosages
Depending on the various studies and formulations, dosages of 250-1000 mg/day are used, followed by dose- and time-dependent increases in the GSH pool. Usually, the situation returns to baseline 1 month after the complete washout. The infusional, sublingual and liposomal forms and, lastly, the simple oral ones are preferred.

Effectiveness

Strength	Resistant strength	Mass	Endurance	Slimming	Concentration	Recovery
+	+	+	+++	–	–	++++

GLYCEROL

Description
Glycerol is a molecule normally present in our body. It is a tricarbonate alcohol (formed by three carbon atoms), which is the hydrophilic part of the fundamental components of our plasma membranes: triglycerides. When the body uses its fat reserves, it first breaks them down into fatty acids and glycerol; the latter is transformed into glucose in the liver, becoming a source of energy for the cellular metabolism. On the contrary, in conditions of high blood sugar (after a large meal), glucose is transferred to the liver deposits, where it is accumulated in the form of glycogen; if the liver reserves have already been saturated, the newly formed glucose will instead be converted into glycerol and it will be used for the synthesis of reserve triglycerides and so on. Currently, the glycerol on the market is exclusively of vegetable origin and is obtained by the hydrolysis of vegetable fats, such as coconut oil.

Properties
As an energy source, it is not very effective, because several hours pass before its degradation and it remains in the body for a long time, but its main feature is that it binds to water and retains it. Dehydration in athletes alters both the cardiovascular and thermoregulatory function. It can inhibit the resistance to exercise if the loss of fluids during performance exceeds 2% of body weight. This hydrosaline loss cannot be prevented, because it is part of our body's normal physiological response to physical exercise.

This aspect is especially critical if the exercise is conducted in climatic environments at high temperatures. To counterbalance this unfavorable situation, athletes can aim to create a kind of hyperhydration state by consuming excess fluids before the competition. With this kind of "hydroelectrolytic supercompensation", individuals have a greater ability to tolerate the loss of fluids resulting from exertion and dehydration. Excess of pre-exercise fluids increases the thermoregulation capacity and the increase in plasma volume favorably modifies the cardiac output.

However, preventive hyperhydration is generally accompanied by an increase in diuresis, which can result in a significant discomfort during a workout that is conducted at a fast pace. Here glycerol comes into play, the infusion and ingestion of which has been used in research for over 60 years, with a very wide range of therapeutic interventions. The most effective actions relate to the body's water balance (treatment of post-stroke cerebral edema, glaucoma, intracranial hypertension, massive rehydration after gastrointestinal disorders, as a laxative). It can be used also in the supplementation field to obtain certain effects on the cardiovascular and thermoregulation capacity, and on the sports performance.

It should be remembered, however, that for some years (precisely since 2010) WADA (World Anti-Doping Association) included glycerol among the diuretics and masking agents. This is because the volume expansion effect can mask the intake of other prohibited substances.

Evidence

As we have said, the effect of glycerol, if we talk about the aspects inherent to its supplementation, is affecting the body's water percentage. The properties and the manner largely depend on the dilution percentage of a given quantity of product in an aqueous solution. This quantity is calculated according to the body weight of the subject (kg). The serum concentration of glycerol is about 0.05 mmol/L at rest, and can increase up to 0.30 mmol/L during periods of marked lipolysis (induced by prolonged exercises or by a significant caloric restriction). The state of the body's reserves in these situations is also fundamental. During fasting, for example, a normal man produces about 18 g of glycerol in 24 hours and this amount increases when there is a significant depletion of the carbohydrate reserves (as occurs in the case of dietary restriction of carbohydrates or following prolonged workouts). When glycerol is consumed orally, it is rapidly absorbed mainly in the small intestine and its plasma concentrations increase in proportion to the ingested dose. It is normally distributed equally among all the fluid compartments of the body (with the exception of the cerebral medulla) and promotes an increase on the osmotic gradient. When administered at doses above 1 g/kg body weight, the serum concentration of this molecule can increase to about 20 mmol/L, causing a 10 mOsmol/kg increase in plasma osmolality and reflexively increasing a retention of liquids up to 700 mL in the bloodstream. We mentioned earlier that a marked increase in pre-exercise hydration produces an increase in renal filtrate and diuresis. There are studies that compare heavy hydrosaline hydration and supplementation with glycerol in order to argue that glycerol can be used effectively in this sense. Some studies even find a better correlation between these approaches and the final results such as the **improvement of thermoregulation and of the overall hydration with the use of glycerol**. Some studies also show an improvement in endurance performances of about 20% (Montner et al., 1996; Hitchins et al., 1999), while others disagree on this point (Murray et al., 1991; Latka et al., 1997). In the kidney, glycerol, through an increase in its concentration gradient in the medullary area, produces an increased reabsorption of water in the nephron and tends to decrease the diuresis, further saving liquids for the athletic performance, with a net decrease in urination. As the experience in the field shows, glycerol has been **able to prevent muscle cramps induced by physical efforts of long duration**, for example in cycling and football, in subjects predisposed to these problems. However, by virtue of its gluconeogenetic metabolism, the plasma concentration of glycerol tends to decrease over time during the performance and the aforementioned advantages gradually decrease too. Studies on the performance and thermoregulation are controversial, but the literature is fairly in agreement on the effect of "moving body fluids".

A 2015 study (van Rosendal et al.) examined the effects of rehydration with different regimens (oral and intravenous), with or without oral glycerol, on hydration indices and the endocrine system. Nine male endurance athletes were dehydrated by 4%, then rehydrated with 150% of the fluids lost through four protocols: (a) oral = oral fluids only; (b) oral glycerol = oral fluids with added glycerol (1.5 g/kg); (c) = 50% IV fluids, 50% oral fluids; (d) = 50% IV fluids, 50% oral fluids with added glycerol (1.5 g/kg), using a randomized crossover design for the study.

The subjects then completed a cycling performance test. The restoration of the plasma volume was higher for the IV oral glycerol> IV> oral> oral glycerol study groups, respectively. Urine volume was reduced in both IV study groups compared to oral. The IV and IV oral glycerol groups resulted in lower aldosterone and cortisol levels during the rehydration. IV administration with oral glycerol resulted in a maximal fluid retention. In summary, IV conditions resulted in higher water retention than oral levels, and lower levels of regulatory fluids and stress compared to both oral conditions.

This study concludes that IV infusion of fluids associated with an oral glycerol intake (both practices prohibited by WADA) achieved a more rapid and complete restoration of plasma volume and net water balance, which was maintained during the following exercise and was associated with lower levels of fluid regulation and lower stress hormone levels. The oral fluid replacement + oral glycerol group also proved more valid than oral fluid replacement alone, confirming the previous studies. These changes were also associated with a performance improvement of 3.5-4.1%.

Therefore, the use of glycerol would allow to obtain a sort of **persistent hyperhydration at least during physical activity** and would consequently provide benefits regarding better thermoregulation and better resistance to stress, especially in hot environments. Despite the small number of studies that correlate glycerol and its relationship with muscular effort, it therefore appears to be an interesting supplement due to its peculiarities and safety.

The last aspect is proven especially in light of the great use that has been made over the years in the medical field, for the management even important pathologies. Side effects from glycerol ingestion during the supplementary protocol are rare, but, in case of too high doses, they include nausea, gastrointestinal disturbances, lightheadedness, blurred vision. For this reason, it is advisable to carry out tests of these approaches during training to see the individual response of each athlete. Glycerol derivatives such as glycerin are used as enemas for persistent constipation, in order to take advantage of the osmotic effect of liquid retention even in this situation.

Dosages

The analysis of studies in this area indicates that the athletes who use this supplement are above all those of resistance/endurance sports. The protocols for these subjects provide for the ingestion of 1.2 g/kg of body weight in 26 mL/kg of body weight of liquid, over a period of 60 minutes, within 30 minutes of exercise. So, for example, a 70 kg person should dissolve 84 g of glycerol (1.2 g × 70 kg) in a solution of about 1.8 liters of water (26 mL × 70 kg) and drink it in 60 minutes, letting the body adapt itself without ingesting anything in the 30 minutes preceding the sporting activity. To prevent the metabolization of glycerol and the decline of the above benefits, a maintenance intake of 0.125 g/kg of body weight in a volume equal to 5 mL/kg can also be programmed during the exercise, which will delay dehydration. Here too, our hypothetical subject of 70 kg will have to dissolve 8.75 g of glycerol (0.125 g × 70 kg) in 350 mL of water (5 mL × 70 kg). In post-exercise, if you want to induce a quick restoration of the hydroelectrolytic balance, you can still take 1 g/kg of glycerol for every 1.5 liters of liquids introduced, then 70 g of glycerol for every 1.5 liters, again in the case of the previous subject. However, it must be taken into account that these protocols should be tried in training, since the increase in water retention caused by glycerol produces an increase in body weight and the athlete must measure themself with this added weight. The properties of glycerol can also be effective in the case of bodybuilding. Here, the desired effect is that of a breakdown agent, favoring hydration at the muscle and not at the subcutaneous level, in order to draw liquids from the interstitial tissue and thus highlight the individual fiber bundles of the subcutaneous muscles.

The doses of intake are similar (about 0.8-1 g of glycerol/kg of body weight), but are accompanied by a smaller volume of liquids (about 500 mL).

Finally, we recall that a 2012 study (van Rosendal et al.) established that doses higher than 0.032 ± 0.010 g/kg of lean mass (much lower than those required for rehydration) lead to a detectable urinary excretion of glycerol. Therefore, athletes under WADA jurisdiction should absolutely avoid the intake of glycerol.

Effectiveness

Strength	Resistant strength	Mass	Endurance	Slimming	Concentration	Recovery
−	+	−	++	−	−	+++

GREEN TEA

Description

Tea is the most popular drink in the world, with more than 4000 years of tradition. It comes from the leaves of the *Camelia sinensis* plant, a small, highly branched evergreen tree with oblong, toothed and sharp oval leaves.

Green tea is obtained from the tea leaves that are directly dried after harvesting, while the leaves that undergo fermentation in a stream of hot air before being dried provide black tea, which is richer in caffeine than green tea. The drying process deactivates the oxidizing enzymes but leaves the antioxidant polyphenols, which are the main ingredients of tea, intact. 80% of the tea consumed in the world is black tea, while 20% is green tea. Black tea is more popular in Western countries, while green tea is mostly consumed in Asia.

The polyphenols in tea are known as catechins, which are also present in chocolate, red wine and apples, and to a lesser extent in black tea due to fermentation.

Properties

Green tea is not only a powerful antioxidant, but it can also help prevent cancer, provide cardiovascular and brain protection, and promote fat loss.

Chen Zang, a famous Chinese pharmacist who lived during the Tang dynasty, said: "Every medicine cures a particular disease, but tea is the medicine that cures any disease."

One of the most interesting research developments in recent years has been the discovery of green tea's extraordinary anti-aging and anti-cancer properties. Countries with high consumption of this product (mainly China and Japan) have been found to have a low percentage of cancer patients. In Okinawa, a Japanese island located between Japan, China and India, affected by the influences of these cultures, there is the highest number of centenarians in the world and scholars believe that this may be partly due to the abundant consumption of green tea and turmeric. In Japan, women who teach the tea ceremony (and therefore drink much more tea than the average person) are known for their longevity; cases of cancer deaths in this group are very rare.

Evidence

In a recent study, the authors concluded that a large daily intake of green tea, about 10 cups, is able to extend the life of people who are 80 years old, but can also extend the life of younger people, avoiding premature death, mainly due to cancer. One experiment found that drinking two cups of tea a day reduced the incidence of lung cancer in 850 male smokers by 66%.

Drinking tea can also protect against skin cancer. In fact, it reduces the production of melanin by limiting its overproduction and limiting the inflammatory reaction to sun exposure. The **caffeine** present in tea is responsible for the stimulating action at the level of the central nervous system, which manifests itself with an increase in the intellectual activities, alertness and mental tone. However, this effect is counterbalanced by **theanine**, which promotes brain relaxation by reducing anxiety and stress, without altering the state of alertness. In addition, green tea protects brain neurons and inhibits the breakdown of the neurotransmitter acetylcholine, necessary for memory and learning, which is lacking in those suffering from the Alzheimer's disease.

From a cardiovascular point of view, green tea appears to be able to lower cholesterol and in an eight-year study of 1,500 middle-aged individuals, it was found that those who drank more than 60 cL of green tea a day had a 65% lower risk of developing hypertension. A recent study of 340 subjects with a history of heart attack, conducted in the US, showed an approximately **50% reduction in the risk of heart attack** among those who consume at least one cup of tea a day, compared to those who do not consume it at all.

But the beneficial actions of green tea do not end there. In fact, green tea has recently been proposed as a supplement to be combined in slimming diets. It has a **thermogenic effect**, as it increases the production of heat, thus making the body burn more calories; but not only: it increases the release of CCK, a hormone of the intestine that **reduces the appetite** and enhances the effect of adrenaline, a powerful fat-burning hormone, inhibits the pancreatic-gastric lipase, which is the enzyme responsible for the digestion of fats, and also inhibits alpha-amylases, thus reducing the absorption of carbohydrates.

In a study of overweight and obese women, Cardoso Gabrielle Aparecida et al. wanted to examine the effects of consuming green tea for six weeks, combined with weight training. The study found that in the green tea group there was an **increase in the resting basal metabolic rate, muscle strength and muscle mass, and a reduction in fat mass, triglycerides and waist circumference, significantly higher than those induced from training only**.

In a double-blind study, 640 mg per day of green tea polyphenols was supplemented to 35 men for four weeks during a weight training program. At the end of the trial, the subjects who had taken the placebo had higher levels of CPK, indicating a greater muscle damage and a lower recovery capacity.

In another study, 12 men took a green tea supplement and after 30 minutes of cycling at 60% of their maximum, they experienced a **17% increase in the rate of fat oxidation**.

The increase in the fat oxidation was also the result of a study published in 2017: the supplementation of 500 mg of green tea per day, taken for 8 weeks, **increased the fat oxidation and the values of GLUT4** (the best known and studied glucose transporter) during the post-recovery period: participants had performed a 60-minute cycling workout (75% VO_{2max}). In 2018, they published the results obtained from a double-blind case-control study started in August 2012 on 73 women, aged between 18 and 65 years, with a BMI ≥27 and with LDL values ≥130 mg/dL. The study shows that the women treated for 6 weeks with green tea extract had **a significant reduction in LDL levels, equal to 4.8%, and an increase, equal to 25.7%, in leptin**, despite not having changed the anthropometric parameters of their body composition.

Several studies on the properties of green tea have been published in recent years. In 2018, a study suggested that the green tea intake combined with exercise (high-intensity interval walking, or alternating between fast and slow walking) caused a **higher reduction of the postprandial glucose concentrations** in a group of 12 sedentary subjects, compared to the group that only exercised and took a placebo.

Regarding sports activity, the importance of green tea was seen in the recovery after the physical activity: 20 untrained men performed exercises with the aim of inducing soreness of the triceps muscle. Blood samples were taken at different times to determine the serum markers of muscle damage, oxidative stress and antioxidants. **It was found that supplementation with green tea (500 mg per day), despite the persistent sensation of pain, had positive effects on the recovery after an intense physical exercise.**

In 2019, a further study divided 16 young crossfit athletes into two groups: one group consumed two capsules containing 250 mg of green tea extract, once a day for 6 weeks, and the second group took placebo capsules. **The consumption of 500 mg of green tea extract after 6 weeks was correlated with a marked increase in the antioxidant capacity in the blood, with significantly higher values of superoxide dismutase.**

Dosages

It can be taken either as a drink or as a capsule supplement. The stimulating effect of the infusion is maximal for a short infusion time. Prolonged infusion results in a higher extraction of tannins; these, in turn, tend to bind to caffeine, which becomes less absorbed. In order not to destroy the active ingredients of green tea, it is recommended that the water that is poured into the cup or teapot (according to the chosen method) is not boiling, but a few degrees lower (about 80° C), and it should be left in the infusion for no more than one and a half to two minutes. As a capsule supplement, the effective dosage is 450-900 mg per day of a mixture containing all polyphenols, half of which must be EGCG (epigallocatechin gallate).

Effectiveness

Strength	Resistant strength	Mass	Endurance	Slimming	Concentration	Recovery
+	+	+	++	+++	++	++

GUARANA

Description

The fruits of this plant, whose scientific name is *Paullinia cupana*, are small red capsules that generally contain only one seed. After being dried in the sun, the shiny ovoid seeds are lightly roasted, in order to free them from the integument and form a paste with water and, often, with cassava flour or cocoa powder. The aim is to obtain a stimulating beverage.

The main components of these seeds are: tannins, polyphenols (catechins and epicatechins), caffeine (3-5%) and other xanthine derivatives (theophylline, theobromine etc.). They also contain saponins, resins, terpene derivatives and guaranine, a compound similar to caffeine, present in considerable quantities, whose stimulating and tonic effects are modulated by the activity of tannins. The action of guarana is basically similar to that of coffee, compared to which it is considerably richer in tannins and caffeine.

Properties
This plant is traditionally used to increase the body's physical resistance in critical situations. Its chronic intake has a stimulating effect on the memory, while it acts acutely at the level of the respiratory system, where it induces a relaxation of the bronchial smooth muscles and reduces the effect of bronchoconstrictive substances. Behavioral and toxicological studies on guarana in repeated administrations excluded toxic effects and activities other than the stimulant and tonic one. Due to the tannin content, prolonged administration of guarana-based preparations can have a slight astringent effect in the intestine. The beverage made from guarana has, other than stimulating, also anti-diarrheal and anti-neuralgic properties.

The effect obtained was found to be superior to that of a similar dose of synthetic caffeine. In the brain, caffeine stimulates the attention and ideation, decreasing the feeling of fatigue. At the cardiovascular level, it stimulates the contractile force of the heart muscle, increasing the myocardial consumption of oxygen, and has a moderate peripheral and diuretic vasodilating action; moreover, it acts by facilitating the burning of fats in all tissues.

Evidence
In 1989, a US study demonstrated the particular property of the substances extracted from guarana seed to prevent the formation of blood clots and to eliminate the clots that are already formed.

Its action determines:

- an excitation of the central nervous system at the cortical (a stimulation of the waking state, a decrease in the sense of fatigue, nervousness, insomnia and tremors) and bulbar (vasomotor and respiratory center) levels;
- a stimulation of myofibrils in the heart, with an increased frequency and a stronger contraction;
- a bronchial spasmolytic action;
- a general vasodilating action;
- a weak diuretic effect;
- a stimulation of the gastric secretion (not recommended for those suffering from gastritis);
- a stimulation of lipolysis.

Furthermore, the tannins present in the extract stimulate the secretion and increase the average life of a lipolytic hormone (adrenaline), thus proving **useful in slimming diets**, while the caffeine content has also proved useful in the lipid metabolism (Lima et al., 2006): a 2018 study by Da Silva Lima et al. has proved how another way of increasing the energy metabolism occurs through an improvement in the mitochondrial biogenesis; finally, the review by Marques et al. (2018) summarizes its properties in this specific field. As for a more in-depth examination of the psychotropic effects, please refer to the chapter on supplementation for concentration.

Dosages
The titrated dry extract is mostly present in commercially available preparations and its dosage varies from 500 mg to 1 g per day. Due to the presence of caffeine, it is preferable to take guarana in the morning or in the early afternoon, and not to exceed the daily dose of 3 g.

Effectiveness

Strength	Resistant strength	Mass	Endurance	Slimming	Concentration	Recovery
+	++	−	++	+++	+++	++

HMB

Description
β-hydroxy-β-methyl-butyric acid (HMB) is a metabolite of the essential amino acid leucine (LEU) and derives directly from alpha-ketoisocaproate acid (alpha-KIC). The importance of leucine in the stimulation of protein synthesis is now known and clear to all: about 80% of this amino acid introduced with the diet is used in the complex mechanism of protein synthesis, while the remainder is converted into alpha-ketoisocaproate and (only 5%) in HMB. This reaction takes place in the cytosol of liver cells and is mediated by the KIC-dioxygenase enzyme. Finally, HMB will first be converted into HMB-CoA and then into HMG-CoA, which will lead to the synthesis of cholesterol through the mevalonate pathway.

Properties
The use of HMB as a sports supplement dates back to 1996, when Dr. Nissen demonstrated how HMB was useful for increasing the lean mass and athletic performance. In fact, HMB, acting like leucine, growth hormone, insulin-like growth factors (IGF-1 and IGF-2), testosterone, etc., directly stimulates the complex machinery of mTOR (mammalian Target of Rapamycin), which in turn leads to an increase in the protein synthesis.

HMB, acting at the level of the MAPK/ERK metabolic pathway, determines the increase in the expression of myogenin and MEF2, in the levels of GH (growth hormone) and in the mRNAs regulated by IGF-1, causing the proliferation of myoblasts and leading to an increase in muscle fibers. It is important to emphasize that HMB not only works in the anabolic phase, but above all in the anti-catabolic phase. HMB would in fact favor of the reduction of the expression of the tumor factor of proteolysis (PIF), which normally leads to the degradation of all nuclear factors and to the activation of proteasomes, those multiprotein complexes responsible for the degradation of proteins. For these reasons, HMB is particularly suitable for sarcopenic subjects or for those affected by cachexia, since, by reducing the catabolic processes affecting the proteins and muscle tissue, it is able to avoid the progression of these diseases and also increase the muscle mass.

The intake of HMB can be associated with that of leucine: the combined action of the two substances could in fact stimulate the anabolism in an excellent way, since leucine mainly induces the protein synthesis, while HMB works in the anti-catabolic phase, which is anabolic. Therefore, this allows you to have a better result in terms of muscle mass gain. Physiologically, it is very difficult to obtain sufficient quantities of HMB from the diet alone, as only 5% of the leucine taken with the diet converts into β-hydroxy-methylbutyrate; therefore, with a calculator in hand, it would take 60 g of leucine to obtain 3 g of HMB (which is the quantity necessary to exert the aforementioned effects), a very difficult amount to reach with the diet alone.

Evidence
As a sports supplement, HMB has multiple qualities, not only aimed at increasing muscle mass, but also at increasing athletic performance. A 2011 double-blind study conducted on male and female trained subjects, showed how a supplementation of 3 g of HMB for 7 weeks, divided into three daily doses, improved all anthropometric and athletic parameters. In the experimental group, there were significant changes in the **increase in FFM or lean mass**, a reduction in fat mass and an **increase in the training loads**. Subsequently, the researchers evaluated the anaerobic capacity of the subjects, verifying how the power expressed by the subjects of the experimental group increased significantly, together with the fatigue resistance index and the aerobic capacity (VO_{2max}). In another study by Matthew Vukovich et al. the effectiveness of HMB has also been demonstrated for its ergogenic effect

on endurance: expert cyclists supplemented with 3 g of HMB per day showed a **significant increase in VO$_{2max}$ and a decrease in lactic acid levels**, unlike those belonging to the control group, who had instead taken only 3 g of leucine. Finally, the researchers measured the main anabolic hormones, the catabolic hormones and the factors that regulate the inflammatory response. The most important results concerned the increase in growth hormone, testosterone and a reduction in the concentration of interleukin-6 and interleukin-1, the inflammatory cytokines.

Another very current research conducted in 2014, highlighted the extraordinary capabilities of HMB in terms of **increasing the muscle strength**: for 12 weeks, the participants of this study took a quantity of HMB-FA (Hydorxy-Methylbutyrate-Free Acid) of 3.4 g/day, divided into three doses. Researchers evaluated squat, bench press, and deadlift ceilings every four weeks and found dramatic changes. For the squat, there was a 25% increase (from week 0 to week 12), for the bench press an 18% increase and for the deadlift the maximum load increased by 16%.

Later, the researchers found that the body composition improved in the experimental group, recording a decrease in fat mass of 5.4 kg (from 17.9 to 12.5 kg), while lean mass increased by a whopping 7.4. kg (67.1 to 74.5 kg). As for hormonal dosages, the researchers recorded a significant **decrease in blood cortisol** of 4.1 µg/dl compared to the initial measurement.

Table 44.5 Changes in ceilings after 12 weeks of HMB administration

	Study weeks				p values
	0	4	8	12	
Total force (kg)					
Placebo	426.7±14.5	444.6±14.5	457.8±14.5	452.0±14.5	0.0001
HMB-FA	426.7±14.5	458.7±14.4	477.6±14.5	503.8±14.5	
Squat (kg)					
Placebo	143.8±5.2	150.4±5.2	155.4±5.2	151.1±5.2	0.0001
HMB-FA	143.7±5.2	154.9±5.2	162.4±5.2	179.9±5.2	
Bench press (kg)					
Placebo	112.9±6.6	116.4±6.6	118.5±6.6	116.7±6.6	0.02
HMB-FA	112.4±6.6	120.8±6.6	123.7±6.6	125.2±6.6	
Deadlift (kg)					
Placebo	170.4±9.2	178.2±9.2	184.3±9.2	184.5±9.2	0.009
HMB-FA	170.3±9.2	182.7±9.2	191.2±9.2	198.4±9.2	
Wingate peak power (W)					
Placebo	879.1±38.3	927.0±38.3	987.2±38.3	982.5±38.3	0.01
HMB-FA	879.7±38.3	936.0±38.3	980.7±38.3	1.038.6±38.3	
Vertical jump power (W)					
Placebo	5.224±73	5.636±73	5.839±73	5.854±73	0.001
HMB-FA	5.219±73	5.835±73#	6.039±73	6.211±73	

A study by Jay Hoffman of the University of Central Florida in Orlando, found that HMB could help prevent the effects of overtraining. Intense exercise, as well as extreme military training or repeated cross-training sessions, often leads to overtraining, depression of the immune system and muscle catabolism. This could lead to an impaired performance, upper respiratory infections and damage to muscle tissues. Supplementing HMB (3 g/day) for 23 days reduced the symptoms of immune suppression, the inflammation and muscle loss in soldiers engaged in intense military training, compared to the placebo group (fake HMB).

Examples of stressful workouts include 6 to 8 hours of night sailing through rough seas, carrying heavy loads for long distances, and severe sleep deprivation.

These quite striking data, may suggest how HMB can be used for all sports, from power to endurance ones, without forgetting the therapeutic and preventive use it possesses against those pathologies that lead to a degeneration of the muscle tissues.

Dosages

At the administration level, the effective dose of HMB is 3 g, divided into three intakes with the main meals (breakfast, lunch and dinner). The dosage can rise to 6 g/day in people who are severely underweight or with debilitating diseases (cachexia, sarcopenia and even cancer). The free form of HMB (HMB-FA) is the most effective and has a higher bioavailability level than the calcium salt form (HMB-Ca). If taken 30 minutes before the training, as in anticipation of a particularly intense and expensive athletic performance in terms of Kcal, it reduces the production of lactic acid and the catabolic processes in the muscles and slows the increase of free radicals.

Effectiveness

Strength	Resistant strength	Mass	Endurance	Slimming	Concentration	Recovery
+++	++	+++	++	++	–	++

7-KETO-DHEA

7-keto-dehydroepiandrosterone (7-Keto-DHEA), also known as 7-oxoprasterone or oxo-dehydroepiandrosterone, is a prohormone produced by the metabolism of dehydroepiandrosterone (DHEA) prohormone. The 7-Keto-DHEA produced by the body derives from the oxidation of DHEA by 7-alpha-hydroxylase and 7-dehydrogenase, in the cells of the reticular zone of the adrenal glands, brain glial cells and skin fibroblasts, hepatocytes and gonads. 7-Keto-DHEA is not converted directly into testosterone or estrogen, so it has been studied as a potentially more manageable "relative" of DHEA, as it does not cause any side effects due to a possible hormonal imbalance caused by an excessive production of testosterone (in women) or estrogen (in men). Around the age of 50 , 7-Keto-DHEA levels drop by 50%. The World Anti-Doping Association (WADA) lists 7-Keto-DHEA as a prohibited anabolic agent.

Properties

The antiaging effects of DHEA are now widely known, while the fact that some of the beneficial actions procured by the administration of this hormone are attributable to hormones derived from the metabolism of DHEA (such as 7-Keto-DHEA), is less known. The reduced production of 7-Keto-DHEA contributes to the so-called immunosenescence phenomenon, which is one of the mechanisms linked to aging.

The progressive decline in the hormone derived from DHEA, together with the possible increase in cortisol levels, is one of the causes of the loss of the immune system function, with the relative predisposition to contract infections and to develop chronic inflammation, autoimmune diseases and cancers. At an immunological level, 7-Keto-DHEA performs its functions by antagonizing the action of glucocorticoids at the receptor level, especially on immune system cells, carrying out an action on the induction of interleukin-2 and of the whole system of TH1-dependent cytokines, with a significant activation of the cell-mediated immunity, controlling the pro-inflammatory cytokines of the TH2 system (interleukin-4, 6, 10) and optimizing the production of the anti-infective antibodies.

7-Keto-DHEA causes fat loss by activating the thermogenesis mechanism, which is characterized by the production of heat from food. Maintaining thermogenesis at good levels allows us to optimize the basal metabolism, which tends to deteriorate with aging, and which decreases every time we undergo a diet. 7-Keto-DHEA activates the thermogenesis through the activation of the mitochondrial thermogenesis, through a strong induction of three liver enzymes that perform a lipolytic action on liver fatty acids (malic enzyme, glycerol-3-phosphate-dehydrogenase, acetyl-CoA- oxidase), and through the activation of the UCP2-3 uncoupling proteins at the mitochondrial level, located in muscle and adipose tissue, which are involved in the production of energy from fat storages.

Both actions seem to be supported by a direct action of 7-Keto-DHEA and by the increased production of T3, which derives from the anti-cortisol action of 7-Keto-DHEA at the hypothalamic level. Furthermore, while not converting into testosterone, it exerts a positive effect on the libido and on the production and mobility of spermatozoa, which would support its use in male reproductive disorder therapies.

Evidence

The most important studies on the effects of 7-Keto-DHEA on the immune system were performed on a group of macaques with SIV and on a group of HIV-infected patients. In both cases, in addition to an improvement in the clinical and prognostic picture, there was a highlight in the optimization of leukocyte levels and in particular of lymphocytes, with a normalization of the CD4/CD8 ratio. A work by Doctor Zenk of the University of Minnesota Research Center, has highlighted how the administration of 7-Keto-DHEA to a group of elderly people optimized all their immunological functions, restoring a youth-like functioning with an increase in neutrophils, CD4 and Natural Killer cells, and a CD8 reduction.

In a double-blind study on 30 overweight patients subjected to a controlled diet (about 1800 Kcal/day) and mild physical activity, the administration of 200 mg/day of 7-Keto-DHEA resulted in an activation of the basal metabolism, with a 5-6% increase in plasma FT3 levels, as well as a weight loss of about 6.5 kg in 2 months (versus 2.1 kg in the control group). This loss was related exclusively to the fat mass, with a preservation and a slight enhancement of the lean mass (as opposed to the control group). This last notable effect would be attributed to its anti-catabolic-antiglucocorticoid effect and to it inductive action on IGF-1 levels.

A 2007 study showed that the administering 7-Keto-DHEA to overweight adult subjects, in combination with a calorie restricted diet, effectively reversed the decline in the resting metabolic rate (RMR), which is normally associated with diets. 7-Keto-DHEA has been shown to possess the ability to increase RMR by 1.4% above baseline levels and has been shown to lead to a daily increase in RMR of 5.4% when administered with a low calorie diet. In a study carried out at the Department of Endocrinology of the University of Prague, they highlighted the ability of 7-Keto-DHEA to moderately reduce total cholesterol and LDL levels, and to increase HDL cholesterol and apolipoprotein A-1, both of which are protection factors for the cardiovascular risk.

At the same dosage, these effects appeared more evident than with the administration of DHEA. The data obtained in a 2015 study published in *The Journal of Steroid Biochemistry and Molecular Biology*, showed that 7-Keto-DHEA is a metabolic modulator that increased the glycolytic flow of Sertoli cells (hSC), which are responsible for spermatogenesis.

Higher concentrations of 7-Keto-DHEA also increased the lactate production, which is extremely important for the successful progression of spermatogenesis *in vivo*, without causing any alteration of the intra-cellular oxidative profile of hSCs. A Phase 1 safety study in humans by Davidson et al. at the Chicago Center for Clinical Research, has shown that dosages up to 200 mg/day for 4 weeks do not cause any adverse side effects, that the peak plasma concentration occurs in about 2 hours and that the half-life is also 2 hours. Primate studies have shown that even prolonged treatment at high doses (500 mg/kg) is free from any toxic effects.

Dosages
It is preferable to use 7-Keto-DHEA alone in patients in whom DHEA is contraindicated (acne, hirsutism, androgenic alopecia, polycystic ovary syndrome, neoplasms or hormone-dependent preneoplastic states), in cases where DHEA has caused side effects or when estrogen and testosterone levels are optimal, and you do not want to change them. The normally recommended dosage is 50-200 mg/day. 7-Keto-DHEA should preferably be taken after the main meals (2 times a day), divided into two equal doses, in order to maintain steady plasma levels. If you want to optimize its thermogenic and muscle mass conservation actions, it is preferable to take it 2 hours before physical activity.

Effectiveness

Strength	Resistant strength	Mass	Endurance	Slimming	Concentration	Recovery
–	–	+	–	+++	+	+

KIC: ALPHA-KETOISOCAPROIC ACID

Description
Strength athletes who also seek muscle hypertrophy turn more frequently to supplements and/or substances with a mainly anabolic function. However, it is important to consider that there are also alternative ways related to anti-catabolism that allow you to preserve and improve your muscle mass. Alpha-ketoisocaproic acid (KIC) is mainly used as a supplement for its anti-catabolic effect, intended for protein and muscle saving, although it is not well known or marketed probably due to the high cost of production (and consequently of sale).

KIC is the keto acid of leucine (an important branched amino acid that controls muscle protein metabolism). Branched chain keto acids (BCKA) are very similar to branched chain amino acids (BCAAs) and among the BCKAs, KIC is perhaps the most important; for this reason, sportsmen in general, but especially those who undergo intense training, could use it or at least take it into consideration. However, alpha-ketoisocaproic acid has an efficacy that does not depend on the presence of leucine, but appears mainly due to its metabolite, HMB.

Properties
KIC is essential for the production of energy in the muscles and for the detoxification from ammonia. During high-intensity exercises, such as weight training, ammonia is produced in high quantities, playing an important role in muscle fatigue.

KIC could increase what is called "anabolic drive" (let's say an aid for protein synthesis) thanks to its stimulation in the secretion of insulin. Both leucine and KIC have been shown to stimulate the secretion of insulin, which increases the transport of amino acids within the cells, thus increasing both the anabolic and anti-catabolic capacity.

If we analyze KIC, we note that it carries out numerous positive actions in the muscle cell, and in fact it is involved in a better nitrogen balance, an antioxidant action and in the elimination of ammonia, but the most significant action concerns its ability to block ACTH and cortisol; therefore, KIC is considered a true anti-catabolic agent which reduces the damage of muscle tissue and accelerates the recovery. The intake of KIC also increases the level of HMB (β-hydroxy-β-methyl-butyric acid), another key metabolite of leucine.

Evidence

A 1984 study on rats, published in the *Biochemical Journal*, reported that leucine is able to stimulate the protein synthesis, but without being able to reduce its degradation (catabolism) in the absence of transamination. From here, we understand that the anti-catabolic effect of leucine, unlike the anabolic one, requires transamination. On the contrary, KIC has anti-catabolic rather than anabolic effects, which means, it can decrease the muscle degradation but cannot stimulate its synthesis.

Indeed, it has been shown that supplementation with KIC, with relatively high doses, shows a decrease in the rate of excretion of 3-methylhistidine (an indicator of contractile muscle degradation) in patients with Duchenne muscular dystrophy.

A recent study conducted at Kingston University (UK) also examined the effects of supplementation with KIC and β-hydroxy-β-methyl-butyric acid (HMB) on parameters and symptoms induced by muscle damage, following eccentric exercises. Six men followed an exercise protocol that induced muscle damage on two different occasions. The subjects took 0.3 g of KIC/kg with a total of 3 g of HMB or placebo for 14 days prior to the exercise protocol. The results showed that HMB + KIC reduced the signs and symptoms of exercise-induced muscle damage.

For years, the effect of KIC has been studied in association with arginine and glycine, so much that a company has created a real patented compound, useful in terms of anti-fatigue and anti-catabolism supplements, which is glycine-arginine-alpha-ketoisocaproic acid (GAKIC). This product promises a better synthesis of creatine by our metabolism, the production of nitric oxide with its effects especially at the vasodilatory level, and a better production of growth hormone, with an improvement in recovery times and in cell regeneration processes.

The first study examining the effects of GAKIC supplementation on performance was published in the prestigious *Medicine & Science in Sports & Exercise* journal in 2000. But what can you expect from GAKIC? The use of GAKIC increases the ability to support exercise capacity in terms of strength and duration, during intense workouts. **It also helps to delay the muscle fatigue, thus increasing the muscle performance.** For an athlete who trains with weights, it can mean doing extra reps with the usual load. In this way, it can put more stress on the body, which will adapt by increasing the protein synthesis and with other mechanisms that will allow the body to improve for subsequent workouts.

One of the first studies on GAKIC was conducted by Dr. Bruce Stevens and his colleagues at the University of Florida and their goal was to quantify the effects of GAKIC supplementation on dynamic muscle performance (strength, total work, fatigue), by measuring parameter variations in acute, exhaustion, high intensity and anaerobic isokinetic exercise conditions. The study subjects (13 healthy men) consumed a low calorie beverage containing either 11.20 g of GAKIC powder or 9.46 g of sugar (control). Both drinks had the same calories. At the end of the experiment, the results showed that the drink with GAKIC significantly increased the performance compared to the control.

What the authors verified is that GAKIC:

- increases the ability to sustain the muscle strength by at least 28% during intense anaerobic exercise;
- has the ability to support total muscle work during intense anaerobic exercise and increases it by about 12%;
- increases the total exercise capacity and performance by decreasing the onset of muscle fatigue, especially in the early stages of anaerobic exercise that lasts at least 15 minutes.

The second interesting study, conducted by Buford and Alexander Koch at Truman State University, focused on determining the effects of supplementation with GAKIC on the anaerobic performance of cyclists who performed repeated sessions over time.

Ten healthy men consumed either a drink with GAKIC or sugar as a placebo, with an identical dose in the first study. This study found that supplementation with GAKIC significantly attenuated the power drop that is usually associated with performing repeated anaerobic sprints. It is thought that this improvement is also due to the ability of GAKIC to **faster remove** the toxins (and especially ammonia) that are produced during intense workouts more quickly, especially if repeated over a short period of time, and which interfere with the normal functioning of the metabolic processes' compounds in the muscle, decreasing its ability to produce more power.

Dosages

The amount of KIC needed to have results in terms of muscle growth is in the order of 15-20 g per day, so it is more convenient and perhaps healthy to use HMB.

As for GAKIC, it is usually recommended to take about 10 g 45 minutes before the training and/or the competition, in order to ensure that its effects are maximal.

Effectiveness

Strength	Resistant strength	Mass	Endurance	Slimming	Concentration	Recovery
++	+++	++	–	–	–	++

L-ALANYL-L-GLUTAMINE

Description

L-alanyl-L-glutamine is a dipeptide formed by glutamine and alanine: it is a much more stable form, resistant to heat and acids, and above all with a greater solubility than the classic glutamine: while classic glutamine tends to be quickly hydrolyzed to glutamic acid in aqueous solutions, L-alanyl-L-glutamine solves this problem.

All fitness and bodybuilding enthusiasts have already heard of it and many have also used it as a supplement, but perhaps not everyone knows the real benefits it can bring.

Properties

Among the characteristics, there is first of all a greater bioavailability: compared to the same L-glutamine in free form, L-alanyl-L-glutamine has a higher absorption through the intestinal wall. Its transport from the intestine to the bloodstream takes place thanks to transporters called PERPT1, expressed in small part also in the colonocytes.

Furthermore, L-alanyl-L-glutamine is more stable than the free amino acid L-glutamine in acidic conditions and at high temperatures. This is an important property, for example, for parenteral solutions used in clinical nutrition: the high temperatures reached with sterilization alter the structure of glutamine in free form, while L-alanyl-L-glutamine is highly soluble in water and temperature resistant, with a solubility rate of 568 g per liter, much higher than that of glutamine in free form, which is 35 g per liter at 20° C.

Evidence

One study reports that following the ingestion of 60 mg/kg of L-glutamine or 89 mg/kg of L-alanyl-L-glutamine (equivalent to 60 mg/kg of glutamine) during a fasting state, over the next 4 hours the mean value of the area under the plasma glutamine curve was 124% higher than that recorded after the intake of single amino acids.

The dipeptide therefore seems to be more effective in increasing the amount of glutamine directed to the muscles, compared to glutamine alone.

Studies in mice that were administered L-glutamine (1 g/kg) or L-alanyl-L-glutamine (1.5 g/kg) for 3 weeks showed higher plasma glutamate concentrations. The same result is not achieved by administering alanine together with free glutamine. To explain the mechanism underlying this evidence, we recall that glutamate, from the bloodstream, reaches the muscle cells, where it is converted into glutamine (glutamine-glutamate cycle). If glutamine increases in the tissues, there may be a lower demand for glutamate, which is therefore not recalled from the bloodstream to support the intracellular stores of glutamine and is therefore detected in greater quantities in the blood. This reflects the greater presence of glutamine in the muscle cells, following the intake of the dipeptide.

The clearance of L-alanyl-L-glutamine is mainly borne by the kidneys, unlike the free form amino acids alanine and glutamine, which are metabolized mainly by the splanchnic tissues (liver and intestine). This preference for the renal elimination of the dipeptide is most likely due to the fact that the enzyme that hydrolyzes the dipeptide (which breaks down L-alanyl-L-glutamine into L-glutamine and L-alanine) is mainly located in the kidneys.

Heat Shock Proteins (HSP) belong to a family of protein molecules that cells produce in case of exposure to stress conditions such as rising temperatures: they prevent the formation of those aggregates that are formed by the folding of proteins, potentially toxic for the cell. This serves to maintain and preserve the functions and its metabolism in the cell. A typical situation in which HSPs are produced and activated is an intense training. Studies carried out so far only on mice, show that after supplementation with L-alanyl-L-glutamine, it increases the expression of HSPs and also increases the hepatic reduced glutathione (GSH), suggesting a protection against oxidative stress.

In animal models, it has been shown that L-alanyl-L-glutamine facilitates the absorption of electrolytes to a greater extent than glutamine. During prolonged physical exercise, in which the dehydration stress is an important factor to consider, this characteristic of the dipeptide suggests its potential use to improve both resistance to fatigue and the performance indirectly, by improving the hydration. In fact, we note that it is often found in pre-workout supplements used in the world of sports, but especially in bodybuilding and fitness, almost always together with other ingredients, in order to maximize not only the hydration and the muscle pump, but also the performance, understood as an expression of strength.

Current evidence suggests that L-alanyl-L-glutamine may be a more effective supplement than glutamine due to its greater stability and water solubility, and also due to its prolonged plasma half-life. Glutamine alone has a half-life of 2 hours, while the dipeptide half-life is almost double. Further research may also clarify the possible uses to improve the performance.

Dosages

Some studies report dosages of 0.2-0.5 g, others dosages of 1 to 3 g per day. To optimize its use, it may be advisable to take it before a workout, in the case of sports such as bodybuilding and fitness, especially together with other molecules that promote the production of nitric oxide, such as citrulline. Instead, in the case of endurance sports, to promote the maintenance of muscle hydration and consequently improve the performance, and to decrease the sensation of fatigue, L-alanyl-L-glutamine can be taken in association with sports beverages containing carbohydrates and minerals, during training sessions and/or competitions.

Effectiveness

Strength	Resistant strength	Mass	Endurance	Slimming	Concentration	Recovery
–	–	++	+++	++	++	++

LEUCINE

Description
Leucine is a very interesting amino acid that has been studied since the 1970s for its properties in regulating protein metabolism. It is one of the famous essential amino acids, to be clear those that we are unable to produce endogenously and that must necessarily be included in our diet. In addition, it is the king of BCAAs (branched chain amino acids - leucine, isoleucine and valine), which have been so lucky in the world of fitness. These branched amino acids are metabolized by specific transaminases (BCAT) at the muscle level. In particular, leucine is transaminated to its alpha-ketoisocaproate keto acid (KIC), which is mostly converted into isovaleryl-CoA, while around 5% is metabolized into β-hydroxy-β-methylbutyric acid (HMB).

Properties
BCAAs are important in sports because they are not metabolized by the liver; their first use, in fact, was linked to the administration to patients suffering from hepatic insufficiency. In this way, muscle catabolism was countered (they are mostly picked up only by the muscle) without further stressing an already strongly altered liver metabolism. They are very important in positivizing the body's nitrogen balance, which is essential for having an anabolic situation. They make up about a third of muscle tissue. In the post-workout compensation phase, 90% of the amino acids used for muscle recovery of damaged fibers are BCAAs. Leucine is the progenitor for the anabolic properties and for the stimulation of mTOR, the characteristics of which are listed in the following table.

Table 44.6 The features and functions of mTor

- mTOR is the metabolic pathway that regulates the eukaryotic metabolism to a greater extent (anabolism and catabolism)
- It is activated by various exogenous factors: growth factors (insulin, IGF), leucine and EAA, cellular oxygen level, energy state (AMPK), inflammatory factors (TNF-α, NF-κB), genotoxic stress
- It has two large catalytic subunits: mTORC1 and mTORC2
- The most important and mostly known is mTORC1, the one that activates the protein synthesis, as well as the synthesis of different cell organelles
- mTORC2, on the other hand, seems to have an influence on the cytoskeletal organization of cells and its function is still under investigation

Not just protein synthesis:
- mTOR regulates numerous other biological reactions
- In the presence of an adequate caloric (high ATP/ADP ratio) and essential amino acids (leucine) intake, this mechanism contributes to the synthesis of mitochondria and, in particular of lipids, which make up the cell membrane (via SREBP1)
- In addition, in the presence of optimal oxygen levels, it regulates the mitochondrial membrane potential and allows the activation of all oxidative processes by increasing the synthesis of mtDNA, resulting in an increase in the oxidation of fatty acids for energy purposes
- If there is a lack of nutrients, mTOR promotes autophagy and the degradation of organelles to recover nutrients for their own sustenance and for cell growth

The foods that are richest in leucine are eggs, cod, parmesan, pork, skim milk, veal, lupins, chicken breast, soy, peanuts and especially whey proteins.

Evidence

The properties of leucine are peculiar both in athlete and elderly, diabetic, sarcopenic and dyslipidemic subjects. The first effect of supplementing with this amino acid is its role in **stimulating the protein synthesis**. While before it was thought that it was the BCAA branched chain amino acid pool to perform this function, then it was seen that even the supplementation of leucine alone already had an effect on protein synthesis. It is believed that this effect is mainly due to the stimulation of the mTOR pathway and due to the concomitant insulin secretion with the increase of leucine in the circulation, although in reality some studies show that the anabolic effect of leucine, which occurs at a dose of at least 3 g, is partly independent of the presence of insulin. The intake of this molecule has also proved to be particularly interesting in fasting states, in line with other processes that leucine supports and which are mainly related to glucose metabolism. But let's go into detail. At high doses, leucine **stimulates the insulin secretion**; the body realizes that the levels of this fundamental amino acid are high and that therefore there is room for protein synthesis. At this point, as a consequence, we have the activation of the mTOR complex and the cascade of its reactions, which lead to an increase in the muscular plastic stimulus. In this case, the increase in the concentration of circulating amino acids and insulin are synergistic in "muscle building". But if the administration is chronic and moreover it is done at high doses, leucine produces a state of hyperinsulinism like diabetes, inducing a decrease in the peripheral sensitivity to this hormone and a decrease in the effect on mTOR (the stimulus on the protein synthesis). On the other hand, in subjects who have already developed type 2 diabetes (or subjects on dexamethasone therapy) in which hyperinsulinism has already been established, low leucine levels have been seen to improve the peripheral insulin sensitivity. This produces a decrease in inflammatory adipokines in the body, improving the underlying pathological picture. Low pulsatile insulin secretions produce anabolism, while chronic stimulations of this powerful hormone slow it down (in addition to increasing, as mentioned before, the inflammatory state of the subject).

Leucine can act by improving both of these aspects depending on the dosage, timing of intake and the general nutritional status of the individual.

We have said that the **anabolic effect of leucine passes through the stimulation of mTOR**, although it is not well known how this happens, but this activation is directly associated with the increase in protein synthesis in two distinct ways. Firstly, by increasing the speed of the protein synthesis, that is, the process by which information at the genetic level results in the formation of a protein, and secondly, by increasing the quantity of proteins that can be formed in a given period of time.

There is also some evidence that **leucine supplementation can produce benefits even when taken together with large doses of proteins**, as if leucine were able to amplify the peak anabolic response to a meal and also extend the duration of the protein synthesis following the same meal. An explanation for this may be the rapid increase in blood concentration of leucine not reachable with a simple protein meal, possibly also based on whey proteins (very rich in leucine), which would take some time to free the leucine from proteins and would never reach the peak obtainable with the administration of leucine in its free form.

In a study carried out on young soldiers, it was shown that 3.5 g of leucine associated with essential amino acids were more effective in stimulating the protein synthesis than 1.87 g of leucine combined with the same amount of amino acids. However, the simultaneous presence of essential amino acids is important in order to build muscle mass, because if there are no building blocks (the amino acids necessary for the formation of proteins), even if there is the activation of mTOR, this does not translate into muscle growth.

In a study carried out in 2011 at Leeds Metropolitan University in Great Britain, it was found that after 12 weeks of weight training combined with supplementation with 4 g of leucine, there was a **greater increase in muscle mass and strength** compared to the placebo group.

Normally, it is believed that the quantity of proteins of high biological value contained in a single meal necessary to stimulate protein synthesis, is around 20-30 g (in about 20 g of whey protein there are 3 g of leucine). In a study conducted by the University of Maastricht in the Netherlands, it was found that in elderly people with an average age of 74 years, a meal containing 20 g of protein supplemented with 2.5 g of leucine produced a greater increase in protein synthesis than a meal without supplementation

Furthermore, as we get older, we become less sensitive to the signal of activation of protein synthesis by leucine and therefore, higher dosages are required.

Although it has now been well established that leucine consumed during and after weight training promotes muscle growth, it is not yet clear how things stand regarding its effect on the physical exercise if consumed before. **If the goal is to increase the muscle mass, taking leucine before the training may not be a good idea**, as muscle growth requires an anabolic situation at the protein level and a catabolic situation at the carbohydrate level, for the purpose of restoring the energy through the glycogenolysis.

Thus, although leucine stimulates the protein synthesis, on the other hand it prevents the splitting of glycogen into glucose by limiting the immediate energy availability necessary for muscle contraction and therefore for optimal power training. The case of endurance training is different, for which the preservation of muscle glycogen in favor of the use of fatty acids can be an advantage in the long term. In a Brazilian study (*Nutrition*, 29: 1388-1394, 2013) on rats, it was found that the administration of **leucine before exercise improved the performance in a maximal endurance test and favored the saving of muscle glycogen to a greater extent, compared to BCAAs**.

Another reason why leucine taken before exercise could have a negative effect, is its ability to modulate some neurotransmitters in the brain. Serotonin is a neurotransmitter with a sedative effect and intense and prolonged physical exercise increases its production in the brain, presumably increasing the feeling of fatigue. In reality, even more than at the level of serotonin, the feeling of fatigue is linked to the relationship of this with another neurotransmitter, dopamine, which instead favors the state of alertness, mental concentration and motivation.

Consequently, a low serotonin/dopamine ratio achieved by decreasing serotonin or increasing dopamine should positively affect the performance. Leucine decreases serotonin with a mechanism of competition with tryptophan at the level of the blood brain barrier, which is the precursor of serotonin. However, on the other hand, it also inhibits the production of dopamine by competing with tyrosine, which is the precursor of dopamine. At this point, if you wanted to take leucine before training or before a competition in order to save muscle glycogen, it would be good to take tyrosine at the same time, in order to avoid the negative impact of leucine on dopamine levels.

Another **less known effect of leucine is the anti-catabolic effect**, which has been hypothesized since the administration of leucine produced a drop in LDH enzyme (cell damage index), measured in the post-workout period. Subsequently, the administration of leucine was also evaluated in frankly hypercatabolic subjects such as sarcopenic, bedridden patients and in patients receiving corticosteroid therapy (such as dexamethasone, which induces gluconeogenesis with a demolition of the lean mass). Leucine has had good results in each of these patient classes. At the moment, there are interesting studies on a leucine metabolite, in particular: β-hydroxy-β-methyl-butyric acid (HMB), which would seem to be the effector of the beneficial results of supplementation with leucine on the muscular anti-catabolism.

Leucine also takes part in other metabolic processes related to lipid metabolism and seems to increase the mitochondrial biogenesis of the cell and the preferential use of fats by striated muscle tissue. This would be mediated by the expression of genes such as *PGC-1α* and by sirtuins that take part in the regulation of the energy metabolism by modulating thermogenesis, the mitochondrial mass (understood as the number of functioning mitochondria) and the consequent increased oxidation of fatty acids. Last but not least, leucine and all BCAAs have a detoxifying function. Not being metabolized by the liver, they produce much less nitrogen waste. In this way, fewer "toxic intermediates" (ammonium and urea) have to be disposed later by the body.

Dosages

Protocols for leucine intake require the proportion of this amino acid to vary from 5 to 10% of a total protein pool and around 50% of a BCAA pool. This is to have the desired effects on body composition. In particular, the leucine intake should be at least 3 g at a time for a total of 45 mg/kg/day in sedentary subjects, with the purpose of achieving a decrease in the catabolism (minimum dose). But if the subject has a greater expenditure, given for example by training with weights, the dose must increase adequately. However, it has been seen that doses from 200 mg/kg/day upwards do not have a further effect on the improvement of the performance and muscle growth, and indeed can create problems of hyperinsulinism that were mentioned above. So, in practice, an optimal dosage should go from 3 to 15 g per day of leucine (divided into several intakes if more than 5 g per day), depending on the case and above all on the degree of training and on the sustained loads.

Effectiveness

Strength	Resistant strength	Mass	Endurance	Slimming	Concentration	Recovery
++	+	++++	++	+	–	+++

LIPOIC ACID (ALA)

Description

Lipoic acid (or alpha-lipoic acid, ALA) is a sulfur molecule that exists in two forms in the nature, as a cyclic disulfide or as an open chain with the name of dihydrolipoic acid.

In recent years, many studies have been carried out on ALA and its multiple functionalities, applied both in the sports and in the clinical field, but also to improve the quality of everyday life of active and sedentary individuals.

A molecule discovered in 1951, it immediately attracted the attention of scientists for its universal antioxidant characteristic, as it has the ability to neutralize free radicals in both aqueous and lipid environments. Moreover, it is the only antioxidant that maintains this property even in the oxidized form.

It is present in foods of plant and animal origin. It is found in abundance in potatoes, broccoli and spinach, but the main source is red meat and liver.

Most of the actions it performs in the body and applications in the clinical (and non-clinical) field are due to this antioxidant property.

Properties

One of the first clinical uses of ALA was in the treatment of type 2 diabetes (non-insulin-dependent), caused by insulin resistance (the pancreas continues to produce insulin which cannot be effectively used at the peripheral level).

This pathology involves both hyperinsulinemia and dyslipidemia, with all the resulting consequences (for example glycation, hypercholesterolemia, hypertriglyceridemia, hypertension, etc.) that are harmful to the body.

Glycation can be considered a form of catabolism, as it is capable of damaging the proteins of all tissues; this happens because with high blood sugar levels, there are many glucose molecules available that can react with muscle proteins, collagen, myelin, skin, nerves, connective tissue, endothelium, compromising their integrity and causing an accelerated aging with a series of pathologies attributable to the complications of diabetes.

In this situation, ALA intervenes in two possible ways: by neutralizing free radicals that damage and occupy cellular insulin receptors and by stimulating carriers (cellular transport systems, GLUT1 and GLUT4) that carry this sugar from the blood into the cells. The result is that the entry of glucose into the cell is improved, and blood sugar levels are reduced, as is the risk of glycation and the organic deterioration. ALA is a very powerful antioxidant capable of exercising its function both inside and outside the cell membrane, since it is an amphoteric substance, that is, both water-soluble and fat-soluble. It is also able to regenerate vitamins C and E and restore glutathione to its reduced form. Its detoxifying action in the liver is also very important: it is able to protect the liver from the damage caused by amanita phalloid poisoning (a fungus) and by all those drugs that, going to overexertion and damage the liver, prevent it from carrying out its multiple functions. ALA is also a substance **capable of chelating heavy metals (mercury)**.

ALA is an enzymatic cofactor of the oxidative decarboxylation of pyruvate and other keto acids, and therefore helps to optimize the metabolic pathways of the energy production.

Let's start with glucose: once in the cell, if energy needs prevail, it enters the process of glycolysis, during which glucose is transformed into pyruvic acid which becomes, in the presence of oxygen, a smaller molecule called acetyl-coenzyme A. This molecule can enter the Krebs cycle in the mitochondrion, binding to an oxaloacetate molecule and forming citric acid (the Krebs cycle is also called the citric acid cycle), which, after undergoing various reactions, gives rise to oxaloacetic acid again, producing numerous ATP molecules plus carbon dioxide and water in the various passages. Acetyl-CoA can also derive from the beta oxidation of fatty acids; among other things, this is the reason why camels or hibernating animals, accumulating fat (the camel in the hump, bears in the body in general), are then able to survive without ingesting water for long periods, using what is produced by the catabolism of acetyl-CoA which derives from fats.

However, at this moment, we are interested in acetyl-CoA which derives from pyruvic acid, which in turn derives from glucose. The enzymatic complex that favors this passage from pyruvate to acetyl-CoA contains our ALA. Thus, by increasing the amount of ALA, we have more acetyl-CoA that comes from pyruvate and that can enter the Krebs cycle, so we can increase the amount and speed of the conversion of glucose into energy. The fact that ALA can increase the energy reserves in the form of ATP in the muscle is very important for the athlete, as a muscle that accumulates more ATP is a muscle capable of doing more repetitions before reaching exhaustion. So, without changing other factors, just adding ALA can make us stronger. But the most interesting thing is that this increase in strength comes at the expense of the accumulation of fat. How does this phenomenon happen?

Normally, in the body, glucose not used as fuel by the muscle or brain is stored in the liver as glycogen, after which it is converted into triglycerides and stored as fat. If your muscles have the ability to transform and accumulate a certain number of calories from carbohydrates in the form of ATP, any excess will be transformed into body fat and accumulated in fat cells.

According to Dr. Hans Tritshler, a German researcher, ALA can increase the conversion and the accumulation of glucose as ATP by about 40%, and this through various mechanisms, including the stimulation of GLUT1 and GLUT4, which are carrier molecules that transport glucose into the muscle cell. Consequently, this increased capacity creates a much higher energy potential for the ATP accumulation in muscle cells, which will promote the performance and, moreover, will take place at the expense of fat accumulation; that is, ALA is able to convert a surplus of carbohydrates into muscle energy rather than into lipids in the adipose tissue.

As for the ergogenic effect of ALA, several studies have shown an improvement in performance, an improvement in lean mass and, above all, a good decrease in the percentage of body fat, all without changing the diet (which is probably already balanced). In particular, for weight loss, it acts as a metabolic accelerator, as it increases the availability of acetyl-CoA (deriving from pyruvate) which enters the Krebs cycle, increasing the production of ATP and providing more energy to the body.

Evidence

We usually think in terms of anabolism and catabolism and, when we think of catabolism, our mind immediately thinks of cortisol and the microtraumas of training; consequently, our efforts are aimed at counteracting cortisol and promoting the tissue regeneration with an adequate nutrition and supplementation. In reality, despite being misunderstood by most, there is another form of particularly insidious muscle catabolism, which does not depend on training but on our main fuel, glucose, which is glycation. Glycation occurs when parts of glucose molecules react with tissue proteins and damage them. ALA reduces the glycation damage and thus, by saving proteins, practically performs an anti-catabolic function.

Generally, the blood is too alkaline to allow glycation, but the production of lactic acid during exercise can acidify the tissues. Excessive intake of acidifying foods may also be sufficient. During these periods of acidosis, these broken glucose chains attack the proteins of the muscles, skin, nerves and connective tissue, compromising their structural integrity. Glycation amplifies the catabolism induced by training and is one of the reasons why, as we age and insulin sensitivity worsens, we lose muscle. Especially in athletes, the glycation of the connective tissue predisposes to injuries and the damage caused by glycation does not induce, unlike those caused by training microtraumas, the release of IGF-1 and therefore does not stimulate the reparative processes.

ALA has an insulin-mimetic hypoglycemic effect, all in the name of regulating the glucose metabolism, now considered a fundamental element both for the muscle growth process and for lipolysis.

Kalliopi Georgakouli et al., in 2018, performed a study to measure the responses on exercise status and redox status following ALA supplementation in subjects with G6PD deficiency.

G6PD deficiency makes cells more sensitive to oxidative stress, while antioxidant dietary supplementation could restore the redox balance and improve the exercise-induced oxidative stress. To examine the effects of ALA supplementation on redox status indices in G6PD deficient subjects, eight adult males participated in this randomized, double-blind, placebo-controlled crossover study. Participants were randomly assigned to receive ALA (600 mg/day) or placebo for 4 weeks, separated by a 4-week washout period. Before and at the end of each treatment period, participants exercised following a comprehensive exercise protocol on a treadmill. Blood samples were obtained before (at rest), immediately after and 1 hour after the exercise, for subsequent analyzes of the total antioxidant capacity (TAC), uric acid, bilirubin, thiobarbituric acid reactive substances (TBARS) and carbonyl proteins (CP). ALA resulted in a significant increase in resting TAC and bilirubin concentrations. In addition, the TAC increased immediately and 1 hour after the exercise, after both treatment periods, while bilirubin increased immediately after and 1 hour after the exercise when they were given ALA alone. No significant changes in uric acid, TBARS or CP were observed at any time. In conclusion, it has therefore been seen that supplementing ALA for 4 weeks can improve the antioxidant status in subjects with G6PD deficiency.

Researchers have highlighted the mechanism by which **ALA triggers fat loss**. Multiple studies have shown that hypothalamic AMPK is important for regulating the food intake and energy expenditure and that ALA exerts anti-obesity effects by suppressing the activity of hypothalamic AMPK. Today it is believed that the energy balance is maintained by the hypothalamus, which receives information related to energy excess or deficiencies. There is a kind of sensor to determine the amount of fuel in the cell and it is activated when its energy is running out. This sensor is AMPK (activated AMP-protein kinase) and it is the main cellular regulator of lipid and carbohydrate metabolism. The AMPK protein kinase is activated by an increase in the AMP/ATP ratio: when a cellular energy deficiency occurs, an increase in appetite is triggered, so that a sufficient level of energy is re-established. ALA decreases the activity of the hypothalamic AMPK, reducing the food intake and improving the energy expenditure.

It is now known that obesity is associated with significant morbidity and mortality rates. Even modest weight loss can be associated with health benefits. ALA is a natural antioxidant. Studies have suggested that ALA has anti-obesity properties, so a comprehensive and systematic literature search identified 10 articles related to randomized, double-blind, placebo-controlled studies involving ALA. A meta-analysis was conducted on the differences in mean weight and in the variation in BMI between the groups that received ALA and placebo. Treatment with ALA coincided with a statistically significant greater weight loss of 1.27 kg (confidence interval 0.25 to 2.29), compared to the placebo group. A significant mean overall difference in BMI of −0.43 kg/m^2 (confidence interval −0.82 to −0.03) was found between the ALA and placebo groups. The analysis of the meta-regression did not show any significance in the administration of ALA on BMI and weight changes. The duration of the study significantly influenced the change in BMI, but not the change in weight, although treatment with ALA showed reduced but significant short-term weight loss when compared to placebo.

When the researchers activated the hypothalamic AMPK, the beneficial effects of ALA supplementation on food intake and energy expenditure were nullified, indicating that ALA increases the weight loss through its direct effects on AMPK.

In fact, at a systemic level, ALA increases the levels of AMPK, which is believed to inhibit the muscle growth; other animal studies have shown that ALA induces a downregulation of the mTOR pathway, which is essential for the activation of the protein synthesis (with a mechanism similar to metformin, which also inhibits the protein synthesis); however, it seems that at the dosages that are normally recommended for human use, this effect does not occur.

In addition, during the physical activity, **ALA facilitates the transition from anaerobic to aerobic glycolysis**, allowing a greater use of fatty acids for energy and less production of lactic acid and toxins, which could cause fatigue and lead to an early termination of the workout.

Another important fact for athletes is that ALA increases the accumulation of energy reserves in the muscle in the form of ATP by 40%, allowing for a more intense and productive workout, with a greater training stimulus and a consequent improvement in the performance.

In light of the fact that creatine absorption is influenced by insulin, Burke et al. examined the effects of combining ALA with creatine monohydrate, in reference to the accumulation of creatine in the muscle. In this study, which involved 16 male subjects, biopsies were performed before and after supplementation to determine the concentration of muscle creatine. The results showed a **greater increase in phosphocreatine and total creatine concentrations** in the ALA + creatine monohydrate + carbohydrate supplemented group (1000 mg/day + 20 g/day + sucrose 100 g/day, respectively), compared to a creatine + carbohydrate or just carbohydrate group. The authors concluded that co-ingestion of ALA and creatine (and an amount of sucrose) can improve the muscle concentrations of creatine compared to an equivalent dose of creatine + carbohydrates, or from carbohydrates alone.

The ability of ALA to allow greater entry of sugars into cells (with a preference for muscle cells) is also useful in high-calorie diets, as not all excess carbohydrates will be stored as fat, but a part of them will replenish and enlarge energy supplies. "Sucking" glucose in the muscles brings with it other nutrients and electrolytes that can penetrate more easily inside the cell: therefore, ALA lends itself to being taken with other supplements whose absorption and efficacy are to be optimized (see: creatine, glutamine, pyruvate, amino acids, carnitine, etc.).

With creatine and glutamine, for example, the recovery process and the increase in muscle mass will be favored; associated with pyruvate and/or carnitine will speed up weight loss; taken with other antioxidants, the antiradical effects of the latter will be enhanced.

Dosages

As for the intake, it would be preferable to take ALA after meals as it could cause heartburn, being careful not to chew the capsules and to drink plenty of water.

If used as a heavy metal chelator, it is best to take it on an empty stomach. Taken after training with carbohydrates and other supplements, it can speed up the restoration of energy supplies and anticipate the muscle rebuilding and recovery.

The doses are usually: 50-100 mg as an antioxidant, 600-1000 mg in the treatment of type 2 diabetes, 600-800 mg to optimize weight loss.

When given in dosages of up to 10 mg/kg of body weight, for long periods of time, no harmful effects were found.

Effectiveness

Strength	Resistant strength	Mass	Endurance	Slimming	Concentration	Recovery
+	++	+++	++	+++	–	++

MAGNESIUM

Description

Magnesium is an alkaline-earth mineral that in its pure state is shiny and silver in color, and becomes opaque in contact with air due to the oxidation process. It is one of the most naturally occurring minerals, just think that 2% of the earth's crust is made up of magnesium and that this element is predominantly present in sea water. It plays a very important role in many reactions that occur within our body and participates in the synthesis of hundreds of enzymes.

99% of the magnesium in our body is localized within cells, of which: 50-60% is concentrated in bones, 24.5% in muscles, 24.5% in the nervous system, myocardium, liver, in the kidneys and other organs with a high metabolism rate; only 1% is present in extracellular fluids (plasma, cerebrospinal fluid). From a dietary point of view, magnesium is present in whole grains, dried fruits, cocoa, meats (both red and white), dairy products and legumes. The amount of magnesium present in our body is about 24 g (0.35 g/kg) and on average our daily requirements are between 300 and 500 mg.

Properties

Magnesium is a fundamental mineral and comes into play in the physiological reactions of metabolic energy production (Mg-ATP complex), as well as in the regulation of the neuromuscular activities of the heart muscle, in muscle contraction, and also in blood pressure and vascular tone regulation. Thanks to these characteristics, magnesium has been shown to be very effective in reducing blood pressure and vascular resistance.

From an energy point of view, magnesium binds to numerous complexes containing phosphate, such as ATP, phosphocreatine and other phosphometabolites, making up the cytosolic and mitochondrial pool that allow the cell to carry out important bioenergetic reactions, especially for the control of the carbohydrate metabolism. In the body, this element comes into play in keeping the amount of liquids inside the cell and in the external environment constant; in fact, magnesium is one of the main minerals present in the cell cytoplasm, together with potassium, sulphates and phosphates.

Magnesium plays a fundamental role in maintaining a constant water balance and above all, in maintaining the charge potential of the cell membrane constant, in order to allow the passage of small solutes and to favor the excitability process of the cell itself, allowing the passage of the nervous signal.

From a purely sporting point of view, magnesium is often associated only with the replenishment of mineral salts after a long session of aerobic sports. In reality, this supplement has a real ergogenic effect, as the improvement of the conduction of the nerve signal, the stabilization of blood pressure and therefore of the electrolyte balance, and the improvement of magnesium-dependent energy processes allow this **mineral to be used for both power and endurance sports**.

Magnesium is essential for the assimilation of phosphorus, calcium and potassium and plays a very important role in regulating the activity of muscles and nerves, influencing the permeability of cell membranes; it promotes the maintenance of the balance and the activity of the nervous system, through a relaxing and calming action with attenuation of the excitability of nerves and muscles, and with the reduction of adrenaline secretion (it is therefore effective in the presence of cramps, migraines, nervousness, irritable bowel, tachycardia).

In the presence of trauma and/or stressful psycho-physical situations, magnesium levels are considerably reduced, leading to the onset of neuromuscular disorders and cardiovascular and gastrointestinal diseases. It serves as an essential cofactor in enzyme catalysis and also functions as a key electrolyte to keep the body fluids in balance. It is also essential in the metabolism of lipids, proteins and carbohydrates, and allows the production of energy.

Evidence

A 2015 study by Kass et al. highlighted how the use of magnesium **improves the cardiovascular parameters (blood pressure, systolic and diastolic pressure) and sports parameters (maximal strength and recovery capacity) with acute and chronic supplementaton**. In this study, subjects were divided into two groups (acute and chronic) and given 300 mg of magnesium three hours before the physical tests. In the chronic group, magnesium was administered for four weeks, while in the acute group only for one week. The acute group showed a greater increase in maximal strength exercises and also in the recovery capacity compared to the chronic group (however, the values were significantly better than the initial tests without magnesium administration or compared to the placebo).

Researchers believe that this increase in strength is due to the improvement of some muscle mechanisms such as the increase in the formation of the Mg-ATP complex, the increase in the expression of troponin through the calcium concentration gradient which improves the energy metabolism and therefore the muscle contraction, following a recruitment of greater quantities of actin. The authors explain this decrease in potency in the chronic group by arguing that continuous high dosages of magnesium can increase its excretion due to the fact that taking a high an amount for a long period changes the water homeostasis and leads to the saturation of magnesium stocks in storage sites, effectively increasing its excretion.

However, the chronic group had the greatest improvements from a cardiovascular point of view, in fact the systolic and diastolic blood pressure was lower than in the acute group and compared to the placebo. This is explained by the fact that the persistence of magnesium in the extracellular environment causes a reduction in blood pressure, due to the vasodilation produced by this mineral.

Regarding sports parameters, although the positive effect of Mg on the muscle function has been widely recognized, studies on the effectiveness of Mg supplementation in young athletes have produced conflicting results, therefore the purpose of the study by Cordova et al. (2017) was to examine the effect of Mg supplementation on muscle damage markers and the association between serum Mg levels with these muscle markers. Twelve men that played elite basketball (PB) from a Spanish professional basketball league team and a control group (CG) made up of twelve college students who regularly practiced recreational basketball and participated in junior college leagues, participated in this study.

The athletes took a supplement of 400 mg/day of Mg in the form of Mg lactate. Blood samples were taken four times during the season, separated by 8 weeks: T1: October, T2: December, T3: March, T4: April. Serum Mg concentrations showed a significant reduction in T3 (1.56 ± 0.03 mg/dL) compared to T1 (1.69 ± 0.04 mg/dL) and T2 (1.69 ± 0.04 mg/dL). At the end of the study, the serum concentration of Mg was significantly higher (T4: 1.79 ± 0.06 mg/dL) compared to T3. Levels of muscle damage parameters remained the same throughout the season (p >0.05), with the exception of creatinine, which decreased significantly after T2, and then significantly increased in T3 and T4 compared to T2. In conclusion, these results suggest that supplementing with Mg during the competitive season, or during the most intense season, can prevent the damage of the associated tissues.

A 2011 study highlighted how magnesium supplementation in young and sedentary athletes increased the **concentration of total and free testosterone**. In this study, the subjects were divided into three groups (sedentary and Mg, training and Mg, training and placebo), two of which were given magnesium in the form of magnesium sulphate ($MgSO_4$) in a dose of 10 mg/kg for four weeks. The workouts had a fairly long duration (90-120 min), while the testosterone measurements were made both before and after the training session.

At the end of the four weeks, the groups taking magnesium, both sedentary and exercised, had significant increases in total and free testosterone, but the group that took the supplement and exercised had markedly higher values. Researchers argue that the positive action of magnesium is carried out in mitigating the catabolic phase induced by the training, as well as in improving the energy functionality by increasing the availability of ATP and the influx of water into the tissues, promoting a better muscle recovery.

Magnesium has been reported to increase bone formation in several studies. Although there is some information regarding the concentrations of magnesium ions that influence the bone remodeling at the cellular level, little is known about the effect of magnesium ions on the cell gap junctions. Therefore, a 2016 a study was carried out with the aim of investigating the effects of different concentrations of magnesium on bone cells and to further evaluate its effect on osteoblast gap junctions. Cultures of normal human osteoblasts were treated with magnesium ions at concentrations of 1, 2 and 3 mmol for 24, 48 and 72 hours.

Magnesium ions induced significant increases (p <0.05) in cell viability, alkaline phosphate activity and osteocalcin levels on the human osteoblasts. These stimulating actions were positively associated with the magnesium concentration and the exposure time. Furthermore, intercellular communication through the osteoblast junction was significantly promoted by the magnesium ions. In conclusion, this study demonstrated that magnesium ions induced the activity of osteoblasts by improving the intercellular communication through the gap junctions between cells and also influenced the bone formation. These results can contribute to a better understanding of the influence of magnesium on bone remodeling and to the advancement of its application in the clinical practice.

Other studies have highlighted the importance of magnesium in high intensity sports. In this type of sport, in which maintaining a good energy level and minimizing the excess stress induced by training is of fundamental importance, magnesium plays a fundamental role in reducing the sense of fatigue and in prolonging the peak performance. A study by Rahman et al. in 2014 showed how **magnesium depletion during high intensity training increased all the markers of muscle damage and overtraining** (AST, ALT, GGT, CPK, LDH, uric acid, creatinine) in mice subjected to high intensity exercise in water. In addition, there was a significant worsening of some indices influenced by an excess protein catabolism, such as blood glucose, pH, triglyceride and LDL concentration, which were significantly higher in these mice.

The excess of muscle catabolism due to the increased production of stress hormones causes an increase in all these indices, with a consequent depletion not only of magnesium, but also of the main electrolytes (K, Na, Ca, Cl, HCO_3).

Leaving the sports world, a recent review (Mooren, 2015) highlighted the positive role of magnesium in the reduction of insulin resistance and in type 2 diabetes. Epidemiological studies have shown that the chronic intake of a quantity of magnesium between 300 and 400 mg improves glucose homeostasis by lowering glycated hemoglobin levels and by reducing blood sugar levels in patients with diabetes mellitus, and we know that improving insulin sensitivity can lead to better use of energy and plasticity substrates by the muscle cell.

In addition to diabetes, magnesium improves symptoms in women with PMS with a dosage of about 300 mg of magnesium or organic magnesium salts (pidolate, gluconate, aspartate, citrate) taken in the preovulatory period.

Wanting to bring back the discourse on the importance of supplementing magnesium in various sports, Cordova et al. conducted a study in 2019, whose main purpose was to analyze the effects of magnesium supplementation in preventing muscle damage in professional cyclists taking part in a 21-day cycling race.

Eighteen professional male cyclists from two teams were recruited to participate in the research. They were divided into two groups: the control group and the magnesium supplemented group. The supplement consisted of an intake of 400 mg/day of magnesium during the 3 weeks of the competition. Blood samples were collected according to WADA rules at three specific times during the competition: immediately before the competition, in the middle of the competition and before the last stage.

Levels of serum and erythrocyte magnesium, lactate dehydrogenase, creatinine kinase, aspartate transaminase, alanine transaminase, myoglobin, aldolase, total protein, cortisol and creatinine were determined. Magnesium levels in serum and in the erythrocytes decreased during the race. Circulating tissue markers increased at the end of the competition in both groups. However, the increase in myoglobin was lower in the supplemented group than in the control group, and this led the researchers to conclude that magnesium supplementation was able to exert a protective effect on the muscle damage.

The fact that a good nutrition and a good supplementation are always associated with physical activity is obviously not a coincidence, in fact the sedentary lifestyle is highly associated with an increased risk of cardiovascular diseases, obesity and type 2 diabetes. Regular physical activity has positive effects on health, but it is also known and several studies have shown that intense exercise can induce the oxidative stress and cause DNA damage. Since magnesium is essential for maintaining the DNA integrity, Petrovic et al. conducted a study in 2018, whose purpose was to determine whether the supplementation of magnesium for 4 weeks in students with a sedentary lifestyle and in rugby players could prevent or reduce the DNA damage.

The study showed that the number of peripheral blood lymphocytes (PBLs) with basal endogenous DNA damage was significantly higher in rugby players than in students with a sedentary lifestyle, but magnesium supplementation was also observed to be able to significantly reduce the number of cells with high DNA damage, in the presence of exogenous H_2O_2, in both students and rugby players, and it significantly reduced the number of cells with average DNA damage in rugby players, compared to the corresponding control group who had not taken the supplement. Consequently, these results suggest that magnesium supplementation for 4 weeks had an effect in protecting the DNA from oxidative damage in both rugby players and young people with a sedentary lifestyle.

Practicing sports, therefore, especially at a moderate and high level, is a form of stress and activates the hypothalamus-pituitary-adrenal (HPA) axis, inducing the body's inflammatory response. Due to current eating habits and due to the increase in energy expenditure, athletes are sensitive to the exhaustion of magnesium ions. The aim of the study by Dmitrašinović et al. of 2018 was to investigate, through the assessment of plasma ACTH, serum IL-6 and salivary/serum cortisol levels, whether chronic magnesium supplementation could reduce the damaging effects of stress in amateur rugby players. Rugby players ($n = 23$) were randomly assigned to the intervention and control groups. Baseline samples were collected before the intervention group began a 4-week supplementation with magnesium (500 mg/day).

Blood and saliva were collected the day before the match (day 1), the morning of the competition (match) and during a 6-day recovery period (day 1, day 3 and day 6), while ACTH, serum and salivary cortisol, IL-6, and total and the differential white blood cell counts were determined at each point. There was a statistically significant increase in ACTH concentration in the intervention group compared to the control group, while reductions in cortisol concentrations between the two groups were the highest at day 1 ($p < 0.01$) and at the competition (game) day ($p < 0.01$). The results also revealed that magnesium completely suppressed the increase of IL-6 levels observed in the control group on day 1 and day 3, compared with day 1 ($p < 0.01$), and also decreased the neutrophil/lymphocyte ratio in the intervention group, compared to the control group ($p < 0.01$).

In conclusion, these results suggest that magnesium supplementation could have an important influence on the change in the parameters of the HPA axis activity and on the reduction of the activation of the immune response, following intense physical exercise such as the game of rugby.

Dosages

Dosages of magnesium vary based on the type of supplement taken. If magnesium is taken in the inorganic salt form, such as magnesium sulfate or carbonate, it is necessary to settle on 500 mg/day, instead of 300 mg which is sufficient for organic salts such as magnesium citrate or pidolate, as the bioavailability is much higher. To promote its absorption during or after the training, it is necessary to take magnesium in a mixture of electrolytes, then associated with potassium, chlorine and sodium, to favor its entry into the cell.

In case of severe deficiencies (difficult to assess), it can go up to 1.5 g/day in three intakes.

Effectiveness

Strength	Resistant strength	Mass	Endurance	Slimming	Concentration	Recovery
++	++	+	++	+	++	++

MALTODEXTRIN

Description

The term *maltodextrin* comes from the composition of the molecule, made up of maltose (two glucose molecules) and dextrose (glucose). They are therefore glucose polymers that can range from a minimum of 4 to a maximum of 20 monomers joined together. These glucose molecules are linked together with glycosidic bonds α (1→4) (between site 1 of one unit and site 4 of the next unit) to form the main linear structure that is also called *amylose*. This main structure there gives rise to lateral, peripheral branches with type α bonds (1→6) called amylopectin. The endogenous amylases (salivary and pancreatic) hydrolyze the α (1→4) bond, residing the peripheral oligomeric compounds which are called *dextrins*. These will then be hydrolyzed by the intestinal border (which has α-1.6 glycosidase) and then absorbed.

The processing of these supplements involves making them from larger starch polymers which are then hydrolyzed to the desired length molecule. The starchy products that are most used for their production come from cereals such as corn, wheat, oats and rice, but tubers such as potatoes and tapioca can also be used. An important concept for evaluating these products is the dextrose equivalent (DE) of a maltodextrin. This is a value that describes how similar a maltodextrin is to the reference sugar, dextrose. Therefore, maltodextrins with very high DE will be those made from short polymers (more similar to glucose), while maltodextrins with low DE will be made from longer polymers (more similar to starch).

The DE scale ranges from a minimum of 3 to a maximum of 20. Generally, a question of interest is whether maltodextrins can cause problems for people that are intolerant to gluten or acutally celiac, since they are often produced from wheat. Normally these products undergo such a process in order to lose all the antigen-like protein part, that could stimulate the immune system of an already sensitized person. However, for these subjects, it is better to prefer maltodextrins extracted from tubers or rice and avoid those derived from wheat. It should also be remembered that these products should be tested during the training because individual responses can vary from one athlete to another. As for their palatability, maltodextrins are colorless and tasteless and are often flavored with fructose or various sweeteners. In particular, the association with fructose gave better results in terms of performance.

Properties

The first property of maltodextrins is the rapid impact on the subject's blood sugar. These products have been designed for the replenishment of carbohydrates during sports activities (mostly prolonged) so as not to have the physiological drops in performance, events that every true sportsperson knows well. In fact, they have a high glycemic index (GI), even higher than that of white sugar, but they have some peculiar differences. Although they are more or less long glucose polymers (one would therefore expect a different absorption by the intestine by virtue of their molecular weight), it should be remembered that they are, however, extremely artificial and refined products and lack the composition of macronutrients (fibers, proteins and lipids) that modulates the GI in natural foods. Even products with very low dextrose equivalence (DE) (see above) create rapid spikes in blood sugar, much greater than normal foods.

The influence on glycaemia has three main effects, which are: the decrease in the perception of fatigue, the anticatabolic effect that allows the sugar to be used for the energy saving muscle, and the anabolic effect related to the insulin peak (useful for replenishing the glycogen and to cotransport amino acids within the muscle during the post-workout period). The osmolarity of these products is different from that of normal carbohydrates and has an advantageous role in prolonged exercise conditions. If we take simple glucose as an example, its osmolarity is five times greater than that of maltodextrins. As we know, the more a carbohydrate is surrounded by water, the simpler its chemical structure.

Each glucose molecule, for example, tends to bind four molecules of water. This sugar therefore causes a retention of the intraluminal fluids that tend to stretch the smooth muscular walls of the stomach, which responds by increasing the tone of the pylorus and lowering the gastric emptying speed. Supplements with a simple glucose substance are never a good idea in an elite sportsperson.

The fluid retention that you have with this practice at the gastrointestinal level can cause abdominal pain and swelling, up to frank diarrhea. It goes without saying that even the most nuanced aspects of this mechanism can affect the hydration of the subject, which is a fundamental parameter to be best controlled during a race. Let's not forget that the dilution, the timing in relation to the effort and the period of intake of maltodextrins (understood as the intake time of the supplement) has very direct implications for the athlete. Consuming maltodextrins outside the scope of physical exertion or during short-term efforts (under 60 minutes) will probably have the only effect of increasing the subject's fat mass and the inert load that the athlete will have to carry during the physical exertion.

Evidence

We all know how carbohydrates are the "source of joy and torment" of every athlete. Whether you do any sport in the wide range from endurance (endurance or resistance training) to resistance training (weight training or counter resistance), the correct management of the carbohydrate intake has always been an essential factor for the performance. On the contrary, an incorrect planning of this step alone can severely affect the result of our workouts and also our body composition. Carbohydrates are an exceptional fuel and their use in the muscle is influenced by many factors, but the main ones are the intensity of the exercise, its duration and the amount of glycogen stored in the body (liver and muscles). Another important factor is the type of carbohydrate that is taken, which can be diversified according to the glycemic index (GI).

The depletion of glycogen reserves during continued sports activities decreases the yield of our performance by 13%. This occurs during the transition from carbohydrate to lipid metabolism (less performing fuel in maintaining an intense exercise). An athlete who typically has to manage this limit is the marathon runner, who has to measure the intensity of the exercise, their pulse and their sensations in order to work purely by burning lipids for the most part of the race. Carbohydrates will be needed for the final sprint.

It is therefore evident that for prolonged activities (purely aerobic, but not limited to them) the re-supplementation of carbohydrates during exercise, especially for an athlete that is not adapted to the metabolic efficiency of the best use of fats for energy purposes, can maintain the performance at the highest possible level for that athlete. Hence the need for supplements that provide a gradual carbohydrate supply during the exercise, without triggering complicated digestive circuits that subtract the blood circulation from the muscles that are used in athletic performance: maltodextrins.

A 1990 study by Davies et al. highlighted the bioavailability and the modulation of insulin after administering various solutions containing different forms of carbohydrates to American students. The administered solutions consisted of 6% maltodextrin and glucose-fructose at various percentages (6, 8, 10%) compared to a placebo (water only). The results showed that the solution containing only maltodextrin increased both blood sugar and insulinemia more than other glucose and fructose solutions, avoiding dangerous glycemic peaks that can lead to a reduction in energy. Also in this study, the 8% glucose-fructose solution had characteristics similar to maltodextrins, but with a higher total concentration. The ability of maltodextrins to bind a smaller number of water molecules, and therefore to have significantly lower osmolarity values, allows it to be better absorbed within the intestine and to obtain an increase in blood sugar levels with a smaller dosage than glucose and fructose, avoiding unwanted effects such as bloating, intestinal cramps and osmotic diarrhea. **Maltodextrin supplementation is much more effective for endurance sports, especially for its ability to restore muscle glycogen stores** and for its stability in the intestinal environment (Davis et al., 1990).

An interesting use could be that of resistant maltodextrins (Resistant MaltoDextrin, RMD), in which the processing of starch acts as a fiber, by stimulating the intestinal peristaltic movements.

Dosages

Maltodextrins must be diluted in water, at a concentration of 60-70 g per liter of water (in this way, we can obtain iso- or slightly hyposmolar solutions) (generally, it is better to get it more diluted than more concentrated). The gradual intake of the caloric drink favors its oxidation at the cellular level (usually 200 cc of liquid every 20 minutes during the effort is a good approach). We tend to prefer to use products with low DE at the beginning of a long endurance race and to keep products with high DE for the final rush. The supply of endogenous glycogen before the competition is very important, but it must be achieved using natural foods (easier to manage). In fact, an error in the calculation of the dose of maltodextrin that is used in order to produce the much sought supercompensation, will have the unique effect of increasing the fat mass as we already mentioned above.

Effectiveness

Strength	Resistant strength	Mass	Endurance	Slimming	Concentration	Recovery
+	++	+	+++	–	+	++++

MCT

Description

Medium Chain Triglycerides (MCTs) are a class of lipids in which three medium chain saturated fatty acids (6-12 carbon atoms) are bonded to a glycerol molecule. In nature we find these compounds in many foods, but the food that is richest in them is coconut oil.

The progenitors of these medium-chain glycerol-binding fatty acids that boast particular characteristics are: caprylic, capric and lauric acid. In medicine, there have been various applications of MCTs: malabsorption, HIV, cachexia, Alzheimer's and Parkinson's diseases, cardiovascular diseases, diabetes and cancer. What is surprising is that they can be used to obtain diametrically opposite results on paper. Traditionally, in fact, as in the examples reported above, they have been used for nutrition protocols in particular cases of physical and organic wasting.

However, in recent years, new trials of these compounds for weight control and for an improvement of the body composition have become increasingly popular in the literature. MCTs, in fact, are rapidly metabolized allowing immediate energy production, especially for those organs that require huge quantities of oxygen, such as the brain and heart; moreover, they are sequestered much less by the adipose tissue to make them fat storage. In order to analyze the influence of the metabolism of these lipids on the sense of satiety, on body composition and on the increase in energy expenditure, we carried out a review of the publications reported in Pubmed and Elsevier between 2000 and 2010.

There were studies that analyzed the supplementation of MCT in the short term and others in the long term. Of these, six showed a decrease in the body mass index (BMI), resulting in weight loss. One showed a positive effect on satiety and four showed an increase in the energy expenditure.

Properties

Unlike long-chain saturated fatty acids (with 14-20 or more carbon atoms), MCTs are poured directly into the portal circulation without first passing through the lymphatic pathway. Long-chain fatty acids (LCTs) must be separated from glycerol by the lipase enzymes in the intestine. Subsequently, they form micelles which are absorbed by the brush border and are reconnected to the glycerol in the enterocytes to form new triglycerides. The latter access the lymphatic stream and then continue to the thoracic duct and pour into the general bloodstream. This whole part is completely skipped when it comes to MCTs.

First of all, the triglycerides that contain them boast a better water solubility than their long-chain counterparts and therefore do not require enzymatic hydrolysis by intestinal juices. They are absorbed intact and flow directly into the portal vein, binding here to the albumin to then reach the target cells. At the cell membrane level, then, MCTs directly access the cytoplasm and even penetrate the mitochondria without the need for the carnitine transporter (necessary for all other fatty acids). Let's now analyze the oxidative side of these nutrients and their relationship with insulin. The dysregulation of lipid beta oxidation plays a fundamental role in the pathophysiology of obesity and insulin resistance.

By virtue of their kinetics in the body, MCTs do not stimulate particular increases in insulin. A dehydrogenase for MCTs called SCHAD (Medium-and short-chain-3-hydroxyacyl-coenzyme A dehydrogenase), NAD^+-dependent, catalyzes the third reaction of beta oxidation. This enzyme is particularly present in the heart, liver, fatty tissue and pancreatic islets of Langerhans. Current data report SCHAD as a key element of thermogenesis. SCHAD-deficient patients present with hyperinsulinism, suggesting that blocking of this reaction may explain the insulin surge. Thus, the metabolism of MCTs and the stimulation of their enzymatic pathway increases the thermogenesis and improves the insulin sensitivity.

Let's now look at the side of the nerve transduction pathways that are stimulated by the use of MCTs. As we know, the central nervous system is responsible for the sense of hunger and the search for food in conditions of energy need. This scale is regulated by the timing of food intake, by their quality and peculiarities and by the storages of fat. The ingestion of certain nutrients can promote a greater sense of satiety by decreasing the search for additional food. It has been suggested that the quality of certain lipids (MCT, in fact) increases the "satiating power".

This would be expressed in particular through a relaxation of the gastric tone (increase in stomach distension) given by lipids in general, specifically more by MCTs, which would induce a decrease in hunger through afferents to the vagus nerve. As for the uptake of MCT by adipocytes, since these are not carried by blood transport lipoproteins (by virtue of their kinetics), they do not come into contact with the lipoproteinlipases of the adipose tissue, which sequester the fatty acids from the blood for storage purposes in the adipose tissue.

Evidence

Given the peculiarities of these fats, an important use would be recommended. But how do they behave *in vivo* in the various studies? The easier metabolization is confirmed by studies that show a low post-MCT insulinemic rise and an absence of the blood lipoprotein rise, with a consequent decrease in the anabolism of the lipid tissue. This has led many studies to agree that replacing some of the dietary lipids with MCTs can led to an improvement in the body composition of normal and overweight subjects. The stimulus of thermogenesis also seems to be confirmed by a study in which oxygen consumption was evaluated after a meal in which 400 Kcal of MCT and 400 of LCT were administered to different groups.

After MCT ingestion, oxygen consumption was 12% higher in the MCT group compared to only 4% in the LCT group. Also on this front, another study even found a correlation between MCT and stimulation of brown fat which, as we know, leads to a reduction in fat mass. If spicy dishes containing capsaicin are associated with MCTs, there is even a synergistic and additive effect of the two substances. There are conflicting opinions on the improvement in cases of diabetes and further studies will serve to clarify this link, although the low insulin stimulus of these fats seems to be confirmed. The combination of a diet containing MCT and exercise further improved the body composition of overweight subjects.

Some theories in the sports field assumed that the use of MCTs preserved glycogen stores in athletes and therefore favored their performance in competitive subjects. However, only one study has shown an improvement in this regard by linking it to the decrease in lactate production on a HIIT (High Intensity Interval Training) protocol. On the contrary, all the other studies which also investigated the performance side, did not find significant post-supplementation differences. Further studies are needed to investigate the glycogen savings during MCT supplementation and any implications on the athletic performance.

A really important contribution from the use of MCTs occurs in conditions that require the immediate use of an energy substrate or in particular diets, such as the ketogenic diet.

Given the success of the ketogenic diet and its effects on the long-lasting aerobic performance, we tried to understand how it was possible to speed up the induction of ketosis in order to limit the time window of discomfort that is derived from the adaptation to ketone bodies. A study published in the *Journal of Nutrition and Metabolism* in 2018 shows that 30 mL of MCT three times a day for 20 days, halved the time it takes for the brain to use ketone bodies, a process known as keto induction.

Supplementation with MCT was also able to improve the mood and probably all the other symptoms related to excess ketone bodies, such as constipation, intestinal irritability, bloating, headache and halitosis. The real advantage of supplementing with MCT lies in the ability to maintain the ketosis even by consuming a quantity of carbohydrates three times higher than the classic 6% expected for VLCKD.

All this allows to avoid the normal adverse effects given by the inversion of the sources of the micronutrients that are used (fats instead of carbohydrates), which cause an immediate change of the microbiota, with a rapid depletion of the communities (for example lactobacilli and bifidobacteria) that previously populated the intestine. As examples we can mention their usage in order to induce a state of ketosis without the negative effects on the mood, derived from the momentary unavailability of beta-ketoacyl-CoA transferase, or the brain enzyme capable of converting vinegar-acetyl-CoA into 2-acetyl-CoA, ready to be used as an energy substrate.

MCTs can be successfully used as a fuel for swimming, cycling or running competition, as their fast metabolization, added to the easy crossing of the blood brain barrier and the absence of insulin peak, allows the maintenance of a stable blood sugar. If you also consider the saving of muscle glycogen, they become a very useful supplement for maintaining lactate levels in optimal ranges that do not affect the performance.

Dosages

The doses of MCTs vary greatly from study to study. The ranges are from 5 to 30 g of MCT per day to promote weight loss in overweight individuals. In the study on the stimulation of thermogenesis, MCT provided 400 Kcal (1 g MCT = 8.3 Kcal), equal to about 48 g of MCT. As for the effects on the induction of ketosis, the optimal dosages are 30 ml 3 times a day, for a period ranging from 5 days upwards. As a pre-workout supplement, especially as a brain fuel, 30 g can always be used together with essential amino acids in order not to increase insulin levels.

Effectiveness

Strength	Resistant strength	Mass	Endurance	Slimming	Concentration	Recovery
–	+	–	+	+++	+	+

MELATONIN

Melatonin is a hormone produced by the pineal gland or epiphysis, located in the back of the brain. From a chemical point of view, it derives from a precursor amino acid, tryptophan, which is hydroxylated to 5-OH-tryptophan and subsequently transformed into serotonin, which in turn, in the absence of light, is converted into melatonin. The main biological function of melatonin is to mark the rhythms of the biological clock and is able to act as the conductor of all the most important hormones in the body. Melatonin is secreted almost exclusively at night, in response to the light-dark alternation and its levels are 10 times higher than during the day, with a peak at around 2 am.

It could therefore be said that the production of this hormone, stimulated by the dark, represents the signal for our body that it is time to sleep. In fact, melatonin has been used for decades to treat sleep-related disorders. In the morning, when we perceive the light, the secretion of melatonin ceases and other hormones take over, such as the adrenal ones (cortisol, adrenaline), which help us get going. Melatonin has a circadian rhythm, with its own specific curve that can be altered, like that of cortisol, by various factors. For example, the melatonin curve can be altered by blue lights (such as those emitted by TV and computer and smartphone screens), benzodiazepines, beta-blockers, and some antidepressants and antipsychotics.

After the age of 30-40, melatonin production drops and around the age of 60 it is about half that of a 20-year-old. This is perhaps one of the reasons why older people tend to sleep less.

Properties

Melatonin promotes sleep, but its action is not limited to inducing sleep (even if this would already be enough to be able to consider it a useful supplement for athletes, who need a greater amount of sleep to recover from intense workouts that can create problems falling asleep, especially if performed late in the evening); in fact, it also acts at other levels. Melatonin is also produced by the mitochondria and consequently it can be said that all cells produce melatonin. This is of particular importance, as mitochondrial density varies from cell to cell and also varies depending on the senescence process affecting the cell, particularly the mitochondria.

Melatonin is one of the most powerful antioxidants in our body, as it fights free radicals, which are chemicals that cause damage to the DNA, cell and mitochondrial membranes, and to proteins, a damage that is at the basis of many age-related diseases and changes, including atherosclerosis and cancer, skin wrinkles and hair loss.

A fundamental characteristic of melatonin is its ability to pass through the blood brain barrier, thus exerting its protective action at the level of the brain structures and helping to prevent some neurological degenerative diseases, such as Alzheimer's and Parkinson's disease. Taken as a supplement, however, it is not able to reach those concentrations at the level of the third ventricle that are reached by the production and direct release of melatonin in the third ventricle by the pineal itself.

Another important action of melatonin is the ability to boost the immune system, both by stimulating the thymus to produce a greater number of T lymphocytes and by limiting the production of cortisol, the stress hormone with an immunosuppressive power; it also has an anti-inflammatory effect, stimulating the production of interleukin-2.

Its regulatory action is expressed on various other hormones, in fact it could be defined as the "hormonal orchestra conductor": it stimulates the production of GH (or somatotropic hormone), the anti-aging hormone that stimulates and maintains the muscle mass, promotes the loss of body fat, decreases the secretion of cortisol, with which it has an inverse relationship, and optimizes the secretion of progesterone; moreover, melatonin modulates the production of thyrotropic hormone (TSH), which stimulates the thyroid to synthesize other hormones, such as T3 and T4, it modulates the insulin production by acting on the beta cell receptors of the pancreas, regulates the production of leptin and ghrelin, hormones related to the sensation of hunger, the first is an anorectic, the second is orexigenic.

Probably, also thanks to these hormonal modulations, melatonin has been shown to be effective in promoting weight loss. Melatonin supplementation appears to promote weight control by also altering the gut microbiota, according to a study conducted on mice by Chinese researchers. In this study, the mice were fed a high-fat diet that altered the gut microbiota leading to weight gain. However, the supplementation of melatonin altered the bacterial colonies of the intestine and caused a reduction in weight, fat storage and adipose tissue.

Other studies have also found that melatonin supplementation is able to reduce the inflammation and normalize adipokines, which are important signaling chemicals. Therefore, melatonin supplements seem to be a valuable aid in promoting the control not only of sleep, but also of weight. Gut microbiota imbalances are linked to obesity, weakened immune system, periodontal disease, cardiovascular problems, cancer, back pain, allergies and it also appears to be a probable cause of autism (*Journal of Pineal Research*, 2017).

Furthermore, melatonin also modulates the production of the sex hormones estrogen and testosterone by the gonads and adrenal glands, so much so that its use at high doses as a contraceptive has been considered to avoid the risks of carcinoma associated with the use of synthetic estrogen.

Melatonin exerts this effect through the inhibition at the level of the hypothalamic GnRH, responsible for the stimulation of FSH and LH by the pituitary, decreasing, the possibility of ovulation and the production of estrogen in women, and the spermatogenesis and testosterone production in men. Conversely, at physiological doses it exerts an effect favoring the normal hormonal secretion. Melatonin acts simultaneously as both SERM (Selecting Estrogen Receptor Modulator, which displaces estrogens from their receptor) and SEEM (Selecting Estrogen Enzyme Modulator, which inhibits the enzymatic pathway that leads to the formation of estrogens or more powerful estrogens).

Consequently, given the increased estrogenic stimulation of breast tissue in hormone replacement therapy, xenoestrogen exposure and obesity, and its correlation to breast cancer, melatonin can be considered an ideal treatment for the prevention of this disease in the population at risk. This molecule is both water-soluble and fat-soluble and this allows it to exert its antioxidant effect both inside and outside the cell. Melatonin in the extracellular space is five times more powerful, as an antioxidant, than glutathione, considered the most powerful water-soluble antioxidant, and within the cell it is twice as powerful as vitamin E, a powerful fat-soluble antioxidant.

At the skin level, possibly also as a topical administration, it has a stimulating effect on the fibroblasts, improving the trophism of the skin.

Another effect is related to the **reduction of lactic acid production**. We know that the excessive production of lactic acid is a limiting factor in sports activity because, circulating in the blood, it prevents you from continuing the activity, causing severe muscle pain. Melatonin is able **to bind to lactic acid**, thus avoiding the appearance of these adverse effects.

Furthermore, melatonin is able to reduce side effects in patients treated with ionizing radiation, so it could be of help as a support in antineoplastic therapies.

Melatonin also exerts a cardioprotective effect through several mechanisms: thanks to its antioxidant power, it inhibits the oxidation of LDL cholesterol; in addition, it has a vasodilating effect, reduces hypoxia, reduces mitochondrial dysfunction, prevents reperfusion damage, and also has an anti-inflammatory, antiarrhythmic and antihypertensive effect.

The best-designed anti-aging strategy to keep melatonin levels high is to reduce the number of calories. If young animals are fed with only 60% of the quantity of food that is normally taken, in addition to maintaining a good production of melatonin, they even live for a 50% longer time than animals that have free access to food. In addition, animals have a lower incidence of all degenerative diseases and look younger even at a very old age.

How can melatonin extend the human life?

Possible mechanisms include several pathways in which melatonin can intervene, which are summarized in the following table.

Table 44.7 Antiaging mechanisms of melatonin

- The reduction of the damage caused by free radicals
- The stimulation of the aging immune system
- The protection of the cardiovascular system
- The stabilization of the body's biological rhythms
- The re-establishment of the night cycle of rest and recovery
- The stimulation of growth hormone production

Evidence

In 1991, prof. Giacomo Zaccone, professor of Comparative Endocrinology at the University of Messina, with his colleagues from San Antonio, measured the melatonin levels of three groups of rats: elderly rats which had been given free access to food; elderly rats raised on a low calorie diet; young rats fed freely. He observed that elderly rats that had a normal diet had significantly reduced melatonin levels compared to juvenile rats (an age-related decline in melatonin production was observed in all animals, including humans, studied up to this moment). The undernourished aged rats, however, produced twice as much melatonin as their well-fed peers; moreover, they produced almost as much melatonin as rats with an age equal to one fifth of theirs.

This suggests that caloric restriction and the maintenance of melatonin production go hand in hand or that in any case the intake of melatonin could simulate the positive effects of calorie restriction without the negative effects that, in humans, can be the decrease in energy and the loss of muscle mass. In 2001 Klinkene et al. reported that the onset of breast cancer in women who had gone blind before the age of 65 was 49% lower than in women who had a normal vision. Since melatonin production in blind women is high throughout the day, these researchers have suggested a possible antitumor role of this substance. According to various studies, melatonin inhibits the proliferation of cancer cells in the breast, uterus and ovary.

In a 2017 study published in *Pineal Research*, melatonin was shown to reduce body weight, fatty liver and low-grade inflammation, as well as improved the insulin resistance in mice that were fed a high-fat diet (HFD). Furthermore, melatonin significantly changed the composition of the gut microbiota in HFD-fed mice. In particular, by decreasing the ratio between *Firmicutes* (associated with obesity) and *Bacteroidetes* (more present in normal-weight individuals), and by increasing the presence of mucin-degrading bacteria of the *Akkermansia* genus, which are associated with a healthy mucosa.

Taken together, the findings suggest that melatonin can be used as a probiotic agent to reverse the HFD-induced gut microbiota dysbiosis and may help us better understand the mechanisms that regulate the various beneficial effects of this substance.

Numerous studies, mainly on hibernating animals, have shown that the supplementation of melatonin and a short photoperiod increase the mass of brown adipose tissue (BAT) which is a thermogenic tissue in mammals. The activation of BAT leads to an increase in energy expenditure which could, at least theoretically, be a possible tool for the treatment of obesity and type 2 diabetes.

A recent study tried to evaluate BAT in patients with melatonin deficiency (radiotherapy or surgical removal of the pineal gland) before and after daily melatonin replacement (3 mg) for 3 months. All four patients had an increase in BAT volume and activity, and there was also an improvement in blood cholesterol and total triglyceride levels, with no significant effects on body weight, liver fat and LDL or HDL levels and. Although not statistically significant, fasting insulin levels and insulin resistance HOMA decreased in all four patients.

Current results show that the oral replacement of melatonin increases the volume and the activity of BAT and improves blood lipid levels in patients with melatonin deficiency, suggesting that melatonin is a possible activator of BAT. Future studies are desirable because hypomelatoninemia is generally present in the elderly and appears as a result of exposure to light at night and/or due to the use of beta-blocking drugs.

A study was carried out in order to evaluate the effect of melatonin supplementation on the antioxidant capacity and DNA damage in high intensity training athletes (HIIT). Two groups of athletes, one that took a placebo (PG) and the other who took melatonin (MG) (20 mg/day) were monitored for a period of 2 weeks of HIIT and strength training.

The total antioxidant capacity (TAC) and glutathione peroxidase (GPx) and superoxide dismutase (SOD) activities were analyzed in their blood samples. DNA damage was measured in isolated lymphocytes before and immediately after the exercise. The supplementation increased the plasma levels of melatonin in the group treated with melatonin ($p < 0.05$) 2 weeks after the surgery. The analysis of the antioxidant status indicated higher values ($p < 0.05$) of TAC and GPx in MG compared to post-intervention PG. DNA damage was reduced in MG ($p < 0.05$) compared to PG in post-training conditions. Antioxidant status was associated with DNA damage ($r = -0.679$; $p = 0.047$) in athletes treated with melatonin. This study suggests that the supplementation of melatonin improves the antioxidant status and may have beneficial effects by preventing DNA damage induced by high intensity training.

A systematic review and meta-analysis of randomized controlled trials (RCTs) was conducted to clarify the effect of melatonin supplementation on the glycemic control. In summary, the current meta-analysis has shown a promising effect of melatonin supplementation on glycemic control, by reducing fasting glucose and increasing QUICKI (insulin sensitivity control index), but further studies are recommended using higher supplementation doses and a longer intervention period, to confirm the impact of melatonin on insulin, HOMA-IR indices (Homeostatic Model Of Insulin Resistance) and HbA1c (glycated hemoglobin expressing the average of glycemic levels for the last three months).

How to increase the body's production of melatonin?

It is possible to do this naturally, by manipulating the foods of the daily diet. Melatonin is naturally present in cherries. The precursor of melatonin, tryptophan, is an amino acid present in foods rich in proteins, such as milk, turkey, legumes and seeds, and therefore the diet must not be deficient in this amino acid. Carbohydrates also have their importance if consumed in the right dose in the evening because they favor the entry of tryptophan into the brain (this is one reason why not consuming carbohydrates in the evening can hinder sleep). As a supplement, it is possible to use **tryptophan** itself or *Griffonia* extracts, which contain 5-HTP, the direct precursor of serotonin, which is also the precursor of melatonin.

However, it is advisable to eat in a measured way as the calorie restriction favors the production of melatonin (and longevity).

The exogenous intake of **magnesium** increases the activity of serotonin-N-acetyltransferase, an enzyme involved in the synthesis of melatonin. Rats that were administered a diet lacking in magnesium had a 33% reduction in melatonin values.

As for **physical activity**, it is good not to train intensely too late in the evening, as it has been shown that an intense workout, even of only 20 minutes, reduces the secretion of melatonin in the following 3 hours due to the production of cortisol and, as you know, cortisol and melatonin are antagonists.

Three more rules

1. During the day, try to expose yourself to intense light for at least a couple of hours.
2. Reduce exposure to light (especially blue light) during the evening hours.
3. Make sure you go to bed before midnight (preferably before 10pm) and with all lights off.

In some cases, however, our bodies cannot produce enough melatonin; the reasons can be various: age, alcohol and caffeine abuse, electromagnetic and radioactive pollution, alterations in the sleep-wake/light-dark rhythm, as in shift workers or night workers or in jet-lag syndrome. In all these cases, the use of melatonin as a supplement may be useful.

Dosages

The production of melatonin already decreases at the age of 40, so its supplementation can be useful in order to compensate for the progressive deficit that occurs with aging. Melatonin is present on the Italian market as a supplement, but only at a dosage of 1 mg; Higher dosages fall within the realm of pharmacology, while dosages up to 10 mg are available as a supplement in the US.

The recommended dosage is from 0.5 to 5 mg depending on age and problems. The antiaging dosage is about 0.5-1 mg; to treat sleep disorders and jet lag (time zone syndrome) it is 3 to 5 mg. It is advisable to start from a low dosage and possibly increase it, if necessary, up to 10 mg/day. In general, the recommended dosage for anti-aging purposes is 1 mg from the age of 40, increasing by 1 mg every decade. It is good to take it about an hour before going to bed, always at the same time. Its effectiveness is less effective when taken on a full stomach, possibly because it is not absorbed well. Melatonin is well tolerated in recommended doses and for limited periods (3 months).

Some people report difficulty in waking up in the morning or lethargy even during the day and in some people it has the "paradox effect", that is, it causes difficulty in sleeping and possibly nightmares. Others have reported a mild headache, upset stomach and a decreased libido, as it can reduce the production of sex hormones. It can increase the risk of blood clotting. Normally, these side effects can occur with dosages higher than 10 mg per day, or when it is combined with other drugs. Those taking 1 mg dosages do not normally report any side effects.

The administration of exogenous melatonin leads to hypnotic and hypothermic responses in humans, which can be linked to immediate reductions in short-term physical and mental performance. Depending on the dose of melatonin, these effects may still be evident 3-5 hours after the administration for some types of cognitive performances, but the effects on physical performance seem to be more short-lived, so **it is not recommended to take the product on the day of the performance** or immediately before the activity, as it may degrade your performance.

Effectiveness

Strength	Resistant strength	Mass	Endurance	Slimming	Concentration	Recovery
–	+	–	–	+++	–	+++

MUCUNA

Description

Mucuna, identified with the scientific name *Mucuna pruriens*, belongs to the *Fabaceae* or legume family, just like beans, chickpeas, peas, lupins and broad beans. These are herbs, shrubs, trees or vines that cling to supports or by means of tendrils.

The characteristic that is common to all the species of the family concerns the fruit, called legume or pod, which contains the seeds, which are the most used part of this plant. In the mucuna, the ripening fruit has a very hairy skin, is about 10 cm long, 1-2 cm wide and produces seven shiny, flattened, black or dark brown seeds.

Mucuna grows spontaneously in tropical African and South Asian regions, particularly in India, from the slopes of the Himalayas to Sri Lanka, and in the Caribbean areas up to South America. Due to its important medicinal properties and industrial needs, this plant is now extensively cultivated for commercial purposes.

Properties

Mucuna pruriens, traditionally used in Ayurvedic medicine, contains levodopa (L-dopa), an amino acid precursor of dopamine. Dopamine is a hormone that also acts as a neurotransmitter and plays an important role for the brain, as it is responsible for activating the sensation of pleasure and well-being; this neurotransmitter also acts at the pituitary level by stimulating the production of growth hormone, whose function is to keep the body young. Several studies have now ascertained that the administration of L-DOPA represents one of the most effective treatments against Parkinson's disease, since the lack of dopamine is responsible for the loss of the control on body movements.

The increase in brain dopamine favors the recovery of impulses and therefore decreases muscle stiffness and tremors. These properties continue to be studied and even confirmed, as demonstrated by numerous studies, including very recent ones (2020). Like *Tribulus terrestris*, mucuna is also traditionally used to increase the body's natural production of growth hormone and testosterone, involved in physical, mental and sexual well-being. In fact, this plant has been used for a long time as an aphrodisiac and especially against erectile disorders, as confirmed by various studies that have proven an increase in the rate of steroid hormones and blood flow in the penile area.

In addition to being effective for men by increasing the productivity of spermatozoa, mucuna promotes the ovulation in women and improves liveliness and motor coordination in both men and women.

From an ergogenic point of view, this product has been discovered and increasingly used also by bodybuilders, who aim to increase the production of growth hormone and testosterone, and therefore to increase their lean mass.

Evidence

As mentioned above, there are numerous studies relating to the use of mucuna in Parkinson's, but they will not be cited because they are not congruent with the purpose of these pages.

Given the potential benefits of stimulating the growth hormone production for both health and fitness purposes, many food supplements have been formulated with the aim of increasing its release.

A 2011 study published in *Nutrition and Metabolic Insights* specifically analyzes the effects of adaptogenic herbs, including mucuna. The purpose of this test was to determine the effects related to the intake of the extract of this plant on the circulating levels of GH in healthy and trained subjects. Fifteen men took this extract; their blood was collected before and after 20, 40, 60, 80, 100 and 120 minutes of ingesting the extract, and was later analyzed using the ELISA method. Further investigations are necessary to confirm the efficacy of mucuna, even if the test results showed an increase in serum GH levels starting 60 minutes after the ingestion, with very variable values from subject to subject.

Moving on to another field, a 2012 study proved how the antioxidant efficacy of mucuna is able to protect the erectile tissues, a very important factor since incorrect lifestyles damage these tissues, with all the consequences we can imagine. Obviously, taking this substance is not enough, but bad habits must also be changed. In 2018, another study was able to demonstrate the efficacy of mucuna on damaged penile nerves of elderly rats, so much so that the authors conclude that "its traditional use for sexual problems is amply justified".

In fact, an interesting research carried out in 2017 had shown, *in vivo* and *in vitro*, how the mucuna extract managed to obtain more than discrete improvements in the synthesis of eNOS and, consequently, in erectile function: of importance is the fact that it was of a private extract of L-DOPA, which led researchers to find the active components in catechol and polyphenols.

Also in 2018, in a study in which mucuna was used in association with *Tribulus* and Ashwagandha, it was shown that it had the ability to elevate the hormone levels and enhance the sexual behavior of rats. Many studies have then confirmed the efficacy of mucuna in the treatment of male infertility. In a 2012 research, a mixture of medicinal plants with aphrodisiac potential was administered orally to albino rats (for 40 days) and to oligospermic patients (for 90 days).

In albino rats, the treatment with this herbal composition for 40 days resulted in a significant increase in body weight, testis and epididymal weight. At the same time, sperm motility and sperm density were significantly increased. In oligospermic patients, after 90 days of treatment with this herbal composition, sperm density and motility increased as a result of an increase in testosterone levels. No side effects were noted for the duration of the trial.

A 2019 study provided interesting indications, showing that rats that took 0.75 g/kg of mucuna extract achieved important results, while those that took doses up to three times higher also reported important side effects. The research had arisen precisely from some similar problems that occurred in Nigeria on men who had taken excessive dosages.

Also in 2019, this time on rabbits, mucuna once again improved several parameters, including the sexual behavior.

Again in 2019, a review confirmed the potential of this phytoextract: 5 g/day for 1 week improved both testosterone levels and the sperm count more than other known substances that were tested concomitantly.

Dosages

These studies used 5 g of dried *Mucuna pruriens* powder for the increase of testosterone and numerous sperm parameters, while for Parkinson's disease the dosages were between 10 and 20 mg/kg even if, as often happens, the standardization of extracts is not always the one advertised and it is therefore difficult to really take the correct dose.

Taking mucuna together with α-GPC can help maximize the GH release during sleep, allowing for a better recovery and a greater muscle growth. In this case, the effective dose of mucuna is equivalent to 600-700 mg of extract (standardized to 15% L-DOPA), taken about 30 minutes before going to bed. If this approach disturbs the sleep, it may be useful to associate it with 500 mg of tryptophan, synergistic in the stimulation of GH and it also mitigates the psychostimulating effect of dopamine.

Effectiveness

Strength	Resistant strength	Mass	Endurance	Slimming	Concentration	Recovery
+	+	+	+	+	+	+

NAD⁺/NADH

Description

NAD, or nicotinamide adenine dinucleotide, is a biological molecule belonging to the class of redox coenzymes, which means that it has the task of transferring electrons, allowing redox reactions.

To be clear, when we oxidize food we produce ATP and "reducing power", i.e. the electrons produced by these reactions are captured by the NAD and FAD (flavin adenine dinucleotide) to be transferred to the mitochondrion.

From a chemical point of view, NAD consists of four different substances, nicotinamide (or niacin or vitamin PP or vitamin B3), adenine (one of the five nitrogenous bases of nucleic acids) and two nucleotides (containing one phosphate group and one sugar group, which usually consists of ribose).

In cells it is present in two forms, depending on its oxidation state; NAD^+ is the oxidized form that regulates the oxidation reactions. When it acquires two electrons and two protons (H^+) to become $NADH_2$ ($NADH + H^+$) it transforms into its reduced form. Hence NAD^+ is the oxidized form and NADH is the reduced form. NAD^+ and NADH play a role in the energy management of the cell. However, there is also NADPH (nicotinamide adenine dinucleotide phosphate), which instead belongs to the class of dehydrogenase coenzymes and is present in all the enzymes that control the deactivation of ROS (reactive oxygen species), such as glutathione reductase and thioredoxin reductase.

NADPH is also used in the anabolic pathways, such as the synthesis of lipids and cholesterol, and for the lengthening of fatty acid chains (see below).

At the biochemical level, NAD assists the main redox reactions of the cell and enters the energy production system of both glycolysis and the Krebs cycle. During these oxidative processes, the released electrons and protons will be received by the oxidized form NAD^+ and FAD^+ (which become $NADH_2$ and $FADH_2$). NAD^+ and FAD^+ are coenzymes that transport electrons to the mitochondrion.

The NADH will then enter the complex system of the mitochondrial electron transport chain, where the transported electrons will be used to produce a proton gradient on the mitochondrial membrane. Subsequently, these protons (hydrogen ions) will be conveyed into the ATP synthetase enzyme to synthesize ATP starting from ADP (mitochondrial respiratory chain).

It can be said that the energy levels of the cell depend on the $NAD^+/NADH$ ratio or on the ADP/ATP ratio. If a cell is in a low energy state (greater presence of NAD^+ or ADP), it will set itself on an "oxidizing metabolism" and will try to increase its energy level (the concentration of ATP) from the oxidation of food. If, on the other hand, the cell is in a state of high energy level (higher intracellular concentration of NADH or ATP), the further ingested glucose will take the pentose phosphate path, a path through which molecules with 6 atoms of carbon become molecules with 5 carbon atoms. This, in addition to forming sugars with 5 carbon atoms (pentosis), produces another reducing power, this time linked to NADP (which becomes NADPH+H).

Despite the fact that it is composed of complicated biochemical reactions, the pentose phosphate pathway does not lead to any production of ATP. The pentoses, on the other hand, are used to produce DNA and RNA (proliferative stimulus), while the reducing power will be used (in conditions of high cellular energy) to produce fatty acids and cholesterol. This is why, if our calorie intake is greater than our consumption, we tend to have a change in the lipid panel and subsequently a weight gain.

NAD is also considered to be the active form of niacin, or vitamin B3, and can be found in many foods, such as red meat, liver, nuts, legumes, fish, poultry, yeast; therefore, a balanced diet should not cause deficiencies in this important cofactor.

Properties

NADH, therefore, plays a central role in the production of ATP. In fact, the oxidation of NADH requires a considerable number of chemical processes and cofactors, ranging from the degradation of glucose into pyruvate in glycolysis, to the subsequent degradation of acetyl-CoA in the Krebs cycle. During this last stage, various reducing molecules are produced (i.e. $NADH_2$ and $FADH_2$), which will enter the mitochondrion to be oxidized. The oxidation of these molecules to NAD and FAD causes an electron transfer between the protein complexes of the mitochondrial crests (electron transport chain) and gradually a gradient of protons is created between the internal and external mitochondrial matrix. These protons then arrive at ATP synthetase, which produces ATP starting from ADP.

It can be seen that NADH plays a fundamental role in maintaining a constant ATP production and in keeping the cell's energy levels high. There are several NADH supplements that would increase the cellular ATP production and improve its performance. Evidence is still scarce in this regard, but it should be emphasized that, if confirmed in more structured studies on humans, the problem of reserving their supplementation for subjects who carry out intense and prolonged physical activity would arise. In fact, high cellular levels of reducing power in conditions of low ATP use could excessively stimulate the pentose phosphate cycle, with an increased cell proliferation and the with the formation of fatty acids and cholesterol.

If NADH works in conditions of high levels of cellular energy, its oxidized form NAD^+ works in conditions of low energy. NAD^+ is an important electron acceptor and takes part in the antioxidant complexes of our organism. It comes into play as a scavenger of free radicals and especially with regard to reactive oxygen species (ROS), since it accepts the unpaired electron of these molecules, transforming them into non-toxic compounds.

For this reason, increasing the availability of NAD^+ improves the antioxidant capacity, but it has also been found to stabilize the mitochondrial function. Increasing the NAD^+ pool could also produce an increase in longevity in humans (there is already evidence on *Drosophila, C. elegans* and mice). With aging, NAD^+ levels drop, leading to mitochondrial dysfunction, a reduction in the number of mitochondria and an increase in oxidative stress. Good levels of NAD^+, on the other hand, stimulate sirtuins (NAD-dependent deacetylases that play a key role in the regulation of many processes related to the body's homeostasis, such as the regulation of metabolism, apoptosis, DNA repair and the inflammatory response).

The activation of sirtuins stabilizes the mitochondrial DNA, favoring an increase in the longevity of the mitochondrion. It also stimulates the factor PGC-1α (coactivator 1α of the nuclear receptor activated by the peroxisomal proliferator γ) which promotes the mitochondrial biogenesis in skeletal muscles and in brown adipose tissue.

We often hear of mitochondrial dysfunction as the basis of aging-related pathologies. The same calorie restriction, which has a voluminous literature on its anti-aging effects, produces an increase in the body's NAD^+ levels.

Exercise would also create a calorie deficit, increasing NAD^+ levels in the same way. Remember that NAD^+ increases in situations where the cell works at low energy (such as after calorie restriction or after the exercise). SIRT1 (the most studied human sirtuin) would be the point of contact between autophagy (remember the 2016 Nobel Prize) and mitochondrial function. Incidentally, in these low-energy situations, AMPK (AMP-adenosine monophosphate kinase) is also activated, which in turn activates the FOXO gene (longevity gene also stimulated by SIRT1).

Evidence

Since we are talking about supplements, we can say that NAD^+ precursors (NAD^+ boosters) can be used to increase the endogenous pool of this metabolite. A 2018 study (Rajman et al.) considered the use of nicotinic acid, nicotinamide (NA), NMD (nicotinamide mononucleotide) and NR (nicotinamide riboside) to increase the endogenous pool of NAD^+ *in vivo*.

There are many effects of NAD^+ found organically. To mention the most important, NAD^+:
- promotes the cognitive and sensory functions;
- stimulates gluconeogenesis in the liver and insulin sensitivity in the muscles;
- stimulates the function of endothelial cells and protects against cardiovascular and cerebrovascular diseases;
- stimulates the oxidation of fats;
- regulates the immune function and inflammation;
- promotes and prolongs fertility in both males and females;
- improves DNA repair (other NAD^+-dependent pathways are in fact those of PARP1-2, involved in DNA repair and in the regulation of gene transcriptions).

The most studied NAD^+ precursor in humans is nicotinamide (NA). Dated studies, recently taken up by Garg et al. (2017) found that high doses (greater than 1 g) of NA can counter hypercholesterolemia (lowering LDL and increasing HDL). Although it has been shown that NA increases NAD^+ levels with at least a partial improvement in the cholesterol profile in humans, these effects are hardly discussed in the literature. Research on the effects of NR and NMN in humans (other NAD^+ boosters) is also gradually being enriched, with a series of clinical studies registered or currently underway.

For example, a randomized, double-blind, three-arm crossover pharmacokinetic study in 12 human subjects showed that NR increases the NAD^+ pool up to 2.7-fold in human blood with a single 1000 mg oral dose (Trammell et al., 2016). Researchers from the University of Washington instead completed a clinical trial with 140 participants, showing that NR administered orally leads to a dose-dependent increase in NAD^+ (with doses from 250 to 1000 mg/day), up to a plateau of approximately 2-fold increase in 9 days (Airhart et al., 2017). Another study reported positive effects of NR on the vascular endothelial function in healthy middle-aged and elderly adults (Heilbronn, 2017).

Other studies have shown how increasing the NAD$^+$ pool can regenerate the functionality of neurons affected by ischemia (it would intervene in mitigating damage from ischemia/reperfusion, a source of free radicals). A 2014 study by Wang et al. demonstrated how the concentration of NAD$^+$ drops dramatically in apoptotic neurons induced by the excitotoxicity of glutamate. The in vitro administration of 15 mmol of NA reduced the number of neurons with the condensed nucleus due to the toxic action of glutamate by 50%, also reducing ROS levels caused by the impaired mitochondrial functionality.

The antioxidant effect of NAD$^+$ protects the mitochondrial membrane from free radicals and prevents the degradation of mtDNA (mitochondrial DNA), with a consequent protection of the mitochondrial biogenesis. According to some authors, sarcopenia is also intimately related to the mitochondrial dysfunction and the decrease in the endogenous NAD + pool. In the future, the administration of NAD$^+$ boosters could therefore prove useful also in the prevention of sarcopenia. Other studies have investigated the possible antiaging effect of NAD$^+$. Experiments on mice show that the expression of sirtuins, in particular of SIRT1, is dependent on the amount of NAD$^+$ available in the cells.

In these mice, a depletion of NAD$^+$ influenced the expression of SIRT1 in the beta cells of the pancreas, resulting in a decrease in the production of insulin by the same cells. Supplementation with NA brought gene expression levels back to normal, resulting in the restoration of pancreatic activity and in a normalization of insulin secretion (Imai et al., 2014).

As for NADH, it enters into many reactions of metabolic energy production and, especially in aerobic conditions, improves the production of ATP. In the sports field, supplementation with NADH has proved particularly useful in the treatment of the chronic fatigue syndrome, typical of overtraining. Some studies have shown how this molecule is able to promote the recovery. NADH is often associated with coenzyme Q10, as they are two of the main components of the energy production mechanisms at the mitochondrial level.

A 2015 study by Castro-Marreno et al. showed how the administration of 200 mg/day of CoQ10 and 20 mg/day of NADH for 8 weeks to subjects suffering from chronic fatigue syndrome, significantly improved the energy production (ATP), reduced some markers of oxidative damage such as lipid peroxidation, reduced the sense of fatigue according to the Fatigue Impact Scale (FIS), as well as improved the mitochondrial function. The authors believe that this supplementation can be very useful in treating the chronic fatigue syndrome by increasing the energy production.

Dosages

The possible uses of NAD$^+$ and NADH have not yet been fully investigated and leave new areas of research open. What is known and evident is the importance of NADH as a metabolic stimulator in the production of energy (ATP) and of NAD$^+$ as an important antioxidant agent in reducing the negative action of free radicals on the cell membrane, for the maintenance of the mitochondrial health and autophagy.

There are no supporting studies that indicate NADH as a factor that increases the sports performance with acute or chronic supplementation (particularly in situations of intense physical activity associated with poor recovery). Therefore, this substance can be useful in those people who frequently play endurance sports and who need more available energy in the long term. NADH can be used to aid the recovery in overtraining situations.

The dosages used in human studies range from 10 to 20 mg of NADH/day, for a period of at least 8 weeks in case of intense and prolonged exertion. It is useful to associate it with CoQ10 to allow a greater energy efficiency and to improve the energy production.

For NAD$^+$ boosters, studies mention dosages of up to 1 g of NA and 250-1000 mg for NR, which would be able to increase the endogenous levels of NAD$^+$.

Effectiveness

Strength	Resistant strength	Mass	Endurance	Slimming	Concentration	Recovery
NADH							
−	+	−	+++	+	−	+++
NAD⁺ BOOSTERS							
−	−	−	−	++	−	−

OMEGA-3

Description

The name of these compounds comes from the position of the first double bond, starting the count from the terminal carbon (carbon ω or carbon n). Counting from carbon ω, the first encountered double bond occupies the third rank, hence the term omega-3.

The main fatty acids of the omega-3 group are:

- alpha-linolenic acid (18:3; ALA);
- eicosapentaenoic acid (20:5; EPA);
- docosahexaenoic acid (22:6; DHA).

The numbers in brackets indicate that these three fatty acids have 3, 5 and 6 double bonds, respectively in their chains composed of 18, 20 and 22 carbon atoms.

Omega-3 fatty acids are present in all the cells of our body, where they contribute significantly to the fluidity of cell membranes and, at a systemic level, they modulate the production of compounds with multiple biological activities: this explains the numerous physiological roles of these compounds.

The production of these fatty acids (EPA and DHA) **depends on the enzymatic activity of desaturases** (delta-6 desaturases) and **elongases** on their precursor, which is the essential alpha-linolenic fatty acid. Unfortunately, delta-6 saturase is often poorly available for this conversion due to a competition between omega-3 and omega-6 (which are too high quantities) and because it is inhibited by stress, viral infections and age.

Therefore, long-chain omega-3 fatty acids (in particular eicosapentaenoic acid, or EPA, and docosahexaenoic acid, or DHA) must in fact be obtained through food or by supplementation.

The use of foods enriched in omega-3 allows among other things to selectively lower the omega-6/omega-3 ratio in the diet to 10:1, currently around 20:1 in our society, which should instead be changed, according to the most modern views, at about 4:1, 2:1.

This imbalance creates a greater formation of type 2 prostaglandins, with an inflammatory action, which can be the basis of most of the chronic degenerative diseases that afflict humans in the modern society. The main sources for the intake of omega-3s such as EPA and DHA remain fish products. Generally, omega-3s can be found in common foods, such as fish, preferably seawater, fish oil, krill oil, shellfish. Currently, the only significant vegan source of DHA are microalgae (phytoplankton) and their supplement is called "algae oil". The DHA component is equivalent to that derived from fish and the safety of use is also similar.

Other plant sources of omega-3 fatty acids tend to have the structure of the alpha-linolenic acid (ALA) precursor and significant plant sources of ALA include hemp seed oil, walnuts and flax seeds, while supplements with smaller amounts ALA include spirulina and chlorella.

Unfortunately, the classic Western diet (European or American) tends to have a highly favorable ratio for omega-6 fatty acids (it is thought that we should normally have an omega-6:3 ratio of about 15-20:1).

In Japan, the ratio is thought to be around 4:1, while in India it varies widely between rural (5-6:1) and urban (38-50:1) areas. If we took the Paleolithic diet as a reference, we could estimate a ratio of 1:1. Fat from wild animals also appears to have a similar ratio, while that from farmed animals has higher amounts of omega-6 than omega-3.

Properties

The biological effects of omega-3s on the body are manifold, but mainly affect three systems: immune, cardiovascular and central nervous system.

In the United States, Dr. Donald Rudin, former director of the molecular biology department of the Eastern Pennsylvania Psychiatric Institute in Philadelphia, and author of the book: *Omega 3 oils: a practical guide*, discovered that the lack of omega-3 fatty acids was at the base of most mental illnesses, as these fatty acids provide the substrate on which niacin and other B vitamins form the Series-3 prostaglandins, which serve to regulate the microcircuits throughout the body.

It is not difficult to understand the importance of omega-3s in the functioning of the central nervous system if we realize that at least 30% of the human brain is made up of DHA. In fact, breast milk is a very rich source of DHA and studies carried out on formula-fed babies that did not contain DHA (all formula milks), showed that these subjects could have a doubled increased risk of having neurological dysfunctions in their adult life.

There is experimental evidence that omega-3s can have a positive influence on insulin resistance and therefore exercise a sort of prevention against the onset of diabetes. In a 1993 study, it was found that insulin resistance is related to the type of fatty acids that make up cell membranes. The more omega-3 and omega-6 are present in cell membranes, the higher the sensitivity to insulin, the more saturated fatty acids, the higher the resistance.

It has been seen that GLA supplements (gamma-linolenic acid, present in borage oil, an omega-6 with particular anti-inflammatory characteristics) regress the symptoms of neurological degeneration present in diabetics and providing omega-3 DHA blocked the degeneration of the retina of the eye, which is the cause of the frequent cases of blindness in severe diabetes. The cause of retinal cell degeneration is due to the fact that DHA is the most represented polyunsaturated fatty acid in these cells, but, in the presence of high levels of glucose in the blood, our body is unable to produce DHA from ALA (alpha-linolenic acid) and it is therefore necessary to take it directly as a supplement or with a diet that is rich in fish.

As for the effects on the cardiovascular system, it is known that omega-3 fatty acids exert an effective antiplatelet action, they control plasma lipids (especially triglycerides) and also the blood pressure. The most recent information on the antiarrhythmic effects of omega-3 fatty acids is also of particular interest, which may explain the protective action of these compounds against sudden cardiac death, frequently caused by severe ventricular arrhythmias. Different studies have shown that EPA and DHA have antiarrhythmic effects on the heart muscle.

The modulation of the biological responses by omega-3s is also of a particular importance, acting on the activation and control of some specific biochemical messengers, **eicosanoids**. Eicosanoids are derivatives of arachidonic acid, a fatty acid with 20 carbon atoms; they are considered "superhormones" and have a mainly signaling function. In the subcategory of ecosanoids we also find **resolvins**, **protectins** and **prostaglandins**, which control every aspect of the human physiology by acting at the cellular level.

Prostaglandins, in particular, manage important functions such as: cell permeability, coagulation processes, sexual and reproductive functions, fat mobilization, capillary fragility, va-

soconstriction, immune and inflammatory responses. Prostaglandins, unlike hormones, are synthesized and work where they are needed. They are normally divided into three groups:
- series-1 (PGE1), considered "good", derive from dihom-gamma-linoleic acid (DGLA);
- series-2 (PGH2), considered "bad", derive from arachidonic acid (AA);
- series-3 (PGI3), considered "good", derive from eicosapentaenoic acid (EPA).

Prostaglandins of series 1 and 3 have vasodilator, anticoagulant and anti-inflammatory effects, lower LDL cholesterol (Low Density Lipoproteins, which mainly transport phospholipids and free cholesterol), increase HDL cholesterol (High Density Lipoproteins, which transport phospholipids and esterified cholesterol to the liver, from where it is eliminated through the bile) and inhibit the cellular proliferation. Series 2 prostaglandins have the opposite effect: they are vasoconstrictors, promote platelet aggregation and are related to the activation of the HPA axis (Hypothalamus-Pituitary-Adrenal) by stimulating the transcription of CRH (Corticotropin-Releasing Hormone) in response to inflammation. Our body needs all three types of prostaglandins, but in the right proportions. If type 2 prostaglandins prevail due to a wrong diet, we will have a predisposition towards chronic inflammatory diseases.

Resolvins are powerful signaling molecules involved in the inflammatory processes, they derived from omega-3 fatty acids and have the ability to "resolve" the inflammatory process. Those that derive directly from EPA (without the need for metabolization into DHA) are indicated as belonging to the E series, while those derived from DHA are cataloged in the D series. Resolvins of the D series have anti-inflammatory properties and act by inhibiting TNF-α, a proinflammatory molecule. Now resolvins are available as supplement.

In moderate doses, fish oil appears to positively influence the bioenergetics of the metabolism through a combination of a better nutrient absorption and a better functioning of mitochondrial enzymes. Many of the antidiabetic effects of fish oil can be indirectly linked to the increased glucose absorption and use in the muscle, as well as to a higher sensitivity to insulin. By having a modulating effect on the permeability and sensitivity of cell membranes to insulin, omega-3 fatty acids can exert ergogenic effects, leading to an improvement in sports performance and making muscle cells more permeable to nutrients such as glucose and amino acids. Furthermore, supplementation with omega-3-s can promote the muscle growth by exerting anti-catabolic effects. Muscle proteins undergo a continuous process of synthesis (anabolism) and destruction (catabolism). In a healthy state, the anabolic and catabolic processes can be modulated to maintain the stability or to promote an increase in muscle mass (as observed with resistance training combined with a correct nutrition and supplementation).

The muscle tissue catabolism can often be found in particular clinical cases (for example, diabetes, kidney failure, trauma), during restrictive diets and during other stressful conditions. During these critical states, muscle protein breakdown (catabolism) overcomes the muscle protein synthesis (anabolism), which results in muscle loss and weakness. It is in this context that fish oil plays an important role, in fact EPA significantly reduces the degradation of muscle proteins in the ubiquitin-proteasome system. Another mechanism through which fish oil exerts its anti-catabolic effect, is the reduction the levels of cortisol, a hormone with a catabolic effect that contributes to a number of other harmful effects on health when it is present at chronically high levels. Finally, the improved membrane fluidity (especially of red blood cells) and the production of anti-inflammatory and vasodilator prostaglandins are of interest to athletes, as they favor the transport of oxygen and nutrients to muscle tissues during the exercise.

Evidence

A link between fish oil intake and health is confirmed not only by scientific research, but also from practical experiences and history, as in the case of the German occupation during the

Second World War, in which the Norwegians, forced to return to their traditional diet based on fish, beans and whole grains, given the limited availability of industrial foods, recorded a 10% decline in diseases such as schizophrenia, cardiovascular disease and cancer.

After the war, the Norwegians returned to consuming commercial and industrially processed foods and the level of the aforementioned diseases immediately returned to the previous values. Another interesting study to verify the effect of omega-3s on the health was the observation of the Inuits of Greenland. Despite having a very high fat diet, they had a very low incidence of cardiovascular diseases. By comparing the blood lipid profile of the Eskimos with that of the Danes (who consume a diet considered "normal"), it emerged that in the Inuits, the levels of total and LDL cholesterol (the proteins that carry bad cholesterol) were much lower and the levels of HDL (which carry the good cholesterol) were higher.

Since the diet of the Inuits is rich above all in fish, seal and polar bear meat (which, feeding on fish, have a very rich omega-3 fat), it was concluded that DHA (docosahexaenoic) and EPA (eicosapentaenoic) were responsible for these findings. In fact, subsequent observations showed that the beneficial effects exerted by omega-3 on the cardiovascular system, as well as in **lowering the levels of total cholesterol and LDL**, consisted in increasing the formation of eicosanoids and consequently of prostaglandins in a beneficial way, by **reducing the blood viscosity**, increasing clotting time and **decreasing blood pressure**. Subsequently, the studies that used linseed oil (very rich in alpha-linolenic acid, the leader of the omega-3s from which DHA and EPA can be formed) gave the same results.

Omega-3s have also come to the fore thanks to the Italian "GISSI" study, in which the Associazione Nazionale Medici Cardiologi Ospedalieri (ANMCO), in collaboration with the Mario Negri Institute (Consorzio Mario Negri sud), examined a sample of 11,324 people affected by myocardial infarction, dividing them into four subgroups. After a 4-year follow-up, patients treated with omega-3 had reduced events of heart attacks, sudden death, strokes and overall mortality compared to those who received no treatment. These data confirm the hypotheses that had been formulated by two important USA studies, the first carried out on volunteer doctors, the second on almost 85,000 nurses. They lasted 16 years and were published in the prestigious *Journal of the American Medical Association* (JAMA).

To be fair, it should be mentioned that a subsequent double-blind randomized prospective study, published on May 9, 2013 by the journal *NEJM*, conducted in Italy in collaboration between IRCCS - Institute of Pharmacological Research "Mario Negri", Consorzio Mario Negri Sud and Italian general practitioners, demonstrates how omega-3 treatment does not show advantages either in terms of mortality or hospitalization due to cardiovascular events. This shows that we must not limit ourselves to the results of a single study, but that we must take into account as many of them as possible.

There are not many studies in the literature on the effects of omega-3s on the sports performance; However, we can cite some of them that nevertheless give positive indications. A study on a football team used a supplement consisting of a blend of fish oils and vegetable oils, which provided GLA, EPA (eicosapentaenoic) and DHA (docosahexaenoic), and a placebo made from olive oil. The group that used the blend achieved a **significant increase (+ 6% *vs.* 1%) in the maximum bench press**.

Another study included four groups of young males. One group served as a control, which means that they continued to follow previous habits, another group was given a fish oil supplement plus a diet rich in salmon, equivalent to the daily intake of 3-4 g of omega-3s. The third group carried out an aerobic training program and the last group followed both aerobic training and omega-3 supplementation. After 10 weeks, the greatest improvements in the aerobic efficiency occurred in the groups subject to the training program, but there were significant improvements also in the group that used only omega-3-based supplements, compared to the control group.

In a 2014 Japanese study at the University of Tokyo, it was shown that supplementing cyclists with 3.6 g of EPA for 8 weeks results in lower oxygen consumption at the same level of exercise intensity and the same metabolic efficiency of an exercise is determined by the cost of oxygen at a given intensity. Subsequently, in 2015, again in Japan, the experiment was repeated by administering 3.6 g of omega-3 (in this case EPA + DHA) and they found an **improvement in the endurance capacity due to the increase in the concentration of nitric oxide** of 8 µmol per liter and a 5% increase in blood flow, compared to the placebo.

From what has been explained so far, it seems evident that polyunsaturated fatty acids and especially omega-3s play an important role for the health of the individual and thanks to their modulating effect on regulatory hormones and on the blood circulation, they can probably exert a beneficial effect both in strength sports and endurance sports.

Fish oil (in this case as EPA) incubated in muscle cells is associated with an increased ability for the muscle cell to switch from using glucose to using fat as the primary substrate for oxidation, a phenomenon known as "Bioenergetic flexibility" of "metabolic switching". In mice subjected to immobilization, fish oil supplementation was found to reduce the rate of muscle degeneration.

If EPA is added to the hospital enteral nutrition, some studies have shown greater maintenance of lean mass after the surgery, although this efficacy has not been confirmed by all studies conducted to date.

As for the ergogenic effect, several studies have directly studied the effect of fish oil on the metabolic pathways that are the basis of muscle growth, with very interesting results. In one study, healthy men and women of young or middle age (25-45 years of age) took 4 g of fish oil per day, providing a daily dose of 1.86 g of EPA and 1.5 g by DHA. The result was a **significant increase in the anabolic response and muscle protein synthesis**, with an improvement in the use of amino acids and in the response to insulin.

The increased anabolic response was also linked to greater activation of the mTOR signaling pathway, which is considered a crucial control point for the muscle anabolism and muscle cell growth.

Fish oil supplementation in the elderly confers anabolic effects on the muscles. The same research group conducted another study, using an identical protocol (1.86 g of EPA and 1.5 g DHA for 8 weeks) in healthy elderly subjects over 65 (mean age 71 years).

The results were the same as for the younger subjects; fish oil supplementation significantly increased (up to 60%) the response to muscle protein synthesis induced by amino acids and insulin. Another property of fish oil could be that of attenuating the anabolic resistance that develops with aging. The researchers were struck by this response and concluded that **high doses of fish oil may be useful for the prevention and the treatment of sarcopenia**.

When it comes to the prevention of muscle mass loss with aging, a fundamental question is whether these beneficial anabolic and anti-catabolic effects on the muscles translate into benefits on the physical performance. A couple of long-term studies show promising effects. A long-term (6-month) study in postmenopausal women showed that fish oil supplementation (which provides 1.2 g of EPA + DHA) was able to improve physical performance indices (such as walking speed) compared to a placebo group (olive oil).

Additionally, during a 90-day resistance exercise program in older women, consuming fish oil supplements (2 g per day) resulted in greater muscle strength gains and in an improved functional capacity compared to a placebo.

More and more studies show that the anabolic effects of nutrients (for example amino acids or proteins), hormones (for example insulin and testosterone) and/or muscle exercise can be improved with long-term fish oil supplementation.

A recent literature review concluded that long-term fish oil supplementation, along with adequate anabolic stimuli such as exercise and proper nutrition, could potentially provide a safe, simple and inexpensive intervention to counteract anabolic resistance related to aging and to the associated loss of muscle mass, strength and performance.

Finally, the inflammatory effects related to sporting activities must be considered based on the resistance of the tissue. The obtained effects depend on the release of arachidonic acid by the membranes that are stimulated by physical exercise, with the consequent formation of inflammatory eicosanoids, which activate the cytokine response and the cellular reactivity. In equilibrium and normality conditions, the reactivity of omega-6s can be balanced with the compensatory anti-inflammatory role of omega-3s and their mediators.

In a study carried out on individuals with low IGF-1 levels (IGF-1 is a powerful anabolic hormone), the administration of 720 mg of EPA and 480 mg of DHA for 8 weeks increased IGF-1 levels. In chronic stressful situations, such as very intense workouts, IGF-1 levels can be too low to allow muscle growth, in addition to the fact that, in this situation, it is very easy to have a high state of inflammation, both at the muscle level and on adipose tissues, which makes it difficult to build muscle and mobilize fats for energy purposes. In this case, omega-3s can prove useful, increasing IGF-1 and decreasing the inflammation.

Evan Lewis of the University of Toronto and his collaborators demonstrated by electromyography that omega-3 supplementation for 3 weeks increases muscle activation and reduces the fatigue during a maximal sprint test on a stationary bike. The subjects who participated in this test had taken 5 mL of seal oil per day, which contains 375 mg of EPA, 230 mg of DPA and 510 mg of DHA. Since these fatty acids are essential, the eating habits of the athletes are of crucial importance to create a balance with an effective and efficient anti-inflammatory effect. Athletes should evaluate their intake of fatty acids (especially omega-3s) to understand if they have anti-inflammatory defenses and if the sporting activity they perform could have caused a pro-inflammatory condition.

A study wanted to analyze the effects of physical exercise alone or in combination with the supplementation of polyunsaturated fatty acids of the omega-3 series (omega-3 PUFA) and oleic acid, on parameters related to the metabolic syndrome (MSyn) and on other cardiometabolic health markers. Thirty-six patients with MSyn followed high intensity interval training (HIIT) for 24 weeks. In the randomized double-blind study, half of the group consumed 500 mL/day of semi-skimmed milk (8 g fat, placebo milk) while the other half consumed 500 mL/day of skimmed milk enriched with 275 mg of omega-3 and 7.5 g of oleic acid (omega-3 + OLE). The results showed that omega-3 + OLE treatment increased plasma levels of omega-3 by 30%, albeit not significantly ($p = 0.286$). In addition, improvements were observed in the VO_{2max} peak (12.8%), in the mean blood pressure (–7.1%), in the waist circumference (–1.8%), in the percentage of total (–2, 9%) and abdominal (–3.3%) fat mass in both groups.

However, insulin sensitivity (measured by intravenous glucose tolerance test), serum C-reactive protein concentration and high-density lipoprotein only improved in the omega-3 + OLE group, by 31.5, 32.1 and 10.3 % respectively ($p < 0.05$). Fasting triglyceride and glucose levels and plasma fibrinogen concentrations did not improve in any group after 24 weeks of treatment. Supplementation with omega-3 fatty acids and oleic acid improves the effects of training in patients with metabolic syndrome. To conclude, lipidomic analysis is necessary to obtain the maximum benefits from any sports activity, by controlling the role of lipid exchange for an effective membrane homeostasis and to be informed in the case of an unsuitable fatty acid composition.

In mice, for quite long periods of time, fish oil can preserve the effects of some hormones (insulin, adiponectin) on muscle cells when an obesogenic diet is consumed daily. This may be due to the DHA component, which seems to be able to partially reverse the reduction in glucose absorption observed in the muscle due to the high amount of palmitic acid, a saturated fatty acid.

It is important to note that the reduction in the omega-6/omega-3 ratio is associated with an increased glucose absorption and an improved glucose tolerance throughout the body.

The omega-6/omega-3 ratio had positive effects if it stood at 0.5:1-1.5:1 (fish oil) compared to 17.5:1-29.7:1 (control), measured in the cell membrane. The muscle cell membrane appears to have a high response capacity to dietary changes. The intake of omega-3s quickly improved the insulin sensitivity *in vivo*.

Supplementation with fish oil in rats (5% of food intake) was able to normalize the stress response. The same situation has been replicated in other animal and human models by making them take DHA daily in high doses (1.5-1.8 g DHA) and it has been seen that the adrenaline response to stress was particularly attenuated. There are still no reliable data on cortisol. In some cases, even high doses of DHA would not seem effective in decreasing it. The EPA is able to modulate some immune functions associated with stress.

Interestingly, a low dose of EPA + DHA, approximately 762 mg per day, can reduce norepinephrine levels even in people considered to be "non-stressed".

It appears that a deficiency of omega-3 fatty acids can reduce the glucose metabolism in the brains of rats and it is hypothesized that this effect is related to the reduction of the GLUT1 receptor.

An interesting study conducted on healthy young individuals who consumed no more than one fatty fish (containing omega-3s) per week, found that adding 450 mg of DHA and 90 mg of EPA to their diet for 12 weeks increased their brain oxygenation during cognitive tests.

Fish oil appears to improve the blood flow to the brain in adults who have a low consumption of fish in the diet.

In response to exercise in already trained men, high-dose fish oil (2224 mg EPA and 2208 mg DHA) for six weeks was able to reduce their inflammatory cytokines (CPR and TNF-alpha) at rest, but it failed to modify exercise-induced changes in their immune parameters.

Natural Killer cells seem to have improved their cytotoxicity two hours after an exercise (after which they return to baseline values) following the intake of fish oil. The intake of 3000 mg of fish oil (1300 mg EPA and 300 mg DHA) per day for 6 weeks in healthy men is able to increase the exercise-induced NK cell activity in conjunction with an increase in IL-2 (no change in IL-4, IL-6, cortisol, or IFN-γ). Possible explanations for this result include an increase in IL-2 levels (known to stimulate the activity of NK cells) and a reduction in the concentration of PGE2, which would seem to attenuate the inhibitory-type regulatory mechanisms of NK cell activity.

The main components of fish oil, EPA and DHA, are polyunsaturated fatty acids, and any unsaturated bond (double bond) can possibly be oxidized; this phenomenon causes a lipid to become an oxidant and to produce other oxidizing substances. It is a fairly common phenomenon in polyunsaturated fatty acids. If, from a certain point of view, there are benefits in the oxidation of a polyunsaturated fatty acid (for example, the production of eicosanoids starts from the oxidation of DHA), on the other hand, a strong oxidation of the polyunsaturated fats can be harmful for the body. Often, supplements contain vitamin E are given precisely to preserve the fatty acids from oxidation.

To assess the degree of lipid peroxidation, TBARS (ThioBarbituric Acid Reactve Substances), malondialdehyde (MDA), 4-hydroxy-2-nonenal or the oxidative metabolites of eicosanoids (for example, 8-iso-PGF2-α) can be measured in the blood. Sometimes we can measure vitamin E levels in the serum, as it is thought that its reduction is due to its "sacrifice" to prevent the lipid peroxidation.

Of these measurements, those of MDA and 4-hydroxy-2-nonenal may be more reliable. However, supplementation with fish oil was able to reduce the value of 8-iso-PGF2-α in the urine (indicative of an antioxidant effect).

The intake of 3 g of fish oil (EPA + DHA = 1600 mg) for seven weeks, which is already oxidized before consumption, has shown an evident lipid peroxidation in healthy subjects.

Some studies have reported increases in 4-hydroxy-2-nonenal following the consumption of DHA in humans and the combination of fish oil and exercise (albeit limited with vitamin E) may increase the lipid peroxidation in animals as assessed by the measurement of TBARS.

DNA can be easily damaged if the body is subjected to stress. Unfortunately, even oxidized lipids are able to damage the DNA and this is the mechanism that links the oxidation and the risk of cancer (inducing damage to the DNA). This is why we must be very careful about the preservation of omega-3 supplements and even more about the foods that contain them, which must not be oxidized and therefore should be stored in the fridge and if possible, away from direct light exposure.

Studies in men have found that high serum levels of omega-3 fatty acids are associated with higher rates of DNA damage, compared to the levels of omega-6 fatty acids; higher, but still not worrying from the health point of view.

Adenosine monophosphate kinase (AMPK) is a signal molecule linked to nutrients that are antagonists of mTOR and is activated in periods of nutrient deprivation; it is also the molecular target of various supplements such as berberine or metformin. Activation of EPA has the property of activating AMPK in adipocytes through an insulin-independent signal and it can decrease the inflammation by activating the AMPK/SIRT1 pathway.

Through the activation of AMPKa1, DHA can increase the expression of SIRT1 and suppress the inflammation by hindering the NF-kB signal (through deacetylation). This could also be the anti-inflammatory process that occurs thanks to the intake of fish oil. It has been seen that EPA modifies inflammatory signals in adipocytes (usually thanks to the suppression of the action of TNF-α).

The activation of AMPK thanks to EPA can be the underlying mechanism for the release of adipokines, for the improvement of the endothelial and hepatoprotective function, and for the improvement of insulin sensitivity (related to the liver) and autophagic action.

In healthy subjects, 3.6 g of EPA + DHA per day were not able to increase the insulin sensitivity if the subjects followed a high-fat diet (37%). However, this study did note the tendency (although not significant) of increasing the insulin sensitivity in individuals who had a high baseline omega-6 to omega-3 ratio.

If fish oil is given to people who constantly exercise, the effect on insulin sensitivity appears to be additive.

Other studies suggest an improvement in the insulin sensitivity of populations that typically have an omega-3: omega-6 ratio which is unbalanced towards the latter. These populations include the elderly, those with metabolic syndrome, the unhealthy and the obese.

Unfortunately, many discrepancies have been found in insulin sensitivity during the supplementation with fish oil. For example, there are no significant improvements in fasting blood glucose levels or in fasting insulin in type 2 diabetic patients.

The mechanism linked to the increase on the insulin sensitivity can be linked to the preservation of the cell fluidity, especially by rebalancing the omega-6: omega-3 ratio in the cell membranes, as demonstrated by a study by Haugaard et al. which correlates the content of PUFAs in the cell membrane with the insulin sensitivity.

An interesting thing is that in those who develop insulin resistance from high fructose consumption, fish oil unfortunately seems to be ineffective in relieving the insulin resistance (even if it reduces triglyceride levels).

This supports the idea that the insulin-sensitizing effects produced by the supplementation of fish oil are at the cell level, while fructose causes resistance to insulin in the liver and pancreas.

Another possible mechanism is the need to counteract an excess of saturated fatty acids which can cause insulin resistance. Palmitic acid, for example, is known to induce insulin resistance in the muscles and an intake of polyunsaturated fatty acids (omega-3 or 6) can reduce its negative effects.

PGC1α can be induced in the adipose tissue of mice through fish oil supplementation and its activation can increase the energy expenditure through the UCP2 expression, and DHA appears to be the main culprit as it is most closely related to weight loss in humans.

In studies that evaluate the metabolic rate, fish oil has not been shown to significantly influence it, despite the increase in fat oxidation rates.

Instead, it can exert a localized anti-inflammatory effect, which could indirectly help the fat metabolism in people characterized by latent and chronic inflammation.

Astaxanthin is a carotenoid that acts as a lipid antioxidant and it is thought to obtain its health benefits through the consumption of red fish (salmon) or krill oil.

The carotenoid from algae, **fucoxanthin**, appears to have synergistic properties with fish oil in mitigating weight gain in obese and diabetic mice. The addition of fish oil in an amount equal to 6.9% of the diet (rather high dose) was able to make a dietary dose of 0.1% of fucoxanthin doubly effective in suppressing fat gain. It was basically like doubling the dose of fucoxanthin.

Interestingly, fucoxanthin can increase liver DHA levels regardless of fish oil consumption.

Supplementation with fish oil appears to have synergistic effects with statins, in terms of improving the cardiometabolic parameters.

Dosages

The recommended dose for preventive purposes for a healthy individual, but also for individuals with a previous myocardial infarction, is 1 g per day; to exert an anti-inflammatory and pain-relieving effect, the required dosage is 2-3 g, and to have a performing effect on the physical activity you will need 3-4 g. Finally, to achieve a slimming effect you will need more than 5 g.

Effectiveness

Strength	Resistant strength	Mass	Endurance	Slimming	Concentration	Recovery
++	++	++	+	+++	+++	++

ORNITHINE

Description

Ornithine is an amino acid characterized by the presence of a basic side chain consisting of three carbon atoms and plays a fundamental role in the urea cycle. Unlike the other standard amino acids, ornithine is not used for protein synthesis, but, being synthesized in the cytosol from arginine at the end of the urea cycle, it is transferred to the mitochondrion, where it plays an important role as an intermediate in different metabolic processes. The transition between cytosol and mitochondrion is intensified especially during periods of prolonged fasting or during diets with a high protein content, when the oxidation of amino acids becomes a very important energy source.

Properties

Ornithine is the perfect complement to arginine, as the combination of these two amino acids promotes the production of hormones, including insulin, and it improves the regenerative capacity of cells. Among the numerous properties of ornithine, we can mention that it acts as a detoxifier of ammonia, the accumulation of which could be highly toxic and could cause an impairment of the health of the individual (a condition particularly frequent in athletes, for which ammonia levels rise significantly during intense physical activities. Ornithine also acts as a stimulator of GH (for this reason ornithine is present in many supplements that in fact favor, the production of this hormone).

OKG is the acronym that indicates the L-ornithine-alpha-ketoglutarate compound. This product not only constitutes a kind of reserve or a warehouse for the transport of glutamine, but it also has its own functions, including that of showing an anti-catabolic action in the protein metabolism. In the muscle tissue, in particular, it prevents the loss of important proteins, such as myosin, which is one of the proteins that allow the muscle to contract. The degradation of myosin occurs physiologically in response to traumatic or stressful events, such as physical exercises.

The OKG, when introduced from the outside, is able to release glutamine, which prevents the aforementioned phenomena. Studies in the literature are numerous. In particular, the research began in the surgical departments, where it was clearly demonstrated that the OKG supplementation was able to slow down the muscle catabolism induced by the stress of the surgery. The interest in the sports field was immediate. OKG also has an energetic action, as, in synergy with vitamin B6, it promotes the synthesis of glucose from non-glucose compounds (gluconeogenesis) and it also activates the Krebs cycle.

Being a storage form of glutamine, OKG promotes the disposal of toxic substances such as ammonia through the kidney filter. Finally, the product seems to have a moderate anabolic activity, in fact some studies have found that it is able to increase the blood levels of insulin and IGF-1, modally but significantly. To summarize, OKG finds indications in the sports field as it prevents the muscle degradation induced by the stress of physical activity, counteracts mental and physical stress, allows you to better deal with physical activities of both strength and endurance nature and gives moderate anabolic and lipolytic effects.

Evidence

Numerous studies have been conducted on the ammonia detoxification and GH stimulation by ornithine. An interesting study is the one conducted by Bucci et al. (1990), where the administration of four different dosages of ornithine (40, 70, 100 or 170 mg/kg) to bodybuilders (three women and nine men) for three consecutive Saturdays, showed **a rise in baseline GH values** 45 and 90 minutes after ingestion, regardless of the administered dose, and a significant rise at 90 minutes, only after taking the highest dosage, 170 mg/kg.

A study carried out by Zajac et al. (2010) analyzed the effects of ornithine and arginine intake on the GH secretion. A group of weight training athletes were given a mix of arginine (3000 mg) and ornithine (2200 mg) twice a day, three times a week. The results of the study showed that in the group that took the mixture, there was a greater elevation of post-exercise GH levels compared to the placebo group. In addition, higher levels of IGF-1, another GH synergistic hormone that is important for the muscle growth, were also found in the group that took ornithine and arginine.

Demura, Morishita, Yamada, Yamaji and Komatsu carried out a study to examine the effects of taking L-ornithine hydrochloride on a maximal intermittent performance with a cycle ergometer. 10 young athletes were studied; the intensity of the activity was based on the body mass of each of them. **The maximum peak of the maximal repetitions was significantly higher** in the group that took OKG compared to the placebo.

A study carried out by Elam (1988) on a group that took a mix of ornithine and arginine, in combination with exercise with weights, showed a greater reduction in fat mass compared to the group that did not take the supplements.

Dosages

There are no significant studies that can provide detailed guidance on the supplementation protocols. From studies carried out on healthy athlete subjects, the dosage that has been shown to reduce the feeling of fatigue was 2 g of ornithine per day, followed by up to 6 g on the day of the sports performance. Several studies have shown how the administration of up to 15 g per day in patients suffering from trauma favors the reduction of catabolism, thus delaying the cachectic effect. Dosages higher than 10-20 g per day cause the onset of gastrointestinal symptoms. As for the OKG, the dosage should be around 2 g per dose, which should be taken on an empty stomach, one dose in the post-workout period and one before bedtime, in the evening.

Effectiveness

Strength	Resistant strength	Mass	Endurance	Slimming	Concentration	Recovery
+	++	+	+	++	+	+

PANAX GINSENG

Description

Panax Ginseng or **Korean ginseng** is a perennial plant of the *Panax* species belonging to the *Araliaceae* family. The term *Panax* derives from the Greek *pan* (all) and *akèia* (cure, remedy), a word from which also derives the Latin and Italian word "panacea", that is, a remedy for all illnesses; this was in fact considered a plant with miraculous properties, capable not only of curing all diseases, but also of fortifying the spirit, cheering the heart and prolonging life; for this reason, in the past, it was so appreciated that it was bartered for gold and precious stones. The term *ginseng*, on the other hand, comes from the Chinese *pinyin*, meaning "man's plant", as its roots have an anthropomorphic appearance, similar to the human figure, in which head, trunk, arms and legs are often distinguishable.

Ginseng is characterized by the presence of a high content of tonic active ingredients, all B vitamins, vitamins C, A, E, K and folic acid. It also contains all the essential amino acids, minerals and important nutritional trace elements such as iron, magnesium, silica, copper, potassium, vanadium, aluminum, cobalt, manganese, phosphorus, zinc, enzymes, polyunsaturated fats and estrogenic and androgenic hormone-like substances.

Properties

The active ingredients of ginseng are saponins, called ginsenosides, to which its adaptogenic properties are attributable. "Adaptogenic substances" are all those substances of natural origin that help the body adapt to stress by improving the physical vigor and the mental concentration, favoring a restorative effect; adaptogens regulate the body's internal balance by stimulating it when depressed and by calming it when excited; in this way, excessive reactions to stressors are reduced.

It is indeed interesting to note how some ginsenosides are able to cause opposite effects, for example **RG1** stimulates the central nervous system and increases the blood pressure, while **RB1** lowers it and exerts a sedative action. Lately, great importance has been given to **RG3**, especially for its ability of mitigating the negative effects related to stress. RG3 is able to decrease the stress-induced excitotoxic and oxidative effect by improving the memory, it decreases inflammation at the microglia level and decreases apoptosis (cell death) of neurons in neurodegenerative conditions such as Parkinson's and Alzheimer's.

In particular, at the level of the central nervous system, there was noted an increase in the electrical activity of the cerebral cortex cells, especially in an area located near the hippocampus, which controls the memory, attention and the brain functions. In addition, ginseng increases the levels of dopamine, adrenaline and noradrenaline in the brain, thus exerting an antidepressant, euphoric and psychostimulating action. Other equally well-known and important actions are those related to the strengthening of the immune system, the reduction of oxidative damage in smokers, the increase in the concentration of blood antioxidants and, especially in postmenopausal women, the reduction of cortisol levels with a reduction fatigue, insomnia, depression etc.

Evidence

A recent study by Korean scientists, published in the *International Journal of Impotence Research* and conducted on 119 men with mild or moderate erection problems, showed that taking four tablets of the extract a day resulted in a significant, although not striking improvement of the **erectile dysfunction** in treated patients and did not show any side effects. According to the authors of the research, this extract would in fact improve all aspects of sexuality by increasing the blood flow into the corpora cavernosa of the penis and exerting a stimulating action at the level of the central nervous system, and therefore it could be used as an alternative medicine to improve the life quality of men suffering from a sexual dysfunction.

Above, it was said that this adaptogenic substance decreases the excitotoxic and oxidative effect induced by stress, improves the memory, reduces inflammation in the microglia and above all decreases apoptosis (cell death); in fact, it is no coincidence that ginseng has always been used all over the world as a traditional medicine for the treatment of cancer and other diseases.

As for the ergogenic effect of ginseng, various researches conducted on athletes have shown a **marked improvement in the efficiency of the aerobic work**, with a decrease in the production of lactic acid and pyruvic acid, a reduction in the levels of free fatty acids in the blood, an increase in the oxygen consumption and respiratory function and a **decreased recovery time after maximal athletic trials**. Supplementation with titrated dry extract of ginseng would be able to preserve the glycogen present in striated muscles and the liver, probably thanks to the ability to induce the oxidation of free fatty acids in place of glucose, with a release of greater amounts of energy.

It also emerged that the titrated dry extract of ginseng would increase the density of capillaries and the intensity of oxidative processes in the skeletal muscles, with a consequent increase in the aerobic potential of the muscle under exertion, even if the effects of its use for sports performance improvements are yet to be proven with certainty.

In a double-blind study conducted by Forgo and Kirk, some athletes were given 200 mg of ginseng extract standardized in ginsenosides at 7% or 200 mg of ginseng extract standardized in ginsenosides at 4% + 400 mg of vitamin E, or a placebo every day for 9 weeks. Using the bicycle ergometric test, significant differences were observed in favor of both ginseng preparations compared to the placebo group, in relation to heart rate, blood lactate levels and maximal oxygen absorption after the exercise. In addition, a double-blind, placebo-controlled study on 28 trained male athletes examined the persistence of the effects after a 9-week treatment (200 mg of ginseng extract with 4% ginsenosides, or a placebo) beyond the treatment period.

Compared to the placebo, the ginseng extract produced significant improvements in the maximal oxygen absorption during the exercise, in the heart rate at maximal exercise, an improvement of the forced respiratory volume, forced vital lung capacity and of the visual reaction time.

In 2016, Bach et al. conducted a meta-analysis to study the effectiveness of ginseng supplements on reducing the fatigue and improving the physical performance. They included randomized trials that examined the effectiveness of ginseng supplements on reducing the fatigue and improving the physical performance compared to placebos. The most significant results were the reduction of fatigue and the improvement of the physical performance. The meta-analysis showed a statistically significant efficacy of ginseng supplements on reducing the fatigue.

An important effect of ginseng could also affect the **resolution of muscle damage and the inflammation induced by exercise**, as shown by a recent study published in *The American Journal of Chinese Medicine*. Eighteen male college students were randomly assigned to an experimental group (RG, n = 9) or a placebo group (P, n = 9); the RG group took, 200 mg/day of Korean red ginseng extract (mixed with 200 mL of water) three times a day in the 7 days prior to the test and for 4 days after the test, while the P group took 200 mL of water containing an extract of *Agastachis herba* with the same frequency.

All subjects then performed the test on the uphill, high-intensity treadmill (two 45-minute shifts at 10 km/h with a 15-degree incline, separated by 5 minutes of rest). Plasma levels of creatine kinase (an enzyme used as an index of muscle damage, abbreviation CK) and interleukin-6 (a protein implicated in the physiology of inflammation, abbreviation IL-6) were measured before exercise and 24, 48, 72 and 96 hours after the exercise. The IL-6 levels were also measured 1 hour and 2-hours post-exercise, while an oral glucose tolerance test (OGTT) was performed 24 hours after the exercise to assess the insulin sensitivity.

The test showed that 72 hours after the exercise, the level of CK in the RG group was significantly lower than that of the P group and that the levels of IL-6, glucose and insulin were also significantly lower. The results of this study suggest that supplementation with ginseng could reduce the muscle damage and the inflammatory responses induced by exercise, with a consequent improvement in insulin sensitivity.

Muscle damage induced by an eccentric exercise causes delayed-onset vascular stiffening. For this reason, the hypothesis was tested with a 7-day supplementation of ginseng and *Salvia miltiorrhiza* (a Chinese plant) before an acute eccentric exercise, to prove if it could alleviate the arterial stiffening. Using a randomized, double-blind, placebo-controlled study, the subjects were randomly assigned to either the Chinese herb (n = 12) or the placebo group (n = 11) and performed a downhill running trial (eccentric exercise). The results showed that the muscle pain increased 1-2 days after the exercise in a similar way in both groups, while the group that took ginseng and salvia showed a faster recovery on the active range of motion.

The plasma concentration of creatine kinase increased significantly at 24 hours in both groups, but the extent of the increase was attenuated in the group that had taken ginseng and salvia. Arterial stiffness as measured by carotid-femoral pulse wave velocity increased significantly at 24 hours in the placebo group, but this increase was absent in the ginseng and salvia group. The plasma concentrations of CRP and IL-6 increased in the placebo group while no such increases were observed in the group assigned to ginseng and salvia. The changes in arterial stiffness induced by eccentric exercise were associated with the corresponding changes in IL-6 (r= 0.46, $p < 0.05$). In conclusion, it was found that the acute supplementation of ginseng and *Salvia miltiorrhiza* can decrease the delayed-onset vascular stiffness induced by the intense downhill running exercise.

Dosages

Today, ginseng root is dried, pulverized and distributed on the market in various forms: powder, liquid extracts, energy bars, capsules, chewing gums, drinks, tablets to dissolve in the mouth, preparations for infusions or food supplements. The recommended daily dose is 0.5-2 g of powder or 100-300 mg of extract no more than three times a day; the dosage, however, is very subjective and also depends on the type of sporting activity and its intensity. RG3, as such, is available as a supplement only in the USA. The recommended dosage is 5 mg twice a day on an empty stomach or in the form of a nasal spray, 1-2 mg/mL twice a day. You have to use the product for 4 weeks to see any benefits.

Effectiveness

Strength	Resistant strength	Mass	Endurance	Slimming	Concentration	Recovery
+	+	–	+++	+	+++	++

PHOSPHATIDIC ACID

Description
Phosphatidic acid or diacylglycerol-3-phosphate is a phospholipid obtained by the esterification of glycerol with a phosphoric acid molecule, and is the precursor of other very important phospholipids such as phosphatidylserine, phosphatidylcholine and phosphatidylinositol. In addition to having a structural role and participating in the formation of the bilayer of the cell membrane, phosphatidic acid is also a "messenger" molecule that plays a critical role in the stimulation of mTOR, which is the most important metabolic pathway for stimulating the protein synthesis. In sports, its use as a supplement is precisely linked to the ability to stimulate the protein synthesis through the mechanisms that induce the musculoskeletal hypertrophy.

Properties
Phosphatidic acid can be synthesized from a variety of other molecules, but it is unclear whether these precursors (glycerol-3-phosphate (G3P), diacylglycerol (DAG)) and some of its products (phosphatidylcholine, phosphatidylserine, phosphatidylethanolamine or phosphatidylinositol) exhibit a similar ability to activate mTOR.

Phosphatidic acid food sources (soy, eggs) may have a different behavior depending on the number and the specificity of the fatty acids present in the phosphatidic acid molecule. In particular, it has been suggested that saturated fatty acids promote its storage, while the presence of a mix of unsaturated and saturated fatty acids promotes the signaling effect. Soy derivative sources of phosphatidic acid are more likely to promote the **cellular signaling events**, such as the activation of mTOR, compared to sources such as eggs, which apparently do not seem to activate this type of signaling. Therefore, for muscle building, it is more efficient to use forms of phosphatidic acid obtained from sources such as those derived from soy.

Evidence
For decades, it has been documented that weight training leads to an increase in the muscle mass, but the mechanism that triggers the muscle hypertrophy due to a mechanical stimulus is only recently being understood. Recent research indicate that phosphatidic acid can be considered (at least partially) **responsible for the translation of the mechanical stimulus induced by training into the chemical signal that leads to skeletal muscle hypertrophy**. For example, a research conducted by O'Neil et al. showed that the cellular phosphatidic acid content of the cell increases following eccentric contractions, and that this effect is associated with a massive activation of mTOR.

The same way the endogenous production could be promoted through power training, exogenous increases in phosphatidic acid can be provided through oral supplementation. Theoretically, the combination of both of them could lead to a bigger skeletal muscle hypertrophy compared to weight training alone. In fact, the findings in a study conducted by Hoffman in 2012 suggest that phosphatidic acid supplementation enhances the strength and power improvements obtained from power training. In this study, Hoffman examined the influence that the phosphatidic acid contained in soy had on muscle growth and strength in 16 individuals subjected to training with significant weights. The subjects were divided into two groups; one group received 750 mg of phosphatidic acid per day and the other group took a placebo. During the experiment, each subject trained with weights four days a week at 70% of their maximum (1RM), for the entire eight-week trial period. Each subject was tested for their endurance and body composition. The results showed that subjects taking phosphatidic acid experienced a 12.7% increase in strength and a 2.6% increase in the muscle mass, while subjects in the second group who took the placebo only showed a 9.3% improvement in strength and a 0.1% increase in the muscle mass. The results of this study indicate that the ingestion of phosphatidic acid combined with specific power training can produce significant improvements, compared to exercise alone, both in strength and in increasing the muscle mass.

A study similar to that of Hoffman, conducted by Joy et al., showed how the use of phosphatidic acid in different dosages (divided by training days and rest days) caused a higher increase in the parameters of strength and muscle mass in these subjects, compared to the control group. In this study, subjects trained 3 days a week for 8 weeks, with training consisting mainly on strength exercises (max leg presses and bench presses). The subjects supplemented with phosphatidic acid (PA), without using other active ingredients, at doses of 450 mg of PA 30 minutes before the workout and 300 mg of PA immediately after the training, while on rest days the subdivision was in 450 mg for breakfast and 300 mg for dinner. The results showed an increase

Table 44.8 Eight-week resistance training protocol

Excercise	Series/Repetitions (RM)
Monday/Thursday	
Bench Press	1.4 x 10 - 12
Incline Press	3 x 10 - 12
Seated Shoulder Press	1.4 x 10 - 12
Uprights Rows	3 x 10 - 12
Lateral raises	3 x 10 - 12
Shrugs	3 x 10 - 12
Triceps pushdown	3 x 10 - 12
Triceps extension	3 x 10 - 12
Sit up	3 x 25
Tuesday/Friday	
Squat	1.4 x 10 - 12
Lunge/Front Squat	3 x 10 - 12
Leg Curl	3 x 10 - 12
Knee Extension	3 x 10 - 12
Calf Raises	3 x 10 - 12
Lat Pulldown	4 x 10 - 12
Seated Row	4 x 10 - 12
EZ Bar Curl	3 x 10 - 12
Dumbbel Curls	3 x 10 - 12
Sit up	3 x 25

of +2.4 kg in lean body mass (LBM) compared to the placebo group (who were supplemented with phosphatidic acid but did not exercise), which achieved an increase of only 1.2 kg in LBM.

Exogenous sources of phosphatidic acid can promote the **activation of mTOR** in ways which appear to be mediated by multiple mechanisms. For example, it has been shown that the addition of phosphatidic acid to fibroblasts determines the activation of mTOR through an indirect mechanism that depends on the metabolization of phosphatidic acid to lysophosphatidic acid, and it also activates its receptors.

In these recent studies, it was also observed a decrease in the rate of body fat, however the loss of fat can be explained by the increase in lean mass. In addition to its ability to promote the muscle hypertrophy, it has been shown that phosphatidic acid has anti-catabolic properties, preventing the degradation of muscle proteins.

The first indication on the **anticatabolic capacity of phosphatidic acid** comes from a study in which it was observed that, by increasing the availability of an enzyme (PLD1) involved in the synthesis of phosphatidic acid in isolated muscle cells, they reached a significant increase in the levels of phosphatidic acid, which rapidly leads to a reduced expression of a series of genes that promote the breakdown of muscle proteins. In this study, it is interesting to note how the expression of some genes involved in the breakdown of muscle proteins can be stopped by reducing the functionality of one of the proteins responsible for muscle catabolism, which is myostatin.

We know how the amino acid leucine is important in promoting the protein synthesis and in this sense, some scientists have carried out studies to evaluate the anabolic effects of a possible "phosphatidic acid-leucine" combination.

Scientists at the University of Auburn tried to find out if phosphatidic acid and whey proteins (a source of leucine) could act synergistically.

In an animal model, mice were given an equivalent dose of 1.5 g per day of soy-derived phosphatidic acid and 10 g of whey protein concentrate (WPC). To one group only phosphatidic acid was given, to a second group WPC + phosphatidic acid.

The results were surprising: both groups showed the ability to activate mTOR, but only **the WPC + phosphatidic acid group produced significant muscle protein synthesis and a reduction in myostatin levels** (even modest reductions in myostatin levels are capable of causing muscle growth).

Another interesting fact from this study is that the intake of the combined WPC + phosphatidic acid resulted in an increase in GLUT4, a glucose transporter, whose increase is found during exercise and which is related to an increase in the insulin sensitivity.

Therefore, the use of this combination as a supplement could help in the treatment of insulin resistance associated with aging or with the metabolic syndrome.

Dosages

The benefits that can be obtained in terms of the increased protein synthesis and a reduced breakdown of muscle proteins are more evident when the use of this supplement is combined with weight training sessions.

The optimal supplementation protocol must include at least 750 mg of phosphatidic acid from soy derivatives, to be taken immediately after weight training, or by splitting the dose between pre-workout (450 mg) and post-workout (300 mg), as suggested by recent studies.

Effectiveness

Strength	Resistant strength	Mass	Endurance	Slimming	Concentration	Recovery
+++	++	+++	−	+	−	+

PHOSPHATIDYLSERINE

Description

Phosphatidylserine (PS) is an **important constituent of the cell membrane**. From a chemical point of view, this molecule belongs to the class of phospholipids and is made up of two chains of fatty acids, associated with a glycerol molecule, with a phosphate group which is bound by means of an ester bond to the alcoholic group of a serine. In addition to phosphatidylserine, the main membrane phospholipids are phosphatidylcholine, phosphatidylethanolamine and sphingomyelin; altogether these four lipid species make up over 50% of the membrane structure of each cell.

Other phospholipids, such as phosphatidylinositol, are present in lower quantities, and mainly perform functions related to the genesis of signals that intervene in cellular communication mechanisms.

It seems that the food sources capable of providing greater amounts of phosphatidylserine are egg yolk, krill oil and soy lecithin.

Properties

Phosphatidylserine, in particular, is mainly present in the inner sheet of the membrane and in humans it has a preferential localization at the level of the brain and nerves. It has various structural and regulatory functions on the cell activity and is able to modulate the functioning of receptors, enzymes, ion channels and signal molecules, becoming, in fact, an essential component of the regulation of all cellular activities.

Phosphatidylserine is also involved in the apoptosis process. The recognition and the removal of apoptotic cells, in fact, seems to be related to the modification of the expression of particular molecules on the surface of cell membranes; in this way, the apoptotic cells are recognized and phagocytized by macrophages. One of these molecules is phosphatidylserine. Normally located on the inner surface of the membrane, during apoptosis, it passes on the outer side of the membrane, acting as a recognition signal for phagocytosis.

Several studies have shown the effectiveness of this active ingredient in reducing the levels of the stress hormone, cortisol. Cortisol tends to bring the body into a catabolic state which for the athlete involves difficulty in recovering and/or losing muscle mass. Furthermore, cortisol negatively affects the production of testosterone, or rather, it counteracts its anabolic effects, promoting muscle and organic catabolism.

Evidence

Phosphatidylserine can be a valid support for **avoiding the catabolic action of cortisol**. In a 2008 double-blind study, 10 subjects took a dose of 600 mg of phosphatidylserine for 10 days. Blood samples were then taken at rest, 15 minutes after a moderate-intense exercise on a cycle ergometer which consisted of five three-minute phases of progressive increase, starting from 65% and ending at 85% of VO_{2max}, and after a passive recovery of 65 minutes.

Cortisol levels were significantly lower (-39%) in subjects who had taken phosphatidylserine, suggesting that PS may be an effective supplement to counteract the training-induced stress.

Some studies show us that phosphatidylserine increases the learning ability and other brain functions in older people, and that it can preserve them in younger people. Due to its effect on cortisol release, two published studies show that it attenuates the ACTH release of the pituitary gland, when subjected to both physical and mental stress. A study aimed at verifying the ability of this substance to control the excessive release of cortisol in bodybuilders undergoing hard training, carried out at the California State University of Chico, showed that PS seems to have value for those interested in making progress in bodybuilding in a safe, effective and natural way.

In another double-blind study conducted at the State University of St. Cloud, trained cyclists were supplemented with 300 mg of phosphatidylserine per day for 15 days. On the 15th day, after a 90-minute run, CPK values, which express the extent of damage to the muscle cell membrane, were measured, and a significantly lower level was found in cyclists supplemented with phosphatidylserine. Taking 400 mg of PS for two weeks in healthy young adults significantly improved the processing speed (20%) and the accuracy (13% more correct answers, 39% fewer wrong answers).

A study by Monteleone et al., Published in *Neuroendocrinology* in 1990, demonstrated how PS can **significantly improve the GH-cortisol ratio** in subjects subjected to physical exercise, compared to a placebo group that performs the same training and consumes the same diet. However, it seems that phosphatidylserine is able to lower cortisol levels only when they are excessively high and does not seem to reduce them below normal values. PS is not only a valuable aid to attenuate the production of cortisol, but it also has an **antioxidant activity**. A recent study also highlights an ergogenic function of PS, whose supplementation tends to bring an improvement in the physical performance compared to the placebo, even though in this test, it did not affect cortisol levels.

This new application in the sports field is confirmed by further studies on athletes subjected to intermittent high intensity exercises and who find benefits in their performance with PS supplementation.

If we look at physical performance, the intake of 750 mg of PS was able to increase the time to exhaustion by 29 ± 8%, during a bicycle test at 85% of the maximum intensity.

Scientific research does not always show positive data on phosphatidylserine. In one study, taking 750 mg of soy-derived phosphatidylserine, compared to a placebo, given daily for 10 days, showed no effects on cortisol attenuation, oxidative stress markers, perceived pain, lipid peroxidation, and muscle damage caused by intermittent exercise. Pre- and post-exercise plasma concentrations of gamma-tocopherol were increased after the supplementation with PS, although supplementation had no effect on plasma concentrations of other non-enzymatic antioxidants (vitamin C, alpha-tocopherol, retinol and beta-carotene).

Another study shows that supplementation with 750 mg of PS for 10 days does not offer additional protection against the delayed onset of muscle soreness and against the markers of muscle damage, inflammation and oxidative stress, following a downhill race.

Dosages

The standard dose for taking phosphatidylserine would seem to be 100/200 mg three times a day, for a total of 300/600 mg.

Studies on children and adolescents for evaluating the improvement in concentration and attention have used 200 mg, while in non-elderly adults they have used daily doses of 200-400 mg.

By comparing the scientific studies on animals in order to have a useful quantity for humans, it rises to about 550 mg of phosphatidylserine to be taken daily.

In the journal *Biology of Sport*, Fahey and Pearl reported that oral supplementation with 800 mg of PS was effective in reducing serum cortisol concentration after an intensive resistance training. A study published in the *International Journal of the Society of Sport Nutrition* reported similar results. In two separate reports published in *Medicine & Science in Sports & Exercise*, the researchers were able to reproduce such a cortisol response. However, they found that subjects supplemented with PS for 14 days had significantly increased the duration of a run before reaching exhaustion.

Effectiveness

Strength	Resistant strength	Mass	Endurance	Slimming	Concentration	Recovery
+	++	+	+	–	+++	++

PYCNOGENOL

Pycnogenol is a mix of substances that is naturally present in pine bark with constant proportions of procyanidins, bioflavonoids and organic acids: procyanidins (70 ± 5%) are the most present component and consist of subunits of oligomeric catechins and epicatechins; the remainder includes phenolic acids, taxifolines and other minor elements, recently discovered by some scholars of the University of Bratislava (Grimm et al.). First of all, it should be emphasized that 95% of more than 300 published studies on pycnogenol used the product with the trade name of Pycnogenol®, and it was necessary to mention it also because there are numerous "similar products" on the market, but extracted from other species of pine, for which there is no guarantee of effectiveness.

In fact, Pycnogenol® is extracted exclusively from the *Atlantic* subspecies *Pinus pinaster*, commonly called the French maritime pine. This tall tree grows in the forest of the Landes de Gascogne (a territory of over 1,500,000 hectares, 66% pine forest, even up to 80% if we count the national park of the same name, one of the largest parks in Europe), where it was already naturally present, but its number has further increased thanks to centuries of reforestation by humans.

Given the success of the product, attempts were made to extract it from trees of the same subspecies planted in other regions (specifically in the Iberian Peninsula and Korea), but the different environmental conditions prevented their success.

The processing phase is now serialized at the highest levels: the constituents described above are extracted from the freshly harvested bark, crushed and cleaned, and the multistage process, patented and observing the GMP (Good Manufacturing Practice) protocol, uses non-toxic solvents such as water and ethanol and requires that the aqueous product, once purified, is dried, becoming a brownish-colored powder with an aromatic odor and a strongly astringent taste; only 1 kg of pycnogenol is extracted from one ton of bark. A review by D'Andrea (2010) summarizes well all the potential of this substance, emphasizing just how the synergistic aspect of the various components is what gives an added value to this phytonutrient.

If you want to investigate all the substances that make up the pycnogenol, the studies by Tanja Grimm et al (2006) and that of Sivonova et al. (2004) are very interesting and in addition to once again highlighting the excellent antioxidant activity of pycnogenol, they hypothesize the different mechanisms through which this function is carried out, concluding however that "the different processes through which the pycnogenol succeeds in expressing its beneficial effects are not fully known yet".

Properties

Pycnogenol is a powerful blend of antioxidants, it is a natural anti-inflammatory, promotes the production of collagen and hyaluronic acid and contributes to the natural dilation of blood vessels, facilitating the production of nitric oxide.

The use of pycnogenol is expanding more and more and currently includes the following indications:

- cardiovascular health: circulation, cholesterol, blood pressure;
- radical damage (antioxidant action);

- skin care: spots, sun protection, skin elasticity, wrinkles, anti-aging;
- fertility and improved sperm quality, erectile deficiency;
- diabetes: blood sugar, diabetic syndrome, retinopathies, ulcers, microangiopathies;
- ocular health;
- cognitive function: memory, ADHD (attention deficit/ hyperactivity disorder);
- inflammatory problems;
- joint health: osteoarthritis, mobility, flexibility, pain;
- menstrual disorders: premenstrual syndrome, endometriosis;
- oral health: gum bleeding, plaque formation;
- respiratory function: asthma, hay fever;
- sports nutrition: energy, recovery, cramps, nitric oxide;
- chronic venous insufficiency, "economy class syndrome", thrombosis, swelling in the lower limbs.

Evidence

A field in which pycnogenol has recently been examined and which still has a modest number of studies is precisely that relating to the sports performance.

One of the first works in this regard is that of Pavlovic in 1999 (double-blind, controlled placebo-cross study), who found an **improvement in the aerobic performance on 21%** of a group of amateur athletes who ingested 200 mg/day of pycnogenol for 30 days and ran a treadmill test at 85% of individual maximum oxygen consumption. In 2002 Buz'Zard et al. tested pycnogenol (and other substances), finding that pine bark extract significantly increases the GH secretion, and we know how an increase in GH can help in a sport setting.

In 2006 Vinciguerra et al. examined the ability of pycnogenol to reduce cramps and post-exercise pain during the physical rehabilitation in particular populations, such as athletes prone to cramps, patients with venous insufficiency or *intermittent claudication*, and in diabetics with microangiopathy: 200 mg of pycnogenol reduced the cramp episodes in each group, with good statistical significance, for example in the first two cases, respectively from 8.6 to 2.4 per week and from 6.3 to 2.6 per week.

The authors concluded that, overall, these results suggested that the **use of pycnogenol prevents the cramps and the muscle pain at rest, and the pain during and after exercise**. In 2007 Mach et al. evaluated the antioxidant effect of pycnogenol in relation to the aerobic capacity, and here the increase was 21%, same for Pavlovic; in 2010, the Anglo-Australian working group, also led by Mach, carried out another study using a similar protocol in which the subjects, after having ingested 375 mg of pycnogenol, had to pedal to exhaustion on a cycle ergometer whose wattage was increased every 3 minutes:

the average increase was 17% in both trained and untrained volunteers.

The discovery that one of the cofactors of ATP resynthesis, NAD, was greatly increased in the treated subjects was of an absolute importance, supporting the hypothesis that the antioxidant activity of pycnogenol, facilitating the redox cycle and the subsequent production of energy substrates, is able to improve the performance through this path.

Still with regard to the aerobic endurance, in 2007 Bentley et al. found a 15% improvement on the cycle ergometer and in 2012 they tested a group of professional cyclists for Time to Fatigue (TTF) after giving them 375 mg of pycnogenol or a placebo. In this latest trial, the athletes pedaled on two occasions for 5 minutes at 50% of their maximum power, for 8 minutes at 70% and finally at 95% till exhaustion: the group that had taken the pycnogenol outperformed the placebo group by 80 seconds.

In 2013, again Vinciguerra et al. analyzed pycnogenol to observe its effects on "training, exercise, recovery and oxidative stress", using the Army Physical Fitness Test (APFT); in the first test, some untrained subjects were evaluated for 8 weeks (100 mg/day of pycnogenol *vs.* placebo), in the second (150 mg/day of pycnogenol vs. placebo) they evaluated some athletes in preparation for a triathlon.

All the subjects at the first test, thanks to the military type training, improved their performances compared to the initial ones, but the group that had taken the pycnogenol obtained much better results (running for 2 miles, +11%; sit-ups, +23%; pushups, +12%). In the second test, the group that had taken the pycnogenol had even more significant increases, as they were obtained on already trained athletes: for example, a decrease of 7 minutes on the total time of a triathlon and also significantly lower oxidative stress values compared to the control group, an important factor for a faster recovery and for the overall health.

In addition, they observed a significant decrease in running cramps and delayed muscle pain; the authors also found **an important decrease in blood free radicals (-26.7%) one hour after the end of the triathlon**, unlike the control group, in which these levels increased instead.

When undergoing high intensity endurance exercise (EEAI), the muscles produce free radicals, resulting in cell damage; the accumulation of free radicals, due to the more relevant use of oxygen associated with EEAI, can worsen the muscle contraction, accelerating the onset of the sensation of fatigue and decreasing the performance, but in the EEAI fatigue can also depend on a reduced blood circulation, due to the muscle working without receiving sufficient oxygen. To remedy this state of affairs, recent research suggests that the performance can be improved through a nutritional protocol that is able to fight the free radical damage and improve the blood flow simultaneously.

Some polyphenols appear to be the most suitable candidates to achieve both results, as they are believed to be able to increase the body's antioxidant capacity to fight the free radical damage and the associated muscle suffering, and they are also able to stimulate the production of endothelial nitric oxide, with the result of encouraging the dilation of blood vessels, a very useful factor in decreasing the problems deriving from excess free radicals.

In fact, several clinical trials (including Green et al., 2002 and Gliemann et al., 2014) have shown that sports activity determines a marked increase in the production capacity of endothelial nitric oxide: nitric oxide (NO) is the main mediator of blood vessel dilation and allows for an optimization of the blood flow determined by the physical exercise: the pycnogenol influences its release, stimulating the endothelial nitric oxide synthase (eNOS) enzyme.

In a research by Fitzpatrick et al. (1998), the facilitating action carried out by Pycnogenol® against the enzyme eNOS which is present in the endothelial cells of the internal wall of the artery, has allowed the **synthesis of a greater quantity of NO**, with a consequent reduction of vasoconstriction: the action it was found to be dose-dependent and the maximum increase in the arterial diameter reached 78.4% of the maximum possible dilation; Nishioka et al., on the other hand, found an eNOS increase of 46% compared to baseline in the forearms of young subjects who had ingested 180 mg/day of pycnogenol for 2 weeks, while the control group did not obtain any results (Forearm Blood Flow response from 13.1 to 18.5 mL/min).

Two trials have also shown that pycnogenol is able to promote the vasodilation and, consequently, it **improves the blood microcirculation** (Wang et al., 1999; Kohama, 2004). Belcaro et al. (2005) completed a study in which, among other investigations, they also included a cardiocirculatory evaluation through the application of specific sensors on the dermis of the legs: after taking 150 mg/day of pycnogenol for 6 weeks, an increased presence of oxygen and a decrease in carbon dioxide were detected by the sensors. This result suggests that pycnogenol facilitates the aerobic endurance, since blood flow plays a very specific role in the supply of oxygen to the muscles, in returning carbon dioxide to the lungs and in the transfer of lactic acid to the liver.

Pycnogenol can significantly contribute to extend the efficiency of the endogenous antioxidant system in athletes during the physical activity, as it is one of the most powerful antioxidants and has been shown to increase the absorption capacity of oxygen radicals by 40% in the blood of human subjects treated with pycnogenol: 25 subjects ingested 150 mg of pycnogenol for 6 weeks and, at the end of the administration period, the levels of polyphenols in the blood were significantly higher, as was the increase in the ORAC (Oxygen Radical Absorbance Capacity, an evaluation measure developed to quantify the protection that antioxidant substances provide against reactive hydroxides and peroxides) value and HDL cholesterol levels vs. a reduction in LDL levels (Devaraj et al., 2002).

Furthermore, numerous scientific works have shown how the picnogenol allows an effective strengthening of the vein wall and of the microvessels, preventing swelling (edema), micro-bleeding and hemorrhages; in addition, clinical studies have shown that pycnogenol **reduces the healing time of the damaged tissues**, so it can be an aid for the recovery processes, especially in contact sports such as football, rugby, martial arts and boxing.

Returning to the specific studies, in 2014 Ackerman et al. tested some volunteers (well trained) to see if pycnogenol could also have an effect on weight training, in this case during the execution of six sets of squats with ten repetitions. The results in terms of potency were more than fair in favor of the group that had taken pycnogenol (expressed in total watts, 6746 vs. 6493) and, very importantly, the decline of the performance was much slower than the placebo group. The same occurred for the average speed of execution, which even reached considerable significance in almost all sets.

Pycnogenol also finds use in erectile dysfunction (ED). In this case, the subjects (being treated for sexual problems) were treated with 120 mg for 3 months. At the end of the test, the patients showed an improvement (determined by the score obtained at the IIEF, International Index of Erectile Function) which brought ED from moderate to mild; at the same time, a truly significant increase in the plasma antioxidant activity was observed. After 3 months of treatment with pycnogenol, total cholesterol decreased from 201 to 193 mg/dL and, more importantly, LDL cholesterol decreased from 133 to 108 mg/dL, while the placebo group did not show any progress.

Sportsmen may be interested in the positive influence exerted by pycnogenol on the joints: the studies by Belcaro, Farid and Cìsar are excellent examples; the first, with an Italian working group, carried out an important project in this regard, the SVOS (San Valentino Osteo-Arthrosis Study). In short, the conclusions we can draw from the results obtained by these researchers are that **pycnogenol is indicated for the treatment of osteoarticular pain, probably thanks to its antioxidant and anti-inflammatory properties**.

The consumption of pycnogenol limits the activation of the proinflammatory factor NF-κB by 15.8% (a fundamental factor for the activation of all proinflammatory molecules, which play a destructive role in arthritis). Consequently, fewer enzymes of the matrix metalloproteinases (MMPs) family are generated by taking pycnogenol, which in osteoarthritis cause the degeneration of the collagen contained in the cartilage.

It is also documented that in humans pycnogenol naturally inhibits the production of COX2 enzymes (an inducible enzyme, present only in tissues affected by inflammation), helping to significantly reduce joint pain, and is also able to lower the levels of C-reactive protein (an inflammatory marker) by 72%, and those of reactive oxygen species (ROS) by 30%.

In recent years (2017-2020) many other studies have been carried out on this substance, but mainly on aspects related to cardiovascular problems (Malekhamadi, 2019), to the reduction of pressure and osteoarthritis problems, as indicated in "Pleiotropic effects of French maritime pine bark extract to promote healthy aging "(Rohdewald, 2019), in which all the benefits of pycnogenol can be observed at various levels which, especially in "otherwise young subjects", can still have positive effects (also) on the sports practice.

Dosages
The standard dosage starts from 50 to reach 375 mg/day, with an average of 100/200 mg.

Effectiveness

Strength	Resistant strength	Mass	Endurance	Slimming	Concentration	Recovery
–	++	–	+++	++	–	++

PROBIOTICS

Description
According to the Food and Agriculture Organization of the United Nations (FAO) and the World Health Organization (WHO), probiotics are live microorganisms (bacteria, fungi) which, when administered in adequate quantities, have a positive action on the organism, defending it from the attack of pathogenic microorganisms.

The most recent guidelines indicate that there are some fundamental characteristics that must absolutely satisfy:

- they must be traditionally used as a supplement for the human intestinal microflora (microbiota) (there must be medical literature in this regard, depending on the proposed strain);
- must be considered safe for use in humans (for example, the used microorganisms must not carry acquired and/or transmissible antibiotic resistance);
- they must be active in the intestine in such quantities, as to multiply there (form colonies);
- the species, strain and number of microorganisms present in each capsule/sachet must be reported (which usually should not be less than 10 billion, the minimum dose for daily consumption and temporary colonization of the human intestine). Lower quantities can be marketed only in the presence of a literature that certifies, however, for that strain, the colonizing capacity at the determined concentration;
- the quantity of live cells guaranteed in the storage mode suggested on the box must be reported.

The probiotics that are normally used are lactobacilli and bifids. A probiotic, to be defined as such, must have the following characteristics:

- be non-pathogenic and of human origin;
- resist the acidity of the stomach and the action of bile;
- survive in the gastrointestinal tract and adhere to the mucosa by reproducing;
- be perfectly tolerable;
- have beneficial effects on the health by antagonizing pathogenic microorganisms and by producing antimicrobial substances.

It is important to highlight that the main bacteria in the yogurt (*Lactobacillus bulgaricus* and *Streptococcus thermophilus*) or fermented foods, which contain live bacteria, are not currently classified as probiotics.

Properties
Probiotics, in addition to counteracting pathogenic microorganisms by competing with them at the level of the intestinal adhesion sites and by producing bacteriocins that destroy them, they also produce vitamins, contribute to the elimination of cholesterol, are effective for di-

gestive purposes, to prevent constipation and diarrhea, as well as to improve the effectiveness of both the humoral and cellular immune systems, by stimulating the action of macrophages; they participate in the development of intestinal microcirculation (Hooper et al., 2001) and in the development of the central and peripheral nervous system (Rhee et al., 2009); they are also able to modulate the production of neurotransmitters (Forshite et al., 2009), important for the mood regulation (Neufeld et al., 2009), thus also influencing the stress response (Sudo et al., 2004) and the appetite control (Fetissov et al., 2008).

Various studies show that the intestinal flora of obese individuals differs from that of people of normal weight. Some scientists speculate that this difference may be due to the fact that a high-fat, low-fiber diet may favor some bacteria at the expense of others.

Evidence

The scientific literature on the microbiota is really abundant now, and some premises must be made before talking about the effect of probiotics. The microbiota is to be considered as a characteristic fingerprint, which varies from subject to subject. It weighs about 1.5 kg in our body, thus configuring itself as the largest organ in our body, an organ with numerous physiological functions that are essential for our life.

In particular, the "good" bacteria prevent the proliferation of pathogenic bacteria (producers of toxins that tend to move into the blood), they help digest the dietary fibers by producing short-chain fatty acids (SCFA, Short Chain Fatty Acid, an important signal of health for our body). These SCFAs (acetate, propionate and butyrate) can be easily used for energy purposes by the cells of the intestinal mucosa, thus implementing the barrier functions of the intestinal epithelium, but not only. In fact, it seems that there is a double link with the sports performance, i.e. it is believed that these substrates can also be used for energy purposes in endurance exercises (Rankin, 2017).

In a 2015 study (Hsu), some mice were subjected to physical exercise and it was observed that their performance was influenced by the type of their microbiota. Those with the worst performance were the "germ free" (non-colonized intestine), followed by those colonized by a single bacterial species, while the best performance was observed at those with a marked biodiversity of the microbiota (many intestinal bacterial species in equilibrium with each other). This observation could agree with the fact that, often, athletes undergoing antibiotic therapy show a decline in their sports performance.

Antibiotic therapy produces damage to the microbiota and leaves sequelae for long periods, so the alarm about the misuse of antibiotics is even more justified if we consider the role of these bacteria in our health. But the link with the sports activity would be twofold, given that other studies have shown that the right amount of exercise (neither too much nor too little, Clarke 2016) would favor an increase in SCFA-producing bacteria. Furthermore, bacteria produce fundamental vitamins such as vitamin K and those of group B, are able to modulate the responses of the immune system (Codella, 2017) and are able to affect the central nervous system in such levels, so that we are now talking about psychobiota and psychobiotics (Dinan, 2013).

Just think that 90% of serotonin (the hormone of well-being and relaxation) is produced by the enterochromaffin cells of the intestine and that the intestinal inflammation depends fundamentally on the microbial barrier.

Bacteria are also very important for the control of body weight: by transplanting the
intestinal flora from lean mice to fatty mice predisposed to become diabetic and obese, the latter maintained a normal body weight despite a high-fat diet. Consuming too many sugars, on the other hand, causes the intestinal flora to develop (which also includes *Candida*) and sends signals to the brain to take in ever greater quantities. Some protocols for rebalancing the intestinal candidiasis, for example, require extremely low levels of carbohydrate intake.

But what is the connection between the physical activity, bacterial flora and the use of probiotics?

In December 2019, was released a review entitled: "International Society of Sports Nutrition position stand: probiotics".

Here are some noteworthy elements:

1. In the populations of athletic subjects, some strains of probiotics can increase the absorption of key nutrients such as amino acids and proteins and influence the physiological properties of several food components.
2. In athletes, the immune system deteriorates when the training load is excessive; psychological stress, disturbed sleep and extreme environmental conditions are the main factors involved and this would contribute to an increased risk of respiratory tract infections.
3. Supplementation with probiotics has been shown to promote a healthy immune response. In athletes, specific probiotic strains can reduce the number of episodes, the severity and the duration of upper respiratory tract infections.
4. It has been shown that intense and particularly prolonged exercise (extreme endurance), especially in hot environments, increases the intestinal permeability and can cause systemic toxemia with the blood translocation of LPS (lipopolysaccharide).
5. Specific probiotic varieties can improve the integrity of the intestinal barrier function in athletes and the administration of selected anti-inflammatory probiotic strains has been linked to a better recovery from strenuous exercise.
6. The minimum effective dose and method of administration of a specific probiotic strain depend on validation studies performed for that particular strain. Probiotics must include the genus, species and strain of each live microorganism on the label, as well as the estimated total amount of each probiotic strain and the CFU (colony forming units), in addition to the shelf life of the product.
7. Human research has shown potential benefits from probiotics for athletes, which include an improved body composition and lean mass, the normalization of age-related drop in testosterone levels, reductions in cortisol levels, indicating better response to physical or mental stress, a reduction in exercise-induced lactate, and an increased synthesis of neurotransmitters related to cognition and mood. However, these potential benefits require validation in more standardized human studies.

In a study carried out on 119 male and female marathon runners during the three months of preparation before the race, the administration of 600 million *Lactobacillus rhamnosus GG* **decreased the duration of gastrointestinal disorders** without avoiding them. In another study involving 84 participating athletes, men and women, they were given a placebo or a probiotic drink that contained 6.5 billion *Lactobacillus casei Shirota* twice a day, for 16 weeks. The results showed that the subjects who had taken the probiotic experienced a **50% lower percentage of infectious diseases of the upper respiratory tract** (URTI) and, in the presence of URTIs, they showed a greater ability to conduct the training.

Toohey et al., In 2018, studied the effects of *Bacillus subtilis DE111* on the muscle strength, body composition and athletic performance of First Division volleyball and soccer athletes, during 10 weeks of endurance training. Both groups consumed a post-workout protein and carbohydrate drink (consisting of 45g of carbohydrates, 20g of protein and 2g of fat). The group that was supplemented with the prebiotic post-workout drink showed a greater reduction in body fat and an increase in lean mass compared to the placebo. Although no performance benefits were observed, Toohey et al. have hypothesized that the supplementation may have favored a better absorption and usage of proteins in the diet, contributing to the improvement of the body composition, increasing the thermogenesis induced by dietary proteins and altering the satiety signal.

It appears that several strains of lactic acid bacteria, including *L. gasseri SBT 2055, Lactobacillus rhamnosus ATCC 53103*, and the combination of L. *rhamnosus ATCC 53102* and *Bifidobacterium lactis Bb12* are effective in reducing the fat mass in obese humans.

Angelo Tremblay of Laval University (Canada) and his collaborators recruited 125 overweight men and women who underwent a 12-week weight loss diet, followed by a 12-week period aimed at maintaining the body weight. During the entire study, half of the participants ingested two pills containing the daily amount of probiotics from the *Lactobacillus rhamnosus* family, while the other half received a placebo. After the 12-week diet period, the researchers observed an average weight loss of 4.4 kg in the women in the probiotic group, compared with 2.6 kg in the placebo group. After the 12-week maintenance period, the weight of the women in the placebo group remained stable, but the probiotic group continued to lose weight, totaling 5.2 kg per person.

In other words, it appears that the women who took the probiotics lost twice as much weight over the course of the study. In this group, the researchers also observed a drop in leptin, the hormone that regulates appetite, as well as an overall lower concentration of the intestinal bacteria linked to obesity. Probiotic bacteria can act by altering the permeability of the intestinal wall and by avoiding the entry of some pro-inflammatory molecules into the bloodstream, which can help prevent the chain reaction that leads to type 2 diabetes and obesity.

For the moment, studies on the relationship between probiotics and the athlete's immune system are few, but the ones that are out there are still interesting: it is known that when you train intensely, there is a large consumption of glucose and glutamine (preferential nutrients for the immune system) and a large production of free radicals that create a sort of inflammation, thus depressing the immune system and predisposing the athlete to infectious diseases, especially in the upper respiratory tract. Well, given that 70% of our immune system resides in the intestine, one of the ways to decrease the infections, which obviously worsen the athletic performance, is to have a particularly "robust" microbiota, capable of boosting the immune system.

Avoiding infections is particularly important for athletes, as any necessary contextual use of antibiotics will only further worsen the microbiota, making the individual even more sensitive to a possible relapse. To have a good microbiota from the nutrition point of view, we have already seen that we must not consume too many sugars and not too many fats as the endotoxins of the bad bacteria that kill the good ones are fat-soluble and therefore are more active in the presence of large quantities of fats. Bacterial endotoxins, among other things, reduce the muscle protein synthesis and exert an inflammatory action that limits the muscle growth. Among the fats, it is better to choose polyunsaturated ones, such as salmon, mackerel and flax seeds, which are rich in omega-3, and monounsaturated fats from sources such as olive oil, avocado, almonds.

But the preferred nutrients to feed the good bacteria are fibers which perform a prebiotic function, such as whole grains, legumes, seeds, nuts, fresh fruits, berries, vegetables, tubers and mushrooms. It is also advisable to limit red meat and dairy products, which worsen the bacterial flora, and to eliminate industrial foods. In addition, fermented foods such as yogurt, sour cream, Kefir, sauerkraut and miso should be consumed, and a probiotic supplement at a dose of at least 10 billion may be helpful.

The following strains/species have been linked to an increased athletic performance and/or recovery:
1. *B. coagulans GBI-30, 6086* (BC30) at 1×10^9 CFU has beneficial effects on the exercise recovery, in combination with proteins.
2. Encapsulated *B. breve BR03*, in combination with *S. thermophilus FP4*, at 5×10^9 CFU each, has beneficial effects on exercise recovery and performance following exercises that damage muscles.

3. *L. delbrueckii* ssp. *bulgaricus* at 1 × 105 CFU can increase VO_{2max} and the aerobic power.
4. *L. acidophilus* spp., *L. delbrueckii* ssp. *bulgaricus*, *B. bifidum* and *S. salivarius* ssp. *thermophilus* at 4 × 1010 CFU, administered in the form of a yogurt beverage, can increase the VO_{2max}.
5. *L. plantarum* TWK10 at 1 × 1010 CFU has been shown to increase the endurance performance.
6. *L. acidophilus*, *L. rhamnosus*, *L. casei*, *L. plantarum*, *L. fermentum*, *B. lactis*, *B. breve*, *B. bifidum* and *S. thermophilus* at 4.5 × 1010 CFU can improve the performance in hot environments.

The following strains/species have been linked to an improved gut health in athletes:
1. *L. rhamnosus* GG at 4 × 1010 CFU in the form of a milk-based beverage.
2. *B. bifidum* W23, *B. lactis* W51, *E. faecium* W54, *L. acidophilus* W22, *L. brevis* W63 and *L. lactis* W58, at 1 × 1010 CFU.
3. *L. salivarius* (UCC118) (but unknown dose).

The following strains/species have been shown to improve the immune health in athletes by reducing the episodes, severity and duration of exercise-induced infections:
1. *L. fermentum* VRI-003 (PCC) at 1.2 × 1010 CFU and 1 × 109 CFU in males.
2. *L. casei Shirota* (LcS) at 6.5 × 109 CFU twice daily.
3. *L. delbrueckii* ssp. *bulgaricus*, *B. bifidum* and *S. salivarius* ssp. *thermophilus* at 4 × 1010 CFU administered in the form of a yogurt beverage.
4. *B. animalis* ssp. *lactis* BI-04 at 2 × 1010 CFU.
5. *L. gasseri* at 2.6 × 109 CFU, *B. bifidum* at 0.2 × 109 and *B. longum* at 0.2 × 109 CFU.
6. *B. bifidum* W23, *B. lactis* W51, *E. faecium* W54, *L. acidophilus* W22, *L. brevis* W63, *L. lactis* W58 at 1 × 1010 CFU.
7. *L. helveticus Lafti* L10 at 2 × 1010 CFU.

Dosages

Normally, a probiotic supplement contains a combination of various bacterial species with an overall dosage ranging from 1 billion to 10 billion and it must be taken for a period of at least 1 month or even continuously. In particular situations, such as during the use of antibiotics, doses of 5 to 20 billion can be used, once or twice a day, for 1 or 2 weeks. If you have ongoing gastrointestinal problems, you can opt for a dosage of 50 to 200 billion for 2 weeks until the situation improves. Later, it is recommended to return to a dosage of 5 to 20 billion as a prevention of the problem flare-ups.

Effectiveness

Strength	Resistant strength	Mass	Endurance	Slimming	Concentration	Recovery
–	–	+	+++	+++	++	++

PROTEIN POWDER

Description

Proteins, from the Greek *protos* = first or main, are a class of biological macromolecules made up of long chains of amino acids. At a biological level, proteins can perform various functions, including: enzymatic function to catalyze chemical reactions, structural function, transport function (carrier), immune function, cellular transmission, regulatory function, detoxifying and also energetic function.

As a supplement, proteins have perhaps been the most widely used supplements in the sports world for several decades now. Essentially, protein supplementation has the function of adjusting the daily protein quota when you are unable to meet your needs with the diet and for an athlete, the protein powder is used to maintain a constant amino acid intake in order to provide nourishment for the muscles or for rapidly assimilated proteins in specific moments, such as close to training, and to make the most of the moment of maximum anabolic predisposition (anabolic window).

The protein requirement is estimated at 0.8 g/kg/day for sedentary people and 1.3-1.8 g/kg/day for athletes. These quantities have been calculated on the basis of urinary nitrogen excretion due to muscle catabolism and represent the minimum quantities to avoid going into nitrogen deficiency. When the goal is to increase the muscle mass, the protein requirement can be increased to 2.3-2.5 g/kg/day.

It is essential to keep the plasma azotemia level constant, as different types of proteins have different turnover rates; for example, enzymes have a turnover rate of about 10 minutes, while structural proteins (collagen and muscle proteins) have significantly longer renewal times (from 180 to 1000 days).

Properties

Proteins are components of a primary importance, as they perform innumerable plastic, structural, protective and regulatory functions. Our body uses them to repair and form new cells and for the production of enzymes and hormones, essential for the protein turnover (anabolic and catabolic process); in addition, proteins provide calories. Obviously, the main role of proteins for sports use is to provide adequate amounts of the amino acids needed to make up for the increased protein turnover.

At an ergogenic level, proteins play a fundamental role in maintaining and increasing the muscle mass. The richness in essential amino acids, and especially in leucine, determines its ability to positively stimulate the protein synthesis process. This process is a complex protein machine called mTOR (mammalian Target of Rapamycin), which is stimulated by both food and mechanical stimuli. Mainly the essential amino acids (above all leucine), insulin and training activate, by different pathways, the mTOR signal, which activates the catalytic subunit mTORC1 which in turn activates the protein kinase S6K1 and the eukaryotic initiation factor 4E. The phosphorylation of S6K1 triggers the actual protein synthesis, through the activation of the ribosomal protein S6 and other components of the transcriptional machine.

There are various types of proteins deriving from different sources, both animal and vegetable, each with different characteristics and properties.

Parameters for evaluating the quality of proteins
Biological value – This term indicates the amount of nitrogen absorbed by a protein that has been retained for maintenance and/or growth, i.e. the supply of protein nitrogen is corrected with the losses that occur through the feces and urine. If no correction is made for endogenous nitrogen losses, the value is called the apparent biological value. The reference protein is the egg protein, whose biological value is considered equal to 100; the biological values of some proteins are: whey protein, 104; milk proteins, 91; fish, 83; beef, 80; chicken, 79; casein, 77; soy protein, 74; Wheat protein, 54. In some recent studies, biological values of 110 to 159 have been proposed for high quality whey proteins, containing all the original

whey protein fractions (whey proteins isolated by ion exchange). However, these values (110-159) are not yet present in the official FAO/WHO literature.

Protein Efficiency Ratio (PER) – This parameter is typically measured on rats under standardized feeding conditions. PER is defined as weight gain per 1 g of ingested protein. The PER values for the following proteins are: whey protein, 3.6; milk proteins, 3.1; caseins, 2.9; soy protein, 2.1; wheat protein, 1.5.

PDCAAS (Protein Digestibility Corrected Amino Acid Score) – It is a theoretical calculation method for evaluating the quality of proteins (FAO/WHO, 1990) based on both the human need for amino acids and the human ability to digest these proteins. According to the definition of amino acid score, the content of each essential amino acid in a protein is expressed as the ratio or percentage of the content of the same amino acid in the same amount of a recommended standard protein (hypothetical or real) that meets the individual's protein requirement. Here are some PDCAAS values: whey protein, 1.81; milk proteins, 1.30; egg white, 1.19; caseins, 1.18; soy protein, 0.92; bean protein, 0.63; wheat protein, 0.40. The best proteins are the ones with the highest score.

Digestibility – Usually digestibility is measured experimentally and consists of the ratio between the absorbed protein nitrogen and the amount of ingested protein nitrogen, corrected for metabolic nitrogen losses in the stool. Some digestibility values: milk proteins, 95%; soy protein isolate, 95%; soy flour, 86%.

NPU (Net Protein Utilization) – This term refers to the ratio of ingested nitrogen to the amount of used nitrogen. The NPU can be calculated by multiplying the biological value (BV) by the digestibility (D) of a protein. The NPU value obtained, in the case of protein isolates, usually does not change the classification of the given protein, based on the biological value (BV).

Egg proteins
They have a high biological value (100) and PER. Whole egg proteins (yolk + egg white) have been shown to slow the gastric emptying and therefore lower the glycemic index of foods containing carbohydrates. They are also recommended for those suffering from intolerance to lactose and milk derivatives in general.

Whey proteins
They are the best proteins available. They have the highest biological value (104) and PER. Whey protein is gaining more and more success on the market due to its effectiveness. In milk, we find two main types of whey proteins: beta-lactoglobulin and alpha-lactalbumin, both of mammary origin. In cow's milk prevails beta-lacto-globulin, while in human milk, alpha-lactalbumin, which has anti-infective properties and a protective role against microorganisms. In the serum we also find: serum albumin (5% of the protein share) with a high content of glutathione precursors; lactoferrin (a phosphorylated glycoprotein responsible for iron transport), with a favorable action in supporting the immune system, which is also an antimicrobial, antiviral and anticancer agent and can have a probiotic activity, stimulating the growth of beneficial bacteria in the intestinal tract; immunoglobulins (give milk immunological properties and abound in colostrum), proteolytic enzymes, oligopeptides (proteosis-peptones, which come from the partial proteolysis of beta-casein) such as glycomacropeptide (GMP), which is a biologically active peptide derived from casein, with antimicrobial and antiviral properties and beneficial for the digestive system, as it improves calcium absorption and the immune function. Whey proteins increase the secretion of insulin by the beta cells of the pancreas; insulin, in fact, is a hormone with an anabolic role on muscle, heart and adi-

pose tissue, favoring the storage of amino acids, carbohydrates and lipids. Insulin, therefore, is not only involved in the metabolism of carbohydrates, pushing glucose into the cells of insulin-dependent tissues, but is also involved in protein anabolism (proteosynthesis) and therefore in the metabolism of amino acids. By consuming a formula of whey proteins, we do not only increase the quantities of proteins available for muscle cells, but we also increase the storage mechanism of the amino acids in the muscles (proteosynthesis) by various hormones, including insulin and GH.

The fraction represented by whey proteins is the one that shows the greatest capacity for the hormonal stimulation compared to casein or complete milk proteins, presumably due to the high content of insulinogenic amino acids. Compared to other protein sources, whey proteins have the highest insulin index, therefore the greatest insulin stimulating capacity. Furthermore, among the types of whey proteins, the hydrolyzed ones (WPH) show an insulin index that is clearly superior to the others, due to the faster assimilation times. Whey proteins, in addition to being the most effective in promoting the protein synthesis, probably thanks to their high content of insulinogenic amino acids and the high concentration of leucine (about 11%), they also bring a whole range of benefits.

Whey proteins are able to improve insulin sensitivity, the worsening of which predisposes to diseases such as the metabolic syndrome, and to lower blood sugar through a peptide fraction called GILP. Although whey proteins significantly stimulate insulin, there are no negative inflammatory effects caused by hyperinsulinemia which would activate the production pathway of inflammatory prostaglandins, because at the same time, whey proteins stimulate glucagon which instead acts in anti-inflammatory sense.

Whey proteins are able to induce a sense of satiety to a greater extent than all other protein sources and a dose of 45-50 g is able to increase thermogenesis by promoting weight loss. Whey proteins are able to lower the blood pressure when consumed regularly, as they contain peptides (lactalbumin and lactoglobulin or lactokinin) that work as ACE inhibitors (ACE is an enzyme that produces angiotensin 2, a vasoconstrictor hormone that raises the pressure); the inhibition of angiotensin limits the muscle fibrosis and increases muscle regeneration after trauma.

Another healthful effect of whey proteins is their ability to lower the levels of cholesterol and triglycerides: a dose of 50 g per day administered to overweight subjects for 12 weeks reduced the values of triglycerides, total cholesterol and LDL cholesterol.

Furthermore, serum proteins limit the systemic inflammation, as evidenced by the reduction in CRP (C-reactive protein) and IL-6 (inflammatory cytokine). Inflammation is now unanimously recognized as the basis of cardiovascular diseases and cancer. Probably, the anti-inflammatory effect of whey proteins is mediated by their ability to increase the levels of glutathione, a powerful antioxidant that is produced in our body starting from cysteine, a sulfur amino acid of which whey proteins are particularly rich.

In a study carried out in India that included men and women with fatty liver disease (accumulation of fat in the liver that promotes the development of cirrhosis), found that those who took 20g of whey protein for 12 weeks showed a reduction in transaminases (ALT and AST) and an increase in glutathione levels. They are also particularly rich in tryptophan, which increases their biological value and, moreover, makes them particularly suitable in the post-workout, as a recovery, but not in the pre-workout, where they could have a negative effect by increasing serotonin levels, a relaxing neurotransmitter associated with the feeling of fatigue.

The manufacturing companies offer whey protein supplements that are very different from each other, both in price and in characteristics. It is therefore important to explain the differences between the various types of whey protein used in supplements.

Concentrated whey proteins - They are obtained by ultrafiltration, have a protein content that varies at origin from approximately 73 to 83% and contain from 4 to 6% of fat. They are the

most used, as they have a low cost. Supplements that contain these proteins typically have a protein content of about 80% and a fat content of over 4%. However, they are good quality proteins.
Whey protein isolated by ion exchange – They have a protein content at the origin of more than 90% and a fat and lactose content of less than 1%. They are of very high quality and are particularly rich in bovine serum albumin (practically the same in its structure as that of humans) and in immunoglobulins. The typical content of the protein fractions of ion exchange whey proteins is: 50% beta-lactoglobulins (containing 50% branched), 22% alpha-lactalbumin, 5% peptones and other minor peptides, such as lactoferrin, lactoperoxidase, lactolin, lysozyme, relassin, gammaglobulins, beta-microglobulin and other micropeptides.

Whey protein isolated by microfiltration – There are two types: 1) with a protein content at the origin of more than 90%, fat less than 1% and lactose less than about 1%; 2) with a protein content of about 80% and fat less than 1%. Both are quality proteins: type 1 (90%) is comparable in quality to ion exchange proteins; however, type 2 (80%) maintains a high quality. Microfiltered whey proteins differ slightly in composition from ion exchange proteins, due to the different extraction process: they are particularly rich in beta-lactoglobulin, glycomacropeptides and lacto-ferrin.
The typical content of the protein fractions of microfiltered whey proteins is: 55.9% of beta-lactoglobulin (containing 50% of the branched ones); 14.9% alpha-lactalbumin; 1.55% bovine serum albumin (BSA); 3% immunoglobulin G (IgG); 20% of glycomacropeptides; 0.125% lactoferrin and other minor peptides, such as lactoperoxidase, lactolin, lysozyme, relaxin, gammaglobulin, beta-microglobulin and other micropeptides.

Hydrolyzed whey proteins – They derive from the enzymatic hydrolysis of whey proteins. The industrial process is similar to what happens in our stomach, in fact the proteins are broken up by hydrolytic enzymes, in particular sites, to form di- or tripeptides (consisting of 2-3 amino acids). Generally, in these supplements we find polypeptides or macromolecules having a number of amino acids that is less than 100 and this significantly reduces the digestion time and improves the absorption, as it seems that the intestine absorbs di- or tripeptides better than single amino acids.
As a quality, hydrolyzed proteins usually have a very low quantity of fats and carbohydrates and, compared to all the others, have a great speed of absorption, as they have a greater insulin-trophic effect with a consequent faster entry of amino acids into the blood stream. This characteristic allows these proteins to be optimal for post-workout (making the most of the anabolic window), since, in addition to the rapid increase in amino acidemia with the consequent better uptake of amino acids, especially in trained areas, they allow the muscle, in association with rapidly absorbed carbohydrates, to synthesize glycogen more quickly and they also speed up the muscle recovery. The rapidity of absorption of these proteins allows to avoid some unwanted effects such as bloating and flatulence, due to the partial digestion and putrefaction of proteins.
The best whey protein supplements contain hydrolyzed, ion exchanged or microfiltered whey proteins, or mixtures of the three types.

Casein
It has an excellent PDCAAS, i.e. 1, which is the maximum, and a sufficient biological value (77) and PER. Casein tends to absorb a lot of water and increases in volume by forming a gel, which makes it suitable for use in meal replacements. A greater volume in the stomach means more efficacy in giving a sense of satiety. Furthermore, solidifying in the stomach, it releases its amino acids on a regular and continuous basis, drop by drop, with the result of a better use and a maximum absorption.

The whole process of absorption of nutritional substances is further enhanced by the presence of elements contained in casein, called caseomorphins. Caseomorphins are chains of unique bioactive amino acids (peptides with a specific biological function) that are released as the casein is digested in the intestine. When released, these protein derivatives play a very specific and specialized role: slowing the release and breakthrough time of the hundreds of growth factors made available by casein digestion. This retarding action essentially indicates that the body is able to optimize the absorption of all available nutrients, thereby increasing the potential for growth and development.

For these characteristics, they are certainly to be preferred when one is forced to delay the splitting of meals by more than 2-3 hours or during slimming diets, where the anti-catabolic effect of casein becomes particularly important. Compared to whey proteins, these have a significant amount of glutamine (a particularly efficient amino acid for muscle repair) which, together with their slow and gradual absorption, makes them particularly suitable to be taken 30 minutes before going to bed in the evening (casein remains in circulation for almost 7 hours), thus being effective in inhibiting the protein catabolism that occurs especially during the second phase of sleep, aimed at maintaining, through gluconeogenesis, adequate levels of blood sugar, which starts to drop.

Furthermore, glutamine is a particularly efficient amino acid with regard to muscle repair (providing high concentrations of this amino acid, especially in its peptide form which is found in casein, can help safeguard muscle mass during intense training) and as a support to deal with the stress to which the body is subjected both by training and by lifestyle.

Casein could be considered the most "stimulating" protein on the market. With a tyrosine-tryptophan ratio of nearly 5:1, it has a higher concentration of tyrosine (the "regenerating" amino acid) and a lower level of tryptophan (the "sleep-inducing" amino acid) than any other pure protein source. Taking a large amount of pure casein can actually increase the excitatory synaptic levels in the brain, stimulating it. This can be useful for having more concentration and alertness during training, delaying the onset of fatigue.

This relationship between the two amino acids also helps those who are undergoing a low-calorie diet because it fights the feeling of fatigue and listlessness that accompanies this poor diet. Let's not forget the concomitant satiating effect which is equally useful when small quantities of food are introduced throughout the day. After having highlighted the tyrosine/tryptophan ratio of 5:1, we reiterate that casein is perhaps the best protein to consume before going to bed, for its anti-catabolic actions (i.e. the ability to prevent muscle breakdown; sleep is one of the moments with the greater muscle loss, because for 6-8 hours you are basically in a state of fasting), but you must not exaggerate in quantities, otherwise the excitatory effect of tyrosine could take over to hinder the sleep.

Casein can also stimulate a greater production of "glucogenic" amino acids that lend themselves to the production of glucose, to provide energy during physical activity; It has also been shown that large amounts of glucogenic amino acids increase the efficiency in the use of the ingested foods.

The preferable form of casein is the **micellar** one, because the production process involves a lower temperature and therefore does not damage the fragile protein fractions. In this way, casein is rich in lactoferrin, an exceptional protein fraction (it is a glycoprotein of the transferrin family) that can reduce the time needed for recovery by half, according to its studies.

Micellar casein has the highest concentration of this factor for tissue growth and reconstruction. Most of the most important benefits of lactoferrin depend on its iron binding activity. The main functional characteristics of lactoferrin are: antibiotic activity; antiviral activity; it acts on inflammation and improves the immune functions as it is a natural antioxidant; increases the transport and absorption of iron (about 70% more); antiallergic modulation; balance of the intestinal flora.

Recent studies have highlighted how the use of foods rich in lactoferrin increases the formation of immunoglobulins (IgA) in the human body (immunoglobulins are "antibodies" with protective/defensive activity against mucous surfaces in general and the gastrointestinal mucosa in particular, with the function of "an antiseptic protective paint" that allows to regulate the absorption of pathogens, bacterial toxins, pollen, etc.).

Meat proteins
They are the last ones that have entered in the supplement market. By analyzing their chemical component, we can compare this protein source to that of the egg for the amino acid profile. In fact, meat proteins, which for protein supplement purposes are derived from beef, have a biological value slightly higher than 80, but as far as absorption is concerned, they are not limited and therefore we can say that a mixture of these proteins is totally absorbed from our organism, exactly like egg proteins. Furthermore, in meat, there is usually a good amount of carnitine and creatine (with values ranging from 1 to 3%), so they would seem to be ideal as a post-workout supplement to promote muscle recovery.

Furthermore, the almost total absence of sugars and fats makes them more digestible and assimilable than other protein sources, as the presence of fats and sugars slows down the digestion of proteins. In a study by Nicholas Burd et al. of the University of Maastricht in the Netherlands, it was shown that 30 g of beef protein taken after weight training produced the same result on protein synthesis as milk-derived proteins. The milk proteins were able to slightly speed up the protein synthesis in the first two hours of the recovery, but by the fifth hour, the effect was comparable. It should also be mentioned that meat, especially beef, contains a small number of possible allergens, so it is particularly suitable for individuals intolerant to milk, eggs, soy and gluten.

Soy proteins
They have a high PDCAAS (1) and sufficient BV (74) and PER. Soy proteins also tend to absorb a lot of water and increase in volume. Compared to animal proteins, they have a deficiency in methionine (one of the essential amino acids), which in the past seemed to limit its quality, but in recent times it has been seen that the deficiency of this amino acid does not limit the amino acid quality of soy proteins too much. For this reason, they are an excellent substitute for proteins of animal origin and are very efficient in maintaining a positive nitrogen balance.

They are extremely suitable for women suffering from anemia, as soy is very rich in iron and calcium, so they are particularly suitable for those who carry out intense and prolonged workouts. They are less suitable for men because of the presence of phytoestrogens, which lower testosterone if they exceed 60 g of soy protein per day. Proteins extracted from soy contain genisteins and other isoflavones, which have been shown to have anticancer effects. Soy proteins are richer in arginine, and this can promote better blood flow in the muscles by promoting the supply of nutrients.

Rice proteins
Rice proteins are a supplement of medium biological value (BV = 69). They come from brown rice and, even if they have a deficiency in lysine (an essential amino acid), their amino acid profile is higher than that of any cereal; for this reason, they do not create particular deficiencies, and the richness of fibers makes them particularly suitable for those suffering from imbalances of the intestinal bacterial flora. Furthermore, rice proteins do not contain gluten or allergens of animal origin (lactose); for this reason, they are particularly indicated in subjects with multiple intolerances.

Hemp proteins
Hemp proteins, deriving from seeds, are the best in the plant world. On a nutritional level, they are very rich in essential amino acids, as well as in water-soluble vitamins and omega-3 fatty acids. In nature, hemp is the only plant to have appreciable dosages of highly bioavailable polyunsaturated fatty acids of the omega-3 series. The richness and completeness in essential amino acids makes it particularly effective as a supplement for increasing the muscle mass and for accelerating muscle recovery. Furthermore, its completeness in micronutrients (vitamins and mineral salts) makes it a really efficient supplement. It does not present any type of allergen and is therefore suitable for those suffering from intolerances or allergies.

Pea proteins
Pea proteins are a viable alternative to animal proteins, especially for digestibility and for the absence of food allergens. Pea proteins have a good amino acid profile, particularly high in BCAAs and glutamine, and being of vegetable origin, they have a reduced acid load, thus being useful in the event of a tendency to acidosis, linked to training or nutrition.

Wheat proteins
They have a low biological value (54) and PER. Wheat proteins could be interesting for their extreme solubility and high glutamine content (over 40% between glutamine and glutamic acid).

Multiphase proteins
Another type of protein supplement recently released on the market are multiphase proteins. This supplement generally consists of various protein sources, essentially milk, with different rates of absorption. They have been designed to provide a gradual release of amino acids into the blood flow, that is constant and lasting over time in order to always maintain optimal blood urea levels. Generally, the protein sources that constitute it are hydrolyzed, concentrated and isolated whey proteins, concentrated milk proteins and caseins in the form of calcium caseinate and micellar (sometimes egg and/or soy proteins are also present in these formulations).

These protein sources are absorbed in the short, medium and long term. Both hydrolyzed and isolated whey proteins have a very rapid absorption, essentially 20 to 30 minutes after ingestion; the concentrated milk proteins, on the other hand, have an intermediate absorption, while the caseins are assimilated in the long term (2-4 hours). Milk proteins can sometimes be replaced by soy proteins, which, despite having a lower biological value, have a slightly higher absorption rate than milk and therefore better complete the time-released mixture with antioxidant properties, compared to those found in whey proteins.

Regarding the fear that the presence of phytoestrogens may decrease testosterone, in a study by Kalman et al., 12 weeks of supplementation with 50g of soy protein during a weight training program has been shown to actually lower estrogen levels and raise testosterone levels, and adding whey protein lowered estrogen levels even more. If whey proteins are able to stimulate immediate post-workout protein synthesis more than casein or soy, a multiphase blend is able to give the same immediate stimulation but to maintain it even in the following hours, you should provide the amino acids necessary for the muscle throughout the anabolic window, when the whey protein alone ends its anabolic action in a short time. They are also very valid to use for breakfast as they provide a fast protein intake that immediately blocks nocturnal catabolism and increases the protein synthesis in the following hours, thanks to the slower absorbed protein fraction.

Collagen peptides

Collagen is the most abundant extracellular structural protein in the human body and accounts for 30% of the total protein content. When we talk about collagen, we refer to a family of molecules formed by three polypeptide chains with an alpha-helical winding. In the human body, in fact, there are more than 20 variants of collagen that differ according to the tissues in which they are found; however, 80-90% of the collagen in our body is represented by types I, II and III. Collagen is found in the extracellular matrix and is the main constituent of connective tissues such as the skin, bones, cartilages, tendons and ligaments, ensuring their structural integrity, flexibility and strength.

In the recent years, there has been a growing interest in collagen supplements, not only from an anti-aging point of view, but also for the possible effects on sports performance, as well as for the protection and support of connective tissues and joints, for the reduction of the risk of injuries and for the muscle recovery.

The most widely used collagen supplements are derived from various animal sources (cattle, pigs and marine species), although there are also some less common sources, such as genetically modified bacteria and yeasts.

These supplements contain high quantities of amino acids like L-hydroxyproline, glycine and L-proline, which represent almost two thirds of the amino acid profile of collagen and, according to some literature, are able to stimulate the fibroblasts to synthesize new endogenous collagen.

Hydrolyzed collagen is currently the most widely used and most effective form of collagen. By means of chemical or enzymatic methods, smaller and therefore more bioavailable protein fractions (peptides) are obtained; the peptides, in fact, are rapidly absorbed in the small intestine, which can be important for the post-exercise recovery in those who practice sports.

There are studies that have shown that some of the peptides present in hydrolyzed collagen, in particular those containing hydroxyproline, due to their size, would even be able to cross the intestinal barrier, reaching the bloodstream directly. Due to the reduced amount of BCAAs and lysine, collagen has a low biological value compared, for example, to whey proteins. However, it seems that the amino acid profile of hydrolyzed collagen is able to maintain a stable nitrogen balance and lean mass during a low-protein diet. Additionally, collagen contains relatively high amounts of arginine and glycine, both of which are known to be important substrates for the creatine synthesis in the human body.

Among the positive effects of supplementation with collagen peptides on the physical performance, we can mention are reduction of inflammation, stiffness and pain in the joints and the protection of cartilage, thus allowing for the prevention of injuries in athletes of all ages.

Numerous studies have reported a lower perception of joint pain after the supplementation with collagen peptides in healthy active subjects or in those with osteoarthritis.

Evidence

Protein supplementation acquires an important value in sports, both in maintaining the muscle mass and in increasing it. Several studies have shown how the intake of at least **20 g of protein during the post-workout period increases the protein synthesis and therefore the muscle mass, promotes muscle recovery and reduces training-induced catabolism**.

A 2010 study (Atherton, et al.) evaluated the post-exercise effect of consuming 20 g of protein on the prolongation of the protein synthesis. In this study, it was seen that 30 minutes after a training session, there is an important increase in the protein synthesis of about three times the normal values, with a maximum peak within an hour and a half from the training stimulus and with a return to the baseline level after around two hours.

This study has shown how the intake of 20 g of high biological value proteins (containing at least 10 g of essential amino acids) is able to prolong the stimulus of protein synthesis by about an hour, compared to the standard situation. It was also noted that the intake of proteins with a high content of essential amino acids is the essential nutrient for increasing and prolonging the protein synthesis, and above all for reducing the muscle catabolism.

Normally, the muscle protein turnover rate is about 1.2% per day (Kumar et al., 2009) and, if not supported by a sufficient daily protein quota, the catabolic phase begins to prevail with a reduction in the muscle mass.

When a subject carries out an intense workout, they initiate metabolic processes that lead to the destruction of muscle fibers and therefore to the loss of proteins; this phenomenon is called **muscle catabolism**. This phenomenon is normal during training, as the mechanical effort, the increased secretion of catabolic hormones such as cortisol, adrenaline and glucagon, and the use of proteins for energy purposes due to the neoglucogenesis process, bring the body into a situation of protein and nitrogen deficiency.

The immediate post-workout administration of rapidly absorbed proteins of high biological value, such as hydrolyzed or isolated whey proteins, promotes a prompt muscle recovery, promotes and nourishes the protein synthesis, allowing for muscle growth.

Other studies have seen how the administration of protein supplements before the training (at least 30 minutes) reduces the catabolic phase. In the same studies, the protocol included the administration of whey protein isolate before and after the training session, and the administered quantity did not drop below 20 g.

In almost all studies, the proteins were combined with a medium and high GI carbohydrate source (maltodextrin, glucose) and in some others, with creatine; this mix provides the right elements to promote the muscle growth and the energy recovery in the post-workout.

A 2009 study by Douglas and Blake showed that 30 g of high biological value proteins taken at breakfast, lunch and dinner, kept the levels of protein synthesis constant over time, compared to the control group that took about 70% of this amount only in the evening, which activated protein synthesis only after the evening meal.

Another 2006 study (Cribb and Hayes) showed that protein synthesis was more stimulated (+46%) with the **intake of 30 g of whey protein before and after the training, compared to the group that consumed the same quantities in the morning and evening**. In addition to the increase in muscle mass, they found a reduction in fat mass and a greater increase in explosive strength in the experimental group, compared to the control group. This increase in muscle mass is due to the fact that the "anabolic window" has been exploited, which is the period of time after the training that allows the body to implement the protein synthesis, as the nutrients are more directed towards the skeletal muscle and used in the synthesis of new muscle proteins.

This period lasts for at least 2-3 hours after the training session. For this reason, by administering a certain amount of proteins (at least 20 g) every 1-1.5 hours, the protein synthesis process is amplified and is made more efficient, since the training stimulus triggers it, stimulating the metabolic pathway of the mTOR, while the intake of proteins with a high biological value stimulates the protein synthesis via phosphorylating (S6K1), and taking them at regular intervals feeds the complex molecular machine to produce new proteins.

It is equally true, however, as demonstrated by an analysis of all the studies on the subject (meta-analysis) carried out by Lehman College at al., that the total amount of daily proteins is more important than the timing of their intake.

In a study conducted at McMaster University, Canada, it was found that hydrolyzed whey proteins accelerate the protein synthesis at rest or after the training better than caseins and soy proteins, thanks to their faster absorption.

A 2014 study (Farup et al.) showed how the intake of hydrolyzed proteins following a workout with an important eccentric component, significantly accelerated the proliferation of satellite cells in the post-exercise phase. Satellite cells are stem cells present in the muscle tissue, that are activated by growth factors following autocrine mechanical and chemical stimuli.

The eccentric contraction by itself activates the recruitment of these cells that repair the micro-lesions caused by the muscular effort, regenerating new fibers and increasing the muscle mass. To this end, post-workout protein intake accelerates this process and allows these cells to grow and mature faster through the stimulation of the protein synthesis. In this way, both the synthesis of new muscle fibers and the muscle recovery that allows to sustain a higher training frequency, are increased.

In this study, two groups were compared; the control group were administered 56 g of carbohydrates six hours after the training and for the following two days, while the experimental group was given a mix of hydrolyzed proteins (28 g) and carbohydrates (28 g). The training included a session of 15 sets of 10 repetitions with the maximum eccentric component. The biopsy examination was performed 45 minutes before each workout, while the supplement was taken immediately, in the second three-hour period after and in the third six-hour period after training. This supplementation was continued the next day, 24 hours later.

Histological and biochemical examinations showed the significant increase in the concentration of satellite cells in the muscle samples of subjects who were supplemented with proteins and carbohydrates, and above all, it was the type II fibers that increased dramatically. In addition, the levels of creatine kinase (a parameter that symbolizes the degree of muscle damage) were significantly reduced in the subjects taking the protein mix with carbohydrates, compared to the placebo.

The researchers deduced that the richness in essential amino acids and especially in branched amino acids, present in hydrolyzed proteins, stimulated the activity of the mTORC1 enzyme, which presides over the protein synthesis and regulates the activity of satellite cells. Normally, these cells are in a quiescent state when mTORC1 and anaerobic energy (ATP and glucose) levels are low. The activation of this enzyme through the intake of hydrolyzed proteins and the concomitant intake of carbohydrates, associated with anaerobic training with particular emphasis on the eccentric component, produced a maximal recruitment and activation of the satellite cells.

In fact, another study, also from 2014, conducted at the University of Maastricht showed that the simultaneous intake of carbohydrates together with proteins, does not further stimulate the protein synthesis in the following five hours after the training (*Journal of Clinical Endocrinology & Metabolism*, 99(6):2250-2258, 2014).

Supplementing with whey proteins during a weight loss diet seems to help preserve the muscle mass. Researchers from the University of Illinois conducted a study involving overweight women in a 6-month weight loss program. The women were given dietary plans that provided for a recommended protein intake of 0.8 g per kg of body weight (about 55 g of protein for a woman of about 68 kg).

The women participating in the study were divided into two groups: the first group received an additional 25 g of whey protein to be taken twice a day, while the second group received the same amount of a carbohydrate supplement. All these women consumed 1400 Kcal per day. After 6 months, the group that were given the whey protein had nearly a double body weight reduction (–8%) compared to the group that consumed carbohydrates (-4.1%).

The researchers then looked at the changes in the women's thighs using MRI. The results revealed greater fat loss and an increased muscle mass in the women who took the whey protein. These results indicate that an increase in the protein intake with whey protein supplementation helped maintain the muscle mass in relation to changes in body weight and body fat during a low-calorie diet.

In a study of healthy men and women, researchers examined the response of protein synthesis under energy deficit conditions. In these dietary conditions, muscle building levels were studied in association with exercise with weights and with or without whey protein supplementation.

By analyzing the results, it emerged that:
- after 5 days of only moderate caloric restriction (with a reduction in caloric intake by one third of the daily caloric requirement), the rate of protein synthesis was reduced by 27%. However, performing a single exercise with weights brought the protein synthesis rate back to a level comparable to that of a normal calorie diet;
- the consumption of 15 g of whey protein immediately after exercising with weights in the regime of a moderate calorie restriction led to a 16% increase in the protein synthesis rate, compared to the normocaloric diet. If 30 g of whey protein were consumed after exercising with weights, the protein synthesis rate went up by 34%.

In conclusion, calorie reduction alone causes muscle loss. However, if exercise with weights is associated with calorie restriction, protein synthesis is restored to normal levels. The best results were achieved with the consumption of whey protein after exercising with weights, with a double effectiveness when consumed 30 g compared to 15 g.

According to the results of a study by Tahavorgar et al., the regular consumption of whey protein before meals can help you lose excess weight. The obese and overweight men participating in the study were provided with concentrated whey protein (65 g) or soy protein isolate (60 g) which provided the same amount of protein (approximately 54 g). The subjects were asked to take the proteins provided in the afternoon 30 minutes before their largest meal, keeping the usual eating and physical activity patterns unchanged.

After 12 weeks of daily protein supplementation, the feeling of hunger was reduced more in the group of people who had taken whey proteins (43%) than in the group who had taken soy protein (25%), and this resulted in a greater reduction in the energy intake, especially at the expense of carbohydrates. The subjects who consumed whey proteins lost almost double the weight (-6.5 kg) compared to the group that consumed soy protein (-3.5 kg). Body fat percentage decreased from 29.6 to 20.4% in the whey protein group and from 28.2 to 25.1% in the soy protein group. Lean mass increased more in the whey protein group (4 kg) than in the soy protein group (0.5 kg).

In conclusion, both whey and soy proteins led to significant improvements in these subjects' body composition. However, these results indicate that taking whey protein 30 minutes before a large meal is more effective than taking soy protein in reducing the appetite and in promoting a greater fat loss.

Collagen peptides reduce the muscle recovery time: A recent 2019 double-blind, randomized, placebo-controlled clinical study published in the *Amino Acids* journal, showed that subjects taking collagen peptide supplementation experienced a 20% reduction of muscle pain in all time intervals (post work-out and after 24 and 48 hours) following intense training, compared to the placebo group.

In the same subjects who had taken collagen peptides, the shorter recovery time also allowed an increase in the sports performance.

Clifford et al. reported a faster recovery from jumping exercise and a tendency to less muscle soreness after collagen supplementation.

A study also reported that creatine kinase activity following an exercise that involved muscle damage was attenuated by supplementation with collagen peptides, and this is indicative of an improvement in the muscle recovery.

Collagen peptide supplements could improve the muscle contraction, as reported by a study published in the *Journal of Nutrition*; as already mentioned, the glycine and arginine of which collagen peptides are made of, seem to help in supporting the synthesis of creatine, improving the performance during explosive strength exercises and increasing the muscle mass.

In addition to the proven positive effects of hydrolyzed collagen on post-exercise muscle recovery, a 2015 study published in *The British Journal of Nutrition* wanted to investigate the effects of collagen peptide supplementation (15 g/day) on lean mass (FFM), muscle strength and bone mass, in association with weight training, in a randomized placebo-controlled study of 53 sarcopenic elderly men. The results showed that the supplementation of collagen peptides led to an improvement in the body composition with an increase in the lean mass and reduction in the fat mass, an increase in the bone mass and greater muscle strength compared to the placebo group.

In a recent double-blind, randomized, placebo-controlled study published in *Nutrients* (2019), the researchers wanted to analyze the effects of weight training in association with the supplementation of specific collagen peptides on the body composition and muscle strength in 77 pre-menopausal women. These women followed a weight training program in combination with the daily intake of 15 g of collagen peptides or a placebo, three times a week, for 12 weeks. The results of the study showed a more significant increase in the lean mass and strength, measured with the hand grip test, in women who had taken collagen peptides. In addition, the same women also showed a greater loss of fat mass and an increase in leg strength compared to the placebo group.

The effects of supplementation with collagen peptides have also been investigated in young healthy people.

In this double-blind, placebo-controlled study, 25 young people (the mean age was 24 years) completed a 12-week, total body training program for hypertrophy, performed three times a week. The recruited subjects took 15 g of collagen peptides or a non-calorie placebo every day.

The results of the study showed a greater increase in the body mass, lean mass and muscle strength compared to the placebo group, as well as an increase in the synthesis of proteins associated with contractile fibers.

Dosages

The dosages of proteins, intended as a supplement, vary according to their use. As a supplement to allow you to reach the daily protein quota of your diet, the recommended dosage is a maximum of 30 g/day, but it can vary according to the protein quantity to be taken daily with the diet, and that you may not be able to obtain (for example, if you normally need 120g of protein per day, and on the normal diet if you get 80, you can take 40g of protein as a supplement to cover the difference).

Everything changes according to the sporting activity. If the goal is hypertrophy, then the proteins can be taken both during the day and in the evening, as a meal before bedtime (30 g of casein), in order to reduce the nocturnal muscle catabolism. In this case, the administration timing involves taking about 30 g of whey protein or a multiphase blend within 30 minutes after the training, with or without carbohydrates.

Alternatively, to maximize the muscle growth, proteins, preferably hydrolyzed, can be taken both before (about 40 minutes) and after the training (within the next half hour). As for caseins, the dosages are around 30 g half an hour before bedtime, to inhibit the catabolism induced by night fasting and to stimulate the repair of muscle fibers. Most data indicate that a daily dose of around 40 g is appropriate to get the maximum health benefits from whey proteins.

Effectiveness

Strength	Resistant strength	Mass	Endurance	Slimming	Concentration	Recovery
+++	++	++++	++	+++	++	+++

REISHI (GANODERMA LUCIDUM)

Description

The *Ganoderma lucidum* species, commonly called reishi (in Japan) or lingzhi (in China), have been used in traditional folk medicine in Asia for thousands of years, but its use has only attracted the interest of pharmaceutical industries in recent times. In fact, mushrooms represent an important source, even if still viewed with some skepticism, and to date almost 10,000 species are known, of which 2000 are safe for humans, and about 300 of them possess medicinal properties.

The *Ganoderma* genus is large and diverse, globally distributed, and includes species that cause white rot on a variety of tree species. References to reishi as a superior herb that improves the human health were present as early as 100 BC (Cao et al., 2012), and still nowadays, members of the *G. lucidum* species complex continue to be prescribed in traditional Chinese medicine. In the genus *Ganoderma*, there are morphological types such as black, light black, red, purple, yellow and white. Each type of *Ganoderma* has its own biological characteristics.

Ganoderma, in the commonly used medicinal form, includes *G. lucidum*, *G. tsuge*, *G. capense*, and *G. applanatum*. Fruiting bodies are typically grown, ground, and processed into tinctures or teas (Stamets, 2000), although, in fact, this mushroom is increasingly being marketed in tablet and capsule form for the Western market. The active constituents of *G. lucidum* include polysaccharides (including beta-D-glucans, heteropolysaccharides and glycoproteins), triterpenes, essential and non-essential amino acids, sterols, lipids, antioxidants, vitamins B1, B2, B6, iron, calcium and zinc (Huie, 2004; McKenna, 2002).

Properties

The fruiting bodies of *G. lucidum* are considered as a panacea for all types of pathologies, perhaps due to their demonstrated efficacy in cases of chronic hepatitis, arthritis, hypertension, hyperlipidemia, insomnia, bronchitis, neoplasms, asthma, gastric ulcers, atherosclerosis and diabetes. It is no coincidence that it is called the "mushroom of immortality" in China, Japan and Korea.

G. lucidum belongs to the group of nootropic substances. This term was coined in 1972 by Corneliu E. Giurgea and refers to compounds that are able to increase the memory and learning ability, enhance cognitive functions in stressful conditions, protect the central nervous system from neurotoxic substances, accelerate and optimize neuronal processes and increase concentration and focusing (focusing on goals), without giving a sedative or stimulating effect and without causing addiction.

Its contribution to the emotional balance (Shen) is known as the "mushroom of immortality", which in traditional Chinese medicine also means mind-emotion balance. Reishi is also used to increase the energy level, improve breathing, optimize heart and cardiovascular functions, recover the functions of the autonomic nervous system and psychophysical fatigue. Its antioxidant and mitochondrial revitalization action make it a substance capable of slowing down the age-related processes. Unlike other nootropic plants, the effect of *G. lucidum* is not immediately noticeable. Its action is of the "adaptogenic" type and its effects are evident after a few weeks: in fact, initially they seem mild, but in reality they are cumulative and increasingly profound. Over time, it generates a sense of inner calm and harmony and a sharpening of both logical and intuitive mental perceptions.

Professionals of traditional oriental medicine have prescribed the use of reishi as a preventive anti-inflammatory treatment or to improve the immunity (Wang et al., 2012; Hennicke et al., 2016). Reishi is a focal point in ancient Chinese and Japanese works of art and has also been associated with royalty, wisdom, sexual prowess and eternal life (Stamets, 2000).

It is considered both medicine and food, as its consumption can bring the body "into balance", it promotes the health, prolongs life, and prevents and treats many systemic diseases (Willard, 1990).

There are some claims that the spores contain higher amounts of active components, thus proving to be more effective in the treatment of the possible problems and diseases mentioned above, but unlike many synthetic medicines, the mode of action of G. lucidum and the guidelines for its use are not well established. The *Ganoderma* mushroom contains pharmacologically active variables and the effects and effectiveness of the entire product are probably different from those of a single component that acts alone. However, most of the data from animal and *in vitro* studies suggest that the constituents, individually or synergistically, produce beneficial antioxidant, anti-inflammatory, anti-perglycemic, anti-atherogenic and immunoprotective effects (Chen, 2004; Lakshmi, 2003).

Based on some recent studies, the researchers suggest that there are two groups of important bioactive components that have effects on the cardiovascular system. These are triterpenes and polysaccharides, and reishi is the only known source of triterpene compounds, which are called ganoderic acids.

It has been shown that the triterpene fraction is able to suppress the inflammatory response in activated macrophages and, specifically, it reduces the secretion of proinflammatory cytokines such as TNF-α and IL-6, regulates nitric oxide (NO) levels, reduces prostaglandins PGE2 and inhibits histamine release by mast cells. In addition to triterpenes, other substances contained in *Ganoderma*, such as oleic acid, have shown a dose-dependent inhibitory activity on histamine release. At the same time, the high amount of insoluble and soluble beta-glucans interacts directly with the intestinal microbiota and with the cells of the immune system. Of the 200 identified ganoderic acids, A, B and C are believed to have hypoglycemic effects (Hikino, 1985; Tomoda, 1986), while F, B, D, H, K, S and Y ganoderic acids are probably hypotensive (Morigawa, 1986).

More precisely, the mode of action of ganoderic acid B on blood sugar, for example, is by inhibiting alpha-glycosidase, the key enzyme in the carbohydrate metabolism. Furthermore, these acids could suppress the sympathetic efferent activity, just as ganoderic acid S has been identified as an inhibitor of platelet aggregation (Shimizu, 1985; Tao, 1990). The hypocholesterolemic properties that have been attributed to reishi derive from the fact that most of the ganoderic acids perform an inhibitory activity on the synthesis of cholesterol (Komoda, 1989).

To date, two of the most addressed issues by the scientific world are oxidative stress and the intestinal microbiota. In the first case, it is a condition caused by the breakdown of the balance between the production and elimination of oxidizing chemical species. In fact, in biological systems, potentially harmful reactive oxygen species (ROS) are produced during normal aerobic metabolism. These species, if in excess, can damage the DNA, react with lipids or even activate cellular apoptosis processes; for this reason, the use of antioxidants has the aim of preventing the generation of ROS or neutralizing those formed. A deficiency of the antioxidant defenses can lead to oxidative stress, which is associated with a variety of ailments such as heart disease, nervous system disorders, diabetes, arthritis and cancer.

It is therefore no coincidence that in the American Herbal Pharmacopoeia, G. lucidum is mainly recommended for its ability to boost the immune system (Upton and Petrone, 2000; Jin et al., 2012); in fact, some recent research has reported that G. lucidum contains bioactive compounds useful for the well-being of our organism (Sanodiya et al., 2009; Basnet et al., 2017) capable of carrying out anti-inflammatory activities, can elaminate ROS and enhance the immune system (Paterson, 2006; Boh et al., 2007; Sanodiya et al., 2009; Jin et al., 2012). More precisely, G. lucidum produces the antifungal protein ganodermin, which has inhibitory effects against common fungi such as *Botrytis cinerea* and *Fusarium oxysporum* (Wang and Ng, 2006) and also produces other chemicals with antibacterial effects (Isaka et al., 2015); Basnet et al., 2017).

As for the other issue, it is interesting to note how *G. lucidum* effects are also linked to its microbiota enhancing activity, both on the small and large intestine. Microbiota studies are known to have made incredible progress in describing the bidirectional interaction between the gut and the brain in recent years, and we are now aware that the microbiota substantially affects the immunity, hormonal balance, brain health, the psycho-neurological balance and behaviors. For this reason, substances such as *G. lucidum* which are capable of improving the microbiota structure, take on even more importance if they are considered as neuromodulators of the psycho-neuro-endocrine-immunological sphere.

Evidence

A double-blind study on 132 subjects with neurasthenia showed that the regular use of *G. lucidum* (1.8 g, three times a day for 8 weeks) significantly improved the feeling of fatigue and well-being in the treated subjects, compared to the untreated control group (Tang et al., 2005). It improves insomnia with a GABAergic mechanism and regulates the sleep rhythms (Chu et al, 2007; Cui et al., 2012).

In a 2015 study, *G. lucidum* was found to improve the physical performance in women with fibromyalgia.

Fibromyalgia is a chronic syndrome described by chronic generalized pain, stiffness, poor physical condition and poor health-related quality of life. More precisely, in this study, *G. lucidum* was compared with carob flour (*Ceratonia siliqua*), a natural antioxidant substance.

Sixty-four women with fibromyalgia participated in the study and were divided into two groups: the first group took 6 g of *G. lucidum* per day, the second group took 6 g per day. After 6 weeks of treatment, the results showed that *G. lucidum* had significantly improved the aerobic endurance and the joint flexibility ($p < 0.05$).

Another 2009 study sought information on the modulating effect of *G. lucidum* capsules on T-cell subgroups in football players during a 28-day Living High-Training Low (LHTL) trial, and their possible mechanism of action.

Forty male football players were randomly assigned to four groups: the control (who lived at sea level), LHTL1, LHTL2, and LHTL3. The three LHTL groups had remained in normobaric hypoxic chambers for 28 days and all four groups trained together at the sea level. Respectively, the LHTL1, LHTL2 and LHTL3 groups were given a placebo, 10 capsules and 20 capsules of *G. lucidum*/day for 6 weeks. The final data showed that 28-day after the study, in the LHTL1 group, a significant reduction was observed in the CD4+/CD8+ ratio (a high value indicates that there are more lymphocytes in the numerator or CD4 that have a stimulating and helping [helper] function on other cells that produce antibodies, on the other hand, CD8 [suppressors] are those that intervene to suppress it), compared to the baseline.

In addition, a significant reduction was observed between LHTL1 and the control groups at 21 days. In the LHTL2 group, the relative change in CD4+/CD8+ ratio was significantly less at 28 days, compared to the preliminary baseline. In general, in the LHTL3 group, there was an increasing trend on the percentage of changes in the CD4+/CD8+ ratio compared to the baseline, higher than the values of the LHTL1 and LHTL2 groups, but this was not significant.

In conclusion, *G. lucidum* polysaccharides have been shown to be active components for the cell-mediated immune function.

In 2014 Rossi et al. evaluated the effects of *G. lucidum* and *Ophiocordyceps sinensis* supplementation in improving the performance in endurance cyclists. A short, 3-month trial of two fungal supplements, *G. lucidum* and *Cordyceps sinensis* (3 capsules of *C. sinensis* and 2 capsules of *G. lucidum* per day), was conducted on 7 healthy male volunteers, aged between 30 and 40 years old, all amateur cyclists participating in the "Gran Fondo" cycling races. This study monitored and compared the following biomarkers before and after the physical exertion: testosterone/cortisol ratio in saliva and the oxidative stress (DPPH free radical scavenging activity).

A reduction of more than 30% in the testosterone/cortisol ratio after the competition, compared to before the competition, was considered as a risk factor for non-functional overcoming (NFO) or overtraining syndrome (OTS). The results showed that, after 3 months of supplementation, the testosterone/cortisol ratio changed statistically significantly, thus protecting athletes from NFO and OTS, and a greater absorption capacity of free radicals was also found in the serum of athletes after the race, thus protecting them from the oxidative stress.

Regarding the antioxidant activity, Xing Guoqing et al. wanted to study the anti-aging effect of the ganoderma polysaccharide on elderly mice. Thirty-six elderly mice were randomly divided into three groups (A, B and C) and were administered respectively 0.3 mL/10 g and 0.15 mL/10 g of solution of a polysaccharide component of *G. lucidum* and 0.2 mL/10 g of a physiological solution by transgastric perfusion. Ten days later, the content of the SOD (Superoxide Dismutase) enzyme was detected in erythrocytes, hepatocytes and brain cells.

The results showed that the SOD content in the erythrocytes and brain cells in group A was significantly higher than in group C ($p = 0.01$). The SOD content in the erythrocytes and brain cells of group B and hepatocytes of both groups A and B was higher than that of group C ($p = 0.05$). For this reason, the researchers concluded that the *G. lucidum* polysaccharide solution was able to increase the SOD content and improve the body's ability to eliminate free radicals, reducing and preventing any cell damage and producing anti-aging effects.

A 2018 study by HuaShuai Li et al. evaluated the effects of *G. lucidum* on mice, in association with a chicken-based supplement, on their physiological adaptation to fatigue and on the improvement of the exercise performance. A busy lifestyle, environmental pressure and a heavy workload often cause extreme fatigue in modern life. In this regard, recent studies have revealed that *G. lucidum* carries out a broad spectrum of biological activities. The mice were divided into dose groups, 0, 833, 1666 and 4165 mg/kg, and followed the protocol for 4 weeks. Physical activities, including grip strength and aerobic endurance, were assessed.

Several biochemical variables associated with fatigue were also evaluated, such as lactate levels, BUN (Blood Urea Nitrogen index) or CK. The hepatic and muscle glycogen levels were measured as an indicator of the energy storage at the end of the experiment. Reishi supplementation, combined with the second supplement, significantly increased the endurance and the grip strength, and demonstrated beneficial effects on lactate production and elimination rate after a tough exercise test. It also significantly lowered the BUN and CK indices after a prolonged exercise and increased glycogen content in the liver and muscle tissues.

Dosages

In conclusion, medicinal mushrooms such as the *G. lucidum* (reishi) species can help prevent and reduce allergic symptoms and various diseases through a complex and articulated series of effects on the body. Its microbiota-boosting action helps maintain the integrity of the mucosa and activates the specific immunity, favoring the body's natural tolerance processes.

In this regard, there is no agreed dosage for the treatment with *G. lucidum*. The recommended dosage, of course, depends on the reason why you choose to use this product and on the condition of the subject; however, the recommended quantities, which are also indicated in most of the supplements on the market, are around 1.5 g of dry extract per day.

Effectiveness

Strength	Resistant strength	Mass	Endurance	Slimming	Concentration	Recovery
+	+	−	+	++	++	++

RHODIOLA ROSEA

Description

Rhodiola rosea is a perennial plant belonging to the *Crassulaceae* family. It grows spontaneously in some cold areas of Northern Europe (Lapland, Scandinavia) and northern Asia (eastern and western Siberia), but can also be found in the Pyrenees and in the Far East. It is a dioecious plant, which therefore has male and female reproductive organs on two different plants. *Rhodiola rosea* grows at high altitudes, between 3000 and 5500 m, and has very developed roots and yellow flowers; the aerial part is used in particular as a food ingredient, while the root is used in medicine.

It was Linnaeus (*Species Plantarium*, 1753) who gave the plant the botanical name *Rhodiola* and the species name *rosea*, alluding to the rose scent of its flowers.

Rhodiola rosea has a long history as a medicinal plant; *Rhodiola rosea* preparations were widely used in traditional Tibetan medicine as early as 300 AD, for the treatment of lung diseases. According to historical sources, *Rhodiola rosea* was also used by the Vikings as a medicine after prolonged physical exertion, due to its invigorating tonic properties.

Ancient Siberian populations handed down its use from generation to generation, considering the plant a valuable aid to increase the physical resistance during cold winters, to treat colds and depression, and to prevent high altitude sickness. This plant (especially the roots) was taken in the form of an infusion or as a hot alcoholic beverage, in order to allow the process of assimilation of its therapeutic nutrients.

Many years ago, it was used only by the people of the territories where it grows spontaneously, while recently it has been sown and cultivated. To date, thanks to numerous experiments in this regard, it is agreed that the properties recognized by the popular tradition are justified by scientific studies.

However, it was mainly in Russia and the former Soviet Union that *Rhodiola rosea* root preparations were recognized and used in mainstream medicine; here, its use in medicine dates back to the early 1960s and several studies have shown its stimulating, anti-fatigue and anti-depressive actions. After the fall of the Soviet Union and with the disclosure of numerous scientific studies conducted by Soviet scientists, the West became aware of this plant, whose properties were even considered a Soviet military secret.

Rhodiola rosea and its active components have a marked and well documented adaptogenic action. Several studies report that this action results in a greater resistance to the harmful effects of various stressors; *Rhodiola rosea* extracts have been shown to protect against the harmful effects of oxygen, cold and strenuous exercises. Its natural principles, as reported by many authors, seem to increase work capacity, the tolerance to anoxia and the resistance to some types of radiation and toxin poisoning; it also reduces the fatigue and regulates brain functions, improving the mental capacity and the memory.

Properties

The therapeutic properties of this plant are to be traced back to the active ingredients contained in it and to their quantitative ratios; inside the rhizome, in fact, there are numerous constituents, such as organic, citric, malic, oxalic and succinic acids, essential oils with the presence of phenylethyl alcohol, cinamaldehyde, citral, macro- and micronutrients, including manganese in a high percentage.

The most important components are phenolic and glycosidic types, such as salidroside and rosavins (rosavin, rosarina, rosin), which characterize it and differentiate it from other species of *Rhodiola*, in which salidroside, p-tyrosol and other substances are present.

As mentioned, *Rhodiola rosea* has an adaptogenic power and allows the body to adapt to stressful stimuli, thus making it more resistant to mental and physical stress. Up to a certain point, the organism is physiologically able to respond and cope with conditions of psychophysical stress, but when this exceeds certain levels or becomes chronic, the body's response mechanisms no longer work properly, with consequences such as hormonal imbalances, decreased physical endurance and intellectual abilities, mood alterations, anxiety, depression, sexual dysfunctions, as well as alterations in the functionality of the cardiovascular system, lowering of the immune defenses, acceleration of aging and facilitation of the onset of some chronic diseases.

Rhodiola rosea turns out to be a valid help in these conditions, since its action causes a gradual and physiological response of the organism, or an adaptation, reducing the impact of stress factors without bringing the system to exhaustion, as happens with other stimulating substances. Many studies have shown that salidroside and tyrosol are among the most active components, while other components appear inactive when taken alone, but show synergistic effects when a certain combination of salidroside, rosavine, rosarin and rosin is used to increase the resistance to stress of various kinds.

Furthermore, *Rhodiola rosea* seems to interfere with various physiological mechanisms: it stimulates the metabolism, promotes the use of fats at the tissue level and, thanks to its ergogenic function, it improves the physical resistance to exhausting physical efforts and has antioxidant and protective effects on the cardiovascular system. There are also studies aimed at demonstrating an improvement in the sports performance with the supplementation of *Rhodiola rosea*.

Evidence

Several studies have shown how *Rhodiola rosea* has beneficial effects on the physical performance, increasing the muscle endurance and energy, and consequently reducing recovery times. In addition to representing a valid help for athletes and sportsmen, the supplementation of this herbal medicine in the diet is useful in all those conditions of psychological stress and depression that involve a decrease in the energy levels and which, indirectly, can still contribute to the worsening of any eventual sports performance. The active ingredients contained in *Rhodiola rosea*, in particular those with a high biological activity, such as rosavine, act by inhibiting COMT (Catechol-O-MethylTransferase), an enzyme that inactivates serotonin, and the transport of 5-HTP (5-hydroxytryptophan) across the blood-brain barrier, which is a precursor of serotonin.

The end result is an increase in blood levels of serotonin, a hormone, which participates, for example, in regulating mood, sleep, behavior, the cardiovascular function and the memory.

Some studies also show how *Rhodiola rosea* supplementation increases, in addition to serotonin levels, even the levels of dopamine and noradrenaline, avoiding the increase in numbness that would be given by the increase in serotonin alone, COMT being an enzyme involved in the metabolism of various neurotransmitters. Several authors also report that the anti-fatigue and anti-stress effect of *Rhodiola rosea* can also be attributed to its ability to modulate the release of cortisol, the "stress hormone" par excellence.

Due to the ability of *Rhodiola rosea* to increase the serotonin levels, numerous studies attribute an antidepressant effect to this adaptogenic plant; serotonin, by acting on the mood regulation, determines, in fact, a reduction in stress response reactions.

A study evaluated whether a chronic treatment with a hydroalcoholic extract of *Rhodiola rosea* containing rosavine and salidroside in different percentages could prevent the alterations induced by chronic stress: the results showed that this extract can hinder the onset of the typical chronic stress disorders, with an efficacy similar to fluoxetine, a powerful antidepressant.

Rhodiola rosea is particularly indicated in cases of intellectual fatigue; the effect is probably due to its ability to activate the endogenous production of creatine phosphate and ATP in brain cells. For this reason, *Rhodiola rosea* seems to be able to stimulate mental activity, by increasing concentration and the memory.

A study was carried out to evaluate the effect of the dry extract of *Rhodiola rosea* titrated in rosavine at 3%, on the mental performance in subjects subjected to psychophysical stress.

161 subjects between the ages of 19 and 21 were enrolled and administered two or three *Rhodiola rosea* capsules or a placebo orally, for 30 days. The evaluation was made using a specific anti-fatigue index and the result of the experiment showed a **significant decrease in fatigue** in the subjects who had taken the extract.

A clinical study evaluated the effect of *Rhodiola rosea* extract in patients suffering from stress-related fatigue. Sixty patients aged 20 to 55 were enrolled and received 576 mg/day of this extract or a placebo, orally, for 28 days. They measured the quality of life index with a questionnaire and also the symptoms of fatigue, depressive symptoms, attention and cortisol levels in pre- and post-therapy saliva. The levels of cortisol in saliva in response to stress were found to be higher in the placebo group, compared to the group that took the extract.

The study indicated that the *Rhodiola rosea* extract has an evident anti-fatigue effect and improves the mental performance, particularly in subjects suffering from stress-related chronic fatigue. Consequently, the cortisol-reducing effect is useful in subjects who have high levels of this hormone, which can have a negative impact on various aspects such as the immune system, the body's ability to metabolize nutrients, weight control and on the memory. The benefits in terms of neurostimulation and on the reduction of cortisol production in athletes, could contribute to possible improvements in terms of performance and recovery. Some research shows, in fact, how this plant can counteract the states of overtraining by increasing the energy levels and the physical endurance.

By increasing serotonin levels, *Rhodiola rosea*, in addition to being a valuable aid in cases of mood disorders, also appears to be useful for weight loss. It has been shown that rosavin, contained in the root of this plant, stimulates the biosynthesis of hormones such as adrenaline, norepinephrine and adrenocorticotropic hormone, which by activating adenylate cyclase in the fat cells, promote the release of fatty acids from the blood.

This effect, therefore, occurs mainly thanks to the mobilization of fatty acids that are accumulated in the adipose tissue, following the stimulation of the lipase. The mobilization of fatty acids from the adipose tissue represents the increase in the substrate for the production of ATP. Clinical studies conducted in this regard have shown that to achieve greater weight loss, physical exercise must be associated with the intake of *Rhodiola rosea* extract, so that the fatty acids put into circulation are used by cellular mitochondria for energy production; in this sense, the supplementation of *Rhodiola rosea* constitutes **a valid aid for a slow metabolism, promoting a slimming effect**. In addition, the increase in serotonin levels suppresses the obsessive desire for carbohydrates (carb-craving), carrying out an anti-anxiety action and, consequently, allowing for a greater weight control. The lack of serotonin can, in fact, lead to the intake of excessive amounts of carbohydrates with a high glycemic index, especially in the evening, as a compensatory action; in this sense, *Rhodiola rosea* supplements could be effective against binges or "nervous hunger". Added to this is the fact that the glycosides contained in the root increase the levels of dopamine, a neurotransmitter that promotes the sense of satiety.

Another effect attributed to *Rhodiola rosea* that is exploited in sports, is the **increase in the resistance to fatigue**. Thanks to the increase in the substrate, consisting of free fatty acids, for the production of ATP, there will be an amount of energy adequate to the needs of the muscles during intense and prolonged physical exercises, with a consequent improvement in the physical performance and an increase in the resistance to fatigue, due to the ability of *Rhodiola rosea* to also allow rapid normalization of lactic and uric acid levels.

A clinical study investigated the effect of *Rhodiola rosea* on the physical capacity, muscle strength, speed of leg movements, reaction times to stimuli and attention. 24 apparently healthy subjects were enrolled in this study.

One hour after ingesting 200 mg of a *Rhodiola rosea* dry extract titrated in 3% rosavine or a placebo, they underwent the measurement of the speed of leg movements, reaction times and attention. The next day, always after taking the same dose of *Rhodiola rosea*, the maximum isometric tension at the knee level and the maximum resistance to effort were measured. After a 5-day interval, the experiment was repeated. The results of the study were as follows: non-significant increase in the resistance to prolonged exertion (time to muscle exhaustion from 16.8 to 17, 2 minutes), VO_{2max} peak passed from 60.0 to 63.5 mL/min, the pulmonary ventilation increased from 115.9 L/min to 124.8 L/min.

All other parameters remained unchanged. The researchers concluded by stating that *Rhodiola rosea* extract promotes the psychophysical performance, albeit moderately. Clinical studies conducted on athletes have also shown an improvement in pulse, blood pressure, lung capacity and heart rate normalization times: after 10 minutes of rest, the pulse had dropped to 67 beats per minute in subjects who had taken *Rhodiola rosea* and at 86 in the subjects of the control group.

A 2007 study showed that *Rhodiola rosea* **shortens the muscle recovery time after submaximal or maximal exercises**, partly because it increases the synthesis of messenger RNA, and therefore of proteins, and partly because it appears capable of promoting the intracellular penetration of glucose and numerous other micronutrients, also favoring their use in cellular metabolic processes, responsible for energy production. In fact, it seems able to increase the levels of adenosine triphosphate (ATP) and creatine phosphate (CP) in the striated muscle tissue, and to protect the organization of mitochondria in the event of hypoxia.

An *in vitro* study has shown how salidroside may be able to stimulate the penetration of glucose into striated muscle cells, based on the dose; this active ingredient contained in *Rhodiola rosea* seems to increase the phosphorylation of AMPK and acetyl-CoA carboxylase (ACC), and increase the activation of AKT (PKB), induced by insulin, and also increase the penetration of glucose.

The activation of AMPK could be involved in the effects of salidroside on insulin sensitivity and glucose transport. A study of about thirty male endurance athletes between the ages of 20 and 30, evaluated the influence of chronic *Rhodiola rosea* supplementation on the perception of fatigue, heart rate, test duration and, in general, on the physical performance. The subjects were divided into two groups (A and B); while group A was given *Rhodiola rosea* for a period of 4 weeks, group B was given a placebo and, after the supplementation period, both groups underwent a depletion test at 75% of their VO_{2max}.

Following a 2-week wash-out, group B was given *Rhodiola rosea* for a period of 4 weeks, while group A received a placebo. Again, both groups underwent a further exhaustion test using the same protocol. The results of this study did not reveal statistically significant effects with regard to the maximum heart rate and VO_{2max} values after the administration of *Rhodiola rosea* for 4 weeks. Significant differences were not found even in the perception of fatigue, which was assessed using a specific scale; however, it is interesting that the athletes who had taken *Rhodiola rosea* were able to prolong the effort for a longer time, compared to the control.

This preliminary study appears to demonstrate a **positive effect of *Rhodiola rosea* on the performance of endurance activities**. However, further investigation is needed to confirm these findings. *Rhodiola rosea* also appears to improve the cardiovascular function. Stress, in fact, is a risk factor for cardiovascular diseases. The adaptogenic action of *Rhodiola rosea* extract probably modulates the release of catecholamines and corticoids in the stress response phase, thus modulating the cardiac response to it.

From some experiments conducted on animals, it seems that *Rhodiola rosea* extract can contribute to the prevention of heart disease and to the protection of heart tissue. Some studies indicate that *Rhodiola rosea* can reduce the increase in oxidative phenomena resulting from staying at high altitudes, making it a valuable aid for those who practice altitude sports. A clinical study evaluated the effect of *Rhodiola rosea* in patients placed at a simulated altitude of 4600 m. These were 15 healthy volunteers, who remained at the simulated altitude for 7 days, treated with titrated dry extract or a placebo for the same period of time.

The evaluation was made by measuring pCO_2, pO_2, the presence of oxyhemoglobin, the presence of serum lipoxides and malondialdehyde in the pre- and post-exposure urine. It was noted that there were no significant differences between the two groups regarding pO_2, pCO_2 and oxyhemoglobin concentration. In fact, in both groups there was a sharp drop in pO_2 (−81%) and a net increase in pCO_2 (+38%) and in the concentration of oxyhemoglobin (+31%). The subjects of the placebo group, on the other hand, showed a notable increase in serum lipoxide and urinary levels of malondialdehyde, which was almost non-existent in the subjects of the group treated with *Rhodiola rosea*, indicating its powerful antioxidant effect.

As we have seen, many studies date back to the times of the "cold war", but *Rhodiola* (also of other species, not only *rosea*) is still being tested recently: in 2018, Anghelescu et al. confirmed the potential of this plant and, in the same year, Jòwko et al. carried out various tests on male students, obtaining good results in terms of mental alertness (and also at the antioxidant level), but only modest in terms of physical endurance, even if, reading the research thoroughly, they do not seem as insignificant as stated by the same authors.

A couple of other works from 2017 reaffirm the proven effectiveness of *Rhodiola rosea* in fatigued subjects, underlining its adaptogenic value; finally, in a very recent study (Ballmann et al., 2019), a dosage of 1500 mg/day of *Rhodiola rosea* plus 500 mg (!) before a Wingate test, allowed to obtain excellent results (with more than discrete statistical significance) on college students.

Dosages

There are different ways of using *Rhodiola rosea*; there is no suitable and valid dosage for anyone, since the daily dose depends on personal needs, the type of preparation, the composition of the product and the reason why it is taken.

Generally, the average recommended dose of the extract is 100-200 mg, two to three times a day, to be taken before meals, for 1-2 months.

Rhodiola rosea appears to be effective against fatigue at a dose of 100 mg, taken orally, while the anti-fatigue effect was noted with an oral intake of 300-700 mg. The recommended dosage in sports in order to improve the performance can also be higher; in any case, it is important that the root extract is titrated in rosavine at a minimum of 3% and in salidrosyl at 1%. Also, it is always best to seek expert advice if you want to take a *Rhodiola rosea* supplement.

Effectiveness

Strength	Resistant strength	Mass	Endurance	Slimming	Concentration	Recovery
−	+	+	+++	+++	++	++

RIBOSE

Description
Ribose is a cyclic monosaccharide with five carbon atoms (a pentose, unlike glucose, which has six and is a hexose). Important and vital molecules of our organism such as DNA and RNA have ribose among their fundamental components. Most of the ribose we need to fulfill our daily needs is obtained by converting the more abundant glucose through the pentose phosphate pathway in the cytoplasm, especially in the liver and adipose tissue. This pathway in its oxidative part allows to oxidize glucose and to obtain ribose as well as a reducing power transporter (NADPH), which at the same time will ensure important antioxidant properties for the cell's cytosol. In the non-oxidative part, on the other hand, the pentoses are converted into hexoses.

Properties
To function, our body can draw energy from the lipid reserves (almost infinite) and from the carbohydrate reserves stored in the liver (about 100 g) and muscles (about 350 g), as well as from phosphocreatine (PC, about 120 g), always taking into consideration a subject weighing 70 kg.

All these elements converge to a single purpose, which is the formation of the "energy currency" of our organism, known as ATP (adenosine triphosphate), whose composition is as follows:

$$adenine + ribose + 3\ phosphates$$

This is the ultimate effector of an infinity of physiological reactions ranging from the functioning of cellular pumps and active transcellular transports, to the more complex contraction reactions between actin and myosin muscle microfilaments. It has been calculated that, in a day, every human being consumes and produces an amount of ATP equal to their body weight, through the mitochondria. Like RNA, DNA, purines and nicotinic and flavinic acids, including molecules used for the energy exchange such as GTP, also ATP has a ribose among its constituents and this can make us understand how the supplementation of this sugar may be indispensable in the conditions in which we need to quickly regenerate the cellular energy pool.

It should be emphasized that the catabolism of purines is of vital importance for the energy homeostasis, as it allows to obtain the ribose that otherwise would have to be produced through the pentose phosphate pathway, with a consequent theft of glucose, essential for the production of ATP. However, in conditions in which physical exertion is prolonged and incessant, the diet does not satisfy the organic needs and we cannot bear all the impending stressors, the ATP shares are not correctly restored and the risk of a metabolic burnout can be avoided if ribose is supplemented at the appropriate time.

The formation of ribose phosphate via the pentose phosphate pathway is a limiting step in the formation of new IMP (nucleoside precursor) molecules. In animal studies, it has been seen that by increasing the supply of ribose to the muscles, the pathway known as the adenine salvage pathway was enhanced, and therefore the formation of ADP, with an increase in the rate of intracellular ATP refreshment as a consequence. The cellular reaction to this supplementation in human models with ischemic heart disease is particularly interesting. The first cardiology study on the use of ribose after myocardial ischemia was published in 1991; the hypothesis first theorized and then demonstrated by the researchers was that the ischemic myocardium had dormant parts that would be activated only after the blood flow was restored.

In case of oxygen deficiency, ATP is completely consumed and the ATP-dependent Na/K pumps are blocked. The cell retains Na (osmotically active) and Ca (which activates the intracellular lytic enzymes). This produces the swelling of the cell and its internal damage up to the explosion, giving rise to the so-called myocardial necrosis. The extent of this cardiac cell death is often leads to a systolic hypofunction, a drop in VO_{2max} and a lower quality of life.

In these cases, the intake of ribose improved the heart function after the cardiac decompensation, restored the previously depleted muscle ATP pool in 12 hours instead of 72 and speeded up the heart function recovery.

Other studies, always on pathological subjects, have found correlation between ribose dosages and quality of life scores in fibromyalgia patients. Given the decline in intracellular ATP during the muscle contraction, these findings have paved the way for a whole series of hypotheses on ribose supplementation. Another fact to consider is that ribose is largely "manufactured" in the adipose tissue, therefore its possible lower production in athletes with a very low percentage of fat can be a contributing cause of the feeling of "low energy" that they often experience.

Foods containing significant amounts of ribose can be dairy products, eggs and mushrooms. However, the quantities needed to improve the sports performance can only be met through supplementation.

Evidence

Ribose is rapidly absorbed from the intestinal tract even at very high doses (>100 g/day) or during exercise. Some studies have tested the induction of organic glycation during supplementation with ribose, but have not found any correlation, suggesting that this supplement, even if it is not ergogenic, is still not harmful for short periods.

Several studies have shown that ATP stocks take about 3 days to return exactly to starting levels after exercises of particular muscular effort and the reason lies in the competition between the pentose phosphate pathway, oxidative phosphorylation and glycolysis. In 2009, John G. Seifert, together with his team, tested the effects of supplementing 7 g of ribose before and after a 25-minute cycle ergometer workout, with a progressive increase in wattage every 3 minutes. The heart rate reached was 80-90% of the max HR, without exceeding the lactate threshold.

The study showed that ribose supplementation, compared to the placebo, was able to maintain the intramuscular glutathione pool and at the same time it limited the peak of malondialdehyde (MDA), a lipid oxidation product related to oxidative stress. Considering that at the muscle level ribose can be used for the resynthesis of a part of the nucleotides that are degraded during the consumption of ATP, some studies have shown a greater and more rapid restoration of the intracytoplasmic ATP pool after the administration of ribose. Although the rate of this refreshment is greater for ribose than for the placebo, this effect is more marked in pathological models (animal or human) and in untrained subjects, compared to trained subjects.

In a study by Seifert et al. (2017), it is clear that the speed of recovery of ATP reserves depends on the "fitness" (state of physical fitness) of the subject in question. Only subjects with a lower than average VO_{2max} peak benefit from the supplementation of 10 g of ribose per day. These benefits are denoted both in the flattening of the muscle damage markers (creatine kinase) and in the perception of physical effort during an interval exercise. Other studies such as that of Van Cammeren et al. in Florida (2002), evaluated the positive effects of ribose supplementation on the performance of 20 bodybuilders, finding that 5 g pre- and 5 g post-workout led to a significant increase of both 1RM and of the total training volume. Further studies, such as those by Raue et al. and Bernardi et al., demonstrated the advantage of supplementing ribose on a cycle ergometer sprint, in which the supplementation of ribose, compared to cellulose, allowed for a greater expressed strength.

Regarding the conflicting evidence, the limitations relating to some aspects of the studies must be recognized: the lack of a heterogeneous group of subjects with the same characteristics and the insufficient quantity of ribose in most cases could have affected the results of the studies, so much so that Seifert et al., in 2017, wanted to investigate the issue by making two different groups take ribose based on their training status, taking into account the VO_{2max} parameter.

Dosages
Ribose can be taken in capsule or powder form: the average recommended dose is 3-5 g once or twice a day in cardiopaths. There are few studies on fibromyalgia and chronic fatigue syndromes, where the recommended dose is 5 g, three times a day. For athletes, on the other hand, the dosages that are used in the literature to evaluate the ergogenic effects were higher, usually 0.2 g/kg of body weight (about 15-25 g in total).

Effectiveness

Strength	Resistant strength	Mass	Endurance	Slimming	Concentration	Recovery
–	+	–	++	–	–	++

SAM-E (S-ADENOSYL-METHIONINE)

Description
S-Adenosyl-Methionine, also known as ademetionine or SAM-e, is a substance that is naturally produced by our body. From a chemical point of view, S-Adenosyl-Methionine (SAM) is a coenzyme involved in several reactions and has exceptional properties for the health and for sports. SAM-e was first described in 1952 by the Italian researcher Giulio Cantoni.

Properties
Each cell in our body synthesizes SAM-e from adenosine triphosphate (ATP) and methionine, with the help of an enzyme called methionine adenosyltransferase. In the body, this coenzyme basically participates in three important types of biochemical reactions: transmethylation, transulfuration and aminopropylation. Transmethylation is the process by which methyl groups (CH_3) are transferred from one molecule to another; transulfuration allows the production of physiological sulfur compounds such as cysteine, taurine, glutathione (one of the body's main antioxidants), CoA etc.; while aminopropylation is the process of producing polyamines, organic compounds that are essential for the cell development, with the function of regulating the protein synthesis, DNA and RNA synthesis and cell division, ensuring the stabilization of the phospholipid structure of the cell membranes, acting as cell growth factors and as regulators of glucose homeostasis of intracellular Ca^{++}.

Through these mechanisms, S-Adenosyl-Methionine guarantees the protection and regeneration of the tissues (in particular of connective tissues and cartilage at the level of the joints), determines anti-inflammatory effects comparable to those of NSAIDs but without the side effects which are characteristic of these molecules, possesses powerful antioxidant capacities and maximizes the hepatic production of glutathione, which detoxifies the body even in the case of alcohol, steroids and drugs in general.

At the brain level, SAM-e has numerous beneficial effects: it is involved in the synthesis of neurotransmitters, membrane phospholipids (such as phosphatidylcholine and phosphatidylserine) and melatonin, it increases the number of neurotransmitter receptors and has a positive effect on neuronal membranes, as, by improving the receptor-neurotransmitter bond, it makes the neurotransmission more efficient. Finally, this molecule intervenes on the metabolism of catecholamines (dopamine, noradrenaline, adrenaline) and serotonin. This and other actions can, at least partially, scientifically explain why the increase in the endogenous availability of sulfo-adenosyl-methionine has an anti-depressant action.

SAM-e, in fact, has been shown to be effective in improving the symptoms in all forms of depression, except manic-depressive diseases, being particularly effective in the types of depression with no apparent cause. A meta-analysis of seven double-blind studies showed that SAM-e is significantly more effective compared to a placebo (74% *vs.* 5%). An analysis of nine double-blind clinical trials confirmed that SAM-e is even more effective (15%) than tricyclic antidepressants in the treatment of depression (76% *vs.* 61%). Furthermore, SAM-e acts faster than antidepressant drugs and is completely free of side effects, thus representing an excellent alternative for those who cannot tolerate prescription drugs; this has been confirmed by multiple studies conducted in Great Britain, Italy and in the United States. Depressed patients who can especially benefit from SAM-e are the elderly and those suffering from cardiac arrhythmia, glaucoma, hypotension, constipation and recent ischemic episodes.

An important epigenetic aspect is the following: SAM-dependent RNA methylations play a critical role in the gene expression. One study analyzed the methylation status of ribosomal RNA (rRNA) and transfer RNA (tRNA) in the *Escherichia coli* strains, in which cellular SAM-e was down-regulated. There, in fact, a serious growth defect of the strain was observed. SAM-e is used as a donor of methyl groups for a wide variety of methyltransferases and is involved in many essential biological processes. In the eukaryote, 5-methyldeoxycytidine (m5dC) is an important epigenetic sign responsible for various processes, including differentiation and reprogramming. SAM-e is also a methyl group donor for the protein and RNA methylation.

Evidence

From an ergogenic point of view, SAM-e is a critical factor during the creatine synthesis process (with an increase in the physical performance, reduced fatigue and increased recovery capacity after the exercise). The precursors of creatine are arginine and glycine, which in the first biosynthetic step form ornithine and guanidoacetate. Subsequently, guanidoacetate, through the intervention of SAM-e, becomes creatine. For this reason, SAM-e can be particularly useful **for the endogenous production of creatine**, as for example in vegetarians or in those who do not tolerate it well in the intestine, as well as for the so-called "non-responders", people who do not benefit from using creatine as a supplement.

Probably for the same reason, creatine supplementation also has a psychotropic effect, determined by the saving effect of SAM-e. By taking creatine as a supplement, we decrease its endogenous synthesis and thus do not consume SAM-e. An important function of SAM-e is to intervene in the synthesis of polyamines (putrescine, spermidine and spermine) which are essential for the cell development, protein synthesis and DNA and RNA synthesis. They regulate the glucose homeostasis and have an anticatabolic effect. Furthermore, in the brain, SAM-e intervenes in the metabolism of catecholamines (adrenaline, noradrenaline and dopamine) and in that of serotonin, thus exerting a nootropic and antidepressant effect.

Furthermore, the antioxidant role of SAM-e has already been underlined. The increase in oxidative stress plays an important role in the asthmatic inflammation of the airways and SAM-e, a powerful methyl donor, is known to protect against tissue injury and fibrosis, through the modulation of oxidative stress. In a study by Ding et al. (2018), the results define a role for SAM-e in acute stress-sensitive gene expression.

Clinical studies have shown that supplementation with SAM-e determines an **improvement in sports and in intellectual performance**, representing an aid for the memory, the immune system and for the maintenance of intellectual faculties, against depression, pain, chronic fatigue etc.

Dosages
The normally recommended dosage ranges from 200 to 1200 mg per day.

Effectiveness

Strength	Resistant strength	Mass	Endurance	Slimming	Concentration	Recovery
+	+	+	++	–	+++	++

SODIUM BICARBONATE

Description
Sodium hydrogen carbonate ($NaHCO_3$), also called sodium bicarbonate, is a derivative of carbonic acid, an alkalizing salt capable of increasing plasma bicarbonate levels. The origin of the name dates back to the eighteenth century, at the time of Lavoisier, when salts were classified as combinations of a metal oxide with a non-metallic oxide. In the case of sodium bicarbonate, to explain the presence of oxides and hydrogen combined with water molecules, it was written with the formula $Na_2O \cdot 2CO_2 \cdot H_2O$, and therefore its name was bicarbonate of soda, later replaced with sodium bicarbonate. It is a salt obtained from the ashes of some types of algae or plants, and from waters that flow from rocks that are rich in sodium; it is also produced by the human body, where it helps maintain a correct pH level on the bloodstream. On the market it is found in the form of a colorless and odorless powder, and being a salt, it is soluble in water but not in alcohol.

Properties
Sodium bicarbonate is a buffer substance; in the presence of hydrogen ions, the carbonate ions are transformed into hydrochloric acid and then into CO_2 (carbon dioxide), which is transported and eliminated in the lungs. It is present in saliva, where, through the neutralization of acids resulting from the decomposition of the bacterial plaque, it carries out a protective action for the dental enamel. It counteracts the aggressive action of stomach acids on the mucous membranes, preventing the onset of ulcers, and finally it intervenes in the respiratory exchanges, transporting carbon dioxide from the tissues to the lungs, where it is expelled. It has an alkaline composition (not acidic) with a 9 pH value and it is for this characteristic that it has wide applications, first of all in the industrial field, as a component of animal foods, in the fumes of fabrics and incinerators to break down the acid components, as a component of detergents, in various pharmaceutical and medicinal applications (for example in dialysis) and as a component of toothpastes, given the neutralizing power and the delicate abrasiveness.

In our homes it is used to wash fruits and vegetables in order to eliminate parasites and impurities, to soften legumes during cooking, for confectionery preparations thanks to its leavening and antacid power, as a deodorant for refrigerators, cat litter, shoe racks, as a color enhancer, and also for foot baths to relieve the sense of swelling and tiredness of the legs and feet. The main use of sodium bicarbonate, given its ability to neutralize acids, is in the presence of heartburn, peptic ulcers and gastritis, and whenever it is necessary to alkalize the urine or other body fluids. In the case of drug intoxication which have weak acid characteristics, sodium bicarbonate makes the urine basic and inhibits their renal reabsorption, favoring their excretion.

In patients predisposed to the formation of uric acid kidney stones, sodium bicarbonate prevents their formation by alkalizing the urine. Regarding indigestion, reflux and, in any case, in all conditions that cause excessive gastric acidity, sodium bicarbonate is used in pharmaceutical preparations with an antacid action, associated with dimethicone to reduce the size of the carbon dioxide bubbles that form in the stomach, thus attenuating the phenomena of flatulence and belching.

Finally, sodium bicarbonate can be used in sports through the use of supplements that allow athletes to prolong their resistance to the lactacid effort, during which considerable quantities of lactic acid are produced and then released into the bloodstream by blocking the muscle contraction, with a subsequent tendency to a slight acidification.

Evidence

Several studies have been carried out to verify the effects of sodium bicarbonate intake in athletes. In June 2015, Krustrup, Ermidis, Mohr (*J Int Soc Sports Nutr*. 2015; 12:25) published a study to verify the effects of sodium bicarbonate intake by young athletes during intermittent high intensity training and the improvement in their sports performance. The intake of sodium bicarbonate has been shown to improve exercise tolerance, but the effects on high intensity intermittent trainings are less clear. Therefore, the goal of this study was to determine the effects of sodium bicarbonate intake on the performance of young athletes. 13 young athletes (23 years old) performed a test (Yo-Yo IR2) on two different occasions in a random order, with or without prior intake of sodium bicarbonate (0.4 g per kg of body weight). During the tests, their heart rate was constantly measured, the perception of exertion was assessed and venous blood samples were often taken. Performance increased by 14% in athletes who took sodium bicarbonate compared to the control group, with a concomitant increase in blood alkalosis and a peak in blood lactate levels. They also had lower levels of fatigue. Brisola, Miyagi, da Silva and Zagatto (*Appl Physiol Nutr Metab*, September 2015) carried out a study to verify the effects of a strong sodium bicarbonate supplementation on a maximum oxygen deficit, accumulated after a single maximal effort in running athletes, and also the correlation with performances during running races of 200 and 400 m.

Two groups were studied: one with a high sodium bicarbonate administration and the other with the administration of a placebo (dextrose), during 200 and 400 m competitions. It was found that, despite the improvement in the maximum accumulated oxygen deficit, the performance did not benefit. Therefore, we can conclude that both the maximum accumulated oxygen deficit and the anaerobic lactic metabolism are modified after a high administration of sodium bicarbonate, but this is not correlated to the performance during the 200 and 400 m running races. A research conducted by Finnish scholars, published in the *Journal International Society Sports Nutrition* in 2013, showed how **sodium bicarbonate supplements improved the swimming performances of less than 60 seconds duration**. The fatigue that is felt during a high intensity training session is linked to the increase in acids that interfere with the chemical reactions necessary to continue the training. Bicarbonate is the most important antacid in the body. A study carried out at the University of Western Australia found that bicarbonate supplementation is able to improve the performance during 20 m sprint repetitions. Most studies **show that bicarbonate supplements improve the performance during high-intensity workouts. However, sodium bicarbonate at effective dosages produces severe side effects, such as diarrhea, abdominal cramps, and nausea**.

In 2019, a study was conducted on 20 healthy young men with the aim of investigating the effects on the performance during HIIT (High-Intensity Interval Training) workouts, given by

6 weeks of sodium bicarbonate supplementation. 10 participants were given a solution containing 0.2 g/kg body weight of sodium bicarbonate for each training day (3 workouts per week), the other 10 participants were given a similar solution, but free of sodium bicarbonate (placebo group). **The obtained data suggested that supplementing with sodium bicarbonate before HIIT training improved the performance and reduced the amount of lactate in the blood.**

In the same year, an article was published in the *Journal of the International Society of Sports Nutrition*, comparing the results obtained by karate athletes during a specific aerobic test (KSAT). This randomized double-blind study examined the effects of supplementing caffeine and sodium bicarbonate, taken together and individually, and compared to a placebo group.

Capsules containing 6 mg/kg of caffeine were taken 50 minutes before the test, while 0.3 g/kg of sodium bicarbonate was consumed starting 3 days before the KSAT and up to 60 minutes before the test. Time to exhaustion (TE), rate of perceived exertion (RPE) and blood lactate levels were measured before, immediately after and 3 minutes after the test.

TE was significantly improved in the group that took separate caffeine and bicarbonate and the group that took them together, compared with the placebo group. Therefore, this study shows that both caffeine and sodium bicarbonate, consumed together or separately, improve the performance of karate athletes.

Dosages

Over the last 60 years, studies on the use of sodium bicarbonate as a sports supplement, given its remarkable properties as a buffer substance capable of counteracting the onset of acidity during sports performance, have given conflicting results, depending on the quantity used. By administering 135 mg/kg of body weight 90 minutes before a sports performance, there are significant benefits in improving the performance, even for long periods, thanks to its buffering action which is capable of counteracting the muscle acidity; on the other hand, this dosage can cause gastric problems. It is therefore preferable to start with dosages of 20 mg/kg of body weight to check the tolerance levels.

As an antacid, bicarbonate can be taken 1-2 hours after the end of meals together with a glass of water, with a dosage of 325-2000 mg, one to four times a day.

Effectiveness

Strength	Resistant strength	Mass	Endurance	Slimming	Concentration	Recovery
−	+++	+	++	−	−	+

SUPER-AMIDE

Description

Super-amide or SuperStarch, is a natural product that represents an innovation in the context of the intake of gluten-free carbohydrates. SuperStarch is a complex carbohydrate (derived from non-genetically modified corn) that uniquely stabilizes blood sugar levels, without causing any reaction from insulin, the hormone that promotes fat storage.

Properties

Energy drinks are undoubtedly among the most consumed supplements by athletes, especially those who practice endurance sports. They normally contain mixtures of fructose, glucose, maltodextrin and glucose syrup, at a total concentration ranging from 6 to 8%. The problem with these products is that, being rapidly assimilated, they raise the blood sugar with a consequent stimulation of insulin, leading to fluctuations in the blood sugar itself, which rises and falls, thus hindering a constant blood sugar level. Furthermore, the insulin stimulus inhibits the oxidation of fats for energy purposes and favors the use of glucose, and this, especially in long-lasting aerobic sports, is a limiting factor for the maintenance of glycogen reserves, which become essential when the aerobic effort reaches its maximum intensity. During aerobic exercise it is undoubtedly better to use fats instead of glycogen for the following reasons:

1. Energy reserves in the form of fat are much higher than those of glycogen.
2. It is physically impossible to consume carbohydrates in sufficient quantities in order to restore the glycogen consumed for efforts lasting more than a few hours.
3. Theoretically, any ingestion of carbohydrates will lead to significant fluctuations in blood sugar and insulin, the so-called "insulin rebound".
4. By taking carbohydrates to restore glycogen, we raise the levels of insulin, which inhibits the use of fats for energy purposes. However, thinking of being able to use only fats as energy during the training is utopian and is probably only possible in athletes who have adapted to a ketogenic diet, a diet based almost exclusively on fats and proteins: about 60 % of fats, 30% of proteins and no more than 10% of carbohydrates (proteins must not be higher, as a high protein consumption would favor the neoglucogenesis, i.e. the transformation of proteins into glucose which will inhibit the ketogenesis). Athletes who follow a diet rich in carbohydrates will undoubtedly deplete their hepatic glycogen reserves after prolonged fasting exercises, and this also affects the brain function, leading to tiredness, fogging and concentrating difficulties.

Hence the use of sports drinks, which contain simple sugars, having these characteristics:

1. High osmolarity (i.e. they draw a lot of water), which leads to a slowed gastric emptying, increased gastric pressure and a limited intake per drink.
2. A rapid increase in blood sugar after ingestion, which entails the risk of "rebound" hypoglycemia and the need for frequent intakes.
3. A rapid increase in insulin levels, which involves the inhibition of the use of storage fats for energy purposes, an increase in the use of glycogen for energy purposes and, over time, a negative impact on health and on the body composition.

The evolution of glucose supplements for sports use starts from the use of glucose and finally arrives at the formulation of products such as Vitargo® (another beverage used in endurance sports, see below), which are simply better than long-chain maltodextrins, but they still stimulate insulin and raise blood sugar levels.

In reality, the goal would be to find a carbohydrate with all the necessary characteristics, such as:

1. A slow glucose release.
2. Minimal insulin stimulation.
3. Complete absorption.

Thanks to a technology developed to save the lives of children suffering from a rare genetic deficiency that causes a disease known as "Glycogen storage disease", in which there is a deficiency in the hepatic glucose-6-phosphatase enzyme (an enzyme involved in the release of blood glucose), it was possible to create a thermally treated product, rich in amylopectin (the equivalent of glycogen for plants) and able to supply glucose continuously, preventing the states of hypoglycemia that in these children often lead to neurological damage and early death. It is practically a super starch with a very high molecular weight, a huge glucose polymer (from 250 to 2000 times larger than all other simple or complex carbohydrates) with a very low osmolarity, a very low gastric impact and a very fast transit at the stomach level, and it is eventually absorbed completely.

Evidence

Obviously, for this product conceived for medical use, as well as for others such as BCAAs that had been studied for patients suffering from chronic liver diseases, the potential use was immediately seen also in the sports field. In a study conducted by Michel Roberts et al., nine trained cyclists (around 30 years old) weighing around 80 kg, after a 10-hour fast, cycled for 150 minutes at 70% of VO_{2max}, ending with an exhaustion ride at 100% of VO_{2max}.

The participants ingested 1 g/kg of super starch or maltodextrin 30 minutes before the exercise and within 10 minutes after the completion of the performance, and blood samples were taken every 15 minutes before, during and 90 minutes after the exercise. The results showed comparable results during the performance, but in the recovery phase there was a higher increase in blood sugar with maltodextrins, a lower insulin level with super starch and, again with super starch, there was an increase in esterified fatty acids and glucose, which indicated a greater oxidation of fats.

This study concluded that the **ingestion of super starch before a prolonged exercise with the cycle ergometer increases the lipolysis, compared to the ingestion of maltodextrin**.

In another study, 10 soccer players were given isoenergetic amounts of dextrose, maltodextrin, Vitargo®, super starch and a placebo (water) in a 7% solution. The experiment noted that blood glucose concentrations 60 minutes after the ingestion were significantly higher in those who took dextrose, maltodextrin and Vitargo®, while for placebo and super starch there was no difference (so for super starch, there was no rapid surge in the blood sugar).

90 minutes after the ingestion of dextrose and Vitargo®, the blood glucose values were significantly higher compared to the placebo, while after 120 minutes, only Vitargo® continued to produce a higher blood sugar than the placebo. The only drink that kept blood sugar consistently higher than the placebo after 180 minutes was waxy corn starch. The conclusions, here, were that the super starch did not cause a rapid increase in the blood sugar (therefore it did not give insulinemic rebounds), but kept it elevated for a much longer period of time, compared to other carbohydrate sources (making it interesting especially in long-lasting sports such as cycling, marathon, triathlon etc.).

For years, super starch was considered a fast-absorbing carbohydrate and this hypothesis, of course, was used by the industry to implement its sales. The aforementioned studies, on the other hand, report the opposite. The "key to the problem" was that the waxy corn starch, used to make super starch, was used for the production of Vitargo®, which instead had a high glycemic index: about 137, synonymous with a rapid absorption. This product, in fact, in order to obtain these characteristics, was heat treated with a particular patent, while raw waxy maize starch shows the kinetics of the super starch described above. Incidentally, since 2005 Vitargo® is no longer even derived from waxy corn starch but from potato starch.

Dosages

The recommended dosage is 25 g 30-45 minutes before exercise, which can be combined with a small snack based on dried nuts. Some, however, also suggest higher dosages, 40 to 60 g pre-workout.

Effectiveness

Strength	Resistant strength	Mass	Endurance	Slimming	Concentration	Recovery
–	++	–	++++	+++	+	+

TAURINE

Description
Taurine is an interesting sulfuric amino acid, found only in the animal kingdom (meat, milk, fish, eggs); in humans it is abundant in the muscles, retina, heart and brain, where it performs important regulatory functions. It is another amino acid considered "conditionally essential" because, even if the body is able to produce it, in certain situations it is easy for a deficiency to occur. Together with glutamine, it is the most abundant free amino acid in the muscle cell. Taurine is synthesized by the liver from two amino acids: methionine and cysteine, in the presence of vitamin B6, but in some cases there may be deficiencies.

For example, taurine deficiency states are common in vegetarians, in people on diets with inadequate caloric or nutritional intake, in pregnant women and in athletes, individuals who need more nutritional intake. Deficiencies of this amino acid, in fact, most commonly appear as the result of a total protein deficiency, a rare occurrence in Western countries.

Properties
The effects of taurine in the body involve various organs and tissues; in particular, the main actions of taurine affect the liver, the eyes, the metabolic system and the cardiac, nervous and muscular systems, where this amino acid plays protective, regulator and antioxidant roles.

At the cardiac level, taurine stabilizes the flow of ions, thus preserving the integrity of the membrane, and it is of considerable importance both in ischemic heart disease and in conditions of poor oxygenation of the heart, in relation to its protective action against the toxic effects of free radicals: for further information, a review by Bkaili et al. (2019) exhaustively summarizes its properties, as can be seen from the title: "Taurine and cardiac disease: state of the art and perspectives".

In the brain, taurine deficiency can cause memory loss, but it has the most important effect on depression. Low serum taurine values can be associated with manic-depressive disorders for a complex range of causes. Obviously, the maximum positive effects occur only if it is taken together with all the other bioregulators (vitamins, folic acid, mineral salts, etc.) which complement and enhance their action. Taurine, being an antagonist of the GABAergic system, which is a sedative system, also promotes the attention and concentration. From a metabolic point of view, taurine plays a fundamental role in the synthesis of bile acids, deriving from cholesterol, produced in the liver and incorporated into the bile, essential for the digestion of fats and for the absorption of fat-soluble vitamins.

In addition, researches have already been conducted for several years, showing **how taurine affects the metabolism of carbohydrates by producing an effect similar to that of insulin, i.e. acting as a hypoglycemic substance**, capable of lowering the amount of sugar in the blood. It is worth remembering that insulin, if produced in excess, remains in the circulation, creating damage to the body, causing a faster aging, raising the blood pressure, inhibiting the weight loss process, etc. If, on the other hand, this hormone is secreted in a suitable quantity, it has anabolic properties and allows the entry of nutrients into the muscle cells, accelerating the recovery processes, energy recovery and protein synthesis.

Evidence
Due to the multiple effects, it exerts both in the body and in sports, taurine can be considered a "wild card" supplement. In fact, in addition to the effects we saw above, it is very important both in the muscles and in the joints. At the muscle level, it improves the contraction by increasing the flow of calcium and potassium, and its deficiency can cause cramps; in the joints, on the other hand, it exerts a protective action by limiting the degeneration of hyaluronic acid.

This amino acid is also useful for slimming, as, by improving the exchange of oxygen between blood and the tissues, it allows the oxidation of fatty acids. Supplementation with taurine **reduces the sense of fatigue and tiredness**, since taurine acts as a mild caffeine-like psychoanaleptic and maintains a high sense of wakefulness and response to stimuli, which are particularly important requirements during sports competitions or intellectual time trials.

This can be translated, as recently highlighted by Waldron et al. (2019), in tangible improvements in a prolonged effort on the cycle ergometer, especially at higher intensities. Waldron himself, in 2018, had compiled a review on the results that can be obtained with taurine supplementation on the endurance exercise, confirming good results. Yatabe et al., in 2003, used mice models to demonstrate how the administration of taurine increased the running time on the treadmill and again, in 2009, how it also reduced the exercise-induced muscle fatigue. Also in mice, it was observed that taurine is able to stimulate the secretion of the growth hormone (GH), probably through an action that affects the opiate peptide system of the hypothalamus.

A point on which we must pay attention is also the ability of taurine to **increase the cell volume**, since it is concentrated above all at the cytoplasmic level and therefore exerts an osmotic effect. We know that the increase in cell volume or the state of hydration works as an anabolic signal, while the decrease in this volume promotes the catabolic processes. All substances that promote this volumizing effect (such as glutamine, creatine and taurine) can therefore be considered protein synthesis stimulants. **The anti-catabolic role of taurine has been confirmed by several studies.** For example, important research has shown that taking three 500 mg doses, distributed throughout the day, resulted in a 20% decrease in 3-methylhistidine (3-MH), a marker used to monitor the muscle breakdown. A study with taurine (2 g) in combination with BCAA (3.2 g), to be taken three times a day for 2 weeks before the physical tests and 4 days after the same tests, showed that only the combination of the two supplements improved the feeling of soreness; on the contrary, neither the placebo nor the substances taken individually were able to reduce the muscle pain.

Dosage

A good time to take taurine is at the end of the training, especially in association with other supplements, to create a highly anabolic mix, or in the evening to promote the secretion of GH at night and to promote an adequate rest. In the first case, it can be associated with glutamine, arginine pyroglutamate and/or lysine HCL, with zinc monomethionine aspartate, magnesium aspartate and vitamin B6, in order to create an anti-stress effect and to stimulate the release of testosterone.

In the second case, it can be taken with calcium and magnesium, elements that support its action to promote sleep and therefore the energy recovery. During meals, it can be taken to modulate the post-prandial glycemic peak. Taking it before the training can promote the concentration, but in people predisposed to hypoglycemia it is not recommended, as a hypoglycemic crises may occur. After the training, thanks to its insulin-mimetic property, it favors the entry of glucose and amino acids into the muscle cell.

Before the training, therefore, to give a hand to concentration, you can take from 1 to 2 g, especially if you follow a vegan diet, but also after the training, always at the same dosages, to create a highly anabolic mix, in synergy with glutamine and other supplements.

Effectiveness

Strength	Resistant strength	Mass	Endurance	Slimming	Concentration	Recovery
–	–	++	–	++	+++	++

TRIBULUS TERRESTRIS

Description
Tribulus terrestris is a plant belonging to the *Zygophyllaceae* family, characterized by branched stems, small leaves and yellow flowers, widespread in Europe, Asia, Africa, Australia and in tropical areas. Traditionally this plant was used in Indian and Chinese medicine for the treatment of a series of pathologies, such as renal, cardiovascular, gastrointestinal and hepatic dysfunctions, while since the late 1970s it has been used as a supplement in the sports field for its effectiveness in stimulating the production of androgens and, for the same reason, for the treatment of sexual disorders.

As for the properties of *Tribulus terrestris*, as for most plant extracts, it is important to consider some fundamental aspects: each plant has a very specific season and cultivation area and its handling requires specific techniques that guarantee the conservation of the active ingredients contained therein. Failure to comply with these protocols can lead to the deterioration of these substances, therefore the loss of the hormone-stimulating effects of the plant itself.

Properties
The effects of *Tribulus terrestris* are essentially linked to a group of organic substances with hormone-like activity called saponins, of which the main one, contained in the seeds of the plant, is protodioscin, a steroid molecule that has the ability to increase the endogenous production of various hormones such as testosterone, dihydrotestosterone, luteinizing hormone (LH), dehydroepiandrosterone (DHEA) and dehydroepiandrosterone sulfate (DHEA-S), resulting in an increased spermatogenesis, increased ejaculatory volume and increased libido. An increase in pubic hair has also been observed in young people with hypogonadism. All these effects make *Tribulus terrestris* an interesting supplement and, as an adaptogen, it brings different results depending on the physical status of those who take it.

Evidence
The athlete in optimal psychophysical conditions does not seem to obtain particular results in body mass or strength from Tribulus terrestris. On the contrary, in exhausted and stressed subjects, this acts as a revitalizer, also promoting an increase in libido, sperm quantity and vitality, which are reduced in the presence of chronic stress.

In a 1981 Milanov study, increases of more than 70% in LH and 40% in testosterone were found, and also El Din et al. (2019) found significant increases in male hormone levels (total and free) and, specifically, in the sexual activity.

An interesting work by Ma et al. (2017) found good anaerobic results on boxers with a supplementation of 1250 mg of *Tribulus terrestris*, but not thanks to an increase in testosterone, but due to a decrease in IGFBP-3.

Wu et al. (2017) achieved excellent results, with an increase in both testosterone and IGF-1, a result that leads them to recommend its use to increase the muscle mass and improve the performance in high-intensity activities. The intake of *Tribulus terrestris* can, in some subjects, also lead to an increase in estrogen and lead to an aromatization of testosterone: therefore, its use must not be indiscriminate!

***Tribulus terrestris* can be a valuable aid to counteract the natural psychophysical and performance decay of men over 40-50 years old or young people subjected to intense training.**

Dosages
As with all substances that modify the endocrinological profile, cyclization is recommended; therefore, after a maximum period of 6 or 8 weeks, it would be advisable to suspend its intake

for an equally long period. An amount that makes the supplement effective must be about 750-1500 mg of pure extract per day. The distribution should be in 3-4 times a day, with meals. Given that the half-life of protodioscin is very low (2.5 hours), a more frequent administration schedule could increase its effectiveness.

Effectiveness

Strength	Resistant strength	Mass	Endurance	Slimming	Concentration	Recovery
++	+	++	+	+	–	+

TURMERIC (CURCUMA LONGA)

Description

In everyday language, when we talk about turmeric we usually mean the *longa* species, although there are many others. *Curcuma longa*, defined as *curcuma* par excellence or *Indian saffron*, due to its color, or more rarely *turmeric*, is a perennial herbaceous plant of the *Zingiberaceae* family, native to Southeast Asia. The plant can reach a maximum height of about one meter and is characterized by large leaves, 30-40 cm long, with an elongated petiole. The component of the greatest commercial interest of the plant is the root, a large cylindrical, branched, yellow or orange rhizome, strongly aromatic.

Turmeric powder is obtained from this yellow rhizome, a spice that has become very popular in recent years and which is still increasingly used in gastronomic preparations. It is added to give flavor and color to salad dressings and is one of the favorite spices of the inhabitants of Okinawa, the island in the south of Japan, known for having the longest life expectancy in the world, and also the longest expectation of incurring aging without diseases such as cancer, cardiovascular disease, osteoporosis, diabetes and autonomic disorders such as Alzheimer's disease.

Obviously, it would be simplistic to trace these results back to the use of turmeric; in reality, the inhabitants of Okinawa, in addition to leading a healthy and stress-free life, follow a low-calorie diet with a low glycemic index, based on foods that do not raise the blood sugar, which are low in saturated fats and rich in soy and fish. Soy contains phytoestrogens, which protect against tumors and act as antiaging substances; fish is rich in omega-3s, which have a protective function at the cardiovascular level and against various degenerative diseases, and also improve brain function by protecting against the pathological aging.

However, in Okinawa, turmeric is used daily, as a spice to flavor foods and the inevitable green tea, or as a medicine. Both the polyphenols in green tea and curcumin (the main active ingredient in turmeric) are able to activate protective genes and thus increase the longevity and improve the health.

In order to obtain the well-known yellow-orange powder, the rhizomes of the plant are boiled and dried in the sun or in the oven.

Curcumin, due to its bitter, spicy and extremely volatile taste, and due to its properties, has also become a very popular ingredient in some food supplements.

The interest in the use of curcumin-based supplements lies in the fact that its use has long been known, in countries such as India and China, also for the treatment of dermatological diseases, infections, stress and depression, liver and gallbladder problems, bleeding, chest congestion, menstrual disturbances, flatulence, bloody urine and toothaches.

Properties

Turmeric is a plant with numerous properties, which are conferred on it by the essential oil and other important substances contained in it, called curcuminoids (and mainly curcumin). David Frawley, the founder of the American Institute of Vedic Studies in Santa Fe (New Mexico), says: "If I had to rely on one herb for all possible health and dietary needs, I would definitely choose the Indian spice turmeric" (in: *Turmeric: the Ayurvedic spice of life*, edited by Prashanti de Jager, 2000). It is a traditional plant of the Ayurvedic medicine, used as a general cleansing and digestive remedy, in the presence of fever, infections, dysentery, arthritis, jaundice and various liver disorders. Some pharmacological studies have highlighted its anti-inflammatory and pain-relieving properties, useful for combating muscle and joint pain, but also rheumatic and menstrual pain and migraine. Curcuminoids have been shown to have antioxidant effects comparable to those of vitamin E. On the contrary, in the presence of high concentrations of free iron or copper, curcumins behave as pro-oxidants and contribute to the formation of ROS and cell death by apoptosis induced by them. This property could be of significant interest for the effect on cancer cells. In fact, in some studies in which the reproductive system was treated, the antitumor property resulted in an antiapoptotic action on normal cells and a proapoptotic effect on cancer cells. Therefore, curcumin, with its anticancer action, plays an important role in the prevention and treatment of various diseases, from cancerous to autoimmune, neurological, cardiovascular and endocrine (diabetes) ones.

A very important aspect to consider, and which cannot be overlooked, is that curcumin is a lipophilic polyphenol, i.e. it is almost insoluble in water, and is unstable at the intestinal pH, which is why it is difficult to absorb and easily eliminated by our body. The metabolic pathway that is mostly involved in the pharmacokinetics of curcumin is glucuronation.

In fact, it has been observed that in the cytosol of the human liver and in the intestinal tissue, there is a capacity of reduction of curcumin from 5 to 18 times higher than in the mouse (Siviero, 2015). Curcumin, in fact, at a pH = 7, is rapidly degraded with a hydrolytic process that produces substances (vanillin, ferulic acid, feruloylacetone) with negligible biological activity compared to the original compound.

Table 44.9 The systemic bioavailability of curcumin following the oral administration

Template	Dosage	Pharmacokinetic data
Mouse	400 mg	No traces of curcumin in the coronary circulation; traces in the portal blood (<5 μg/mL)
Mouse	2% of the diet	Plasma levels: 12 nmol
Mouse	50 mg/kg	Plasma levels: 0.2927 ± 0.065 μg/mL
Mouse	2 g/kg	Moderate serum concentrations
Human	2 g/kg	Not detectable or very low serum concentrations
Human	36-180 mg/die	Not detectable in plasma up to 29 days of treatment

To address this problem, some strategies have been developed in recent years to increase its bioavailability. Numerous methods have been proposed, including the use of adjuvants such as:

- an association with piperine: the latter is a powerful inhibitor of the metabolism of nutrients and dietary ingredients, and by inhibiting the hepatic and intestinal glucuronidation, it can slow down the metabolism of curcumin and increase its bioavailability. Some supplements, in fact, contain a compound called **bioperine**, which works just like piperine and increases its absorption;

- an association with other compounds: alpha-lipoic acid, bromelain, cyclodextrin, epigallocatechin-3-gallate (EGCG) etc. This blend gives rise to a chemically high profile phytotherapeutic product, with an absorption and bioavailability that are 5-7 times higher than those of curcumin;
- phytosomal formulations (curcumin phytosome): in this case, curcumin is complexed with phospholipids (phosphatidylcholine) or other lipid carriers (phosphatidylserine). If piperine is added, there is a further increase in its bioavailability;
- liposomal formulations: liposomes are made up of microscopic artificial vesicles; phosphatidylcholine is used for the creation of liposomal curcumin;
- nanocurcumin: in this case, the active ingredient of turmeric, encapsulated in polymeric nanoparticles, is soluble in water and shows an increase in its bioavailability (Bisht, 2006);
- structural analogues of curcumin: they have a chemical structure formulated without the more unstable portion of curcumin.

Evidence

In a **1992 study by Soni et al.**, curcuminoids have been defined as powerful scavengers of superoxide and hydroxyl radicals; in addition, they favor the maintenance of glutathione (GSH) levels and decrease the concentrations of the end products of radical oxidation. Curcumin also protects against lipid peroxidation, the inactivation of glutathione peroxidase (GPx) and oxidative attack on DNA. As for the sports field, there are many studies in the literature regarding the anti-inflammatory action of curcumin in the case of DOMS (Delayed Onset Muscle Pain).

Drobnic et al. (2014) and Nicol et al. (2015) wanted to study the possible attenuation of DOMS following curcumin supplementation. More precisely, the aim of the first study was to verify the ability of curcumin to attenuate the damage from oxidative stress and from the inflammation related to acute muscle injuries, induced by continuous eccentric exercise. DOMS, due to eccentric muscle activity, is associated with inflammatory responses and the production of reactive oxygen species (ROS) that support both inflammation and oxidative stress. Subjects in the curcumin group reported less pain in their lower extremities than subjects in the placebo group, although significant differences were observed only for the right and left anterior thighs. The increase in the markers of muscle damage and inflammation tended to be lower in the curcumin group, but significant differences were only observed for IL-8, two hours after the exercise.

In the second study, however, we wanted to observe whether it was possible to obtain improvements in the period following the training with a supplementation of 2.5 g of curcumin twice a day. Twenty-four and 48 hours after exercise, curcumin caused significant reductions in pain during single-leg squat (VAS scale −1.4 to −1.7; 90% CL: ± 1.0) and small reductions in creatine kinase activity (−22-29%; ± 21-22%). In addition, a small increase in one-legged jumping performance was observed to be associated with a reduction in pain (15%; 90% CL ± 12%). Regarding the anti-inflammatory activity in this second study, curcumin decreased the levels of IL-6 24 hours after the exercise.

Also in **2015, Sciberras et al.** investigated the effect of turmeric supplementation on cytokine and inflammatory marker responses after 2 hours of cycling. Resistance exercise induces the production of IL-6 by myocytes, which is believed to compromise the intracellular defense mechanisms. Eleven male athletes (35.5 ± 5.7 years; W_{max} 275 ± 6 W; 87.2 ± 10.3 kg) who consumed a low-carbohydrate diet of 2.3 ± 0.2 g/kg/day underwent three double-blind trials with curcumin supplementation, placebo supplementation and no supplementation (control), to observe the response of serum interleukins (IL-6, IL1-RA, IL-10), cortisol, C-reactive protein and for the subjective evaluation of the training stress.

The serum concentrations of IL-6 one hour after the exercise were: 2.0 for curcumin, 4.8 for the placebo, 3.5 for the control group. Participants reported "better than usual" scores in the subjective assessment of psychological stress during supplementation with curcumin, indicating that they felt less stressed during the training days (p = 0.04), compared to the placebo.

We have already talked about the association of curcumin with piperine: its effectiveness was demonstrated in a study in which by maintaining the ratio of 20 mg of piperine to 2 g of curcumin, the absorption of the latter was 20 times higher and its brain concentrations increased by 48% (Shoba, 1998).

Delecroix et al., In 2017, also wanted to analyze the effects of an oral consumption of the combination of curcumin and piperine on the kinetics of recovery after exercise-induced muscle damage. Forty-eight hours before and after exercise-induced muscle damage, ten elite rugby players consumed curcumin and piperine (experimental condition) or a placebo, according to a randomized crossover design. Some physical performance, creatine kinase concentration and muscle soreness were assessed immediately after the exercise, and at 24-hours, 48-hours and 72-hours post-exercise. From the results obtained by the group who took a combination of curcumin and piperine, it was possible to deduce that this form of supplementation before and after the exercise can attenuate some aspects of muscle damage, such as the production of proinflammatory cytokines.

Also, **Jäger et al.**, in a study published in July 2019, wanted to determine whether with a high dose of curcumin supplementation it would be possible to mitigate the decrease in the performance, following the muscle damage induced by downhill training. Sixty-three physically active men and women were randomly assigned to supplementation of 50 mg and 200 mg of curcuminoids or a cornstarch (PLA) placebo, for 8 weeks, in a controlled, double-blind, randomized, parallel group study. At the end of the supplementation period, the subjects completed a downhill protocol intended to induce muscle damage. The muscle function, measured by isokinetic dynamometry, and the perceived soreness, were assessed before and after 1 hour, 24 hours, 48 hours and 72 hours from the activity.

Compared to the changes observed in the placebo group, a dose of 200 mg of curcumin
resulted in reductions in soreness after the completion of the training protocol. Furthermore, it was observed that doses of 50 mg did not appear to offer any advantage over the changes observed in the group that took 200 mg.

As has already been said above, the intake of curcumin-based supplements would seem to be of great importance not only in the sports field. The use of this substance in everyday life, in fact, can help us fight the most feared and studied problem in the recent years: chronic inflammation.

The already known correlation between inflammation and chronic diseases has given rise to a multitude of diet programs, nutritional supplements and guides on the correct lifestyle, many of which allow you to improve your health by counteracting the inflammation. In this regard, **Shimizu et al., in 2019**, evaluated the anti-inflammatory action of curcumin, since chronic inflammation plays a significant role in lifestyle-related diseases, such as cardiovascular disease, obesity and diabetes. The mechanisms underlying this action include the inhibition of **NF-κB** and of the Toll-like 4 receptor signaling pathway, and also the activation of the PPAR-γ pathway, a receptor mainly expressed in adipose tissue, where it plays a key role in the regulation of adipocyte differentiation, fatty acid uptake and storage, glucose metabolism and inflammation.

Type 2 diabetes (T2D) is an established risk factor for cardiovascular diseases
(CVD) and is associated with an impaired lipid and lipoprotein metabolism. Curcuminoids are natural products with antidiabetic and lipid-modifying actions, but their effectiveness in improving the dyslipidemia in diabetic subjects has not been sufficiently studied.

For this reason, in **2017 Panahi et al.** studied the effectiveness of curcuminoids supplementation, associated with piperine as an absorption enhancer, in improving the serum lipid levels in patients with T2D.

A comparison between the different groups in the study revealed significant reductions in the total serum cholesterol levels and an increase in serum HDL levels.

Therefore, the supplementation with curcuminoids could help reduce the risk of cardiovascular events in patients with dyslipidemia and T2D. Other studies conducted on humans have shown a drop in blood sugar levels in diabetic subjects, an increase in HDL ("good") cholesterol at the expense of LDL ("bad") and, in subjects with atherosclerosis, a decrease in the levels of fibrinogen in the blood, resulting in a lower risk of blood clots.

Due to their high incidence, the absence of optimal treatments and the growing economic impact, these metabolic pathologies represent one of the main areas of interest for biomedical research.

Stress is another intensively studied topic. To what extent can both nutrition and supplementation affect the production of cortisol (the stress hormone)? The answer is to a great extent.

It is known that a high-protein diet stimulates the production of cortisol and that, conversely, carbohydrates, through the stimulation of insulin, by inhibiting the 11HSD1 enzyme, which regenerates cortisol from cortisone in the adipose tissue and in the liver, reduce the levels of cortisol.

Consequently, if you want to keep cortisol levels under more control, it is advisable to consume carbohydrates before and during the training. The modulation of cortisol receptors is probably the reason why turmeric exerts a pain relieving effect. In fact, this substance improves the sensitivity of receptors to cortisol and, consequently, keeps the levels of this hormone lower and limits the premature aging caused by its excess.

Turmeric reverses the effects of chronic stress on the behavior and on the HPA axis; in fact, in animals subjected to chronic stress for 20 days, there was an increase in the thickness of the cortex and a decrease in cortisol receptors (dosage 5-10 mg/kg) (**Department of Pharmacology, Faculty of Basic Medical Disciplines, Beijing University**). In conclusion, it is essential to carry out other clinical studies on humans to further analyze and confirm curcumin's ability to act in pathologies of a metabolic nature. Further methods are needed to increase the oral bioavailability of the polyphenol.

In this way, it will be possible that in the near future, we can use this natural product as a strong therapeutic agent for diabetes and related diseases.

Dosages

According to an **FAO** (Food and Agriculture Organization of the United Nations)/**WHO** (World Health Organization) **report** on food additives, the maximum recommended daily intake of curcumin is 0-1 mg/kg of body weight, without any adverse effects. Curcumin chronic toxicity studies have shown that it can be safely administered at oral doses that reach up to 8 g per day.

The simplest and most natural way to take turmeric is by using curry powder more often, as the multiple variations of this aromatic condiment lend themselves to different types of meat, fish and vegetables, as well as to other spices (coriander, cumin, fenugreek, ginger, cinnamon, etc.) which are beneficial to health.

If you want to take turmeric as such, you can take a dose from 3 to 10 g, up to 3 times a day, or in the form of curcumin in capsules, 500 mg two-three times a day, and it is better to be always combined with piperine.

Effectiveness

Strength	Resistant strength	Mass	Endurance	Slimming	Concentration	Recovery
–	–	–	+	+	+	++

TYROSINE

Description

Tyrosine is a non-essential aromatic amino acid that is synthesized by the body under normal conditions from another amino acid, phenylalanine. The tyrosine synthesis site is represented by the adrenal glands, from where, once the production from phenylalanine starts, it takes subsequent conversion pathways. It should be remembered that the tyrosine synthesis process starting from phenylalanine requires, in addition to phenylalanine hydroxylase enzyme, the cofactor tetrahydrobiopterin, which is also necessary in the processes of converting tyrosine itself into its main target products. Tyrosine is an essential component for the production of some important brain chemicals, including catecholamines: adrenaline, noradrenaline and dopamine.

Neurotransmitters help nerve cells to communicate and influence the mood. All three catecholamines exert effects in numerous parts of the body: within the brain, they exert their effects as neurotransmitters, while in the periphery they act as hormones. Tyrosine is also involved in the synthesis of melanin, the pigment responsible for the hair and skin color. Finally, tyrosine represents the synthesis substrate for the thyroid hormones. In addition to influencing the function of other organs responsible for the production of other hormones, tyrosine is one of the most involved amino acids in the structure of almost all proteins in the body. The majority of tyrosine that is not incorporated into proteins is catabolized for energy production.

Properties

- Traditionally, L-Tyrosine has been used to treat a variety of clinical conditions, such as attention deficit disorder (ADD), some forms of depression, to alleviate jet lag fatigue or to improve the cognition, such as during an exam preparation period.
- By stimulating the dopaminergic-adrenergic systems, L-tyrosine presumably causes an appetite suppression, an increased energy expenditure at rest and an increased fat oxidation.
- Furthermore, L-tyrosine is also converted into thyroid hormones which can contribute to the stimulation of the metabolism by increasing the energy expenditure at rest.
- Some research in sports science suggests that tyrosine may have the same energy-boosting effects as branched chain amino acids (BCAAs).
- The increase in plasma levels of these amino acids and the relative increase in the brain determine as a first consequence the decrease in the levels of another amino acid, 5-hydroxytryptophan (5-HTP), an inducer of fatigue, through its transformation into serotonin, while tyrosine increases the production of dopamine, since the feeling of fatigue is mainly determined by an increased serotonin/dopamine ratio. Therefore, tyrosine supplementation in athletes could decrease the feeling of fatigue and maintain the mental focus through the increase of dopamine.

In conclusion, from the scientific literature available today on the actual benefits deriving from tyrosine supplementation, we can say that this amino acid can certainly represent an excellent supplement to improve cognition and mental concentration during acute stress, and to improve the perception of stress. As for the rest of the potential benefits, especially the ones related to the improvement of fatigue management, the increase in energy expenditure and the induction of fatty acid oxidation, the scientific evidence, in some cases, is contradictory. Most of the L-tyrosine mechanisms are linked to the fact that it is a precursor of the catecholamine synthesis, therefore the most important effects of this amino acid at the neuronal level are expressed through the modulation of the synthesis of these neurotransmitters.

Evidence

A study carried out on rats has shown how the intake of L-tyrosine (200-400 mg/kg) can increase the concentrations of norepinephrine in the hippocampus, thus avoiding the acute reduction induced by stress in rats subjected to cold stress. This could demonstrate how the intake of L-tyrosine has the ability to reverse the cold stress-induced memory loss in humans. In another study, it was observed that taking 150 mg/kg of L-tyrosine before a cognitive test in a room where the temperature had been reduced from 22 to 4° C, was able to reduce the time required to response and to increase the number of correct responses, compared to individuals who had taken a placebo.

It has certainly been shown that the administration of tyrosine can accelerate the synthesis and the release of catecholamines, thus representing a useful agent in the treatment of central or peripheral disorders, associated with an insufficient release of catecholamines.

There is currently no evidence that supplementation with L-tyrosine can improve the memory compared to the subject's baseline level, but it may be able to attenuate a memory decrease associated with acute stress.

Tyrosine supplementation can improve the cognitive performance during sleep deprivation without significantly altering the sleep function. One study combined L-tyrosine supplementation with an "extended wakefulness" state and found that the administration of 150 mg/kg of L-tyrosine was able to mitigate the decline in the cognitive performance associated with this deprivation. Studies conducted on mice exposed to very low temperatures have shown a dose-dependent decrease in the immobility time from injections of L-tyrosine (200-400 mg/kg).

Therefore, supplementation with tyrosine can reduce the negative effects of cold stress, and some tests also confirm this in humans. In particular, in a study on humans in high altitude conditions, a protective effect against acute stress was noted thanks to the supplementation of 100 mg/kg of L-tyrosine (divided into two doses, taken one hour apart). The protective effect was manifested by fewer headaches, stress, fatigue, anguish, drowsiness, muscle pain, and with a better cold tolerance; however, such evidence is based on an assessment in an individual questionnaire. This study also noted improvements in mood, compared to a placebo.

Still on the subject of the stress response, we now introduce the concept of hormesis. A concentration-dependent response to an external stressor has been defined as hormesis. The concept of hormesis implies an adaptive process in which, at low doses, a chemical or physical agent that is harmful at higher doses, exerts a beneficial and protective effect in the body. Thus, hormetic processes must be considered fundamentally as adaptive responses. The response occurs when mechanical, chemical or biological insults exceed the body's capacity for homeostasis.

In fact, under stressful conditions, mitochondria release low levels of reactive oxygen species (ROS), which trigger a cytoprotective response called "mitochondrial hormesis". In the study in question, from 2020, we wanted to show that N-acetyl-L-tyrosine (NAT) functions as an intrinsic factor responsible for this activity in animals. N-acetyl-L-tyrosine is an acetylated form of the L-tyrosine amino acid. Acetylation ensures that tyrosine is soluble in water and it is the most bioavailable form of tyrosine on the market. NAT is present in the blood of healthy animals and its concentrations increase in response to stress.

What has been observed is that the pretreatment with NAT significantly increases the heat stress tolerance in tested insects and mice, and this is due to the effects triggered by the transient perturbation of the mitochondria induced by NAT, which causes a small increase in ROS production and leads to responses such as the activation of FOXO (a transcription factor implicated in longevity, resistance to oxidative stress and protection from neurodegenerative diseases), then an increase in Keap1 and also in antioxidant enzymes, with protective effects from cellular stress. In summary, it is proposed that NAT may be a vital endogenous molecule, as a trigger of mitochondrial hormesis.

From the above, it is clear that the N-acetyl-L-tyrosine metabolite works as an endogenous trigger for the mitochondrial hormesis in mammals and insects.

- The low levels of ROS released by mitochondria in difficulty have been deemed important for the induction of "mitormesis".
- Acetyl-L-tyrosine transiently disturbs the mitochondria, causing a slight increase of ROS production and leading to a triggering of mitormesis, allowing the cell to adapt to momentary states of stress.

In a study carried out in the United Kingdom (*European Journal of Applied Physiology*, 115: 373- 386, 2015), it was found that the **supplementation with tyrosine is able to improve the mental clarity and attention in soccer players** during a match simulation in conditions of high ambient temperature.

A pool of scholars from different Dutch universities in recent years, directed according to the occasion by Jongkees or Colzato, has carried out numerous researches that have shown good results at the cognitive and decisional level, but please refer to the chapter on concentration to avoid excessive repetitions.

In anti-aging medicine, the belief that increasing the levels of L-tyrosine in the brain can become an effective pharmacological method to alleviate neurological decline is growing stronger; this belief arises from the fact that catecholamines generally undergo a sharp decrease in states of dementia.

Surprisingly, catecholamines can act as antioxidants in the brain and be neuroprotective, although we are still at the level of preliminary studies. Finally, remember that tyrosine is the precursor of dopamine, which represents the "chemistry of mood" and the main regulator of the processes from which our thoughts arise. Supplementing with tyrosine could therefore increase the mental alertness, concentration level and above all the feeling of well-being, thus compensating for the physical and mental fatigue that can result from intense training or a low-calorie diet, strategies that are often adopted for weight loss.

It is also necessary to mention the etiology of the chronic headache, which is not yet well understood. A hypothesis on its genesis involves an abnormal metabolism of tyrosine. Tyrosine is usually metabolized into L-DOPA via hydroxylation, but another pathway involving its decarboxylation can lead to the accumulation of amines such as tyramine. It is this anomalous accumulation of amines that is suspected by some researchers to play a role in migraines. So, it is possible that higher L-tyrosine intake in migraine sufferers could fuel this process or make it worse.

Dosages

Regarding the recommended daily dosage, clinical studies indicate that tyrosine can be consumed in doses up to 12 g per day. Of course, taking such high doses is not recommended, except in special cases and on the advice of a doctor. A good dosage appears to be between 1 and 5 g, which can also be split into multiple doses throughout the day to maintain a steady supply of tyrosine to the system. Even a single dose, however, can improve the brain function on the spot.

The main side effects can be headaches, stomach pain and intestinal disorders, however they only occur with the highest doses, which, if necessary, must be achieved gradually.

There are some diseases or conditions that make the supplementation with tyrosine problematic: those who suffer from hyperthyroidism or Graves' disease should not take this supplement, as well as those who take drugs such as monoamine oxidase inhibitors or levodopa.

Effectiveness

Strength	Resistant strength	Mass	Endurance	Slimming	Concentration	Recovery
−	+	−	+	++	+++	−

VITAMIN C

Description
Vitamin C (VC), also called ascorbic acid, is a water-soluble vitamin and an essential nutrient (it must be strictly included in the diet). Many animals produce it endogenously, while humans, during evolution, have lost this ability. VC is mainly contained in fresh plant foods such as fruits (oranges, strawberries, mandarins, kiwis, lemons) and vegetables (spinach, broccoli, tomatoes, peppers, etc.). However, since VC is both sensitive to oxidation and thermolabile, these foods must be kept for not too long and must be eaten raw or in any case undercooked (cooking, in fact, reduces their content by up to 75%).

Properties
VC is a water-soluble antioxidant that protects against the free-radicals attack in the intracellular fluid and plasma. As an antioxidant, it is also important because it takes part in the regeneration of other important antioxidants such as glutathione and vitamin E (VE). It is important for the correct formation of connective tissue, in particular collagen (since it is its main structural protein). It is therefore essential for the skin, blood vessels, bones and for tissue repair. It supports the integrity of cell membranes, which is important in the defense barrier against viruses and bacteria.

It promotes the maturation, function and chemotaxis of phagocytes, but also that of T lymphocytes (cytotoxic CD8, in particular, but also the antibody-producing humoral line). At high dosages, it promotes the immune function of complement proteins and the production of IFN-γ. It also appears to take part in the cytokine modulation inherent in the production of histamine (by decreasing it). VC is essential in stressful situations because it is essential for maintaining optimal levels of cortisol, adrenaline and noradrenaline. The adrenal glands have the highest concentration of VC in our body and during a period of stress, they release it from their deposits, favoring a greater production of cortisol.

VC is a powerful antioxidant, which directly eliminates oxygen free radicals and restores other cellular antioxidants, including tetrahydrobiopterin and alpha-tocopherol. Therefore, VC can improve the virus-induced oxidative damage. Studies on the prevention of viral diseases seem conflicting, but instead agree that high doses of VC shorten the period of convalescence during infections. VC is essential for the absorption of other substances such as iron (iron supplementation is often associated with VC in deficient states of this mineral), but also for folic acid and VE, as well as for metabolism of some amino acids such as phenylalanine and tyrosine.

Evidence
A 2019 review (Righi et al.) investigated the evidence in the literature on the effects of VC supplementation on oxidative stress, inflammatory markers, muscle damage, soreness, and musculoskeletal function, in healthy volunteers after an exercise session. This study showed that the supplementation of VC immediately reduces the lipid peroxidation and the inflammatory response (IL-6-mediated), and this up to 2 hours after exercise, compared to the placebo.

However, it appears to have no effect on the muscle damage, cortisol levels, CRP (C-reactive protein, an inflammatory marker), pain and muscle strength. The modulation of lipid peroxidation can be explained both with the direct effect of VC on RONS (oxygen and nitrogen free radicals), and with the restoration of alpha-tocopherol (vitamin E, another actor in defusing the lipid peroxidation with an indirect effect).

The effective doses against peroxidation were above 500 mg. VC would be bioavailable in the bloodstream 40 minutes after taking it by mouth (obviously, the sublingual forms are faster). Based on the results found during sports competitions, vitamin C supplementation can be adopted by athletes as a strategy to promote the recovery after exercise or, in the case of beginner athletes, to aid in the recovery and continuity of regular physical exercise.

However, there is an obligation to point out that transient increases in the production of RONS, as well as the inflammatory response itself and the resulting damage, are necessary stimuli for the muscle adaptation and remodeling. Supplementing with antioxidants negatively interferes with the supercompensation and with the muscle remodeling, and it should be reserved for situations in which a prolonged performance is required and it does not provide for an appropriate recovery (marathon, triathlon, crossfit, etc.). Regarding strength exercises in the elderly, one study (Bobeuf et al., 2009) considered medium-high doses of VC (1000 mg) and VE (600 mg), noting how they produced a lean mass gain (probably by modulating the characteristic excess of free radicals in the elderly).

Dosages

The estimated daily VC requirement is about 90 mg/day for men and about 70 mg/day for women. This rate can be increased if the individual is in a particular condition (pregnancy, infections, prolonged physical exercise). To deal with the dosage topic, we must necessarily introduce the concept of micro-deficiencies. The aforementioned daily requirement depends on the RDA (Recommended Dietary Allowance), which corresponds to the amount of vitamins that protect against hypovitaminosis, such as scurvy. However, the amounts needed for the maximal effect of these vitamins can greatly exceed the RDA level. The spectrum of micro-deficiencies is identified precisely by the range between the RDA and the optimal quantity for the individual subject and can obviously differ from case to case. Many factors, in fact, can influence the state of micronutrients at the level of the organism, for example the lack of VC or certain food groups in the diet (due to a scarce availability or possibility of finding organic food, which has higher levels of vitamins). Some lifestyle choices (for example vegetarianism or veganism) can also affect the micro-deficiencies, in addition to voluptuous activities such as smoking, which requires higher doses of VC. A stressful lifestyle is often accompanied by a lack of sleep and a reduced physical activity. All of this can increase the oxidative stress and, therefore, the need for VC. Pathological conditions such as diabetes and obesity, infections or autoimmune diseases have a negative effect on the state of micronutrients, as well as some genetic assets. Seasonal changes or prolonged physical exercises can reduce the levels of micronutrients at the endogenous level (due to a drop in supply or an increased consumption). In this context, micro-deficiencies are very frequent and the evaluation of the supplementation with VC should be "tailored according to the subject" and should take into account all these aspects. There is no known lethal dose for humans. However, very high doses can induce the appearance of transient gastrointestinal disorders, such as diarrhea, flatulence and bowel movements, due to the acidity of the VC. Most commercially approved supplements go up to 180-1000 mg/day, with 2000 mg/day as the maximum daily intake limit. In general, doses <500 mg are adequate in healthy subjects, while in the pathological subjects with comorbidities and perhaps smokers, and in competitive athletes, it can reach 1 g per day. Some data, however, suggest that chronic high-dose VC supplementation may have a pro-oxidant rather than an antioxidant effect.

Effectiveness

Strength	Resistant strength	Mass	Endurance	Slimming	Concentration	Recovery
–	–	–	++	–	–	++

VITAMIN D

Description
Let's start by saying that vitamin D (VD) is not a vitamin, but a real steroid hormone like estrogen, testosterone and cortisol. As such, it derives from cholesterol and acts on its intracellular receptors (VDR) by modulating the gene expression. It is produced for the most part (80-90%) by the skin after being exposed to ultraviolet radiation, UVB in particular. The remainder is absorbed with food and, once it has passed the intestinal barrier, it reaches the blood by means of chylomicrons and through the lymphatic circulation. However, provitamin D that arrives in the bloodstream, produced through sun exposure or absorbed by food, must undergo two hydroxylations (addition of OH group) to become active, first by the liver and then by the kidney. At this point, the activated vitamin D molecule (1-25 dihydroxycholecalciferol or, for short, calcitriol) is formed.

Properties
In recent years, the work on VD has multiplied exponentially, greatly enriching the knowledge on the biochemical processes that involve it. It therefore seems wrong to attribute only the activity on the homeostasis of calcium and the mineral balance between plasma and bone tissue to this molecule. A good level of VD in our body has implications for the immune system, for the cardiovascular risk, sleep and an infinity of other very important functions. However, the concentration of VD and its receptors tends to decline with age. Daily life, made up of indoor jobs and indoor hobbies, limits the normal photometabolism of VD. Even the ingestion of foods that would favor its assimilation is severely deficient in today's diets, which are based on cereals. Over the years, these habits have produced an endemic hypovitaminosis with regard to VD, and many of the most common diseases of aging could be limited by a good control of this hormone. The ancient Egyptians spoke of the Sun God and the effects that his rays have on humans, "making them capable of expressing the strength of an entire crowd on their own". As for foods, fatty fish, cod liver oil, eggs, butter, vegetables, mushrooms are particularly rich in VD. It should be intriguing how the latter are the basis of nutrition for those populations who do not live in a latitude favorable to prolonged sun exposure. This is to understand that, if VD were not so fundamental, perhaps nature would not have provided in such a balanced and timely way to supply it.

Evidence
The first effect of VD is related to the mineral balance, of calcium and phosphates, between plasma and the skeletal system. VD, by binding its receptors at the gastrointestinal level, favors the greater absorption of calcium and phosphate from the intestinal lumen, thus raising their plasma concentrations. This plasma structure favors an inhibition of bone resorption, mediated by the parathyroid hormone and a stimulus on the secretion of calcitonin, which deposits these minerals in the bone, making it more resistant. It is therefore evident that a good level of VD is essential to avert and reduce the risk of fractures, especially with an advancing age. For many years, this was the only physiological mechanism recognized and

described in medical books. However, doctors used to never measure this hormone except in full-blown cases of osteoporosis/osteomalacia and therefore too late. But the VDR receptor for RV has been discovered in almost all tissues of the body and this has spurred scholars to investigate its other possible physiological roles. But let's follow the order. A decrease in type II muscle fibers was observed in muscle tissue biopsies of subjects with VD deficiency. Classically, this was attributed to muscle disuse resulting from bone depletion in the aforementioned pathological conditions. In fact, the supplementation with VD had reversed this trend and improved the number and trophism of type II muscle fibers (fast fibers with anaerobic metabolism). One study showed that **individuals with a VD deficiency can improve their strength and muscle mass even without exercising, only by taking this vitamin**. Other studies had shown a decrease in the percentage of falls in elderly subjects supplemented with VD, a percentage that further decreased if the association with calcium was made. These studies went in the same direction. The fibers that came to be reconstituted with the supplementation were in fact fast fibers, therefore the first to be activated during the "parachute maneuvers" that we implement in a reflex way after tripping. So, **VD directly affected the muscle tissue**, but to what extent and how? Subsequent tests with the handgrip dynamometer (measurement of hand grip strength) had shown a certain influence of the plasma concentration of calcitriol on the quality of muscle contraction. This is mainly because the VD muscle receptors allow a higher passage of plasma calcium into the muscle cells and its storage in the sarcoplasmic reticulum. The amount of calcium that escapes from this organelle into the muscle cell following a spike of the motor neuron, mediates the quantity and quality of the bonds between actin and myosin and their interaction during muscle contraction (one of the first symptoms of osteomalacia is, in fact, the muscle weakness). So, to put it simply, **VD is involved in the formation of muscle fibers and in the contraction quality**. But what is the evidence in athletes? Well, athletes and subjects in catabolism are perhaps more deficient in VD than the general population, already endemically affected even at favorable latitudes. Research on athletes suggests that optimal levels of VD can reduce the systemic inflammation, protect against stress fractures, stimulate the immune system, ensure optimal muscle function and help in the post-injury recovery.

In support of this concept, many athletes reach their peak physical fitness during the period of the year when VD (and sun exposure) is at its highest (summer and autumn). VD also seems to play a role in muscle anabolism. This effect would depend on IGF-1 (a metabolite of GH which must be free in the blood, in order to perform its anabolic role on the muscle). Most of the circulating IGF-1 is bound to a transport protein called IGFBP-3. This serves as a deposit for the IGF-1, which once unattached, can perform its functions. However, once free, it then undergoes a rapid clearance by the body. The blood concentration of this "IGF-1 reservoir protein" depends on many cofactors and, among these, one of the most significant is the presence of adequate quantities of calcitriol.

Lots of literature directly correlates the treatment with VD with an increase in the plasma concentration of IGF-1. The synergistic associations of VD with HMB or with leucine were also investigated. These associations resulted in an increase in the protein synthesis and lean mass.

VD also acts by controlling the gene expression that regulates the insulin receptors, increasing their sensitivity: since insulin stimulates the muscle growth, VD plays a fundamental role in this function. In a study by Salles et al. vitamin D3 has been shown to increase the ability of leucine to activate the insulin signal, thus increasing protein synthesis, and this occurs mainly by increasing the expression of the gene that codes for the insulin receptors.

VD would even play a role in the aerobic performance, where statistically significant improvement in VO_{2max} has been seen in athletes supplemented with this vitamin. In a review of the scientific literature, Rachela Podjednic and Lisa Ceglia of Tufts University in Boston, reported that low VD blood levels are associated with a lower aerobic capacity and a higher body mass index (weight/height ratio). In addition, a study of men and women aged between 20 and 76, conducted by Paul Thompson of Hartford hospital, found that **individuals with the highest VD levels were endowed with a greater strength**, both in the lower part and the upper part of the body, when compared with individuals of the same age and gender.

In addition to muscles, the VDR receptor is also widely represented in the adipose tissue. In particular, those who are very overweight, those with type 2 diabetes and those with metabolic syndrome have much lower VD levels than the control population. This aspect is explained by some authors with the fact that, being liposoluble, VD would tend to be sequestered by the fat, decreasing its bioavailability.

Some authors, in fact, suggest that supplements should be made by indexing them by body weight, underlining how higher doses are needed for an overweight person in order to fall within the blood range of an optimal concentration. Then, once the weight loss is established, less hormone will be enough because the adipose tissue will tend to release it spontaneously. This correlation between body fat and VD partly explains the possible correlation of this vitamin with testosterone. In overweight males, there is a greater activity of the aromatase enzyme, which converts testosterone into estrogen. This mechanism creates a vicious circle, as estrogen further facilitates the accumulation of fat at the visceral level, promoting the insulin resistance.

VD improves the insulin sensitivity, but more abdominal fat means less VD activated, because it is sequestered within the adipose tissue. So, there is a correlation between high estrogen levels and low testosterone and VD levels.

A study published in 2010 measured VD and testosterone in 2,229 men. A directly proportional correlation was found between total testosterone levels and VD levels, as well as a better ratio of free to bound testosterone in subjects with higher VD levels.

In another study, 54 overweight non-diabetic men took about 3,000 IU of VD per day or a placebo for 1 year. At the end of the study, only the group that had actually taken VD experienced a **considerable increase in the level of total, free and bioactive testosterone**, while the placebo group did not see any improvement. While supplementation with VD appears to be effective in overweight and elderly subjects, there is currently no evidence in favor of a positive effect on the performance with its supplementation in athletes, but it is reasonable to assume that a deficiency may have negative effects, which was verified in a study that correlated vitamin D3 deficiency and laryngeal spasms in elite athletes, 39 situation sports male athletes (football and basketball), aged 15-19 years, assessed with basic spirometry, maximal exercise test and serial spirometry at the end of the test.

Bronchoconstriction was confirmed when the expiratory flow in the first minute was reduced by 10% and laryngoconstriction when it was reduced by 25%. Baseline spirometry was normal for all athletes and, for VD deficiency, this was mild for 12, moderate for 21, and severe for 6 athletes. After the exercise test, 14 athletes were negative, 12 showed only laryngospasm, 4 had bronchospasm and 9 showed both pathological conditions. Laryngospasm was associated with severe VD deficiency, but bronchospasm was not. This suggests a possible negative influence of this deficiency on the athletic performance in predisposed patients (Mozzone, et al. *Exercise bronchospasm and laryngospasm and vitamin D deficiency in elite athletes.* Turin Institute of Sports Medicine, FMSI, Turin).

Research shows that VD protects against colds, flu and other respiratory diseases. A daily dose of VD was particularly useful, however even a weekly dose helps prevent the common cold and flu, while it should be noted that the occasional consumption of high doses of VD did not produce better benefits. Those who are deficient in VD will especially benefit from a regular intake of this vitamin. Several studies have suggested the action of this vitamin in various biological mechanisms, such as nociceptive sensitivity and the modulation of the sleep cycle.

Sleep is an important biological process regulated by different regions of the central nervous system, mainly the hypothalamus, in combination with different neurotransmitters. Pain, which can be classified as nociceptive, neuropathic and psychological, is regulated by both the central and peripheral nervous systems. In the peripheral nervous system, the immune system participates in the inflammatory process that contributes to hyperalgesia. Sleep deprivation is an important condition linked to hyperalgesia, and has recently also been associated with low VD levels. Ineffective sleep and sleep disturbances have been shown to play an important role in hyperalgesia and to be associated with different VD values. Researchers from the Department of Psychobiology of the Federal University of Sao Paulo, Brazil, have analyzed several clinical studies that reported the levels of VD in the blood of subjects with both sleep problems (sleep apnea and insomnia) and suffering from chronic pain (fibromyalgia and rheumatoid arthritis).

The results revealed insufficient levels of VD in the blood (less than 30 ng/mL) in both subjects with sleep disorders and in those with chronic pain. The daily intake of VD improved the quality of sleep and reduced the perception of pain; enriching the diet of the subjects suffering from insomnia with salmon and VD caused a reduction in the time taken to fall asleep, while the patients with sleep apnea, who, in addition to the VD deficiency, also had a high BMI, following the treatment of apnea with CPAP (constant pressure ventilation method in the airways) had benefits as regards both the quality of sleep and the levels of vitamin D in the blood, after only 7 days. Subjects suffering from fibromyalgia, rheumatoid arthritis and osteoarthritis, with the daily intake of VD, showed less hyperalgesia and a better sleep. It seems, therefore, that VD is able to suppress the proinflammatory response and to stimulate the anti-inflammatory one, as well as being a sleep modulator.

Hypovitaminosis D would also favor the chronic inflammatory state by means of an increase of PTH, correlated with the insulin resistance. The chronic increase in insulin leads, as has now been clarified, to an increase in acute phase cytokines and silent organic inflammation that leads to diabetes and cardiovascular problems. It is evident that all these are part of a vicious circle that regenerates itself at the expense of the health of the individual. Many studies have confirmed that **VD supplementation associated with a proper nutrition promotes weight loss in a way that is directly proportional to its circulating levels**. A mechanism for reducing the fat mass would be mediated by the regulation of adipocyte apoptosis induced by calcium and VD supplementation. This would also inhibit the adipogenesis, leading to a negative balance of the fat mass. But a weighted supplementation of VD also improves the cardiovascular risk picture, lowering the blood pressure and triglycerides. So, to summarize, some of the most important effects of VD on our body are related to the skeletal health, the maintenance of lean mass (in particular anaerobic II fibers), the decrease in fat mass and the strengthening of the immune system.

Early research regarding the relationship between VD and athletic performance was conducted by Russian and German researchers, who were the first to report the positive effects of exposure to sunlight in improving the athletic performance and in reducing the sports-related pain. In particular, significant improvements were found in speed, cardiovascular fitness and strength tests. Conversely, low VD levels in athletes have been linked to a decreased muscle strength, poor balance, and an increased risk of injury.

Increasing VD levels reduces the inflammation, pain and myopathy and increases the muscle protein synthesis, ATP concentration, strength and power. Research has shown that the administration of VD increases the anabolic effect of leucine: research conducted by researchers at the University Clermont Auvergne, in France, has shown that the higher the concentration of VD, the greater the anabolic effect of leucine. The study shows that VD increases the insulin receptors sensitivity and the activity of post-exercise cellular anabolic mechanisms.

A review published in 2014 on VD, analyzed several studies conducted on sports subjects. The data show that athletes have a high risk of VD deficiency, especially in winter when sun exposure is scarce; athletes who practice outdoor sports have a lower risk of incurring this deficiency. From the analysis of various researches, it emerged that supplementation with VD improves the sports performance in deficient athletes. Its effect seems greater when vitamin K2 is taken together with the VD, which is very important for delivering calcium to the right body areas (bones and muscles) and for avoiding dangerous deposits in the arteries, which could cause calcifications in the blood vessels.

Two studies reported a significant improvement in muscle strength following the intake of VD: a research conducted on male and female dancers showed a 18.75% increase in muscle strength of the subjects. The same results were reported in a study involving young soccer players. Another study has shown that VD supplementation increases the contraction force of the muscles on maximal bench press and squat exercises. The same results were reported by a study conducted on nineteen year-old swimmers: 12 female and 17 ,male, following supplementation with VD, showed improved strength parameters (measured with the hand-grip test). Scientists reported that the higher the levels of VD in the blood following the supplementation, the greater the muscle strength.

Another study analyzed the effects of VD supplementation on the muscle recovery: the participants were involved in a 30-minute high-intensity training program three times a week; the experimental group took VD, the second group took a placebo. At the end of the study, the two groups were compared and the scientists stated that the experimental group showed less muscle damage (lower levels of AST and ALT in the blood) after the exercises.

Finally, a large meta-analysis compared seven studies with a total of 792 participants. The studies were classified into two groups: Group 1 compared supplementation with VD and exercise versus exercise alone (describing the synergistic effect of RVVD combined with weight training) and group 2 compared VD supplementation alone to a placebo (describing the additional effect of exercise with weights, when combined with vitamin D supplementation). The analyzes of the studies of group 1 found that the muscle strength of the lower limbs was significantly improved in the intervention group; all other results showed positive but not significant effects, so further studies will be needed.

Dosages

The dose should be individualized and adapted to the blood levels found in laboratory tests. VD deficiency is often defined as <20 ng/mL (50 nmol/L), insufficiency as 20-32 ng/mL (50-80 nmol/L), and optimal levels as> 50-70 ng/mL (100 nmol/L). The intake can be done daily or with loads, but the former is preferable for its better manageability. In general, between 2000 and 5000 IU of VD could be taken daily, depending on the initial framework. As a load, however, a commonly prescribed treatment to quickly correct the VD deficiency is a weekly dose of 50,000 IU for 8 weeks. In the case of higher dosages and continuous use, it is good to associate it with vitamin K2, in a vitamin D/vitamin K2 ratio (IU/mg) of 10: 1, in order to avoid the atherosclerotic plaques because of an excessive calcium absorption, as vitamin K2 favors the deposition of calcium in the bones.

Effectiveness

Strength	Resistant strength	Mass	Endurance	Slimming	Concentration	Recovery
+++	+	++	++	++	–	+

VITARGO®

Description

Vitargo® is the registered name for a maltodextrin formulation designed and patented in Sweden at the Karolinska Institutet in Stockholm. As we explained in the part concerning maltodextrins (MD), these are carbohydrate supplements designed for their physicochemical qualities to provide a gradual supply of this macronutrient to the body. We have seen, however, that these supplements have a high glycemic index, almost comparable to that of white sugar. However, unlike what happens with the latter, glucose recovery takes place without triggering complicated digestion and absorption mechanisms that would damage the individual's hydration. So, even if the properties concerning a different absorption kinetics as a function of their polymerization have been somewhat reduced, they are still supplements that can be taken, with the appropriate precautions, during the physical activity. The production of MD derives from the treatment of starchy precursors and the rate of hydrolysis that is set, accounts for a whole series of different properties and kinetics in the body. In this way, it was possible to offer a wide range of products adaptable to the needs of each individual sport. The formulation of Vitargo®, in particular, has advantageous characteristics compared to the other formulations and now we will go on to explain them in an analytical way.

Properties

The properties to be taken into account when choosing a maltodextrin, in order of importance, are:

1. The nature of the starch that is used for the formulation.
2. Dextrose equivalence (DE), i.e. how similar it is to glucose (low DE = slightly similar, high DE = very similar).
3. The molecular weight, which is an index of the osmotic pressure it exerts in the body.
4. The glycemic index, which is a measure of the molecule's absorption rate.

Vitargo® derives from the hydrolysis of corn or potato starch, so it can also be safely used in celiac athletes or athletes with gluten sensitivity. Usually the formulation of MD such as this one still provides for quite complex enzymatic steps that tend to lose the protein part responsible for the immune response towards the product. However, if you want to be sure that aspects of this type do not affect the performance of the subject, this formulation (deriving from naturally gluten-free starches) is very safe. The ED of Vitargo® is very low; this means that the polymer is very complex from a structural point of view (therefore very dissimilar from simple dextrose).

In fact, the molecular weight of Vitargo® ranges from 500,000 to 700,000 daltons, while for example that of a normal MD ranges from about 1000 to 10,000 daltons. As we have already illustrated in the general part on MD, glucose (or dextrose), being a very small molecule, tends to surround itself with water. In particular, every single molecule of glucose attracts four molecules of water. The complexity of the structure of the Vitargo® molecule in terms of glucose chains is therefore high. This being the case, the number of molecules per dose in a solution will therefore be much lower than that of a glucose solution (made up of single dextrose monomers).

The osmolarity and the osmotic pressure exerted by Vitargo® in the intestinal lumen will therefore be very low. Recall that the osmotic pressure of two solutions at different concentrations on the sides of a semipermeable membrane produces a displacement of liquids which is directly proportional to the number of molecules of the hypertonic solution (the most concentrated, with the greatest number of particles).

Since Vitargo® is basically a hypotonic solution, like all hypotonic solutions, it will have few molecules in the solution and will not cause a fluid retention in the stomach and intestines. This aspect favors the rapid assimilation of the macronutrients in question. The latter is a fairly unique feature for hyperenergetic solutions, which, being usually based on dextrose, often create a high osmotic pressure in the intestine and gastrointestinal symptoms in the athlete if taken during the competition.

Like all MDs, Vitargo® has a high glycemic index (137 against the glucose value, which is 140, while 100 is referable to white bread), so it is absorbed quickly. The reason is that being a highly refined compound, it lacks those organic parts that modulate the absorption of nutrients in normal food. In general, the rapid restoration of the muscle glycogen and the supply of a much more efficient fuel during sports activities are therefore favored.

Evidence

We have already talked about the properties of MDs in the reference paragraph. A further concept that can be added is given by the properties deriving from the amylose-amylopectin ratio of these products. **Amylose** is the main starch chain, made from glucose monomers joined by α (1→4) bonds, while amylopectin forms the side chains joined by α (1→6) bonds. **Amylopectin** is the most attacked part by heat and enzymes. Amylose, on the other hand, is the least digestible part, so much that there are products called resistant starches (RS, Resistant Starches) which are almost completely made of amylose and have very low GI. Once a starch is attacked by heat or enzymes, it tends to lose parts of amylopectin in the solution, which gel (become more viscous). The lower the amylose/amylopectin ratio of a form of starch (therefore the more amylopectin is represented), the more this happens. Under these conditions, the dextrose monomers end up in solution and can more easily be absorbed. The manufacturers of supplements had therefore postulated an inverse relationship between the glycemic index of an MD and its amylose/amylopectin ratio. In particular, a lot of amylopectin → high glycemic index; a lot of amylose → low glycemic index. But some studies on waxy maize starch (**WMS**, Waxy Maize Starch), formed almost entirely of amylopectin, have shown that this carbohydrate had a low glycemic index. The apparent contradiction lays in the fact that in the first years of production, Vitargo® (high GI) was extracted from waxy corn starch (later replaced by potato starch in 2005). The explanation was soon given, as the amylopectin-rich molecules of the WMS were treated in vitro with enzymes, for a later use. So it was during this refining that the glycemic index rose, giving Vitargo® the properties described above. A "take home message", therefore, is to remember that the kinetics of foods and the kinetics of supplements can be profoundly different, even if they have the same origin. Untreated waxy maize starch has completely opposite kinetics, and it is used as a super starch in cases of glycogenosis or in endurance sports, to keep the blood sugar stable (see above, *Super starch*).

In 2000, in a study by Aulin et al., 13 healthy and well-trained men ingested carbohydrate solutions (respectively a glucose and a Vitargo® solution) after particularly intense exercises that depleted their glycogen stores. Glycemia and insulin were measured every 30 minutes during the post-exercise period and muscle biopsies were performed at the end of the exercise, and after 2 and 4 hours of recovery. The average muscle glycogen content after the exercise was higher in the group that had taken Vitargo®.

Also in 2000, the same group wanted to study the gastric emptying times of a glucosate compared to Vitargo®, finding that the latter had much better emptying kinetics.

A subsequent study (Stephens et al., 2008) demonstrated an improvement in the performance in those who took Vitargo® compared to a glucose solution, during a high-intensity cycle ergometer exercise.

In summary, the studies reported by the manufacturer show that, compared with normal carbohydrates, Vitargo® has a **70% faster glycogen recovery**, a gastric passage speed greater than 80%, an **improvement in performance by 23%** and an insulin response greater than 78%.

Dosages

The manufacturer recommends dissolving 30 g of the product in 400 mL of water and taking it during the day (therefore the threshold of 14% of solution should not be exceeded). However, this formulation should be adapted to the goals of different athletic performances and it should be combined with other macronutrients or supplements in order to achieve maximum results. In the case of endurance or mixed performances, a part of this solution should be taken in the pre-workout, perhaps together with BCAA 1:1:1 (5 g), so as not to have a reflex hypoglycemia, a part during the activity to maintain the level of performance and a part in the post-workout, to promote the recovery.

The dosage will obviously be individualized with respect to the glycogen stores and the diet, the type of effort and its duration. In the case of purely lactacid performance aimed at potency and hypertrophy, an identical pre-workout (Vitargo® + BCAA 1:1:1) and a post-workout with Vitargo® and leucine (3-4 g) can be used directly.

Effectiveness

Strength	Resistant strength	Mass	Endurance	Slimming	Concentration	Recovery
–	+++	++	+++	–	–	+++

WAXY MAIZE (WAXY CORN STARCH)

Description

Corn starch is well known above all for its uses in the kitchen and for its presence in many industrial products that exploit its properties and characteristics, which depend on the composition of amylose and amylopectin. In corn starch we find about 30% of amylose, while the remaining 70% is made up of amylopectin: the first is a linear polymer of glucose and gives a harder consistency than the second; amylopectin, on the other hand, is a branched polymer of glucose and tends to form a gel, making the products more viscous. The percentages in which these two polymers are present can be modified, in order to have a product that adapts as much as possible to the needs of the producer and/or consumer.

The two polymeric structures have a different timing of assimilation: the branched chains are digested first, while the linear ones are digested more slowly, which is why starchy sources that have more amylose than amylopectin generally have a lower glycemic index and a longer digestion time.

Table 44.10 The proportions of amylose and amylopectin in the starch molecule from different sources

Foods	Amylose (%)	Amylopectin (%)
Wheat	25.0	75.0
Corn	24.0	76.0
Rice	18.5	81.5
Potatoes	20.0	80.0
Tapioca	16.7	83.3

Waxy maize starch (WMS, Waxy Maize Starch) is a polysaccharide consisting of 90-99% amylopectin, and for this reason it has a high glycemic index. It is actually the "basic" form of Vitargo®, which is derived from it. It is characterized by a high molecular weight and a low osmolarity.

Properties

Given the composition, waxy corn starch should, at least in theory, have a glycemic index that is very similar to glucose, given its high digestibility. Hence, it was assumed that it could replace glucose as a post-workout carbohydrate source. Therefore, based only on its structure, it was proposed that the potential characteristics of this molecule were: a rapid stimulation of the plasma insulin production, a rapid blocking of catabolic mechanisms (gluconeogenesis), an anticortisolemic effect, being a promoter of glycogenosynthesis and a vehicle of amino acids and other molecules taken with it, favoring a better assimilability.

All this without forgetting the potential advantage of not promoting a water retention, which is caused by glucose. These interpretations led to generalizations, stating that all high molecular weight carbohydrates, even if more complex and with longer glucose chains, were assimilated faster than simpler structured carbohydrates and also led to greater glycogen storages. It was 2009 when these alleged effects of WMS were denied, and opposite characteristics were proven: a gradual release of glucose as a long-lasting and sustained glucose source.

Evidence

In one study, 50 g of carbohydrates from white bread, waxy maize starch or a mixture of maltodextrin and sucrose (approximately 3:1 ratio) were administered over 3 different days. The response given by blood glucose and blood insulin, calorie expenditure and appetite were therefore measured for 4 hours. After 2 hours:

- the mix of maltodextrin and sugar = glycemic index 163;
- waxy maize starch = 63;
- white bread = 71.

The insulin response measured in the first hour was 3.5 times higher (and even faster) with maltodextrin and sugar, and 1.6 times higher with white bread, when compared with waxy corn starch. These results, like those of numerous other studies, even led to the supposition that it would be more suitable as a long-term source of glucose, in endurance exercises or for individuals who need to control their blood sugar fluctuations.

The misunderstanding about the potential short-term effect probably arose from an erroneous assimilation of the waxy corn starch to Vitargo®, which was produced by it, without taking into account the patented process that distinguishes the latter and which gives it its special characteristics.

We therefore understood how the amylopectin content is not necessarily synonymous with a rapid digestion or absorption.

Dosages

It is recommended to take 30 to 50 g of waxy corn starch dissolved in 500-1000 mL of water. It is more suitable for those who need to take more energy from carbohydrates, looking for a slow but prolonged release of glucose into the blood. As for its use in sports such as bodybuilding and fitness, it could be useful as a possible substitute for the carbohydrate portion of a meal, as an alternative to food, preferably in the hours preceding the physical activity, rather than in the following ones, when we can consume more indicated molecules such as cyclodextrins.

Effectiveness

Strength	Resistant strength	Mass	Endurance	Slimming	Concentration	Recovery
–	+++	++	+++	–	–	+++

YOHIMBINE

Description

Pausinystalia yohimbe is a tree belonging to the *Rubiaceae* family that is widespread in the West African regions (Nigeria, Cameroon, Congo). From the innermost part of its bark, the drug "yohimbe" is obtained, in which we find various active ingredients, including yohimbine, the indole alkaloid most represented in the plant and also the one that is most studied. The quality and quantity of yohimbine within the cortex is highly variable, and the optimum qualitative-quantitative ratio is found at the level of the cortex of the main stems. Furthermore, the concentration of the active ingredient is subject to seasonal variations, being at its maximum during the rainy season and at a minimum during the dry season.

Properties

The use of yohimbine is very widespread in traditional Chinese medicine, where it is widely used for the preparation of infusions and herbal teas considered beneficial for male impotence and sexual desire, but also for the strengthening of physical and intellectual abilities, to support the athletic performance, for weight loss, to lower the blood pressure and, finally, for states of anxiety and depression. Basically, it is considered an aphrodisiac and a stimulating substance, capable of bringing various benefits to the body and mind, up to producing psychedelic effects at high doses.

In scientific literature there are several studies to support the fact that the oral intake of yohimbine can exert a positive effect in the treatment of erectile dysfunction (ED) in men, in the increase of sexual desire and in the resolution of sexual problems of different natures (for example, due to stress, use of drugs or pathologies). Its aphrodisiac properties are due to the ability to interact with the α_2-adrenergic receptors, which regulate the release of neurotransmitters by the nerve endings. In particular, yohimbine acts as a potent and selective adrenergic antagonist of α_2 receptors.

These receptors act as a kind of thermostat, able to sequester part of the released noradrenaline and to inhibit its release. Thanks to the action of yohimbine, the inhibition "negative feedback" control exerted by the α_2-adrenergic receptors is therefore lacking, with a consequent increase in the noradrenergic activity, which results in greater dilation of blood vessels in the corpora cavernosa and an increase in the nerve impulses, improving the sexual performance (greater vasodilation and greater blood flow to the male sexual organ supports the erection, improving the sexual performance and increasing desire).

Recently, in the western world, yohimbine is known and appreciated in the sports field also for its ability to optimize the weight loss process and to improve the athletic performance; these properties are also mediated by the blockade of adrenergic receptors. The latter can be of type α and type β, they are distributed differently in our organism and perform different functions. In particular, in areas where the fat is stubborn, there is a greater presence of α_2-adrenergic receptors, which are considered anti-lipolytic, as they are less responsive to the action of adrenaline and noradrenaline. The blockade of α2 (anti-political) receptors induced by yohimbine results in an increase in lipolysis.

This leads to the inhibition of the synthesis of the adipose tissue and, at the same time, to an increase in its mobilization. What type of adipose tissue are we talking about? We mainly refer to the fat located in the thighs and hips, precisely where there is a greater concentration of α_2-adrenergic receptors. Consequently, the use of yohimbine-based supplements could prove to be particularly useful in the hypolipolytic individual, or in the ginoid one, who accumulates adipose tissue right at the level of the thighs and hips (typical pear shape) and who wishes to decrease the "stubborn" fat precisely in these critical areas.

The use of yohimbine in sports has been documented in several studies, from which it emerged that the intake of the active ingredient before the training is able to improve the sports performance, an effect due to its stimulating properties on the nervous system, the increase in the blood flow and the usage of reserve triglycerides (stored in the adipose tissue) for energy purposes.

Some evidence suggests that yohimbine may also be useful in the treatment of orthostatic hypotension, or the "jolt to the head" that can occur in people with low blood pressure levels. Finally, some studies argue that the use of the drug may be useful in the treatment of anxiety and fear related to phobias, however further research is needed to validate its effective use in combination with other therapies.

Evidence

Most of the research concerning Pausinystalia yohimbe was carried out on yohimbine which, as mentioned, is the most represented indole alkaloid. Once in circulation, it quickly crosses the blood brain barrier and when it reaches the central nervous system, it acts as an antagonist of the α_2-adrenergic receptors. This direct action on the adrenergic receptors has several consequences: human studies have shown that yohimbine is able to influence the sexual behavior: the alkaloid acts as a vasodilator and, by blocking the a_2-adrenergic receptors, it increases the blood flow to the level of the corpora cavernosa, maintaining its filling and therefore the erection. The aphrodisiac action of yohimbine can be enhanced by the simultaneous intake of arginine or citrulline, which are involved in the production of nitric oxide, a powerful vasodilator.

Other studies have shown that yohimbine is able to improve the sports performance: it, in fact, is able to increase the motor activity, to increase the muscle excitement and contraction, and induce the release of the antidiuretic hormone, ADH; the release of ADH in turn determines a fluid retention, an increase in the blood pressure and heart rate. This results in a better blood circulation to the muscles, which can lead to an improved sports performance. In particular, a study conducted on humans analyzed the effects of administering the active ingredient before the physical activity: scientists reported that yohimbine taken pre-workout promotes the sympathetic activity of the central and peripheral nervous system and increases the serum levels of free fatty acids (FFAs, Fat Free Acids) during the exercise.

The release of fatty acids in the plasma allows their use for energy purposes, and this has two consequences: the improvement of sports performance due to a greater availability of energy substrates and, secondly, the promotion of localized weight loss by stimulating the mobilization of stored triglycerides in the adipose tissue.

The effect depends on the dosage used, but it is important to consider that some studies have reported the appearance of some side effects (such as anxiety, hypertension, tremor, sweating) at doses above 30 mg/day. Furthermore, yohimbine is effective in reducing the body fat. An interesting study was conducted on professional soccer players; the athletes were divided into two groups: the study group took yohimbine orally (tablets containing 10 mg of the active ingredient, two separate intakes per day, for a total of 20 mg/day). The control group, on the other hand, took an equal number of placebo tablets. The supplementation protocol, lasting 21 days, was conducted in a context of a controlled diet and hydration for each subject.

At the end of the study, the changes in body composition in terms of lean mass and fat mass in each athlete were analyzed. As for the lean mass, including the muscle mass, no significant changes were identified, while there was a significant reduction in the body fat percentage (from an average of 9.3% to an average of 7%). It can therefore be concluded that the supplementation with yohimbine in combination with resistance training (i.e. strength training or weight training) may be suitable as a strategy for a localized fat loss in sports subjects.

Dosages

Normally, for the preparation of the drug, the chopped bark is dissolved in water or alcohol. Yohimbe or yohimbine supplements are commercially available. It is important to keep in mind that the concentration of yohimbine in the extract of the tree bark can be variable and it is therefore appropriate to refer to the amount of active ingredient, namely yohimbine, which is responsible for the pharmacological and therapeutic properties that we described. You can buy yohimbine-based supplements, in the form of yohimbine hydrochloride, on websites that freely sell "smart drugs".

In addition, supplements are available on the market in which yohimbine is associated with other compounds such as ginseng, guarana, Muira Puama, arginine, citrulline, caffeine, which act synergistically to produce the desired therapeutic effect. Studies show that taking yohimbine in the form of a food supplement (yohimbine HCL) is safe and free of side effects at a dosage of 0.2 mg/kg of body weight.

At such quantities, a stimulating and/or aphrodisiac effect is obtained without significant implications on the heart rate, blood pressure and anxiety states. Given the short half-life of the compound, the dose should be divided into several daily intakes, preferably taken on an empty stomach (as its effects would seem partially canceled by the concomitant food intake). Since the intake of yohimbine is associated with an increase in the postprandial insulinemia, it is essential that the supplement is taken between meals in those wishing to lose weight. Dosages higher than 30 mg/day can cause palpitations, nausea, tremors, sweating, stress or anxiety, therefore they are not recommended.

Effectiveness

Strength	Resistant strength	Mass	Endurance	Slimming	Concentration	Recovery
+	++	–	++	++++	++	–

ZMA

Description

ZMA is a completely natural product that contains zinc monomethionine aspartate, magnesium aspartate and vitamin B6. Tests and analyzes carried out on a significant sample of people have found that it is quite common for the body to suffer from low amounts of zinc and magnesium. This situation, especially frequent in athletes, affects the immune system, sleep quality, metabolism and the sports performance. ZMA supplementation is therefore recommended both for those facing a particular period of stress and for athletes who want to improve their physical performance.

Properties

ZMA is considered a mineral formula with anabolic properties as, through scrupulously conducted clinical studies, it has shown an increase in the level of anabolic hormones and muscle strength in trained athletes, with improvements in free and total testosterone levels. Another important property of this supplement is that linked to the improvement of the quality of the night sleep: a better and deeper sleep, for the athlete and not only, means more rest, less stress, a faster recovery from heavy workouts, therefore an improvement in the performance.

An interesting study on wrestlers has shown how zinc supplementation for 4 weeks can avoid the decrease in the values of thyroid hormones and testosterone, typical of subjects subjected to intense training. **Zinc** is therefore essential to support the production of thyroid hormones, which, among other things, are also involved in maintaining the metabolic rate at adequate levels. Research confirms that when the diet is low in zinc, thyroid hormone levels are low, resulting in a decrease in the burned calories. Another important aspect of zinc supplementation is that of maintaining leptin levels, a hormone responsible for improving the sense of satiety: South Korean researchers have found that zinc deficiency significantly reduces the circulating leptin levels.

In zinc-L-monomethionine, zinc is therefore associated with methionine, a sulfur amino acid essential for the body. This amino acid itself is important for the functioning of the liver and for the production of antibodies. In addition, it prevents the accumulation of fat in the liver and participates in the formation of some non-essential amino acids. It has been shown that the zinc-L-monomethionine compound does not simultaneously cause interference with the absorption of iron or copper, minerals of fundamental importance. This form of zinc is able to reduce the absorption of heavy metals such as, for example, lead, unlike other forms of chelators. In addition to this extreme ease of absorption, zinc-L-monomethionine has a strong antioxidant capacity thanks to the presence of methionine. In fact, this compound is able to inhibit the activity of oxygen free radicals and superoxide radicals, through both enzymatic and non-enzymatic processes. These capacities were evaluated by in vitro experiments and it was shown that at the cell membrane level, this compound has an activity similar to that of vitamin E, but much higher than that of vitamin C and beta-carotene. Even in diabetic patients, an increase in zinc is noted when taking composed zinc formulas, unlike the intake of simple zinc. Magnesium has already been treated and in a specific way but magnesium aspartate is particularly bioavailable and can also boast the properties of aspartic acid which increases tolerance and physical performance in sports activities by promoting fat oxidation and reducing fatigue or depression.

A supplementation of zinc and magnesium, even taken individually, also allows you to maintain lower levels of training induced cortisol (the stress hormone).

Evidence

The ergogenic action of the ZMA has been proven by numerous researches. A study of eight male subjects showed that the muscle endurance and total work capacity decline rapidly with zinc deficiency and that the degree of decline correlates with the reduction in the plasma concentrations of this mineral.

The following study is considered the most significant of all those carried out on this supplement.

Lorrie Brilla, a sports performance researcher at Western Washington University, recently reported that ZMA significantly **increased the free testosterone levels and the muscle strength in NCAA football players**. The results extrapolated from this study were presented by Dr. Brilla on June 2, 1999 at the 46th Annual Meeting of the American College of Sports Medicine in Seattle, and were officially published in the ACSM journal, *Medicine and Science in Sports and Exercise*, vol. 31 n. 5, May 1999.

Specifically, Brilla reported that a group of competitive football players who took ZMA in the evening during the 8-week training program in the spring, had a 2.5-fold increase in their muscle strength compared to a group that took a placebo. After the training period, in the ZMA group, the strength of the legs (measured by an isokinetic dynamometer) increased by 11.6% compared to only 4.6% in the placebo group. In addition, these athletes recorded an increase in free and total testosterone of 30%, compared to the 10% decrease found in the placebo group. Finally, the ZMA group had a slight increase in insulin-like growth factor (IGF-1) levels, compared with a 20% decrease in the placebo group. Many other studies have shown similar results.

The effect of regulating the thyroid hormone production is confirmed by a study by the University of Massachusetts (Amherst), which showed that subjects who followed a low-zinc diet had significantly lowered metabolic rates. The intake of 25 mg of zinc per day for 20 days raised their metabolic rate to levels higher than those prior to the diet.

It is now known that zinc is essential for the immune function; in particular, zinc participates in many aspects related to the immune system. Research confirms that the incidence of acute lower respiratory tract infections significantly decreases following a zinc supplementation. Zinc has also been found to help significantly reduce the duration of fever and the severity of pneumonia and other serious lower respiratory tract infections. Research has shown that people who receive zinc at the onset of cold symptoms have a shorter duration and a lower severity of the cold.

Dosages

The dosages and the proportion between the various constituents of the ZMA are very important. The most effective ZMA supplements provide 11 mg of vitamin B6, 450 mg of magnesium aspartate and 30 mg of zinc monomethionine aspartate.

Effectiveness

Strength	Resistant strength	Mass	Endurance	Slimming	Concentration	Recovery
++	+	++	+	+	−	+++

Acknowledgments

It has been a long time since, for the first time, I considered the idea of writing a book on sports nutrition and especially on supplements. As a doctor, but above all as a "gym addicted" and sports fan in general, I have always tried to be as updated as possible on new discoveries in the field of nutrition and supplementation. For this reason, over the years, I have collected and cataloged a lot of material from studies, research and scientific articles, consulting books, magazines, cutting-edge websites and participating in workshops, conferences and training courses, at home and abroad. All this has allowed me to become aware of how the current panorama in the field of food supplements is becoming increasingly vast, being supportive not only in the sports field, but also establishing itself in the field of traditional medicine and in antiaging and functional medicine.

If, on the one hand, all this has contributed to broadening my sphere of interest, on the other hand, it has made it increasingly difficult to find the time to organize the collected material. Only with the collaboration with a team of professionals with whom, in the meantime, I was related through a great work of research, data analysis, translation and homogenization, I was able, today, to achieve my goal. For the realization of this project, I must therefore thank my collaborators, professionals who follow the motto "we practice what we preach" and who personally observe an adequate diet, train constantly and take supplements.

At this point, I feel that it is my duty to present one by one, in strict alphabetical order, all those who have collaborated in the creation of the second edition of this volume.

Andrea Angelozzi. Degree in Biological Sciences. He practices freelance both in Parma and Teramo. He is a COM Diet® Advisor and Antiaging Advisor, has acquired the AFFWA AMFPC (Metabolic and functional approach in clinical practice) certification and is part of the AFFWA teaching staff. He practices powerlifting at a competitive level and is a fitness and bodybuilding instructor.

Alex Ardenti. Director and photographer, based in Los Angeles, to whom I owe the numerous photo shoots over the years. The cover photograph and my photos on the inside pages are taken by him. He was a European junior bodybuilding champion (NABBA).

Antonella Berardi Nazzarena. Degree in Nutrition Sciences; Master's degree in Nutrition Science. She has obtained several degrees, including "Biotype-specific training and diet" and "The role of circadianity in the onset of diseases and its influence on the body composition" at the Open Academy of Medicine in Switzerland; particularly attentive to the world of women, her studies continue to focus on the delicate female world. She was classified second in the bikini category, Grand Prix Palaeventi Alessandro Grassi in Rossano in 2013, and fifth at the Grand Prix city of Taranto-Grand Slam Open Tour 2013, Miss Body Fashion category (NBBUI).

Anella Serena Borzacchiello. Three-year degree in Quality Control with a nutraceutical focus and a specialization course in "Safety and Quality in the agri-food sector"; Master's degree in Human Nutrition Sciences. Operator in natural food education and nutrition, teacher of HACCP courses. Thanks to her studies on human nutrition, she has acquired over the years the passion for a proper nutrition and sport, which she practices personally.

Alessandra Cascone. Bachelor's degree in Biological Sciences; Master's degree in Biology and Biomedical Applications; advanced training course at the University of Salerno in Dietetics and Nutrition for Wellness, Sport and Physical Performance; training course in Ketogenic Diet, COM Diet® Advisor (AFFWA); training course in Advanced and Sports Basic Nutrition (SIFA). She has always had a passion for sports, carrying out artistic gymnastics at a competitive level for 12 years. She currently practices sports regularly.

Marco Tullio Cau. Degree in Clinical Psychology at the La Sapienza University of Rome and subsequently in Communication Sciences and Sociology at the same university. He also attended numerous Masters, including the Master's in Clinical Nutrition at the Niccolò Cusano University, Rome, the two-year Master's in Sport Psychology (Higher School of Sport Psychology, Rome), the Master's in Psychology of Food Behavior SPICAP, all in Rome. He participated in the advanced training course in Antiaging and Antistress Methodology at La Sapienza University, in the "Lifestyle Expert over 60" course at the University of Bari, in the two-year course as a sexual consultant (ISC-Rome) and obtained various certifications such as AMFPC (Metabolic and functional approach in the clinical practice) AFFWA, ECPS (EFS-ESSM Qualified Psycho-Sexologist, first world certification, Istanbul, Turkey) and others in the USA, where he also attended university courses at the Faculty of Psychology and Sociology of the University of California, Santa Barbara. He teaches AFFWA, AMIA, Sanis, Issa-Italia, Nabba, for the Coni Sports School and for the training course "Wellness and lifestyles", held at La Sapienza University. Marco was an Italian junior bodybuilding champion (NABBA) in 1983 and, in accordance with the motto "we practice what we preach", he still engages in discus throwing, a discipline in which he competes for the Principality of Monaco, after being Italian master champion and record holder multiple times.

Paolo Conforti. Degree in Medicine and Surgery, specialist in Sports Medicine. In 2012 he collaborated on a project with the Italian Space Agency (ASI) on "Cerebrospinal venous return in microgravity". He has acquired the AMFPC (Functional Metabolic Approach in Clinical Practice) AFFWA certification. Course in Regenerative, Anti-Aging and Environmental Medicine – Association of Italian Anti-Aging Doctors (AMIA). Course in Functional and Regulatory Medicine – Italian Society of Functional Medicine (SIMF). Lecturer at the Master of Systemic Functional Medicine – Guidonia Montecelio, Rome. He wrote the "Squilibri della funzionalità cardiovascolare" chapter of the *Guida alla Medicina Funzionale*. Black belt 1st Dan of karate and already a competitive karate athlete.

Laura Crugnola. Degree in Biology; Master's Degree Course in Food Sciences and Human Nutrition. Lifestyle Medicine and Functional Medicine Advisor. COM Diet® Advisor. She works as a nutritionist biologist in Parma with Dr. Spattini and in Milan, where she works for SIFA Srl. She practices fitness and functional training. She is the testimonial of the Lacertosus sports equipment company.

Fabrizio D'Agostino. Degree in Exercise Science and Biotechnology for Health; Master's degree in Human Nutrition Science. He attended the Master's "Dietetics Applied to Lifestyle: from Sedentary to Sports Activities". President of SIFA Srl. He works as a nutritionist biologist and kinesiologist. Lecturer at the Masters of the Federico II and Vanvitelli Universities of Naples, Bicocca of Milan and Unisa of Salerno. Organizer and scientific director of the national congresses. He is the creator of the SIFA Dieta nutritional software and of the FitnessPlay training software.

Fernando Finardi. Lifestyle Medicine and Functional Medicine Advisor, Personal Trainer, Nutrition educator with a Master's in Antiaging Nutrition (AFFWA Academy). Over time he has practiced judo, athletics, cycling, jogging and pilates, but it is bodybuilding, the sport that after 38 years he still carries on with passion, which combines a healthy diet, anti-aging integration and proper lifestyle. He is a great "devourer" of books and scientific papers dedicated to health and well-being. He collaborated in the correction of the texts and in maintaining relations with the various co-authors and with the editorial studio.

Valeria Galfano. Degree in medicine and surgery; food science specialist; Lifestyle Medicine and Functional Medicine Certification (AFFWA). For many years she has been interested in nutrition and sports supplementation, teaching at SIFA on the course "Training, nutrition and supplementation for women". She teaches OPES and CSEN for basic, advanced and elite level personal trainer courses. She holds two Masters for the SISDCA, dealing with topics related to eating disorders. She is the author of the chapter "The diet in cardiovascular diseases" of the book *Prevenzione e terapia dietetica*; she is the author of scientific articles for the journals like *The Endocrinologist and Pharmanutrition and Functional Foods*. In 2015, she became passionate about bodybuilding and since then she has competed regularly in the bikini category. She is the winner of "Miss Etruria BBF 2015" and of the "BBF World Championship 2015", she currently competes in the IFBB federation qualifying among the top positions and obtaining the qualification for the Italian Championship for 3 consecutive years. She obtained the title of competition judge for bodybuilding.

Acknowledgments

Jessica Garsone. Degree in Pharmaceutical Sciences applied to herbal techniques; Master's in Health Biology. She is a COM Diet® Advisor. She has acquired the AFF-WA AMFPC (Metabolic and Functional Approach in Clinical Practice) Certification. She was an athlete at a competitive level of artistic roller skating and subsequently qualified from 2011 to 2017 as a manager and coach at the Rinascita Figure Skating Society of Ravenna. She currently practices fitness consistently, even if no longer with competitive goals, and she is also an expert in functional cooking.

Francesco Guardato. Graduating in Sports Science; FIPE-enabled personal trainer, specialized in the preparation of training programs for women, based on the assessment of body composition; internship at "Progressive Calisthenics Instructor Certification Workshop - New York". He is also a Fipav coach and has attended courses in: Postural Gymnastics with ATS; Functional recovery training and resistance training (FTC); Gluteus Shape Project; Loop Band Trainer. He collaborates with the surgeon and phlebologist Estephan Elias Fares on the problems of microcirculation. Bachelor's Degree in Motor Sciences.

Marco Guercioni. Bachelor's degree in Nutrition Biology; Master's in "Biological sciences - Nutrition and Functional Food". Member of the National Order of Biologists – Ordine Nazionale dei Biologi (ONB). Elite personal trainer (FIF) and member of the Vitamincenter Scientific Committee. He is an active coach in the national and international panorama of Natural Bodybuilding athletes (WNBF-ICN-AINBB-NBFI-FCFN).

Barbara Hugonin. Degree in Biological Sciences; genetic biologist, pediatric researcher; science popularizer and journalist; ESPEN European Diploma in Clinical Nutrition; training in Genetic Counselling and Rare Diseases at Children's Hospital Nationwide in Washington; Medical & Surgery Degree, Harvard Medical School; Fellowship in Lifestyle Medicine and Physical Activities Prescription, Institute of Lifestyle Medicine, Boston; Leadership program in Global Pediatric Clinical Research, Boston.

Ivan Martellato. Degree in Sports Science; degree in Food Science. Bodybuilding and Fitness Instructor. He is scientific director and co-founder of the VitaeDNA genetic testing company. His passion for dissemination allowed him to be a speaker at various conferences and as a teacher at the Master of Functional Systemic Medicine - Guidonia Montecelio, Rome. In 2019, he obtained the AFMPC (Applying Functional Medicine in Pratical Clinic) IFM (Institute of Functional Medicine) certification and in 2020, the course entitled "Peptides Therapy: Modules I and II" at A4M (American Academy of Anti-Aging Medicine), in California. He is also the author of two scientific articles on the muscle physiology, one of which is titled "Mechanical, Molecular Myofibrillar and Proteomic Modifications in Muscle Aging: A Pilot Study". He was second place in Northern Italy IFBB junior Bodybuilding in 2015, third place in the Italian IFBB Bodybuilding Championships in 2016, first place in the Italian WABBA Bodybuilding Natural Championships 2019.

Anna Merusi. Bachelor's degree in Biotechnology; Master's in Food Sciences and Human Nutrition. Since 2016 she as collaborated with Dr. Spattini as a nutritional biologist and she is his assistant and head of the COM Diet° service. In recent years, she has obtained the AMFPC certification (Functional Metabolic Approach in Clinical Practice) AFFWA, Antiaging Advisor (AFFWA Diplomate), COM Diet° Advisor and Food Educator, Course in Regenerative, Anti-Aging and Environmental Medicine (AMIA). Higher Education School "Epigenetics, Biophysics, Nutrition, the evolution from the multidisciplinary approach to salutogenesis, in the era of pollution" (U.P.A.I.Nu.C). She has participated as a speaker at conferences and events and has always been passionate about fitness and cooking, firmly believing in nutrition and physical activity as a medicine.

Giovanni Montagna. Degree in Dietetics, obtained the post-diploma qualification in "Professionals, managers, consultants of wellness, sport and free time" FSE of the Lombardy Region; in 2007 he attended the post-graduate Master's in "Nutrition, Pharmacology and Doping" at the University of Camerino and in 2012 the training course "Wellness and lifestyles" at the La Sapienza University of Rome. Author of the book *Tutto sulla "dieta a Zona" in breve*, he was a teacher at the courses of the AFWA (Functional Academy of Fitness Wellness and Antiaging), of "Profession Fitness", the SANIS school (School of Nutrition and Sports Supplementation) the CONI Emilia-Romagna course for coaches, the FISI cross-country ski instructor course, the Tirrenia Rugby Academy, the Faculty of Motor Sciences of the University of Verona and the Faculty of Pharmacology of the University of Pavia. He was a food consultant for the National Cross-Country Skiing Team, the Senior and Under 20 Rugby National Team, the Vittoria Alata competitive swimming team and the Fiamme Oro Padova sports group. He has also been a speaker at various national conferences.

Caterina Negro. Master's degree in Civil Engineering; Bachelor's degree in Biology; Bachelor's degree in Human Nutrition with thesis on "Bibliographic study on supplements able to improve insulin sensitivity". Lifestyle Medicine & Functional Medicine Certification (AFFWA). Advanced training course in Chronomorphodieta. Technogym Master Trainer.

Antonio Paoli. He is currently Full Professor of Exercise and Sport Sciences at the Department of Biomedical Sciences of the University of Padua. Graduated from ISEF (Higher Institute of Physical Education) of Padua in 1989, in 2004, also in Padua, he graduated in Medicine and Surgery and subsequently (2008) specialized in Sports Medicine in Pavia. In 2011 he became a university researcher and subsequently, in 2013, Associate Professor. In August 2018 he became Full Professor of Exercise and Sport Sciences again at the University of Padua, Department of Biomedical Sciences, where he currently heads the Laboratory of Nutrition and Exercise Physiology. Since 2015 he has been the Rector's Delegate for Sport and Wellness and since 2017, he has been President of the Bachelor's Degree Course in Motor Sciences, also at the University of Padua. Since February 2018 he has held the position of President of SISMES (Italian Society of Motor and Sport Sciences) and since October 2017, that of President of ESNS (European Sport Nutrition Society). Fellow of the European College of Sport Science and the American College of Sport Medicine, he is also Catedrático Extraordinario de Entrenamiento de Fuerza y Nutrición Deportiva y Director de Cátedra at UCAM, Catholic University of Murcia (Spain), and Leading Foreign Scientist at N.I. Lobachevsky State University of Nizhny Novgorod (Russia). Author of more than 160 articles published in international peer-reviewed journals, of three monographs and several book chapters, he is Associate Editor of the Journal of Human Kinetics and is on the editorial board of the *Journal of Translational Medicine*, of the *European Journal of Translational Myology, Journal of Functional Morphology and Kinesiology, Aging Clinical and Experimental Research, Medicine* (Baltimore) and *Nutrients and Sport Science for Health*. His research fields are mainly the physiology of exercise and skeletal muscle, training aimed at weight control and hypertrophy, the biomechanics of exercises, the effects of physical exercise on health and nutrition, with particular reference to the ketogenic diet and fasting.

Antonio Squillante. Antonio earned a Degree in Physical Education graduating summa cum laude from the University San Raffaele (Rome, Italy). He earned a Master's in Sports Performance and Orthopedic Rehabilitation from A.T. Still University (Measa, Arizona) and a Master's in Sports Science from the University of Southern California (Los Angeles, California). He is a Register Certified Strength and Conditioning Specialist (NSCA RSCC CSCS*D) with more than a decade of experience working with high school and collegiate athletes competing at national and international level. He is considered one of the foremost experts in the field of strength training for sport. He has authored the book "Strength Training for Sport" (ATS, Giacomo Catalani Editore) and "Power. The Training of Champions" (UAC, Ultimate Athlete Concepts. He is a Ph.D. student at the Clinical Exercise Research Center (CERC) under the Department of Biokinesiology and Physiotherapy at the University of Southern California (Los Angeles). He is a Registered Certified Sport and Exercise Nutritionist (SENr, CISSN). Former track athlete and American football player, Antonio now competes in powerlifting. He was placed third in the 100 kg raw category at the 2019 USPA California State Championship, qualifying for Nationals. He is a faculty member at Setanta College.

Giorgio Terziani. Visiting Professor in "Discipline del Benessere" at the Saint George School. Organizer of the higher education school "Epigenetics, Biophysics, Nutrition, the evolution of the multidisciplinary approach to salutogenesis, in the era of pollution" (U.P.A.I.Nu.C). Owner of the Eurodream company, which markets Cellfood® products and the Cellwellbeing S-Drive diagnostic methodology

Vittoria Troianiello. Bachelor's degree in Biotechnology; Master's in Biology Applied to Nutrition Sciences. COM Diet® Advisor; Master's in Nutrition and Wellness at the University of Milan; Master's in Drivers of Immune System and Mitochondrial Dysregulation at The American Academy of Anti-Aging Medicine (A4M), USA. Yoga teacher Alliance Certified. Cellulite expert. Mindfulness Educator.